Clinical Topics in Infectious Disease

Clinical Topics in Infectious Disease

Series Editor: David Schlossberg

Infections of the Head and Neck
Tuberculosis, *Second Edition*
Orthopedic Infection
Infectious Mononucleosis, *Second Edition*
Infections of the Nervous System

David Schlossberg
Editor

Infections of the Nervous System

With Foreword by Louis Weinstein

With 75 Illustrations in 134 Parts

Springer-Verlag
New York Berlin Heidelberg London
Paris Tokyo Hong Kong Barcelona

David Schlossberg M.D., F.A.C.P.
Professor of Medicine
Medical College of Pennsylvania
Director, Department of Medicine
Episcopal Hospital
Philadelphia, Pennsylvania 19125-1098, USA

Library of Congress Cataloging-in-Publication Data
Infections of the nervous system / David Schlossberg, editor.
p. cm. — (Clinical topics in infectious disease)
Includes index.
ISBN 0-387-97332-X, — ISBN 3-540-97332-X
1. Nervous system—Infections. I. Schlossberg, David.
II. Series.
[DNLM: 1. Bacterial Infections. 2. Central Nervous System Diseases. 3. Meningitis. 4. Virus Diseases. WL 300 I428]
RC359.5.I54 1990
616.8—dc20
DNLM/DLC
for Library of Congress 90-9864
CIP

Typeset by Kachina Typesetting, Inc., Tempe, Arizona.
Printed and bound by Edwards Brothers, Inc., Ann Arbor, Michigan.
Printed in the United States of America.

9 8 7 6 5 4 3 2 1

ISBN 0-387-97332-X Springer-Verlag New York Berlin Heidelberg
ISBN 3-540-97332-X Springer-Verlag Berlin Heidelberg New York

This volume is affectionately dedicated to
Uncle Mike and Ben, who have always been there,
and, I hope, always will be.

Foreword

I am honored by Dr. Schlossberg's invitation to write the *Foreword* to this monograph. Neurologic disorders may, with varying frequency, complicate the clinical course of many infections. Although these are primarily in the province of the specialist in infectious disease, it is important to point out that they often first come to the attention of the general internist or pediatrician, the surgeon, the radiologist, the epidemiologist, or the expert in Public Health.

The discussion in each chapter of this monograph is directed to a specific area of the nervous system—the meninges, brain, spinal cord, and peripheral nerves—and is presented in great detail. While the information discussed in some chapters is repeated in others, this is advantageous since it eliminates the need to keep referring to chapters in which the same information has been presented. The number of etiologic agents responsible for the diseases described in this monograph is very broad and covers the entire gamut from parasites to prions. Discussions of therapy include not only descriptions of the effective "old" antimicrobial agents, but also those developed most recently. Most advantageous to the reader who may wish to survey the literature related to a specific disease are the extensive bibliographies attached to each chapter. In most instances, these include 100 or more references; in one (Radiology) over 300 are cited.

This monograph makes a signal addition to the medical literature. It brings very important information to all physicians, regardless of their specialty, who may come in contact with patients experiencing infectious diseases of the nervous system, permitting them to establish etiologic backgrounds, anticipate complications, and establish potentially effective antimicrobial therapy.

LOUIS WEINSTEIN, M.D., Ph.D.

Series Preface

Why another series on infectious disease? The question is a fair one in view of the proliferation of monographs, texts, and periodicals on the vast subject of infectious disease. The goal of this series is to provide an additional service to the clinician in the form of clinical information not usually assembled in one convenient volume.

One type of monograph presented in this series will cover a specific infection, detailing microbiologic, research, and clinical aspects. It is hoped that such a compilation will be helpful in both its thoroughness and breadth to the clinician interested in this particular problem. The other type of monograph that this series will provide will discuss a clinical presentation that comprises many possible specific etiologies.

Volumes in the series will be multiauthored, giving us the opportunity to invite authorities in each specific area to contribute their expertise and experience. Regular revisions are planned so that each volume will remain as current as it is thorough.

We hope that our goals are met and that the present series of monographs establishes its own identifiable and valuable niche in the growing compendium of resource material available to the clinician.

Preface

Infections of the nervous system are a fascinating group of syndromes. They have in common dramatic presentations and a gratifying treatability. All classes of organisms may be etiologic, and all parts of the nervous system may be affected.

From a clinical standpoint, these infections are challenging. A differential diagnosis of entities such as brain abscess, neurosyphilis, transverse myelitis, and Jakob-Creutzfeldt disease requires a degree of comfort with infectious processes, neuroanatomy, and medicine in general.

Interrelationships abound in nervous system infections. Cerebellitis may complicate the same viral infection that is later followed by Guillain-Barré syndrome. Lyme disease may cause both radiculopathy and encephalitis. Also, new diseases and information continue to accumulate: improved imaging techniques, the mischief of prions, unforseen manifestations of AIDS, and perils of progress like shunt infection, all challenge our acumen and overview of medicine.

We hope this presentation of nervous system infections will provide an applicable and timely guide for the clinician.

Contents

Contributors

Barry G. W. Arnason, M.D.
Department of Neurology, University of Chicago, Chicago, Illinois, U.S.A.

Fred F. Barrett, M.D.
Medical Director, Department of Administration, Le Bonheur Children's Medical Center, Memphis, Tennessee; Professor of Pediatrics, Department of Pediatrics, University of Tennessee, The National Health Science Center, Memphis, Tennessee, U.S.A.

Michele Barry, M.D.
Department of Medicine, Yale University School of Medicine, New Haven, Connecticut, U.S.A.

Morven C. Barwick, M.D.
Assistant Professor, Neurology, Department of Neurology, University of Connecticut Health Center, Farmington, Connecticut, U.S.A.

Jacqueline A. Bello, M.D.
Division of Pediatric Neurology and Neurobiology, Columbia-Presbyterian Medical Center, Neurological Institute, New York, New York, U.S.A.

Joseph R. Berger, M.D.
Associate Professor, Department of Neurology and Internal Medicine, University of Miami School of Medicine, Miami, Florida, U.S.A.

Frank J. Bia, M.D., M.P.H.
Associate Professor, Medicine and Laboratory Medicine, Department of Infectious Diseases, Yale University School of Medicine, New Haven, Connecticut, U.S.A.

Brian C. Bowen, M.D., Ph.D.
Assistant Professor, Radiology, Division of Neuroradiology, Department of Radiology, University of Miami School of Medicine, Miami, Florida, U.S.A.

Rebecca A. Clark, M.D.
Assistant Professor of Medicine, Tulane University Medical Center, New Orleans, Louisiana, U.S.A.

Bruce A. Cohen, M.D.
Department of Neurology, Northwestern University Medical School, Chicago, Illinois, U.S.A.

Burke A. Cunha, M.D.
Chief, Infectious Disease Division, Vice-Chairman, Department of Medicine, Winthrop-University Hospital, Mineola, New York; Associate Professor of Medicine, State University of New York at Stony Brook, Stony Brook, New York, U.S.A.

Darryl C. De Vivo, M.D.
Divisions of Pediatric Neurology and Neuroradiology, Columbia-Presbyterian Medical Center, The Neurological Institute, New York, New York, U.S.A.

Mark J. DiNubile, M.D.
Assistant Professor, Medicine, Department of Medicine, Division of Infectious Disease, Cooper Hospital/University Medical Center, Camden, New Jersey; Assistant Professor of Medicine, Division of Infectious Disease, UMDNJ/Robert Wood Johnson Medical School of Camden, Camden, New Jersey, U.S.A.

Richard Dix, Ph.D.
Assistant Professor of Microbiology and Ophthalmology, Departments of Ophthalmology, Microbiology, and Immunology, Bascom Palmer Eye Institute, University of Miami School of Medicine, Miami, Florida, U.S.A.

Jerrold J. Ellner, M.D.
Director, Division of Infectious Diseases, Department of Medicine, University Hospitals of Cleveland, Cleveland, Ohio; Professor of Medicine and Pathology, Department of Medicine, Case Western Reserve University, Cleveland, Ohio, U.S.A.

Nicholas J. Fiumara, M.D., M.P.H.
Clinical Professor of Dermatology, Tufts University School of Medicine, Medford, Massachusetts; Adjunct Professor of Dermatology, Boston University School of Medicine, Boston, Massachusetts; Physician, Department of Dermatology, New England Medical Center, Boston, Massachusetts, U.S.A.

Alejandra C. Gurtman, M.D.
Fellow, Division of Infectious Diseases, Mount Sinai Hospital, New York, New York, U.S.A.

John J. Halperin, M.D.
Associate Professor, Neurology, Department of Neurology, State University of New York at Stony Brook, Stony Brook, New York; Vice-Chairman, Department of Neurology, University Hospital, Stony Brook, New York, U.S.A.

Paul D. Hoeprich, M.D.
Professor of Medicine, Chief, Section of Medical Mycology, Department of Internal Medicine, University of California Davis Medical Center, Sacramento, California, U.S.A.

Karen K. Hsiao, M.D.
Department of Neurology, University of California School of Medicine, San Francisco, California; Professor of Virology in Residence, University of California at Berkeley, School of Public Health, Berkeley, California, U.S.A.

Newton E. Hyslop, Jr., M.D.
Professor of Medicine, Chief, Infectious Diseases Section, Principle Investigator, Tulane University Medical Center, Tulane-LSU AIDS Clinical Trials Unit, New Orleans, Louisiana, U.S.A.

John E. Kasik, M.D., Ph.D.
Professor of Internal Medicine, Department of Internal Medicine, Veterans Administration Medical Center, Iowa City, Iowa; Professor of Internal Medicine for College of Medicine, University of Iowa, Iowa City, Iowa, U.S.A.

Shubha Kerkar, M.D.
Fellow in Infectious Diseases, Hahnemann University School of Medicine, Philadelphia, Pennsylvania, U.S.A.

Robert M. Levy, M.D., Ph.D.
Assistant Professor, Neurosurgery and Physiology, Northwestern University Medical School, Chicago, Illinois, U.S.A.

Howard L. Lipton, M.D.
Department of Neurology, University of Colorado School of Medicine, Boulder, Colorado, U.S.A.

Miguel Mateos-Mora, M.D.
Department of Infectious Disease, Mount Sinai Medical Center, Miami Beach, Florida; Fellow, Division of Infectious Disease, Jackson Memorial Hospital, Miami, Florida, U.S.A.

Richard D. Meyer, M.D.
Director, Division of Infectious Diseases, Department of Medicine, Cedars-Sinai Medical Center, Los Angeles, California; Professor of Medicine, UCLA School of Medicine, Los Angeles, California, U.S.A.

Burt R. Meyers, M.D.
Department of Infectious Diseases, Mount Sinai Hospital, New York, New York; Professor of Medicine, Mount Sinai School of Medicine, New York, New York; Attending Physician, Division of Infectious Disease, Mount Sinai Medical Center, New York, New York, U.S.A.

Abdolghader J. Molavi, M.D.
Director, Division of Infectious Diseases, Associate Professor of Medicine and Surgery, Hahnemann University School of Medicine, Philadelphia, Pennsylvania, U.S.A.

Douglas R. Nordli, M.D.
Division of Pediatric Neurology and Neurobiology, Columbia-Presbyterian Medical Center, The Neurological Institute, New York, New York, U.S.A.

Jan E. Patterson, M.D.
Department of Medicine, Yale University School of Medicine, New Haven, Connecticut, U.S.A.

Thomas F. Patterson, M.D.
Department of Medicine, Yale University School of Medicine, New Haven, Connecticut, U.S.A.

M. Judith Donovan Post, M.D.
Department of Radiology, University of Miami School of Medicine, Miami, Florida, U.S.A.

Stanley B. Prusiner, M.D.
Professor of Neurology and Professor of Biochemistry and Biophysics, Department of Neurology, University of California School of Medicine, San Francisco, California, U.S.A.

Kenneth R. Ratzan, M.D.
Chief, Division of Infectious Disease, Department of Infectious Diseases, Mount Sinai Medical Center, Miami Beach, Florida; Associate Professor of Medicine, University of Miami School of Medicine, Miami, Florida, U.S.A.

Louis Reik, Jr., M.D.
Associate Professor of Neurology, Department of Neurology, University of Connecticut Health Center, Farmington, Connecticut; Attending Physician, Neurology, John Dempsey Hospital, Farmington, Connecticut, U.S.A.

Edgar F. Salazar-Grueso, M.D.
Department of Neurology, The University of Chicago Medical Center, Chicago, Illinois, U.S.A.

Merle A. Sande, M.D.
Chief, Medical Service, San Francisco General Hospital, San Francisco, California; Professor and Vice-Chairman, Department of Medicine, University of California School of Medicine, San Francisco, California, U.S.A.

David Schlossberg, M.D., F.A.C.P.
Director, Department of Medicine, Episcopal Hospital, Philadelphia, Pennsylvania; Professor of Medicine, Medical College of Pennsylvania, Philadelphia, Pennsylvania, U.S.A.

Richard T. Sokolov, Jr. M.D.
Clinical Fellow, Division of Infectious Diseases, Cedars-Sinai Medical Center, Los Angeles, California; UCLA School of Medicine, Los Angeles, California, U.S.A.

Tarvez Tucker, M.D.
Department of Neurology, University Hospitals of Cleveland, Cleveland, Ohio, U.S.A.

Jay H. Tureen, M.D.
Associate Clinical Professor, San Francisco General Hospital, Medical Service, San Francisco, California, U.S.A.

Robert E. Van Scoy, M.D.
Consultant, Division of Infectious Diseases and Internal Medicine, Mayo Clinic and Mayo Foundation, Rochester, Minnesota; Associate Professor of Medicine, Mayo Medical School, Rochester, Minnesota, U.S.A.

Louis Weinstein, M.D., Ph.D.
Senior Consultant in Medicine, Brigham and Women's Hospital, Boston, Massachusetts, U.S.A.

Janara J. Younger, M.D.
Assistant Professor of Pediatrics, University of Tennessee College of Medicine, Chattanooga, Tennessee, U.S.A.

Part I
Meningitis

1
The Diagnosis and Therapy of Acute Bacterial Meningitis

BURKE A. CUNHA

Bacterial meningitis is an acute or subacute infection of the leptomeninges and is associated with chemical and cellular changes in the cerebrospinal fluid (CSF). A clinical syndrome associated with a characteristic CSF profile, the main clinical problem in meningitis is arriving at a working diagnosis on which to base empiric therapy. The clinician's diagnostic dilemma is to differentiate bacterial from viral meningitis as well as from mimics of acute bacterial meningitis. Clinical findings must be combined with CSF results to determine quickly the most probable pathogen upon which initial antimicrobial therapy can be based.[6,33,43,46]

The purpose of this chapter is to provide a clinical diagnostic and therapeutic approach to the treatment of bacterial meningitis. It is not a review of the many manifestations of each specific etiologic agent causing meningitis, but rather, offers a clinical basis for determining the differential diagnosis and empiric therapy for a patient presenting with "meningitis."

The Meningitis Syndrome: Clinical and Laboratory Features

Classically, pyogenic meningitis is a life-threatening acute infection manifested by fever and leukocytosis. Except in very young children and the elderly, nuchal rigidity is the cardinal manifestation of meningeal irritation. In addition to a stiff neck on physical examination, other physical findings suggesting meningeal irritation are usually present, such as Kernig's, Brudzinski's, and Hoyne's signs.[43,46] In very young children, irritability, failure to thrive, and a bulging fontanelle may be the only clues.[30,41] Nuchal rigidity in the elderly must be carefully evaluated since many older people have cervical arthritis, which, in the appropriate clinical setting of fever and mental confusion, may erroneously suggest meningeal irritation. Furthermore, the many causes of meningismus need to be taken into account and should be differentiated on physical diagnosis from true nuchal rigidity in adult patients.[19] Dermatologic manifestations of meningitis are associated with specific organisms and are very helpful when present. Mental confusion is not a feature of bacterial or viral meningitis. The clinician must be careful to exclude the mental changes associated with acute febrile illnesses, particularly in elderly patients, before assuming that mental confusion is part of the pathologic process. Mental confusion without nuchal rigidity suggests encephalopathy or encephalitis. Certain organisms may present primarily as a meningitis with an encephalopathic component, such as meningoencephalitis; conversely, many of the organisms responsible for encephalitis may have a meningeal component.[26] As a general rule, a stiff neck in the absence of other findings suggests meningeal irritation caused by a bacterial or viral process. whereas encephalopathy is primarily due to viral infections of the central nervous system (CNS).[33,37]

Most patients with acute bacterial meningitis present with acute illness. However, some organisms present in a subacute fashion (i.e., *Listeria* meningitis in an elderly patient), as a slowly progressive or indolent meningitis (e.g., tuberculous meningitis), or hyperacutely with an extremely fulminant course (e.g., meningococcal meningitis). The rapidity of onset and the severity of the illness are important clinical clues in ascertaining the probable infecting organism in patients presenting with the meningitis syndrome. Similarly, patients presenting with recurrent meningitis or chronic meningitis have specific disease associations with limited diagnostic possibilities.[43] For example, recurrent meningitis suggests an immunologic deficiency or CSF leak, whereas chronic meningitis suggests tuberculosis or fungal meningitis as well as noninfectious CNS involvement—for example, sarcoidosis, systemic lupus erythematosus (SLE), Behçet's syndrome.[4,40,47] The age of the host, the concomitant medical or surgical problems, and epidemiologic clues are all important in arriving at a working diagnosis and predicting the likely pathogens in the meningitis patient. (Table 1.1) While appearances may be deceiving in the very young and the very old, as a general clinical principle, patients with pyogenic meningitis appear "sicker" than do patients with nonpyogenic meningeal inflammation, which includes most viral meningitis.[43,46]

The diagnostic approach to meningitis rests not only on the probable organism suggested by the various features of the clinical presentation, but also as critically on the CSF profile. Demonstration of the specific etiologic organism by Gram stain or culture in the CSF is necessary for a definitive diagnosis of bacterial meningitis. Therefore, staining and culture are the most important tests that can be obtained on the CSF. The opening pressure of the CSF is usually elevated and so is unhelpful except in special situations, such as a low opening pressure attributable to tuberculous meningitis and cord block. Extreme elevations of opening pressure suggest brain abscess with leakage into the CSF circulation. As a general rule, opening pressures in bacterial meningitis are in the 200–300 mm of water range, and the opening pressures in viral meningitis are usually normal or only slightly elevated. The CSF glucose is important in suggesting groups of specific etiologic agents that are associated with hypoglycorrhachia in the CSF. One must remember that CSF glucose levels are commonly low in very young children and are reflective of their low peripheral blood glucose levels. Similarly, in adult patients with hyperglycemia, CSF levels may appear to be normal or even elevated. It must also be remembered that CSF glucose equilibration lags two to six hours behind the peripheral circulation, and the immediately antecedent but not simultaneous peripheral blood glucose should be taken into account before looking for the typical decrease in CSF glucose to less than 50% of the peripheral blood glucose.

Table 1.1 Host-pathogen associations in meningitis.

Host	Organism
Sinopulmonary infection	*S pneumoniae* *H influenzae* *N* meningitidis
Elderly	*H influenzae* *Listeria* Endocarditis Brain abscess 2° dental focus
Sickle cell disease	*S pneumonaie* *Salmonella* *N meningitidis* *H influenzae*
Splenectomy	*S pneumonaie* *N meningitidis* *H influenzae* DF-2
AIDS	HIV Cytomegalovirus Toxoplasma *Listeria* *Nocardia* *Cryptococcus* Tuberculosis Lymphomas
Complement deficiencies	*S pneumonaie* *N meningitidis*
CSF leak	*S pneumonaie*
IV-drug abuser	*S aureus* Gram-negative bacilli
Alcoholism/cirrhosis	*S pneumonaie* *Klebsiella* Enterococcus
Hypogammaglobulinemia	*S pneumoniae* *H influenzae* *N meningitidis* Enteroviruses (especially echoviruses)
V-A/V-P shunts	*S epidermidis* *S aureus* Gram-negative bacilli
Recurrent meningitis	*S pneumonia*, *H influenzae*, *N meningitidis* usually secondary to immune/anatomic defects *Noninfectious CNS diseases* SLE Parameningeal infections
Endocarditis	*S pneumoniae* Enterococcus *S aureus* *Bacteroides*
Brain abscess	Anaerobes *Citrobacter* (children) *S aureus* Gram-negative enteric bacilli

As a general clinical principle, pyogenic meningitis usually decreases the CSF glucose to less than 50% of the peripheral glucose concentration even when the two determinations are taken simultaneously.[11,46] Although red cells in the CSF, certain viral infections, and other processes such as meningeal carcinomatosis can lower the CSF glucose, it is a useful principle and should suggest bacterial meningitis until proved otherwise. Conversely, normal CSF glucose may be seen very early in acute bacterial meningitis, in early tuberculous or fungal meningitis, or with pyogenic parameningeal infections. The presence of red blood cells (RBCs) in the CSF after a traumatic tap or bleed has been considered and sharply limits diagnostic possibilities to relatively few illnesses. Thus, their presence affords an important diagnostic clue. However, it is the cellular response of the CSF to meningeal irritation that causes the most diagnostic confusion for clinicians. In pyogenic meningitis, there are typically 100–10,000 white blood cells (WBCs) with a polymorphonuclear predominance of more than 90%. Bacterial meningitis may be present with less than 100 cells or up to 100,000 WBCs in the CSF. Although there are exceptions—for example—herpes meningoencephalitis may have over 90% polymorphonuclear cells (PMNs) in the cellular differential—the 90% figure is most useful in separating bacterial from viral meningitis. Conversely, parameningeal infections or partially treated bacterial meningitis may be associated with less than 90% PMNs in the CSF.

The usual clinical problem that causes much concern is the presence of a few cells that are predominantly PMNs.[18] Noninfectious-disease physicians are always asking, "How do you explain those PMNs if not by the presence of bacterial meningitis?" It cannot be stated too strongly that no single CSF parameter, with the exception of the CSF lactic acid, can be utilized with such certainty. It is useful to remember that meningitis is a clinical and CSF syndrome requiring both a clinical assessment compatible with the presumed putative agent and a CSF profile that is "suggestive" of and compatible with the clinical diagnosis. One does not have to explain the presence of two or 22 lonesome PMNs if the clinical presentation and the remainder of the CSF profile militate against the diagnosis of bacterial meningitis. By far the greatest number of errors are committed in overinterpreting solitary CSF findings. Less frequent but equally important is the problem of failing to recognize important clues to the diagnosis such as provided by CSF, red cells or eosinophils, increased bilirubin, malignant cells, or "motile lymphocytes." CSF protein measurements are on index of CSF inflammation and blood–CSF barrier permeability and have importance in predicting CNS penetrability of many antibiotics. Diagnostically, however, the CSF protein is elevated in so many CNS disorders that it is usually unhelpful in suggesting a specific etiologic diagnosis. CSF protein levels in the range of 100–500 ml/dl are usual in bacterial meningitis, and very high levels suggest meningeal carcinomatosis, tuberculous meningitis with subarachnoid block, or brain abscess. A normal or decreased protein has no diagnostic significance in the CSF.[29]

In differentiating bacterial meningitis from viral meningitis, the CSF lactic-acid determination is second only to the Gram stain in diagnostic importance. The CSF lactate is the most underutilized and undersppreciated test in the CSF profile.[5,7] This test has been misapplied and incorrectly interpreted in the medical literature as a nonspecific and nonhelpful determination.[11,19,25,28,29] The reasons for this are the modest levels of lactic-acid elevation; 3–6 mmol/L are present in a whole range of inflammatory CNS disorders and are in no way specific for any particular pathogen. This statement is true if one considers the many noninfectious mechanisms of producing a CSF lactic acidosis.[25,28,33] It has also been said that the test provides no information in addition to the information that the other CSF parameters provide, which is equally untrue. The CSF lactic acid should be applied only in differentiating bacterial, partially treated, and viral meningitis.[36,43] It should not be used in diagnosing parameningeal infections, brain abscesses, brain tumors, strokes, multiple sclerosis, and the like. In over ten years of extensive experience with this test, it has never failed me in differentiating among these three clinical conditions, and it has sometimes been helpful in suggesting an infectious versus a noninfectious etiology, such as tuberculous versus sarcoid basilar meningitis.

The medical literature is also unequivocal in assessing the degree of CSF lactic acidosis, which is critically important if one is to draw the correct diagnostic assumptions from this determination. While viral meningitis is invariably associated with CSF lactic-acid levels of less than 3 mmol/L, bacterial meningitis uniformly results in levels above 10 mmol/L, and partially treated meningitis, as well as tuberculous/fungal meningitis, produces a range of intermediate values. However, as mentioned previously, the test is most useful and is the best way, aside from the Gram stain, to differentiate viral from bacterial meningitis.[5,7]

The concept of typical CSF cellular and chemical profiles thus has evolved to the point that we speak of a bacterial CSF profile versus a viral CSF profile. The bacterial CSF profile means the CSF has a positive or negative Gram stain for organisms, but usually a positive, albeit later, CSF culture, a greater PMN predominance with a variable number of WBCs, a decreased CSF glucose to less than 50% of peripheral glucose levels, and a variably elevated protein and highly elevated CSF lactic acid. By contrast, the typical "aseptic" or viral meningitis CSF profile is that of a negative Gram stain and subsequent CSF culture, a normal CSF glucose, variably elevated CSF protein, usually a lymphocytic predominance but not uncommonly an initial PMN predominance (but nearly always with less than 90% MPNs), and always a CSF lactic acid of less than 3 mmol/L. Although other diseases produce interesting combinations and permutations of these values, they remain important clinical parameters to be weighed and evaluated with deference to the clinical presentation. As with the clinical syndrome of meningitis, CSF parameters should not be interpreted alone or out of the context of the CSF profile, and must not be at variance with the clinical features.[43,46]

Clinical Diagnostic Approach

While specific host-pathogen associations are useful in suggesting a specific etiologic organism in the patient with presumed meningitis, they are not helpful in determining whether the patient has meningitis or a related condition. The clinician, therefore, must adopt a syndromic approach to the adult patient with presumed meningitis. It is useful to consider the patient on initial evaluation in terms of the severity of the illness. As has been mentioned, patients with viral meningitis, in general, appear less ill than do those with bacterial meningitis. The difference in the degree of illness can only be appreciated with experience, but nevertheless it is as helpful as any CSF parameter in differentiating viral from pyogenic meningitis. Therefore, patients who are not terribly ill, with meningeal signs and extra-CSF findings that are present but mild, suggest entroviral meningitis, Lyme disease, lymphocyte choriomeningitis (LCM), partially treated meningitis, brain abscess, tuberculosis (TB) fungal meningitis, or sarcoid meningitis. In contrast, the patient who is moderately ill with meningeal signs but prominent extra-CNS findings is likely to have Rocky Mountain spotted fever, leptospirosis, Mycoplasma, meningoencephalitis, or pyogenic meningitis from acute bacterial endocarditis (ABE). The most frightening clinical presentation is that of a critically ill patient with predominantly meningeal signs and few or no extra-CNS findings. Until proved otherwise, this suggests meningococcal, pneumococcal, or *Hemophilus influenzae* meningitis. Patients with a brain abscess and a ventricular leak causing meningitis may also present in this fashion. This approach illustrates the importance of assessing the severity of the illness and the presence of extra-CNS signs in limiting diagnostic possibilities.[33,43,46]

Patients presenting predominantly with encephalopathic signs, with little or no neck stiffness, represent a special subset of patients. The differential diagnosis of primarily encephalopathic presentation is human immunodeficiency virus (HIV) encephalitis, bland emboli from subacute bacterial endocarditis (SBE), herpes encephalitis, arboviral encephalitis, lupus cerebritis, meningeal carcinomatosis, or amebic meningoencephalitis. Clearly, herpes encephalitis would be the most common presentation in this category, followed by HIV encephalitis. Other clinical clues may suggest other conditions, such as a heart murmer or SBE, or specific epidemiologic information may be of use, as in arboviral encephalitis or amebic meningoencephalitis.

The patient presenting with rash and fever who has meningitis is another difficult exercise in differential diagnosis. Once again, it is useful to classify patients by severity of illness to make rapid and intelligent diagnostic assumptions. The cause of a patient's being critically ill with rash and fever and meningitis is usually *Meningococcus, Pneumococcus,* or *Staphylococcus aureus*. While meningococcal disease is the most frequent cause of asymmetrical petechial lesions, *Pneumococcus* may present with the same syndrome, especially in children or in asplenic individuals. *S aureus* endocarditis may result in showers of emboli to the extremities, resulting in distal petechial lesions resembling meningococcemia. Patients with *S aureus* sepsis severe enough to produce impressive petechial lesions on the extremities usually have a recognizable focus of staphylococcal infections—that is, intravenous (IV) line sepsis, ABE, abscess, and so on. Patients who are moderately ill with rash and fever are likely to have leptospirosis or Rocky Mountain spotted fever. The associated clinical findings and epidemiology are useful in separating these two disease entities; patients with leptospirosis and Rocky Mountain spotted fever will have abnormal liver-function tests but the bilirubin is elevated in leptospirosis and not usually in Rocky Mountain spotted fever. The patient with Rocky Mountain spotted fever has bilateral periorbital edema, characteristically an edema of the hands and feet. The patient with leptospirosis is characterized by the absence of these findings and the presence of conjunctival suffusion with or without jaundice. The mildly to moderately ill patient with a rash may have enteroviral meningitis characterized by a central rash that commonly involves the face, but occasionally may be petechial causing diagnostic confusion with *Neisseria meningitidis*. Patients presenting with a rash and drug fever during the course of treatment for meningitis—that is, partially treated meningitis—may appear relatively well but have a symmetrical maculopapular rash that is usually puritic. The characteristic rash of Lyme disease, erythema chromicum migrans, cannot be confused with much else and makes the diagnosis of Lyme disease easy when present. Early patients with the acquired immune deficiency syndrome (AIDS) have a maculopapular rash resembling that of infectious mononucleosis. The AIDS patients tend also to exhibit mental-status changes, changes in personality, or mild encephalopathy, in contrast to the patient with early infectious mononucleosis. Tuberculosis or sarcoidosis meningitis may be associated with erythema nodosum, and so find its way into this diagnostic category.[28,33,36,43] (See Table 1.2.)

Complications may occur early or late in the clinical presentation. If they occur early at the time of presentation, then they become diagnostic clues in the syndromic approach to the patient with meningitis. For example, acute hearing loss early in the course of the disease suggests *H. influenza,* the *Meningococcus,* or Rocky Mountain spotted fever as the most likely organisms associated with this complication. Again, other factors in the clinical presentation, as well as the CSF profile, will help to confirm or rule out specific pathogens associated with deafness. Similarly, seizures that occur early in

Table 1.2. A syndromic approach to adults presenting with "meningitis."

CNS	Differential diagnosis considerations
Patient critically ill	
Meningeal signs predominate	*N meningitidis* *S pneumonaie* *H influenzae* Brain abscess with ventricular leak
Patient moderately ill	
Meningeal signs moderate Extra-CNS findings prominent	Rocky Mountain spotted fever Leptospirosis (Weil's syndrome) *Mycoplasma* meningoencephalitis ABE
Patient ill	
Meningeal signs mild Extra-CNS findings mild	Enteroviral meningitis Lyme disease LCM Partially treated bacterial meningitis Brain abscess TB/fungal basilar meningitis Sarcoid meningitis
Encephalopathy with minimal meningeal signs	HIV encephalitis SBE Herpes encephalitis Arboviral encephalitis SLE cerebritis Meningeal carcinomatosis Amebic meningoencephalitis
Rash and fever with meningitis	
Patient critically ill	*N meningitidis* Asymmetrical extremity trunkal petechial lesions *S pneumoniae* Asymmetrical extremity trunkal petechial lesions *S aureus* Symmetrical petechial extremity lesions
Patient moderately ill	Rocky Mountain spotted fever Symmetrical wrist/ankle petechial lesions Leptospirosis Conjuntival suffusion, jaundice
Patient ill	Enteroviral Facial, truncal, maculopapular, occasionally petechial

(continued)

Table 1.2. *(continued)*

CNS	Differential diagnosis considerations
Patient ill *(cont.)*	Partially treated meningitis with drug fever Symmetrical truncal maculopapular rash, may involve palms/soles pruritic +/–
	Lyme disease Single/multiple ECM lesions near tick-bite site
	AIDS Maculopapular rash resembles EBV, erythroderma, severe seborrhea/psoriasis
	Tuberculosis/sarcoidosis Erythema nodosum of lower extremities

the course of pneumococcal and *H influenzae* meningitis are also associated with a variety of other CNS pathogens, such as herpes histoplasmosis and tuberculosis. Seizures occurring well into the course of meningitis suggest a complication such as cortical-vein phlebitis/thrombosis. Seizures are not usually due to high concentrations of antibiotics in the CSF. The patient with initial seizures who rapidly develops a dense neurologic-deficit encephalopathy leading to coma nearly always has herpes meningoencephalitis. The clinician should be wary of other conditions that may mimic bacterial meningitis, such as mass lesions that may also eventuate in seizures. Clearly, computed-tomography/magnetic-resonance-imaging (CT/MRI) scans are useful in the diagnosis of cortical-vein thrombosis and parameningeal infections.

Subdural effusions commonly are seen in the course of *H. influenzae* meningitis, but also are seen with pneumococcal meningitis. Patients usually present with a recrudescense of fever after an initial improvement, and the diagnosis is made by CT/MRI scans. These effusions generally resolve with treatment and do not need to be drained. Cranial-nerve abnormalities not infrequently complicate pyogenic meningitis. Abnormalities of the sixth, seventh, and eighth cranial nerves in a critically ill patient should suggest meningococcal meningitis. Classically, a seventh-nerve palsy in a fairly well patient suggests sarcoidosis, whereas a unilateral or bilateral abducens palsy suggests tuberculosis in the same setting. Meningeal carcinomatosis is characterized by cranial-nerve abnormalities, but their distribution is variable and so not specifically diagnostic. However, unexplained cranial-nerve abnormalities in the absence of basilar meningitis or the *Meningococcus* should suggest meningeal carcinomatosis.

Many organisms may produce shock and disseminated intravascular coagulation as part of their clinical picture. The patient presenting with purpura and shock in the setting of meningitis usually has meningococcal or pneumococcal meningitis, but the clinician should not forget that *Listeria* may present in precisely this fashion. Another interesting clinical point is that herpes labialis is peculiarly associated with meningococcal and pneumococcal meningitis. Herpes labialis may be seen in a variety of other conditions, but in the setting of meningitis may suggest either of these two pathogens. Patients with herpes meningoencephalitis usually give an antecedent history of herpes labialis and, rarely, fever blisters may be present simultaneously with CNS invasion.[19,43,46,47] The complications of meningitis and associated findings are presented in Table 1.3.

Mimics of Bacterial Meningitis

The main clinical dilemma for the clinician is to tell bacterial from nonpyogenic meningitis. Included in this differential are a wide variety of orgnisms and conditions that mimic bacterial meningitis. A presumptive diagnosis is usually possible taking into account the age of the person and epidemiologic clues, the severity of the illness, clinical findings, and the CSF profile. Each illness commonly associated with a specific disease entity is presented in Table 1.4. Using such information, the majority of clinical problems can be resolved quickly based on key clinical and laboratory clues.

In the differential diagnosis between pyogenic and viral meningitis, the severity of the illness and the CSF profile are the two most important parameters. In differentiating partially treated from viral meningitis, the clinical findings, trunkal rash, pharyngitis, diarrhea, and a normal CSF lactic acid are most helpful.

Herpes encephalitis has a noneasonal distribution and is characterized by a progressive downhill course over several days, with a significant encephalopathic component. The electroencephalograph (EEG) is most useful early in the disease before MRI or CT scans are positive in pointing to a temporal-lobe focus characteristic of this particular disorder. Herpes encephalitis is the viral disease that may most closely mimic a pyogenic process and give the

Table 1.3. Acute complications of meningitis.

Conditions	Usual associated organisms/conditions
Deafness/hearing loss	*H influenzae* *N meningitidis* Tuberculosis Rocky Mountain spotted fever Mumps
Seizures	*S pneumoniae* (early onset) *H influenzae* Group B streptococci Sarcoidosis Herpes Histoplasmosis Tuberculosis Mass lesions Cortical-vein phlebitis/ thrombosis
Subdural effusions	*H influenzae* *S pneumonaie*
Septic arthritis	*N meningitidis* *S aureus*
Hemiplegia	*S pneumoniae*
Cerebral-vein thrombosis	*H influenzae* (associated Jacksonian seizures)
Hydrocephalus	*H influenzae* Tuberculosis Group B streptococci
Cranial-nerve abnormalities	*N meningitidis* (CN VI, VII, VIII) Tuberculosis (CN VI), unilateral → bilateral Sarcoidosis (CN VII) Meningeal carcinomatosis (variable)
Herpes labialis	*N meningitidis* *S pneumoniae*
Panophthalmitis	*N meningitidis* *S pneumoniae* *H influenzae*
Purpura, petechiae, shock	*N meningitidis* *S pneumoniae* *Listeria*

clinician the greatest degree of diagnostic difficulty. Unlike other viruses, herpes meningoencephalitis may result in over 90% PMNs in the CSF as well as a decreased glucose. It is regularly accompanied by red cells in the CSF that may increase the lactic acid, further compounding diagnostic confusion. The negative Gram stain, as well as the encephalopathic factor, is of great value in arriving at a presumptive clinical diagnosis. It should be remembered that red cells in the CSF are associated with relatively few diseases, and they are not usually confused with herpes meningoencephalitis. Importantly, red cells

Table 1.4. Mimics of bacterial meningitis.

Meningeal process	Differential features and diagnostic clues
Enteroviral meningitis	Seasonal distribution: summer Clinically, not as ill May have sore throat, facial/ maculopapular rash, diarrhea CSF: Gram stain (–) Lactic acid: <2 mmol/L
Partially treated bacterial meningitis (usually secondary to *H influenzae*)	Previous antibiotic therapy Subacute onset and severity both viral/bacterial presentation CSF: Gram stain (+/–) Lactic acid: 4–6 mmol/L
Herpes encephalitis	Nonseasonal Dense/prolonged neurologic defects Encephalopathic/coma Antecedent herpes labialis EEG: temporal-lobe focus MRI/CT scan: Unilateral/bilateral temporal-lobe lesions CSF: Gram stain (–) RBCs (+) PMNs may be >90% Glucose may be decreased Lactic acid increased two degrees to RBCs
Meningeal carcinomatosis	Patient usually afebrile with known carcinoma, or elderly without known primary neoplasm Lymphomas most common CNS malignancy, usually stage IV Clinically not severely ill; nuchal rigidity (+/–) Mental-status changes common 80% have cranial-nerve involvement, 3,4,6,7,8 most common CSF: Gram stain (–) RBCs (+/–) Protein very elevated Lactic acid variably elevated Abnormal cytology in 90%
Amebic meningoencephalitis (*N fowleri*)	History of fresh-water swimming one to two weeks prior to presentation Extremely rapid onset leading to death in less than 72 hours

(continued)

Table 1.4. *(continued)*

Meningeal process	Differential features and diagnostic clues
Amebic meningoencephalitis *(N fowleri) (continued)*	Olfactory/gustatory abnormalities may provide early clue CSF: RBCs elevated and low glucose Lactic acid variably elevated Gram stain (–), but mobile ameba on wet preparation
Brain abscess with ventricular leak	Source of septic emboli usually clinically apparent; i.e., mastoiditis, ABE, dental abscess, etc. MRI/CT scans should demonstrate lesions CSF: Mimics bacterial meningitis exactly with ventricular leak except protein highly elevated in abscess Without leak <200 WBCs With leak up to 100,000 WBCs
Leptospirosis	Usually associated with severe disease, i.e., Weil's syndrome Clinically CNS features may be intensified by hepatic failure (encephalopathy) Patient is clinically ill; jaundice, conjunctival suffusion, abnormal LFTs, nausea/vomiting, myalgias, etc. CSF: Bacterial profile CSF bilirubin elevated RBCs(+)
Tuberculosis/fungal meningitis	Some have evidence of primary disease elsewhere. Lung lesions not always apparent (CXR negative in 50%) Subacute clinical presentation of basilar meningitis Fundi may have characteristic choroidal tubercles Tuberculosis classically associated with unilateral (CN VI) abducens palsy May have basilar arterial stenosis, hydrocephalus, or arachnoiditis on MRI/CT scans
Tuberculosis/fungal meningitis *(continued)*	CSF: PMNs initially, leading to lymphs usually less than 500 WBCs Glucose decreased (but may be normal) Lactic acid variably elevated RBCs +/– (RBCs prominent with histoplasma) TB smear/culture diagnostic in 80% Important to obtain serial CSF samples that show decreased glucose and increased protein
Sarcoid meningitis	Usually evidence of systemic sarcoidosis elsewhere, i.e., skin lesions, uveitis, erythema nodosum, arthritis Clinically patients not severely ill and nuchal rigidity mild Cranial-nerve II, VII, VIII, IX, X palsies occur but unilateral/bilateral facial nerve palsy most common/characteristic CSF: Resembles TB/fungal profile, but TB culture negative Usually <100 WBCs
Lupus cerebritis	Obvious evidence of SLE elsewhere, i.e., pneumonitis, nephritis, skin lesions, etc. Nuchal rigidity not impressive, but patient may have seizures/encephalopathy CSF: Resembles TB/fungal profile but TB culture negative Decreased CSF C_4 diagnostic
Lymphocytic choriomeningitis	Seasonal distribution: fall History of hamster/mouse contact in youth/adolescent Biphasic illness: "flulike" illness followed by recovery, then headache, fever, mental confusion, prominent myalgias, aslo decreased WBCs, decreased platelets

Table 1.4. *(continued)*

Meningeal process	Differential features and diagnostic clues
Lymphocytic choriomeningitis *(continued)*	CSF: Resembles viral meningitis Glucose normal/decreased WBC may be >1,000 lymphs Rarely peripheral/CSF eosinophilia
Rocky Mountain spotted fever (RMSF)	Seasonal distribution: spring/fall, with woods/animal exposure Sudden onset with severe headache, but only mild nuccal rigidity Myalgias, periorbital and extremity edema, petechial rash on wrists, ankles, decreased platelets, abnormal LFTs CSF: Resembles viral meningitis WBCs usually <100 lymphs Lactic acid variably elevated Glucose normal/decreased Protein variably elevated
Mycoplasma meningoencephalitis	Clinically severe *Mycoplasma* disease with high, cold agglutinin titers Pharyngitis, otitis, pneumonitis, diarrhea, neuro/cardiac abnormalities, but CNS findings usually less prominent CSF: Resembles viral meningitis profile CSF culture *Mycoplasma* culture (+/–)
Lyme disease	Seasonal distribution: summer, and history of tick exposure Clinically antecedent/concurrent "flulike" illness in summer! ECM helpful when present Cranial/peripheral-nerve abnormality common but unilateral/bilateral facial nerve (CN VII) palsy most characteristic CSF: Resembles viral meningitis CSF cross-reaction with VDRL Lyme CSF IgG titer (+) CSF *Borrelia* culture +/–
Meningovascular syphilis	Subacute clinical presentation with evidence of syphilis elsewhere MRI/CT scans in secondary syphilis may show multifocal, asymmetrical brain lesions CSF: Gram stain (–) Glucose decreased Protein elevated Typically 100–1,000 WBCs = PMNs—early Lymphs—later Lactic acid variably elevated CSF VDRL (+)

are not a feature of pyogenic meningitis. A brain biopsy is not necessary to make the diagnosis if the factors mentioned are all present and in agreement.

A brain abscess with a ventricular leak and associated meningitis closely mimics acute bacterial meningitis. The most important clinical clue is that the patient has an underlying condition that is associated with brain abscess, such as mastoiditis or ABE. A very high number of WBCs in the CSF also suggests a brain abscess, as does a highly elevated protein. Parameningeal foci—that is, localized areas of meningitis or brain abscess—present great diagnostic difficulty to the clinician, or did before the advent of MRI and CT scans. While the lumbar puncture should always take precedence over the CT scan, the CT scan nevertheless is an important diagnostic tool whenever a parameningeal focus is suspected.

In summary, a variety of diseases may mimic meningitis, but most of these have associated findings pointing to the diagnosis, as in SLE. Using the information provided in Table 1.4, the clinician will have a useful diagnostic profile with which to consider or rule out the various mimics of bacterial meningitis.[4,26,34,43,40,47]

Laboratory Diagnosis

Since bacterial organisms most commonly reach the CSF hematogenously, three blood cultures should be obtained in all patients with presumed bacterial meningitis. Subsequent positive blood cultures may provide the earliest specific diagnosis of the organism causing meningitis. In most cases, culture of the nares or pharynx is of no value and may provide misleading information in the patient acutely ill with meningitis. Lumbar puncture should be performed as soon as the diagnosis of meningitis is entertained. Unless a parameningeal focus is suspected, the lumbar puncture should be done immediately and before the CT scan. More patients have died as a result of delays in obtaining the lumbar puncture, or of the physician's insistence that the CT scan precede the lumbar puncture, than have died from a lumbar puncture in the presence of increased intracranial pressure. The CSF appearance should be appreciated. A "milky" appearing CSF should immediately suggest an acute pyogenic meningitis. A Gram stain of such CSF fluid usually reveals a PMN predominance with many organisms. Occasionally, in an acutely ill patient with meningitis and a cloudy CSF, no organisms are seen on the Gram stain. The two organisms usually associated with this type of presentation are the *Meningococcus* and, to a lesser extent, the *Pneumococcus*. Rarely, patients may have a cloudy CSF attributable to organisms with little or no PMNs if the infection is hyperacute and there has not been time to develop a CSF pleocytosis—a fulminant pneumococcal meningitis in an asplenic person.[38,43]

Patients with viral meningitis, parameningeal infections, or chronic or relapsing meningitis usually have clear CSF fluid. Alternatively, the CSF may be clear early in acute bacterial disease, but other parameters will be abnormal; that is, the Gram stain is positive and the CSF lactic acid elevated. A grossly bloody appearing CSF suggests traumatic tap or subarachnoid hemorrhage. Similarly, the presence of xanthochromia suggests recent CSF low-grade bleeding. Red cells are not ordinarily a feature of bacterial or viral meningitis. Their presence in the absence of xanthochromia or a grossly bloody fluid should suggest the possibility of herpetic meningoencephalitis, amebic meningoencephalitis, *Listeria,* leptospirosis, tuberculosis, or CNS malignancy.[4,25,29,33,34,36,37,43]

Microbiologic Evaluation

Microbiologic examination of the CSF by Gram stain provides immediate confirmation of the diagnosis of bacterial meningitis and suggests specific etiologic agents. CSF Gram stains are positive in more than 90% of patients with acute bacterial meningitis. Patients presenting with gram-positive cocci on CSF Gram stain usually have pneumococcal meningitis if they are adults and group B streptococcal meningitis if they are infants. The arrangement and morphology of the organisms seen on the Gram stain of the CSF provide additional useful information. For example, if only pairs of organisms are seen (i.e., diplococci), then *Streptococcus pneumoniae* is the most likely pathogen. If pairs and short chains are observed, then nonpneumococcal streptococci are the most likely organisms to present in this configuration. And last, if the organisms are seen in pairs and clusters, then staphylococci are the most likely organisms. Again, isolated CSF parameters are best analyzed in the associated clinical context, such as *S aureus,* would be the most likely explanation for gram-positive cocci in clusters in the CSF in an IV drug abuser with ABE, whereas *Staphylococcus epidermidis* would be likely in a patient with an infected ventriculoatrial (V-A) shunt.[15] In a patient with petechial lesions resembling meningococcal disease, gram-positive diplococci on CSF Gram stain confirm the clinical impression of pneumococcal meningitis.[43,46] Excessive decolorization of pairs of gram-positive cocci may suggest the *Meningococcus,* which usually presents as gram-negative diplococci on CSF smear. Similarly, *Acinetobacter,* a rare meningeal pathogen, may resemble the *Meningococcus* and lead to diagnosis confusion. However, *Acinetobacter's* clinical presentation and epidemiology in no way resemble those of the *Meningococcus,* which again underlines the importance of not overinterpreting isolated CSF findings.

Gram-negative bacilli, which are small and pleomorphic, suggest *H influenzae,* especially if seen in children under six years of age or in elderly adults. Gram-negative aerobic bacilli are uniform in shape and larger and do not contain a capsule; therefore, the CSF Gram stain serves to differentiate *H influenzae* from all of the other gram-negative meningeal pathogens. Since non–*H influenzae* gram-negative bacilli cannot be differentiated on the basis of the Gram stain, culture is the only way to make a definitive diagnosis and obtain susceptibility data. Gram-positive bacilli should suggest *Listeria monocytogenes* until proved otherwise (Table 1.5). Reports of diphteroids from the CSF should always be suspect and a request made for definitive identification of the organism. Rapid identification may be

Table 1.5. CSF Gram stain in meningitis and associated organisms.

Purulent CSF/no organisms seen	**Clear CSF/no organisms seen**
N meningitidis	Viral meningitis
S pneumoniae	tuberculosis/fungal meningitis
	Sarcoidosis meningitis
Cloudy CSF/without WBCs	Meningeal carcinomatosis
S pneumoniae	Brain abscess
	Parameningeal infection
Gram-positive bacilli	Septic emboli secondary to endocarditis
Pseudomeningitis (*Bacillus* sp., Corynebacteria)	Lupus cerebritis
	Lyme disease
Listeria	Rocky Mountain spotted fever
	LCM
	Viral meningitis
	Listeria
Gram-negative bacilli	HIV
Hemophilus influenzae (small, encapsulated, pleomorphic)	Syphilis
	Leptospirosis
Non-enteric/enteric aerobic bacilli (larger, unencapsulated)	Very early bacterial meningitis
	Partially treated bacterial meningitis
	Meningitis in leukopenic host
Gram positive cocci	**Gram-negative cocci**
Group A, B, D, streptococci (pairs and chains)	*N meningitidis*
	Mixed organisms/ Polymicrobial
S pneumoniae (pairs)	Psuedomeningitis
S aureus (pairs and clusters)	Anaerobic organisms (brain abscess with meningeal leak)
S epidermidis (in shunt infections)	Iatrogenic infection
	Neonatal meningitis
	Meningitis secondary to penetrating head trauma

achieved by doing a hanging-drop preparation of the CSF for motility, since *Listeria* exhibit a peculiar longitudinal tumbling motility not seen in the immotile corynebacteria or propionibacteria. On culture, *Listeria* may be differentiated from corynebacteria by their characteristic hemolysis. If other unusual organisms are seen on the Gram stain, or if other gram-positive bacilli are grown, then the diagnosis of pseudomeningitis should be entertained. Pseudomeningitis has been increasingly reported in the medical literature and should be suspected when unusual organisms or meningeal pathogens are cultured from the CSF with an atypical CSF profile and are incompatible with the clinical situation. It is important to recognize pseudomeningitis since there have been over a dozen case reports since it was initially described in 1973.[10] All sorts of organisms have been described in the literature and have been recovered from the CSF Gram stain or CSF culture (Table 1.6). The usual source of these pseudopathogens is their introduction into the staining or culture process. The clinician suspects pseudomeningitis on the basis of discordant clinical and CSF findings. For example, a patient may present with an "aseptic" viral meningitis and yet grow *Bacillus* sp. from the CSF. Clearly, *Bacillus* would be an unexpected finding in a "viral" CSF profile that is incompatible with the clinical presentation. The discrepancy between CSF findings and the clinical presentation is an important diagnostic clue often overlooked by those who place undue reliance on isolated CSF findings instead of drawing conclusions from all parameters.

Therapeutically, it is important to recognize pseudomeningitis since many patients have received needless and potentially harmful therapy on the assumption that bacterial meningitis did indeed exist. As the awareness of pseudomeningitis increases, the clinician will see more representation of this problem in the literature and recognize it in clinical practice.[10]

CSF Gram stain with mixed morphology suggests a polymicrobial process. Since meningitis is almost always due to one organism, except for neonatal meningitis, the finding of organisms of different morphology should suggest other diagnostic possibilities. First, pseudomeningitis should be ruled out and iatrogenic infection considered in patients receiving multiple lumbar punctures. Polymicrobial organisms of the CSF suggest meningitis secondary to penetrating head trauma or a brain abscess with a meningeal leak. Brain abscess is particularly suggested by finding anaerobic organisms on subsequent culture of the CSF.[33,43] The most complex differential diagnosis is generated by the CSF that is clear, with a negative Gram stain, if the patient does not have viral meningitis. The most important disease not to miss in this situation is a parameningeal infection, or it should alert one to the possibility of emboli from endocarditis.[26,33] The various other causes of a clear CSF with a negative Gram stain that is not viral are usually suggested by specific CSF abnormalities, such as lupus cerebritis, evidence of extra-CNS disease elsewhere (Rocky Mountain spotted fever, HIV, syphilis), or other specific CSF findings, such as meningeal carcinomatosis or Lyme disease.[34,37,43]

Table 1.6. Pseudomeningitis

Author (year)	Microorganism contaminants	Positive CSF Gram stain	Positive CSF culture	No. of patients involved	No. of patients receiving treatment
Musher and Schell (1973)	Gram-negative cocci	4	0	4	0
Joyner et al (1974)	Gram-positive cocci	1	0	1	1
Weinstein et al (1975)	Gram-negative cocci Gram-positive cocci	5	0	5	1
Coyle-Gilchrist et al (1976)	*Flavobacterium Meningosepticum*	0	1	1	1
Ericsson et al (1978)	Gram-negative bacilli	10	0	10	5
Hoke et al (1979)	Gram-negative bacilli	2	0	2	2
Centers for Disease Control (1983)	Gram-negative bacilli	1	0	1	1
Harris et al (1983)	*Salmonella typhimurium*	0	2	2	1
Ullman et al (1985)	*Acinetobacter* CDC group VE-1	1	1	1	1
Strampfer et al (1987	*Aspergillus*	0	1	1	0
Lettau et al (1988)	*Bacillus*	3	13	16	3
Penn et al (1988)	Gram-negative bacilli	15	0	15	3
Cunha and Cohen (1989)	*Bacillus*	0	1	1	1
Gelfand and Cunha (1990)	Fungal elements	1	0	1	1

Therefore, the Gram stain provides important negative diagnostic information that is useful in ruling out a viral process, and if is positive, in suggesting a specific organism upon which to base empiric therapy.

WBC Response

The clinician frequently is confronted with the problem of a CSF pleocytosis with a normal or decreased glucose with a negative Gram stain. This represents an area in which the astute infectious-disease clinician can be of real assistance as a consultant in narrowing diagnostic possibilities. In a situation where predominantly PMNs are seen in combination with a decreased CSF glucose, then partially treated bacterial meningitis or a *Listeria* meningitis would be a reasonable possibility in a patient with a subacute onset of meningeal symptoms. In a patient who has rapidly become encephalopathic with dense neurologic defects, herpes encephalitis should be considered, especially in the presence of CSF RBCs. Care must be taken to exclude a parameningeal infection and not miss the patient with endocarditis and embolic phenomena presenting as a "septic/aseptic" CSF profile. Hemorrhage into the CSF or after neurosurgery (e.g., posterior fossa syndrome) also presents in this fasion. In many instances, associated clinical findings external to the CSF may provide important clues to explain the CSF profile, such as syphilis or sarcoidosis. If the patient presents with predominantly lymphocytes with a normal CSF glucose, then partially treated meningitis again needs to be considered, as well as Lyme disease; HIV; parameningeal infection; tuberculous, fungal, or parasitic meningitis; and meningeal carcinomatosis; in addition to the most common cause, viral meningitis.[28,33,37,40] If a lymphocytic pleocytosis occurs in association with a decreased CSF glucose, then the differential is narrowed somewhat, and in addition includes LCM, mumps, and some cases of enteroviral meningitis, as well as *Listeria*,

leptospirosis, sarcoid TB, and fungal meningitis. Tuberculous meningitis may initially have a normal CSF glucose, but on serial CSF determinations, the glucose will decrease over time, usually accompanied by an increase in CSF protein, which is a clue to the diagnosis of TB.[43,47]

WBCs are predominantly PMNs in acute bacterial meningitis and in some subacute/chronic meningitides. An initial PMN predominance may be observed in early TB, syphilis, and viral, particularly echo and herpes, encephalitis. Rapidly, the PMN predominance is replaced by a lymphocytic response, which also occurs during the treatment of bacterial meningitis. PMNs may be present in the CSF as the result of peripheral blood contimination, and so low numbers of PMNs alone do not suffice for a diagnosis of meningitis. Again, caution must be exercised in interpreting values in a vacuum and out of the clinical context. Pleocytosis of the CSF may persist for weeks or months following CNS infection. Therefore, if additional information from subsequent lumbar punctures is available, the persistence of white cells should not be misinterpreted as an abnormal finding. As long as the numbers of white cells are decreasing and the PMN response is shifting to a lymphocytic response, then the persistence of WBCs in the CSF should not be of undue concern, especially if accompanied by the more important parameters of rising CSF glucose, normalizing lactic acid, and negative culture.[19,43]

The CSF Glucose

As mentioned previously, the CSF glucose must be analyzed in relation to the peripheral blood glucose. Bacterial meningitis decreases the CSF glucose, which may be due to decreased entry into the CSF by glucose, as well as to glycolic utilization by bacteria/PMNs or phagocytizing white cells. Because CSF glucose is one of the primary parameters in differentiating bacterial from viral meningitis, it is important to understand that in certain types of "aseptic" meningitis, it may be lowered, thus leading to diagnostic confusion, among enteroviral meningitis, herpes encephalitis, mumps meningitis, and LCM. Furthermore, CSF glucose regularly is lowered by RBCs in the CSF (CSF eosinophilia). Among other causes of lower CSF glucose are fungal, tuberculous, or amebic meningitis, as well as many of the organisms responsible for recurrent or chronic meningitis, such as SLE and sarcoidosis. CNS malignancy and parameningeal infections should also not be overlooked as a cause of decreased CSF glucose.[37,43]

The CSF glucose is important prognostically since it and the lactic acid are the earliest parameters to normalize after successful treatment of bacterial meningitis. In the common clinical situation where PMNs persist on repeat lumbar puncture in a patient with bacterial meningitis, the clinician can be confident that improvement is being made on the basis of the normalization of the depressed CSF glucose.[5,7]

CSF Lactic Acid

The CSF lactic acid results from a reduced clearance of lactic acid from the local acidosis of the CSF attributable to the pyogenic process. The presence of cells in the CSF account in part for increases in CSF lactic-acid levels; that is, the mechanism of CSF lactic-acid production is not clear, although the significance and usefulness of this determination are clear in terms of its diagnostic and prognostic importance. The CSF lactic acid is a rapid diagnostic test with meaningful results that are available almost immediately. The CSF lactic-acid level is most useful in differentiating viral meningitis, excluding herepes, from partially treated or bacterial meningitis (Figure 1.1). The CSF decrease in lactic acid parallels the increase in the CSF glucose as the bacterial meningitis resolves (Figure 1.2). A return to normal levels of less than 3 mmol/L is a good test of cure if serial lumbar punctures are performed. CSF lactic-acid levels between 3 and 6 mmol/L are uninterpretable since virtually any CSF disease or RBC contamination may provide these values. Only in selected situations—as in fungal versus sarcoid meningitis—may such intermediate values be of assistance. Most researchers reporting in the literature have looked at lactic acid in terms of being normal or elevated and have not fully appreciated the quantitative implications of the test.[5,7] (See Table 1.7).

Other CSF Tests

In my experience, other *c*erebro *s*pinal *f*luid (CSF) tests (limulus lysate assay, CPK, LDH, nitro blue tetrozolium, *c*ounter *i*mmuno *e*lectrophoresis (CIE), antigen) have little or no usefulness in the diagnosis of bacterial meningitis or in differentiating it from viral meningitis. CSF CIE/antigen tests are not comparable to the Gram stain in diagnostic useful-

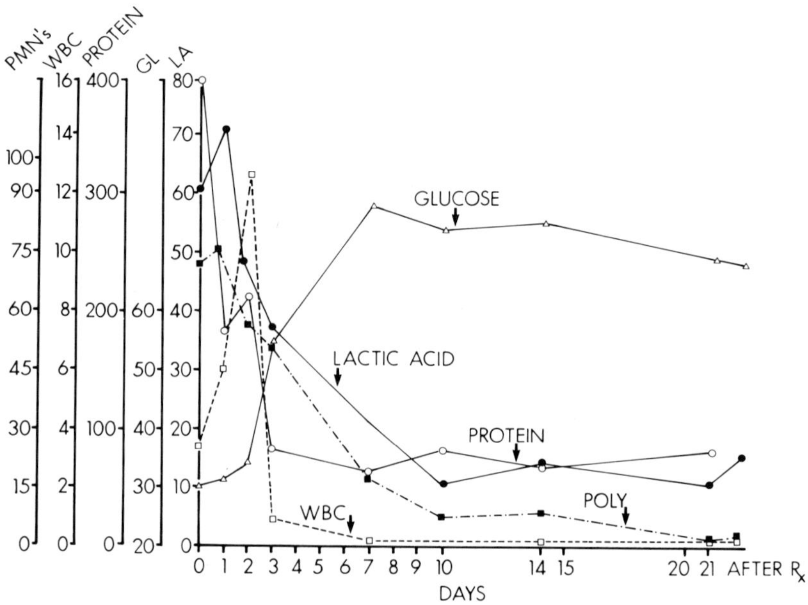

Figure 1.1. Temporal relationship of lactic acid compared with other CSF parameter in a patient with resolving pyogenic meningitis. [Reprinted with permission from Brook, Brecknell, and Overturf[7] (1978).]

ness and should not be relied on unless the results agree with the Gram stain and the clinical presentation. Furthermore, there particularly are problems with CSF CIE determinations, which only exist for a limited number of organisms. There are problems with sensitivity and specificity. It has long been appreciated that there is cross-sensitivity among the allergens of *Escherichia coli,* K-1 strains, and group B streptococci, which further limits the usefulness of this test. Urinary antigens are more helpful than CSF antigens for meningeal pathogens since infections are followed by delayed but prolonged bacterial antigenuria. A positive urinary antigen suggests recent infection but does not localize the infection to the CSF or any other tissue. Therefore, a child with antecedent otitis media may have a urinary antigen positive for *S pneumoniae,* but may currently have *H influenzae* meningitis. It is my view that these tests do not provide any additional useful information and are frequently misleading, and so should not be part of the chemical evaluation of the patient with meningitis. Of value may be the CSF C-reactive protein (CRP) determination in differentiating viral from bacterial meningitis. The CSF CRP is elevated in patients with viral meningitis analogously to the CSF lactic-acid test. Since virtually all clinical problems can be solved by com-

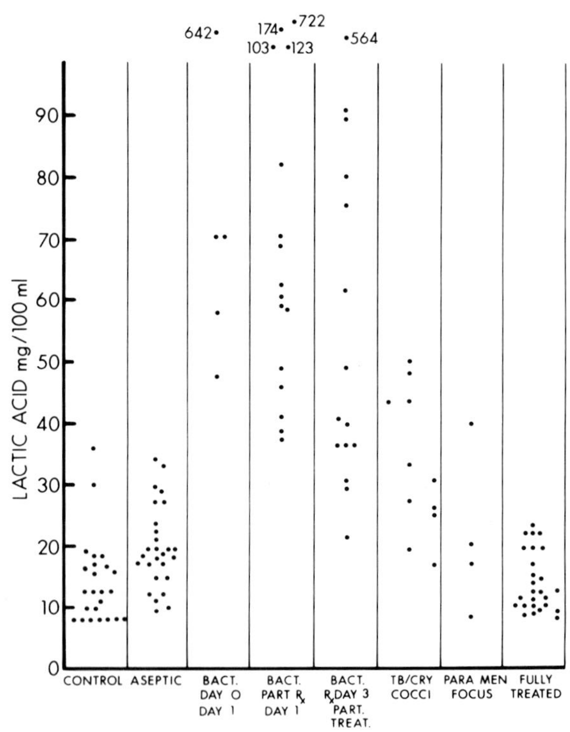

Figure 1.2. CSF lactic-acid values in a variety of CNS disorders. [Reprinted with permission from Brook, Brecknell, and Overturf[7] (1978).]

Table 1.7. Syndromic approach to CSF clues.

Purulent CSF/negative gram stain	**Red blood cells**
N meningitidis	Traumatic tap
S meningitidis	CNS bleed/tumor
Predominantly PMNs/ decreased glucose	*Listeria*
Partially treated bacterial meningitis	Leptospirosis
Listeria	Tuberculous meningitis
Herpes encephalitis	Amebic meningoencephalitis
Tuberculosis (early/beginning therapy)	Herpes encephalitis
Sarcoidosis	**Predominantly lymphs/ normal glucose**
Parameningeal infection	Partially treated bacterial meningitis
Septic emboli secondary to endocarditis	Sarcoidosis
Amebic meningoencephalitis	Lyme disease
Syphilis (early)	HIV
Posterior-fossa syndrome	Leptospirosis
CSF lactic acid	Rocky Mountain spotted fever
<3 mmol/L	Viral meningitis
Aseptic "viral" meningitis	Parameningeal infection
Parameningeal infections	TB/fungal meningitis
<6 mmol/L	Parasitic meningitis
RBCs	Meningeal carcinomatosis
TB/fungal meningitis	**Predominantly lymphs/ decreased glucose**
Herpes encephalitis	Partially treated bacterial meningitis
Partially treated meningitis	TB/fungal meningitis
Parameningeal infection	Sarcoidosis
Tumor	LCM
Any CNS inflammatory process	Mumps
>10 mmol/L	Enteroviral meningitis
Bacterial meningitis	*Listeria*
CSF protein	Leptospirosis
Elevated—	Syphilis
any CNS infection/ inflammation	Meningeal carcinomatosis
Very highly elevated	**CSF eosinophilia**
Brain tumor	Coccidioidomycosis meningitis
Brain abscess	Parasitic infections
TB with subarachnoid block	CNS lymphomas
	Ibuprofen
	V-A/V-P shunts
	Contrast materials
	CNS vasculitis

bining the clinical presentation with a careful analysis of the CSF profile, including lactic acid, there is little to be gained from additional CSF tests and, therefore, they are not recommended.[25,43]

Clearly, other laboratory tests are of use in selected patients with the diagnosis of "meningitis." CT/MRI scans are useful in ruling out mass lesions, in diagnosing HIV encephalopathy, and in ruling out parameningeal infections. These tests should be made when these diagnoses are being entertained, but are not particularly useful in the usual patient with bacterial meningitis. Similarly, an EEG in a patient with suspected herpes meningoencephalitis may provide important diagnostic information if a unilateral or bilateral temporal lobe abnormality is present. In herpes meningoencephalitis, the EEG frequently is abnormal before abnormalities are discernible on the brain or CT scan. Since any patient with a lung or CNS lesion may develop the syndrome of inappropriate antidiurectic hormone (ADH) secretion (SIADH), the finding of a decreased serum sodium has no diagnostic significance in the patient with meningitis.[33,43]

Obviously, in situations where CNS malignancies are suspected, cytologic examination of the CSF often provides the definitive diagnosis. The most common metastatic cancers to the brain are from breast, colon, and lung. Lymphomas frequently provide positive CSF cytologies and are not primary CNS lymphomas. Primary CNS lymphomas are usually seen in AIDS patients where the diagnosis is suggested by the clinical setting. Eosinophils of the CSF are locally produced and are not reflective of eosinophilia in the peripheral blood. CSF eosinophilia suggests a drug reaction, as to ibuprofen or radio-opaque contrast materials. Any CNS vasculitis or lymphoma may also result in CSF eosinophilia. The classic infectious disease associated with CSF eosinophilia are parasitic infections of the CNS and coccidioidal meningitis. Foreign-body material in the CSF may also result in an eosinophilia of the CSF, as with ventricular shunts.[15,37,47]

In addition to antimicrobial susceptibilities done on the CSF, special testing is required for *H influenzae* and the *Pneumococcus*. All blood and CSF pneumococcal isolates should be tested for relative/absolute penicillin resistance by the use of a 1-μcg oxicillin test disk. Similarly, all isolates of *H influenzae* from blood/CSF should be tested for beta-lactamase production by any of a variety of rapid methods. CSF antibiotic levels should be obtained in patients with organisms that are traditionally difficult to treat—non-*H influenzae* gram-negative bacillary meningitis, for example—or in patients who are not improving on seemingly appropriate antimicrobial therapy. Minimum inhibory concentrations and *m*inimum *b*actericidal *c*oncentrations should be obtained on usual CSF isolates to be certain that concentrations of antibiotic in the CSF are more than ten times the MBC of the infecting organism.[3,8,17,21,24,35] Serial lumbar punctures are usually necessary in gram-negative bacillary meningitis and in fungal, syphilitic, or tuberculous meningitis.

Repeat Lumbar Puncture

A repeat lumbar puncture should be obtained, if a specific etiologic diagnosis is in doubt, to monitor an improvement of CSF parameters during therapy, and to obtain CSF samples for antibiotic levels in selected patients. The usual clinical question is whether a follow-up lumbar puncture should be otained in a patient with bacterial meningitis who is improving on appropriate therapy. The answer is that repeat lumbar puncture is not ordinarily indicated in this setting. However, if the patient is not improving as predicted, or if there is a question about the diagnosis (i.e., viral versus bacterial), then relumbar puncture within 72 hours is advisable. Another useful way to differentiate viral from bacterial meningitis is to keep an extra tube of CSF after the initial lumbar puncture, incubate it for six to 12 hours, and re–Gram-stain the specimen. If the patient has bacterial meningitis, sufficient time will have elapsed during the incubation period for the organisms to multiply so that they will be visible on Gram stain of the CSF. If the patient is not deteriorating clinically, this avoids needlessly "covering" patients with aseptic meningitis out of fear, and saves the patient a subsequent repeat lumbar puncture. This simple and reliable procedure is as underutilized as is CSF lactic acid in differentiating viral from bacterial meningitis.

Therapy of Bacterial Meningitis

General Considerations

Empiric treatment of patients acutely ill with bacterial meningitis is critical to survival since the CSF lacks sufficient phagocytes, complement, or antibody to eradicate neuropathogens. Empiric therapy is based on using information from the CSF Gram stain and CSF profile in concert with the clinical presentation.[39,44] (See Table 1.8.) With the exception of meningitis in the neonate and the comprised host, it is usually possible to cover for only one or two probable meningeal pathogens. Effective treatment depends on the antibiotic's being sensitive against the infecting organism, and its penetration of the blood–CSF barrier to provide bactericidal concentrations of the antibiotic in the CSF more than ten times the MBC of the organism. Very few antibiotics penetrate noninflamed meninges, and the efficacy of the most antibiotics in meningitis depends on the increased permeability of the blood–CSF area associated with meningitis. Hematogenously derived bacteria induce increased permeability of the blood–CSF barrier, permitting entrance of the organisms and serum proteins into the CSF. Therefore, the prime protein in the CSF is albumin, since the prime protein serum is also albumin. In acute meningitis, the CSF protein correlates with the degree of inflammation and provides an index of hydrophilic antibiotic CSF penetration.[22] In chronic meningeal inflammation, the CSF albumin reflects the local disease process rather than altered blood–CSF barrier permeability and is not predictive of CSF antibiotic penetration, as in meningovascular syphilis.[6,17,24,29,39,45]

The parameters that determine a drug's penetration into the CSF are numerous, but the most important are the degree of blood–CSF barrier inflammation barrier, lipid solubility, and molecular size.

Table 1.8. Empiric therapy for bacterial meningitis.*

Host	Usual organism	Preferred regimen	Alternative regimen
Neonates ≤2 mo	E. coli Group B streptococci Gram negatives *Listeria*	3rd-generation cephalosporin plus ampicillin	Ampicillin plus gentamicin
Children 2 mo–6 yr	*H influenzae* *S pneumoniae*	3rd-generation cephalosporin	Ampicillin plus gentamicin
Adults and chilren ≥6 yr	*S pneumoniae* *N meningitidis*	Penicilin or ampicillin	3rd-generation cephalosporin or chloramphenicol
Partially treated meningitis	*H influenzae*	3rd-generation cephalosporin	Chloramphenicol
Elderly adults	*S pneumoniae* *H influenzae* *Listeria*	3rd-generation cephalosporin plus ampicillin	Chloramphenicol or TMP-SMX

*Not recommended for meningitis in compromised hosts, shunt-related meningitis, that associated with endocarditis, non–*H influenzae* Gram-negative meningitis, or HIV patients.

Other parameters, such as ionization potential (pKa) are less important.[22] Antibiotics that are hydrophobic and possess good lipid-solubility characteristics (e.g., minocycline and chloramphenicol) penetrate the blood–brain barrier as well as the blood–CSF barrier, even in the absence of meningeal inflammation. Drugs that are not lipid soluble include the beta-lactam group of antibiotics as well as aminoglycosides.[39,45] Even given in meningeal doses, less than 1% of peripheral serum penicillin levels are achieved in the noninflamed CSF. Incredibly, one has almost to die with acute bacterial meningitis for meningeal doses of penicillin to reach less than 5% of simultaneous serum levels in the CSF, resulting in rather meager concentrations of ~2 μ/ml. Fortunately, such low levels are sufficiently in excess of the MBC of the *Meningococcus* or *Pneumococcus* to be effective in treating meningitis resulting from these organisms. As a general rule, most beta-lactam compounds, including third-generation cephalosporins, achieve levels in the CSF that are 10–20% of simulataneous serum levels. Third-generation cephalosporins are effective in treating gram-negative meningitis, not because their CNS penetrability is superior, but because they are exquisitely active against gram-negative bacilli and concentrations in the CSF are well in excess of ten times their MIC 90.[3,17,32] (See Table 1.9.)

All drugs used to treat meningitis must be used in "meningeal doses," which means the drug is given in high enough concentration to assure that the CSF concentration is adequate against presumably susceptible neuropathogens. Gram-negative bacillary meningitis traditionally has been a difficult therapeutic problem.[35] Gram-negative enteric organisms are relatively resistant to most antibiotics and are usually susceptible to aminoglycosides as well as third-generation cephalosporins. Before third-generation cephalosporins were introduced, aminoglycosides and chloramphenicol were the two drugs most commonly used to treat gram-negative meningitis not cause by *H influenzae*.[16] With the exception of the neonate, with a unique blood–CSF barrier, aminoglycosides need to be given intrathecally as well as systemically to treat gram-negative CNS infections. Most frequently, an Omaya reservoir is used for this purpose since the aminoglycosides must be administered into the ventricles as the flow

Table 1.9. CSF concentrations of meningeal doses of antibiotics in adults with meningitis.

Antibiotic	Meningeal dose	Approx. CSF Concentrations	Percent of simultaneous serum levels
Penicillin G	2 μm (IV) q.2h. or 4 μm (IV) q.4h.	~2 μcg/ml	<5%
Ampicillin	1 g (IV) q.2h. or 2 g (IV) q.4h.	~4 μcg/ml	<10%
Nafcillin	1 g (IV) q.2h. or 2 g (IV) q.4h.	~1 μcg/ml	~10%
Antipsuedomonal penicillins	2 g (IV) q.2h. or 4 g (IV) q.4h.	~9 μcg/ml	~20%
Cefotaxime	2 g (IV) q.4h.	~10 μcg/ml	~20%
Ceftizoxime	2 g (IV) q.4h.	~8 μcg/ml	~15%
Ceftazidime	2 g (IV) q.2h.	~8 μcg/ml	~15%
Ceftriaxone	2 g (IV) q.12h.	~9 μcg/ml	~15%
Gentamicin	5 mg/kg (IV) in 3 divided doses q.8h.*	~1 μcg/ml	~10%
Amikacin	15 mg/kg (IV) in 3 divided doses q.8h.*	~3 μcg/ml	~20%
TMP-SMX	10–20 mg/kg (IV) in 4 divided doses q.6h.	~1/20 μcg/ml	~50/70%
Chloramphenicol	1–2 g* (IV) q.6h.	~10 μcg/ml	~65%
Vancomycin	500 mg (IV) q.6h.	~2 μcg/ml	~20%
Minocycline	100 mg (IV) q.12h.	~2 μcg/ml	~50%

*Must also be given IT (gentamicin 10 mg/day, amikacin 30 mg/day). Decrease to 1 g after 72 hours.

of CSF is cephalocaudad. Installation of aminoglycosides at the lumbar level results in inadequate intraventricular concentrations and was found to be an inadequate route of administration. Aminoglycosides penetrate the CSF much better than penicillin G, but do not achieve adequate CSF levels when administered systemically, given the relatively high MICs of gram-negative bacilli.[32,35,45]

The problem of treating gram-negative meningitis by aminoglycosides intrathecally has virtually been eliminated with the advent of the third-generation cephalosporins. Cefotaxime is perhaps the best of these for treating gram-negative bacillary meningitis not attributable to *Pseudomonas* because of its superior CSF pharmacokinetics. Cefotaxime produces the highest and CSF levels most rapidly, which is critical in treating patients with bacterial meningitis.[13] Ceftriaxone has a longer half-life in the CSF, as well as in the peripheral compartment, but has not been shown to be superior to cefotaxime or ampicillin/chloramphenicol regimens and is more expensive than other third-generation cephalosporins.[3,16] If ceftriaxone is being used to treat adults with meningitis caused by susceptible organisms, then it should be administered as 2 g intravenously (IV) every 12 hours.[14,32] In addition to high cost, other problems with ceftriaxone include an unacceptably high incidence of diarrhea, especially in children and in adults with acalculous cholecystitis.[12,17] Other third-generation cephalosporins used to treat meningitis should be administered as 2 g (IV) every four hours, or 12 g/per day, which usually results in CSF concentrations of more than 8 μcg/ml. Unusual neuropathogens, such as *Salmonella, Flavobacterium, Serratia,* and *Acinetobacter,* may also be treated with meningeal doses of TMP-SMX. CSF penetration is good but variable, and CSF levels of Trimethoprim-sulfamethoxazole (TMP-SMX) should be obtained during therapy.[27] *Pseudomonas aeruginosa* meningitis is unusual but has always been a difficult therapeutic problem. Traditionally, intrathecal aminoglycoside therapy was used. At the present time, ceftazidime in meningeal doses in combination with intrathecal aminoglycosides, or preferably with a parenteral antipseudomonal penicillin given in high doses, provides a rational therapeutic approach.

Staphylococcal meningitis traditionally was treated with intrathecal bacitracin or with chloramphenicol for susceptible strains. At the present time, high-dose nafcillin is the usual approach, and in selected cases, TMP-SMX, minocycline, or intrathecal vancomycin may be useful. V-A CNS shunt infections are usually due to *S epidermidis* or *S aureus,* While V-P shunts are frequently associated with gram-negative enteric pathogens. Eradication of the infection almost always is impossible with antimicrobial therapy alone, and almost invariably the shunt must be removed and replaced. Suppressive therapy pending surgery for V-A shunts includes meningeal doses of nafcillin or IV/intrathecal vancomycin therapy. Gram-negative shunt meningitis should be treated empirically with meningeal doses of a third-generation cephalosporin pending shunt removal.[15,43]

Beta-lactam antibiotics are not neurotoxic unless present in very high concentrations. This may be seen in patients in whom antibiotics are administered directly into the CSF, such as penicillin intraventricularly, as was sometimes done in the past, or if CSF levels are inordinately high as a result of altered blood–CSF barrier permeability and/or renal insufficiency. In treating patients with meningitis, the presence of seizures should not be ascribed to a beta-lactam antibiotic, and a careful search should be made with CT/MRI scans for a septic complication of the meningitis. Specific dosing regimens for meningitis in children are presented in Table 1.10.

The treatment of the unusual causes of meningitis—syphilis, fungal (e.g., cryptococcal), or tuberculous meningitis—is beyond the scope of this chapter and the reader is referred elsewhere in this text for treatment details. Pharmacokinetics of amphotericin in treating CNS fungal disorders is difficult to comprehend since only 10% of parenterally administered amphotericin reaches the CSF. Fluconazole offers great promise in treating fungal meningitis, particularly cryptococcal meningitis, since it may be administered orally and achieves high CSF levels of more than 80% of simultaneous serum levels. Fortunately, all of the antituberculous drugs penetrate the blood–CSF barrier in the treatment of tuberculous meningitis, and so it is not a problem from a pharmacokinetic standpoint.

Neither the optimal duration of therapy nor dosing frequency in the treatment of bacterial meningitis has been determined.[17,22,42,45] In experimental animal models, preliminary data suggest that infrequently, very high CSF levels may improve outcome as compared with the lesser, every-four-hour traditional regiments. More data will be needed before applying this to dosing in humans.[45] It is customary to treat acute bacterial meningitis for a period of two weeks of effective antimicrobial therapy.

Table 1.10. Antibiotic doses for treatment of meningitis in children.

	Dosage/day		
Antibiotic	≤7 Days	≥28 Days	Neonates, infants, and children
Penicillin G	100,000–150,000 U/kg in 2 ÷ doses q12h	150,000–200,000 U/kg in 4 ÷ doses q6h	250,000–400,000 U/kg in 6 ÷ doses q4h
Ampicillin	100–150 mg/kg in 2 ÷ doses q12h	150–200 mg/kg in 4 ÷ doses q6h	200–300 mg/kg in 6 ÷ doses q4h
Nafcillin	100–150 mg/kg in 2 ÷ doses q12h	150–200 mg/kg in 4 ÷ doses q6h	
Anti-pseudomonal penicillins	150–225 mg/kg in 2 or 3 ÷ doses q12h or q8h	225–300 mg/kg in 3 or 4 ÷ doses q8h or q6h	300 mg/kg in 6 ÷ doses q4h
Cefotaxime	100 mg/kg in 2 ÷ doses q12h	150 mg/kg in 3 or 4 ÷ doses q8h or q6h	200 mg/kg in 6 ÷ doses q4h
Ceftizoxime	—	—	200 mg/kg in 6 ÷ doses q4h
Ceftazidime	60 mg/kg in 2 ÷ doses q12h	90 mg/kg in 3 ÷ doses q8h	
Ceftriaxone	—	—	150 mg/kg in 2 ÷ doses q12h
Gentamicin	5 mg/kg in 2 ÷ doses q12h	7.5 mg/kg in 2 ÷ doses q12h	
Amikacin	15–20 mg/kg in 2 ÷ doses q12h	20–30 mg/kg in 3 ÷ doses q8h	
Chloramphenicol	25 mg/kg once daily	50 mg/kg in 2 ÷ doses q12h	100 mg/kg in 4 ÷ doses q6h
Vancomycin	20 mg/kg in 2 ÷ doses q12h	30 mg/kg in 3 ÷ doses q8h	40–60 mg/kg in 4 ÷ doses q6h

Certainly, shorter treatment regimens will be introduced in the future, but these cannot be recommended at this time.

An important caveat in treating bacterial meningitis with beta-lactam antibiotics is that the dose should not be reduced as the patient improves. This cannot be emphasized too strongly since it is commonly observed that recovering patients with pneumococcal meningitis relapse as the dose of penicillin is decreased. It must be remembered that as the patient improves, permeability of the blood–CSF barrier decreases and "inflammation-dependent antibiotics," such as the beta-lactams, penetrate the CSF less well as the infection resolves.[39,45] Therefore, "meningeal doses" of penicillins or third-generation cephalosporins must be maintained throughout the entire treatment period and not tapered as the patient improves. Very low concentrations of antibiotic are available after only a few days in the treatment of meningitis with a beta-lactam antibiotic, and decreased doses frequently result in inadquate CSF levels and subsequent relapse or therapeutic failure. Of course, third-generation cephalosporins should not be used to treat *Listeria* meningitis in either adults or children.[2] Recently, cefuroxime has been associated with treatment failure in children with *H influenzae* meningitis, which may be inoculum effect in the CSF/suboptimal dosing regimens. If CSF concentrations of more than ten times MIC_{90} of the organism are achievable with the agent chosen for empiric therapy, then there is no advantage to switching to specific therapy (Table 1.11). Furthermore, certain antibiotics—including the quinolones, imipenem, and polymyxin B—are not useful in the treatment of meningitis regardless of dose or degree of meningeal inflammation. Gram-positive coccal infections of the CSF being treated with vancomycin, except in the neonate, require concurrent parenteral and intrathecal administration. Ordinarily, two weeks of therapy with a beta-lactam antibiotic given in meningeal doses is sufficient for most patients with bacterial meningitis. Therapy beyond two weeks may be necessary in patients with gram-negative bacilli, enterococci, or *S aureus*.[1,31,39,43] Obviously, prolonged therapy is required for patients with tuberculous or fungal meningitis. In acute bacterial meningitis, there is no place for oral therapy following two weeks of parenteral therapy with meningeal doses of a beta-lactam antibiotic. Repeat lumbar puncture is not necessary as a test of cure in most patients with acute bacterial meningitis, but is necessary in patients with meningitis caused by unusual organisms, as well as in patients with tuberculous or fungal meningitis.

Aside from the epileptogenic potential of antibiotics in high concentration in the CSF, and the potential nephrotoxicity of aminoglycosides, TMP-SMX, and vancomycin, side effects are relatively uncommon with the drugs used to treat bacterial meningitis, except for ceftriaxone. The most common side effect of the beta-lactam antibiotics in

Table 1.11. Specific therapy for known bacterial pathogens in meningitis.

Organisms	Preferred regimens*	Alternate regimens
Group B streptococci	Penicillin or ampicillin	Chloramphenicol
Listeria	Ampicillin	Chloramphenicol or TMP-SMX
S. pneumoniae	Penicillin or ampicillin	Chloramphenicol or 3rd-generation cephalosporin
N meningitidis	Penicillin or ampicillin	Chloramphenicol or 3rd-generation cephalosporin
H influenzae	3rd-generation cephalosporin	Chloramphenicol or TMP-SMX
Gram-negative enteric bacilli	3rd-generation cephalosporin	Chloramphenicol or TMP-SMX
P aeruginosa	Ceftazidime 2 g (IV) q.4h.	IV/IT amikacin or antipseudomonal penicillin
S aureus	Nafcillin	3rd-generation cephalosporin, or vancomycin, or chloramphenicol

*To be given intravenously in meningeal doses.

treating patients with meningitis is drug fever,[6,17,43] which is not uncommon in patients receiving prolonged therapy. The longer the patient is on the medication, the more likely it is that an allergic reaction will ensure. Therefore, drug fevers usually are seen after the first week of therapy in patients who are clinically improving and look well, except for the unexplained fever. Repeat blood cultures are negative for such patients, who may have a temperature of 102–106°F, with 102–104°F the most common. Patients with a temperature above 102°F who are not neonates, who are not on beta-blocker medications, or who have pacemakers invariably have a pulse-temperature deficit, which is a clue to the diagnosis. Laboratory findings suggestive of drug fever include an abrupt increase in the erythrocyte sedimentation rate (ESR), mildly abnormal elevations in the alkaline phosphatase/serum transaminases, and low-grade peripheral eosinophilia. Drug fever is a diagnosis of exclusion and is the most common cause of noninfectious fever in the meningitis patient. If the drug fever occurs within a day or two of the end of therapy, the therapy may be continued if the antibiotic is a beta-lactam. If drug fever arises early in the treatment course with a beta-lactam antibiotic, then TMP-SMX or chloramphenicol is a treatment option. If the patient is receiving high-dose TMP-SMX, the hypersensitivity reaction is invariably to the sulfamethoxazole component and the drug should be stopped immediately since serious reactions such as the Stevens-Johnson syndrome may follow. Usually, steroids are not required to treat mild to moderate drug reactions characterized by drug fever.[9]

Nonantibiotic Treatment

Supportive care of the meningitis patient is important. Decubitus ulcers, line sepsis, and pulmonary toilet need special attention and should be carefully monitored.[6,20] Intravenously administered fluids should not be hypotonics, as these may exacerbate cerebral edema and further compromise local blood flow; parenteral fluids should be isotonic to avoid this problem. Recently, it was shown that in *H influenzae* meningitis in children, parenterally administered steroids decreased the incidence and severity of sensorineural hearing loss.[23,31] Further investigation is required before steroids can be recommended as standard adjunctive therapy in the treatment of acute bacterial meningitis in adults, but clearly the use of steroids in patients with neurologic complications seems reasonable.

References

1. American Academy of Pediatrics Committee on Infectious Diseases: Treatment of bacterial meningitis. *Pediatrics* 1988;81:904–907.
2. Arditi M, Herold BC, Yogev R: Cefuroxime treatment failure and *Haemophilus influenzae* meningitis: Case report and review of the literature. *Pediatrics* 1989;84:132–134.
3. Ball AP: Cephalosporins in bacterial meningitis: necessity or luxury? *J Infect* 1987;15:119–123.
4. Bia FJ, Barry M: Parasitic infections of the CNS. *Neurol Clin* 1986;4:171–205.
5. Bland RD, Lister RC, Ries JP: Cerebrospinal fluid lactic acid and pH in meningitis. *Am J Dis Child* 1974;128:151–157.
6. Bolan G, Barza M: Acute bacterial meningitis in children and adults: A perspective. *Med Clin North Am* 1985;69:231–241.
7. Brook I, Brecknell KS, Overturf GD, et al: Measurement of lactic acid in cerebrospinal fluid of patients with infections of the central nervous system. *J Infect Dis* 1978;137:384–390.

8. Cherubin CE, Eng RHK: Bacterial meningitis in the 1980s, or one drug or many?, editorial. *West J. Med* 1987;147:330–331.
9. Cunha BA: Drug fever. *Postgrad Med* 1986;80:123–129.
10. Cunha BA, Cohen S: Pseudomeningitis. *Heart & Lung* 1989;18:418–420.
11. Dagbjartsson A, Ludvigsson P: Bacterial meningitis: diagnosis and initial antibiotic therapy. *Pediatr Clin North Am* 1987;34:219–230.
12. Dankner WM, Connor JD, Sawyer M, et al: Treatment of bacterial meningitis with once daily ceftriaxone therapy. *J. Antimicrob Chemother* 1988;21:637–645.
13. Feldstein TJ, Uden DL, Larsen TA: Cefotaxime for treatment of gram-negative bacterial meningitis in infants and children. *Pediatr Infect Dis J* 1987;6:471–475.
14. Frenkel LD: Once daily administration of ceftriaxone for the treatment of selected serious bacterial infections in children. *Pediatrics* 1988;82:486–491.
15. Gardner P, Leipzig T, Phillips P: Infections of the central nervous system. *Med Clin North Am* 1985;2:297–312.
16. Girgis NI, Abu el Ella AH, Farid Z, et al: Ceftriaxone compared with a combination of ampicillin and chloramphenicol in the treatment of bacterial meningitis in adults. *Drugs Exptl Clin Res* 1987;13:497–500.
17. Haburchak DR: Bacterial meningitis. *Compr Ther* 1988;14:45–50.
18. Hayward RA, Oye RK: Are polymorphonuclear leukocytes an abnormal finding in cerebrospinal fluid? *Arch Intern Med* 1988;148:1623–1624.
19. Kaplan SL, Feigin RD: Clinical presentations, prognostic factors and diagnosis of bacterial meningitis, in Sande MA, Smith AL, Root RK (eds): *Bacterial Meningitis,* New York, Churchill Livingstone, 1985, pp. 83–94.
20. Kaplan SL, Fishman MA: Supportive therapy for bacterial meningitis. *Pediatr Infect Dis J* 1987;6:670–677.
21. Kaplan SL, Fishman MA: Update on bacterial meningitis. *J Child Neurol* 1988;3:82–93.
22. Kadurugamuwa JL, Hengstler B, Zak O: Cerebrospinal fluid protein profile in experimental pneumococcal meningitis and its alteration by ampicillin and anti-inflammatory agents. *J Infect Dis* 1989;159:26–34.
23. Lebel MH, Freij BJ, Syrogiannopoulos GA, et al: Dexamethasone therapy for bacterial meningitis. results of two double-blind, placebo-controlled trials. *N Engl J Med* 1988;319:964–971.
24. LeFrock JL, Smith BR, Molavi A: Gram-negative bacillary meningitis. *Med Clin North Am* 1985; 69:243–256.
25. Leonard JM: Cerebrospinal fluid formula in patients with CNS infection. *Neurol Clin* 1986;4:3–11.
26. Lerner PI: Neurologic complications of infective endocarditis. *Med Clin North Am* 1985;69:385–397.
27. Levitz RE, Quintiliani R: Trimethoprim-sulfamethoxazole for bacterial meningitis. *Ann Intern Med* 1984;100:881–890.
28. Lewin EB: Partially treated meningitis. *Am J Dis Child* 1974;128:145–151.
29. McGee ZA: Bacterial meningitis: current status and directions for the future—an overview, in Sande MA, Smith AL, Root RK (eds); *Bacterial Meningitis*. New York, Churchill Livingstone, 1985, pp 253–264.
30. Meade RH III: Bacterial meningitis in the neonatal infant. *Med Clin North Am* 1985;69:257–267.
31. Nelson JD: *1989–1990 Pocketbook of Pediatric Antimicrobial Therapy,* ed 8. Baltimore, Williams & Wilkins, 1989.
32. Neu HC: Use of cephalosporins in the treatment of bacterial meningitis, in Sande MA, Smith AL, Root RK (eds): *Bacterial Meningitis,* New York, Churchill Livingstone, 1985, pp 203–217.
33. Overturf GD: Pyogenic bacterial infections of the CNS. *Neurol Clin* 1986;4:69–89.
34. Pachner AR: Spirochetal diseases of the CNS. *Neurol Clin* 1986;4:207–221.
35. Rahal JJ: Therapy of gram-negative bacillary meningitis in adults, in Sande MA, Smith AL, Root RK (eds): *Bacterial Meningitis*. New York, Churchill Livingstone, 1985, pp 193–201.
36. Ratzan KR: Viral meningitis. *Med Clin North Am* 1985;69:399–413.
37. Reik L Jr: Disorders that mimic CNS infections. *Neurol Clin* 1986;4:223–248.
38. Rubin RH, Hooper DC: Central nervous system infection in the compromised host. *Med Clin North Am* 1985;69:281–295.
39. Schaad UP: Treatment of bacterial meningitis. *Eur J Clin Microbiol* 1986;5:492–497.
40. Sheller JR, Des Prez RM: CNS tuberculosis. *Neurol Clin* 1986;4:143–157.
41. Stutman HR, Marks MI: Bacterial meningitis in children: diagnosis and therapy. A review of recent developments. *Clin Pediatr* 1987;26:431–438.
42. Stutman HR, Marks MI: Therapy for bacterial meningitis: which drugs, and for how long? *J Pediatr* 1987;110:812–814.
43. Swartz MN, Dodge PR: Bacterial meningitis. A review of selected aspects. *N Engl J Med* 1965; 272:727–734.
44. Talan DA, Hoffman, JR, Yoshikawa TT, Overturf GD: Role of empiric parenteral antibiotics prior to lumbar puncture in suspected bacterial meningitis: state of the art. *Rev Infect Dis* 1988;10:365–367.
45. Tauber MG, Sande MA: Use of animal models of meningitis in developing therapeutic strategies, in Sande MA, Smith AL, Root RK (eds): *Bacterial Meningitis*. New York, Churchill Livingstone, 1985, pp. 141–157.

46. Weinstein L: Bacterial meningitis: specific etiologic diagnosis on the basis of distinctive epidemiologic, pathogenetic, and clinical features. *Med Clin North Am* 1985;69:219–229.
47. Wilhelm C, Ellner JJ: Chronic meningitis. *Neurol Clin* 1986;4:115–141.

Bibliography

Booss J, Thornton GF (eds): Infectious diseases of the central nervous system. *Neurol Clin* 1986;4(1):1–325.

Fishman RA: *Cerebrospinal Fluid in Diseases of the Nervous System*. Philadelphia, WB Saunders co, 1980.

Molavi A, LeFrock JL (eds): Infections of the central nervous system. *Med Clin North Am* 1985;69(2):217–435.

Sande MA, Smith AL, Root RK (eds): *Bacterial Meningitis*. New York, Churchill Livingstone, 1985.

Thompson RA, Green JR (eds): *Infectious Diseases of the Central Nervous System*. New York, SP Medical & Scientific Books, 1984.

Wood M, Anderson M: *Neurological Infections*. London, WB Saunders Co, 1988.

2
Complications of Bacterial Meningitis

JAY H. TUREEN AND MERLE A. SANDE

Acute bacterial meningitis remains an important problem in contemporary medical practice, marked by continued significant mortality and morbidity in spite of antibiotics that are very active against the common pathogens. The age of the patient, infecting organism, and time to diagnosis are the most important determinants of outcome, with death occurring in 3–70% of patients and neurologic residua affecting 10–50% of survivors.[1] While survival and level of neurologic function remain the primary considerations when one deals with the complications of meningitis, it is important to recognize that the disease process is a dynamic one, and that different phases present the clinician with varying problems that commonly occur at those times. In order to optimize care, the clinician must manage the patient in an anticipatory fashion, with a thorough understanding of the evolving illness.

For the purposes of this chapter, we have divided the common complications into *acute*, those that are likely to occur within the first one or two days of admission; *intermediate*, which become manifest during hospitalization and may persist after discharge; and *long-term* residua of the infection. This scheme is not meant to rigidly compartmentalize aspects of the disease, but rather to provide guidance regarding those problems that should be anticipated in certain phases.

Acute Complications of Meningitis

Acute complications of meningitis result from the intense disruption of normal brain function. In addition to the local effects of the infection, there may be systemic consequences that can potentiate the disturbance within the central nervous system (CNS). Although the precise mechanism by which bacterial meningitis produces complications is not completely delineated, recent evidence supports the concept that there are synergistic effects among the infecting organism or bacterial products, the host inflammatory response, and alterations of normal brain physiology that result in brain injury.[2] This section will focus on the pathophysiologic changes that accompany acute meningitis, and point out how these disturbances may play a role in the development of the adverse consequences of infection.

Pathophysiologic Changes

Brain Edema

Brain edema has frequently been noted in clinical and experimental studies of meningitis.[3,4] Much has been learned recently through the use of animal models about the relative contributions of bacterial and host factors in the genesis of edema in this disease. Studies by Täuber and colleagues[5] demonstrated that brain edema was more marked in rabbits with *Escherichia coli* meningitis when treated with rapidly bactericidal antbiotics and that endotoxin concentration in spinal fluid correlated with the degree of edema. These studies suggested that rapid release of endotoxin by lytic antibiotics led to an accentuation of brain dysfunction. In addition, Tuomanen and colleagues[6] showed a similar effect induced by pneumococcal cell-wall fragments. Furthermore, these investigators have demonstrated similar attenuation in the development of edema either by inducing neutropenia[7] or by blocking the entry of white blood cells to the subarachnoid space,[8] suggesting that the host response (the polymorphonuclear leukocyte) to infection may potentiate or mediate damage initiated by the bacterial products.

Recognition

As brain edema may contribute to increased intracranial pressure, the signs and symptoms suggestive of edema will, in part, be those of intracranial hypertension. In extreme situations, signs of impending herniation may be present (anisocoria, abnormal respiratory pattern, absent pupillary reflexes), or the patient with milder degrees of increased pressure may simply complain of severe headache or have a decreased level of consciousness. Brain-imaging studies—cranial computed tomography (CT) scan or magnetic-resonance imaging (MRI) scan—may be used to confirm this diagnosis.

Treatment

The deleterious aspect of brain edema is more likely to be from the contribution to intracranial hypertension than from edema *per se,* and consequently specific therapy to reduce edema should be administered with the goal of intracranial-pressure reduction. Fluid therapy, particularly fluid restriction, must be handled carefully in patients with meningitis, as overzealous restriction or overuse of osmotic diuretic agents may lead to inadequate circulating volume and compromise cerebral perfusion.

Intracranial Hypertension

Increased intracranial pressure is common in meningitis[9] and is probably caused by a combination of brain edema,[4] increased cerebrospinal fluid (CSF) volume,[10] and increased intracerebral blood volume.[11] Intracranial hypertension may create problems by inducing herniation[12] or by reducing cerebral-perfusion pressure (CPP) and contributing to ischemic injury. A recent series in children, where pressure was measured in sequential patients, indicates that virtually all patients had elevated intracranial pressure at the time of diagnosis. We believe that any patient with purulent meningitis should be suspected of having some degree of increased intracranial pressure and should be closely observed for signs suggesting that it is present.

Recognition

The symptoms and signs of intracranial hypertension include worsening headache in the conscious patient, cranial-nerve palsy (especially involving cranial nerves VI, III, and IV), bulging fontanelle in infants, declining level of consciousness, and anisocoria or abnormal pupillary reflexes, which suggest brain-stem compression and impending herniation.

Treatment

Most information about acute treatment of increased intracranial pressure in bacterial meningitis has been derived from animal studies[4,5,7,11,13] and from individual anecdotal experience with patients.[9] A recent clinical study has evaluated changes in intracranial pressure with dexamethasone therapy in the first 24–48 hours of meningitis and determined that form of therapy to be beneficial in lowering intracranial pressure.[14] If dexamethasone is not used initially, it may still be of some benefit as in intracranial hypertension from other causes. If intracranial hypertension is refractory to dexamethasone, or if its use is contraindicated, it would seem prudent to follow guidelines applied to other patients with intracranial hypertension, and apply measures that lower pressure in those settings; that is, either hyperventilation or cautious use of osmotherapy, with a goal of maintaining CPP (mean arterial pressure minus intracranial pressure) at a level of 50–70 torr.

Abnormalities of Cerebral Blood Flow

Cerebral blood flow has been observed to be reduced in both animal[11,15] and human studies[16] in meningitis. The precise mechanism probably involves many factors, including decreased CPP caused by either intracranial hypertension, systemic hypotension, or a combination of the two; cerebral vasculitis, vasospasm, or thrombosis; or possibly decreased brain metabolism. In addition, loss of cerebrovascular autoregulation places the brain at great risk to even minor decreases in CPP, as the normal regulatory mechanisms for maintaining blood flow are impaired.

Recognition

Cerebral ischemia is rarely documented, as quantitative flow studies are invasive and generally not performed in the critically ill patient. However, ischemia is probably frequently present in meningitis, as indicated by increased CSF lactic acid, which occurs commonly.[17] The principal sign of cerebral ischemia would be a decreased level of consciousness; however, this is by no means specific in this setting.

Treatment

There is no specific therapy to improve blood flow, and in fact, augmentation of blood flow could lead to further increases in intracranial pressure by increasing intracerebral blood volume. As so little is known about this in the clinical setting, at this time it seems most prudent to attempt to maintain CPP as in other forms of CNS injury, with minimum CPP from 50 to 70 torr. To monitor this parameter effectively, intracranial pressure monitoring may be necessary in selected patients, particularly those with a rapidly declining level of consciousness or who present in coma.

Specific Complications

Syndrome of Inappropriate Antidiuretic Hormone Release (SIADH)

This syndrome occurs in approximately 30% of children with purulent meningitis.[18] Antidiuretic hormone is released by neurons in the supraoptic nucleus of the hypothalamus and is stored in the posterior lobe of the pituitary gland. Under normal conditions, it is released in response to decreased circulating volume, and acts to increase free-water absorption from the collecting ducts of the nephron. In some patients with meningitis, it may be released in excessive amounts, leading to free-water excess and water intoxication.

Recognition

One should have a high degree of suspicion that SIADH may be present in all patients with meningitis. When it occurs, it is usually within the first 24 hours of admission to hospital. Patients will demonstrate oliguria in spite of absent clinical signs of dehydration and ongoing fluid administration. All patients with meningitis should have serum and urine electrolytes and osmolality measured as part of admission laboratory studies. SIADH is present when hyponatremia is present in the face of concentrated urine with elevated U_{Na} and urine osomolality greater than serum osmolality. One must be cautious, however, as hyponatremia with low U_{Na} suggests decreased circulating volume and is not due to SIADH. Correct interpretation of this study is essential in applying appropriate fluid therapy.

Treatment

If SIADH is present, fluids should be restricted, once intravascular volume depletion is repaired, to approximately two thirds of maintenance requirements (1,000 ml/M^2 every 24 hours). Serum electrolytes should be monitored every six hours until serum sodium returns to normal, at which time fluids can be liberalized.

Seizures

Seizures are present in 15–25% of patients with meningitis and may be *generalized or focal*. Most seizures occur early in the infection and may be caused by increased intracranial pressure or the irritative effects of the infection and resultant inflammatory response. Late-occurring seizures may indicate an intracranial mass lesion, such as empyema. Generalized seizures within the first 24 hours of infection usually do not have poor prognostic significance; however, if they persist or are refractory to anticonvulsants, this may indicate more serious brain pathology, as these patients have a higher incidence of significant sequelae.

Focal seizures may also be due to increased intracranial pressure, or could be indicative of either arterial or venous infarcts. If they are transient and easy to control, they have limited prognostic significance. However, those that indicate a more permanent pathologic lesion are likely to be harder to control, and in general do not have as benign a prognosis as do generalized seizures.

Treatment of seizures in meningitis is with appropriate anticonvulsants. One should also attempt to identify an underlying cause that may be amendable to specific therapy. It is particularly important to control seizures, as the hypoxia and hypercarbia that accompany seizures may potentiate other forms of ongoing brain injury or pathophysiologic abnormality.

Ventriculitis

Ventriculitis occurs in about 30% of patients with meningitis; however, it is seen in up to 50% of neonates with infection caused by gram-negative enteric organisms. There is no way to diagnose this condition routinely without examining ventricular fluid, a procedure that poses added risk and is not usually done. Ventriculitis may be suspected in the appropriate clinical setting, particularly when the patient has seizures that are difficult to control. It may be a cause of CSF cultures that are persistently positive despite appropriate antibiotics.

Intermediate Complications of Meningitis

Some of these problems may have been present earlier in the course of infection, but, because of the patient's instability, might not be recognized until the patient has been in the hospital for a few days. Others may not become manifest until the disease process has gone on for several days.

Subdural Effusion

This is a common complication in children with meningitis, which has been increasingly recognized since the advent of routine CT scanning. Sterile effusions are present in up to 25% of children with *Hemophilus influenzae* meningitis.[1] In almost all cases, these effusions do not require specific therapy, and they resolve spontaneously. In a minority of cases, they cause pressure phenomena that require serial subdural taps.

Recognition

Most effusions are found at approximately five to seven days of hospitalization. Patients may have recrudescence of fever or a decreased level of consciousness, infants may develop a bulging fontanelle, and a rare patient may have a significant increase in intracranial pressure causing cranial-nerve palsy or loss of upward gaze. These symptoms must be differentiated from other causes of increased intracranial pressure, such as subdural or epidural empyema or hydrocephalus. Diagnosis is made by CT or MRI scan.

Treatment

Treatment in most instances is by observation. These effusions rarely cause a significant clinical problem, but they can be troublesome in that they must be differentiated from more serious intracranial events, and if fever is present, they can raise concern about recrudescence of meningitis. When the increase in pressure is significant, fluid must be evacuated. In the infant with an open fontanelle, this is accomplished in a relatively straightforward manner with subdural taps. In the older child or adult, it would involve a neurosurgical procedure. Fortunately, this is rarely necessary.

Subdural or Epidural Empyema

These empyemas are far less common than sterile effusions, occurring only about 1–2% of the time. The mechanism is thought to be the penetration of organisms across the arachnoid or dural membranes; however, it is not known why there appears to be a predilection for this to happen with certain organisms. They are far more likely to occur in meningitis due to *Streptococcus pneumoniae*[19] than with other pathogens such as *H influenzae* or *Neisseria meningitidis*. These are serious complications that require surgical drainage in addition to antibiotic therapy.

Recognition

Signs and symptoms may be similar to those for subdural effusions because of the pressure effect, except that fever is almost universally present. Seizures may take place, and are usually focal. Epidural empyema tends to remain more localized because its spread is relatively impeded by the dura's adherence to the inner surface of bone. Neurologic findings suggest a focal lesion with unilateral weakness or seizures on the contralateral side.

Treatment

Diagnosis is made by CT or MRI scanning or by radionuclide brain imaging. These focal collections of purulent material must be surgically evacuated. Following surgical therapy, treatment with appropriate antibiotics should be continued for two to three weeks.

Fever

Most patients with purulent meningitis will have resolution of fever within the first three to four days of therapy. About 10% of children with meningitis attributable to *H influenzae* will continue to have fever for seven to eight days with no localizing finding. While this is worrisome, it should be recognized that for some patients, delayed defervescence does occur. *Secondary fever* describes the situation where fever has resolved and returned later in the hospitalization. In this situation, patients must have a rigorous evaluation for recrudescence of disease[20] (which is uncommon), as well as for secondary foci that may be evidenced in the form of infected intravenous devices, intracranial empyema, pleural empyema, purulent pericarditis, endocarditis, or septic arthritis. As mentioned previously, subdural effusions may cause fever. By the end of the first week of therapy, drug fever may occur, although this is most typical after 10–14 days. Evaluation should include an examination to identify obvious foci of infection, repeat lumbar puncture and CSF examination and culture, and appropriate radiographic studies.

Brain Abscess

Brain abscess is an unusual complication of meningitis, except with disease attributable to *Citrobacter* sp, where abscess(es) develop in approximately 50% of cases, and, rarely, *Listeria*. These may be present as early as the second week of disease, but most present in the third or fourth week.

As with brain abscess in other situations, patients have fever and signs and symptoms of an intracranial mass lesion. Therapy should be guided by principles applied to brain abscess in general—single, peripheral lesions greater than 2 cm are probably best approached with a combination of surgical and antibiotic treatment, whereas deep lesions or multiple small lesions should be treated with antibiotics alone. Periventricular lesions are particularly troublesome as they are difficult to approach surgically, but intraventricular rupture has a high mortality rate.

Hydrocephalus

Hydrocephalus as a complication of meningitis can be caused by at least two mechanisms: *obstructive hydrocephalus* where there is obstruction to CSF resorption as a result of postinflammatory injury of the arachnoid granulations, and *hydrocephalus ex vacuo* as a consequence of diffuse brain injury with resultant brain atrophy.[21] Obstructive hydrocephalus may arise while the patient is in the hospital, and would be manifest by signs of increased intracranial pressure. Short-term treatment for acute hydrocephalus can be with the removal of CSF by sequential lumbar punctures and acetazolamide. Definitive therapy is by placement of a ventriculoperitoneal-shunt catheter.

Long-Term Complications of Meningitis

Long-term complications range from subtle forms of cognitive impariment to devastating neurologic handicaps. Findings include cranial-nerve injury (particularly deafness caused by injury to the eighth cranial nerve), impairment of cognitive function or behavioral problems, ataxia, hemiparesis, hypertonicity, and residual seizures. Some of these injuries are clearly evident upon hospital discharge, whereas others may take years to become evident. Conversely, many neurologic handicaps that are present at discharge will improve with time.

Impairment of Cognitive Function

Impairment may range from milder forms ("learning disabilities") to global developmental delay. While the actual incidence of milder forms of injury is not known, some suggestion can be generalized by sibling-matched studies of children with enteroviral meningitis in the first year of life, which showed below-predicted-performance scores in 25% of the children with meningitis. The age of the patient is a critical determinant of ultimate outcome, with more serious sequelae occurring in the young. The incidence of more serious forms of injury is probably in the 2% range.

Deafness

Deafness is the most common significant long-term injury in meningitis, with from 5 to 25% of survivors suffering some form of hearing impairment.[22] Once again, there is age and pathogen specificity, with neonates and children with infection with *S pneumoniae* having the highest incidence. It is not known whether the injury is due to vascular damage to the eighth nerve or to inner ear structures; however, it does appear to be a relatively early complication[23] that is frequently diagnosed only after discharge.

Motor Handicaps

These handicaps, may range from isolated paresis to global injury leading to quadriplegia. Weakness may be confined to a single muscle group or nerve distribution, as in an isolated ptosis, or reflect central injury, as would explain hemiparesis, hemiplegia, or quadriplegia. These findings, when present at discharge, may improve with time, as indicated in a clinical study that showed that only 20% of the serious neurologic motor handicaps present at discharge persisted at one year follow-up.

Conclusion

In summary, bacterial meningitis remains an important medical problem with a significant incidence of mortality and morbid sequelae. As most of the cases involve the very young, this results in a great loss of productive years for the patients and a very significant economic burden on the family to provide care for the most seriously injured. At present, our understanding of the pathogenesis of brain injury is incomplete, but much has been learned through the use of animal models and the clinical trials that have been generated from those basic observations. Future studies will be directed at more precisely defining the role of bacterial and host factors, arachidonic-acid metabolites, cytokines, excitatory neurotransmitters, and the pathophysiologic consequences of the infection with a goal of specifically intervening with adjunctive forms of therapy. This, combined with improvements in intensive care for the patient with serious CNS disease, holds the greatest promise for these patients.

References

1. Klein JO, Feigin RD, McCarcken GH Jr: Report of the Task Force on Diagnosis and Management of Meningitis. *Pediatrics* 1986;78:959–982.
2. Sande MA, Scheld WM, Täuber MG, et al: Pathophysiology of bacterial meningitis: Report of a Symposium. *Ped Infect Dis J* 1989;8:929–933.
3. Swartz MN, Dodge PR: Bacterial meningitis: A review of selected aspects. *N Engl J Med* 1965; 272:725,779,842,898,954.
4. Täuber MG, Khayam-Bashi, Sande MA: Effects of ampicillin and corticosteroids on brain water content, cerebrospinal fluid pressure, and cerebrospinal fluid lactate levels in experimental pneumococcal meningitis. *J Infect Dis* 1985;151:528–534.
5. Täuber MG, Shibl AM, Hackbarth CJ, et al: Antibiotic therapy, endotoxin concentration in cerebrospinal fluid, and brain edema in experimental *Escherechia coli* meningitis in rabbits. *J Infect Dis* 1987; 156:456–462.
6. Tuomanen EI, Tomasz A, Hengstler B, et al: The relative role of bacterial cell wall and capsule in the induction of inflammation in experimental meningitis. *J Infect Dis* 1985;151:535.
7. Täuber MG, Borschberg U, Sande MA: Influence of granulocytes on brain edema, intracranial pressure, and cerebrospinal fluid concentration of lactate and protein in experimental meningitis. *J. Infect Dis* 1988;157:456.
8. Tuomanen EI, Saukkonen K, Sande S, et al: Reduction of inflammation, tissue damage, and mortality in bacterial meningitis in rabbits treated with monoclonal antibodies against adhesion-promoting receptors of leukocytes. *J Exp Med* 1989;170:959–968.
9. Minns RA, Engleman HM, Stirling, H: Cerebrospinal fluid pressure in pyogenic meningitis. *Arch Dis Child* 1989;64:814–820.
10. Scheld WM, Dacey RG, Winn HR, et al: Cerebrospinal fluid outflow resistance in rabbits with experimental meningitis: Alteration with penicillin and methylprednisolone. *J Clin Invest* 1980;66:243
11. Tureen JH, Dworkin RJ, Kennedy SL et al: Loss of cerebrovascular autoregulation in experimental meningitis in rabbits. *J Clin Invest* 1990;85:577–581.
12. Horwitz SJ, Boxerbaum B, O'Bell J: Cerebral herniation in bacterial meningitis in childhood. *Ann Neurol* 1980;7:524.
13. Tureen JH, Stella FB, Clyman RI, et al: Effect of indomethacin on brain water content, cerebrospinal fluid white blood cell response and prostaglandin E_2 levels in cerebrospinal fluid in experimental pneumococcal meningitis in rabbits. *Ped Infect Dis J* 1987;6:1151–1153.
14. Lebel MM, Freij BJ, Syrogiannopoulos GA et al: Dexamethasone therapy for bacterial meningitis: Results of two double-bling placebo-controlled trials. *N Engl J Med* 1988;319:964–970.
15. Smith AL. Pathogenesis of *Haemophilus influenzae,* type b meningitis, in Deusch G, Wadstrom T (eds.): *Experimental Bacterial and Parasitic Infections.* New York, Elsevier Science Publishing, 1983, p 295.
16. Paulson OB, Brodersen P, Hansen El et al: Regional cerebral blood flow, cerebral metabolic rate of oxygen, and cerebrospinal fluid acid-base variables in patients with acute meningitis and with acute encephalitis. *Acta Med Scand* 1974;196:191.
17. Brook I, Bricknell KS, Overturf GD, Feingold SM. Measurement of lactic acid in cerebrospinal fluid of patients with infections of the central nervous system. *J Infect Dis* 1978:137:384.
18. Feigin RD, Kaplan S: Inappropriate secretion of antidiuretic hormone (ADH) in children with bacterial meningitis. *Am J. Clin Nutr* 1977;30:1482–1484.
19. Tureen JH, Sande MA: Acute bacterial infections of the central nervous system, in Aminoff MJ (ed): *Neurology and General Medicine.* New York: Churchill Livingstone, 1989; pp 559–575.
20. Whitecar JP Jr., Reddin JL, Spink WW. Recurrent pneumococal meningitis: A review of the literature and studies on a patient who recovered from eleven attacks caused by five serotypes of *Diplococcus pneumoniae. N Engl J Med* 1966;274:1285–1289.
21. Kirkpatrick M, Wngleman H, Minns RA. Symptoms and signs of progressive hyrdrocephalus. *Arch Dis Child* 1989;64:124–128.
22. Finitzo-Hieber T, Simhardi T, Hieber JP: Abnormalities of the auditory brainstem response in postmeningitic infants and children. *Int J Pediatr Otorhinolaryngol* 1981;3:275–286.
23. Dodge PR, Davis H, Feigin RD, et al: Prospective evaluation of hearing impairment as a sequela of acute bacterial meningitis. *N Engl J Med* 1984; 311;869–874.

3
The Aseptic Meningitis Syndrome

Burt R. Meyers and Alejandra C. Gurtman

The aseptic meningitis syndrome is characterized by a set of symptoms and clinical signs in association with certain laboratory evidence of meningeal inflammation manifested by changes in the cerebrospinal fluid (CSF). It is traditionally assumed that the etiology is nonbacterial in nature and secondary to a viral agent.

The classical symptoms include headache, photophobia, meningismus (often with nausea), vomiting, and occasionally changes in mental status, including irritability. Clinically, the patient appears nontoxic without evidence of hypotension; a morbilliform rash not usually petechial may be present in association with clinical signs of meningitis, including stiff neck, with or without Kernig's sign or Brudzinski sign. There may be other signs of viral infection, including pharyngitis, adenopathy, and evidence of hepatitis.

Examination of the peripheral blood usually reveals a normal white-blood-cell count without a left shift, though the white count can be elevated or a left shift occasionally present. Sedimentation rate may be normal or elevated. Various causes for this syndrome have been described (see Table 3.1), including those of an infectious nature (i.e., bacteria and higher-order bacteria such as mycobacteria), fungi, rickettsia, parasites, and spirochetes. Collagen vascular diseases (i.e., lupus erythematosus) or granulomatous arteritis,[1,2] sarcoidosis,[3] chemical meningitis,[4–6] cerebral vascular lesions,[7] epidermal cysts,[8] drug ingestion,[9–16] meningeal carcinomatosis,[17–19] serum sickness,[20] focal central-nervous-system (CNS) lesions, and specific syndromes (i.e., Mollaret's meningitis)[22] may produce this clinical picture. Since most patients with viral meningitis will not be candidates for therapy, it behooves the physician or health-care worker to recognize the treatable causes of the aseptic meningitis syndrome.

Pathophysiology

Viruses may initially cause infection or passively enter through the skin or the respiratory, gastrointestinal, or urogenital tract.[23] Viral growth in extraneural tissues depends on the ability to infect susceptible cells requiring receptors for absorption of the virus and the ability to replicate viral particles within those cells. Viruses may spread through nerve endings with retrograde transmission via neuronal axons (i.e., polio virus); in experimental models, herpes simplex virus has spread by this route. The virus can multiply within the axon, as well as within lymphatic or interstitial tissue between nerve fibers.[24] Viruses can enter via the olfactory route, cause infection of the submucosa, and directly invade the subarachnoid space.[23,24] Herpes simplex virus probably enters by this route, since infection has occurred in this way in experimental models. Most viruses, however, probably enter the CNS following viremia of sufficient magnitude and duration that allow CSF penetration by either growing in the choroid plexus or passing directly through it.[23–25]

It is believed that the enteroviruses, lymphocytic choriomeningitis virus, mumps, and arthropod-born viruses replicate initially in muscle cells or mesodermal cells.[26] Viruses may enter the CNS or may enter the spinal fluid directly following viremia.[24,25] Other agents, such as bacteria, mycobacterium, and fungi, usually enter the body by the respiratory route (i.e., pharynx, sinuses, or lung) and are then disseminated by the bloodstream to the CNS. In some cases, an antecedent pneumonitis followed by fungemia or bacteremia occurs. The bloodstream is usually the source for spirochetes such as *Treponema pallidum* and the agent of Lyme disease,

Table 3.1. Differential diagnosis of aseptic meningitis

Infectious	
Bacterial:	*L monocytogenes*
	Brucella sp
	S pneumoniae (uncommon)
	N meningitidis (uncommon)
	H influenzae (uncommon)
Fungi:	Histoplasma capsulatum
	Cryptococcus neoformans
	Coccidiodes immitis
	Candida Sp.
	Aspergillus Sp.
Mycobacteria	*M tuberculosis*
Rickettsia	*R rickettsii*
Mycoplasma	*M pneumoniae*
Spirochetes	*T pallidum*
	B burgdorferi
	Leptospira Sp.
Parasites	Angiostrongylus
	Cysticercous
Viruses:	
Enterovirus	Polio virus
	Echovirus
	Coxsackie virus
	"New enteroviruses"
Herpes virus	Herpes virus 1 and 2
	Varicella zoster virus
	Epstein-Barr virus
	Cytomegalovirus
Paramyxovirus	Mumps virus
	Measles virus
Togavirus	Rubivirus—rubella virus
Alphavirus	Eastern equine encephalitis virus
	Western equine encephalitis virus
	Venezuelan encephalitis virus
Flavivirus	Japanese encephalitis virus
	Murray Valley encephalitis virus
	St. Louis encephalitis virus
Bunyavirus	California encephalitis virus
	LaCrosse encephalitis virus
Reovirus	Colorado tick fever virus
Arenavirus	Lymphocytic choriomeningitis virus
Rhaboovirus	Rabies virus
Retrovirus	Human immunodeficiency virus
Noninfectious	
Drug ingestion	Nonsteroidal anti-inflammatory agents
	Antineoplastic agents
	Antibiotics
	Immunosuppresants
Chemical	Contrast agents
	Disinfectants, glove powder, etc.
Neurologic disorders	Cerebral vascular lesions
	Epydermal cysts
	Brain tumors
	Epidural–subdural abscess
Miscellaneous	Sarcoidosis
	Serum sickness
	Mollaret's meningitis
	Subacute bacterial endocarditis
	Meningeal carcinomatosis

Borrellia burgdorferi. Mechanisms whereby meningeal carcinomatosis, collagen vascular disease, brain tumors, and brain epidural or subdural abscess cause changes in the chemistries of the CSF have not been fully elucidated. While certain drugs, including nonsteroidal anti-inflammatory agents,[9–11,14] antineoplastic agents,[6,12] immunosuppressants (i.e., Orthocline OKT3—Orthopharmaceutical),[27] and occasionally either trimethoprim alone[13] or in combination with sulfonamides,[16] may produce the aseptic meningitis syndrome, the pathophysiology is not known.

The diagnostic approach to patients who present with this syndrome places emphasis on the history and physical and spinal-fluid examination. Most viral infections are seasonal in nature, occurring during late summer or early fall. Enteroviruses (i.e., echo, Coxsackie) are the most common; others, including mumps and varicella, are less common. A history of exposure to patients with known viral illness is often suggestive. Exposure to pets (i.e., mice or rodents) suggests infection with either lymphocytic choriomeningitis (LCM) virus or, less commonly, *Leptospira* sp. Eliciting a history of sexual contacts is mandatory; herpes simplex virus (HSV-2), and in the appropriate risk group, human immundeficiency virus (HIV-I) may present with this syndrome. Patients must be carefully questioned about risk factors for HIV infection, including intravenous-drug use, sexual promiscuity, sexual preference, and transfusions with blood or blood products. The geographic location of the patient's domicile, as well as travel, must be considered to rule out infection with fungi (i.e., *Histoplasma capsulatum* and *Coccidiodes immitis*) or spirochetes (i.e., *B burgdorferi*). If a patient had pet contact or had been camping, infection with *Rickettsia* or *B. burgdorferi* related to a tick bite must be considered. Rabies, though rare, should be considered if there was contact with or a bite from a sick animal (i.e., skunk, racoon, fox, dog, or bat). Drinking water on backpacking trips may be associated with ingestion of Leptospira; ingestion of unpasturized milk and cheeses may be suggestive of brucellosis.

Since the aseptic meningitis syndrome is associated with other medical conditions, including collagen vascular diseases (i.e., lupus erythematosus), a careful physical examination looking for a typical malar rash or other stigmata is necessary. Other vasculitidies, often found in patients of Mediterranean origin, include familiar Mediterranean fever[28] or Bechet's syndrome,[29] and may also produce this syndrome. Since certain drugs, including nonsteroidal anti-inflammatory agents and anti-immune compounds such as OKT3[27] have been associated with the syndrome, a history of their use must be questioned. If there is a history of upper-respiratory-tract infection (i.e., otitis media, sinusitis) or an intraoral infection of the teeth or gums, a brain/epidural or subdural abscess must be considered; appropriate tests, including a computed tomography (CT) scan, may aid in making these diagnoses. Since subacute bacterial endocarditis[30] has been associated with this syndrome, physical stigmata (i.e., conjunctival petechiae, retinal lesions, cardiac murmur, or evidence of embolic phenomena) must be searched for carefully. The presence of infection with either mycobacteria or fungi or a past history of cancer must be considered.

Equine-associated meningoencephalitis outbreaks occur seasonally, usually in late summer and early fall; there usually is an association with infections in horses.[31] Avian or equestrian sources with spread via mosquitoes is the route of infection to humans. A history of recurrent bouts of meningitis with a benign clinical picture and unknown etiology should suggest the diagnosis of Mollaret's meningitis.

Physical Examination

A nontoxic, febrile patient with or without evidence of meningismus is often noted. Pulse and respiration are usually within normal limits or only slightly elevated, and low-grade fever may be present; on occasion, the temperature may be elevated beyond 103–104°F. Examination of the skin may reveal a morbilliform or vesicular rash or evidence of infection such as a tick bite. The scalp should be carefully examined, as well as the area behind the ears, to look for evidence of tick infestation. Petechial lesions, particularly the hands and feet, suggest Rickettsial infection. There may be other evidence of fungal infection as manifested by papular or papular squamous involvement. Examination of the eyes may reveal conjunctival petechiae or evidence of iritis. A fundascopic examination may reveal either vascular disease or the typical lesions seen in infectious endocarditis. Other lesions include cytomegalovirus (CMV) retinitis or toxoplasmosis; in the appropriate risk group, this suggests the possibility of HIV infection.

Examination of the oral cavity may reveal a mild pharyngitis, and occasionally evidence of vesiculopapular lesions on either the buccal mucosa or the gum margin. Cervical adenopathy may be present. Chest examination is usually normal but a radiograph is necessary to rule out pulmonary infiltrates. The presence of a murmur in this setting suggests the possibility of endocarditis. A pericardial rub is more in keeping with collagen/vascular syndromes. Hepatomegaly, splenomegaly, or adenopathy may be noted. Examination of the groin and genitals is necessary; evidence of a vesicular or ulcerative lesions suggests either viral or spirochetal infection. Ulcerative lesions in the vagina have also been noted in vascular syndromes such as lupus erythematosus. Joint inflammation, particularly monoarthritis, is suggestive of mycobacterial infections. A careful neurologic examination may reveal evidence of neck stiffness on flexion, a positive Brudzinski and/or Kernig's sign. The presence of focality or involvement of multiple cranial nerves is suggestive of central lesions, such as a brain subdural or epidural abscess; embolic phenomena from infectious endocarditis also may produce these lesions.

Laboratory Data

When the spinal fluid is examined, the opening pressure should be recorded; it may be slightly elevated and the fluid is usually clear without sediment. Cell count reveals a predominance of mononuclear cells, usually lymphocytes, though early in the course of certain viral infections (i.e., "echovirus" (ECHO), polio, mumps, and herpes viruses), a predominance of polymorphonuclear leukocytes can be observed.[32–34] The cell count is usually less than 100 lymphocytes per milliliter. Pleocytosis may be absent in 25% of patients with enteroviral infection.[35] Abnormal cells secondary to meningeal carcinomatosis may be seen; large endothelial cells with indistinct cytoplasm suggest a diagnosis of Mollaret's meningitis. Fat droplets may be seen in the CSF following epidermoid cyst rupture.[36] It may be appropriate to make a wet prep of the spinal fluid to look for the parasite Toxoplasma gondii. Gram stain is necessary to rule out bacteriologic causes (i.e., *Listeria monocytogenes*),[37] which may present with a predominance of lymphocytes; among other stains are an acid-fast stain to rule out mycobacterial infections and India-ink stain for cryptococcal infection. Indirect immunofluorescent staining of CSF may show evidence of varicella zoster antigen.[38] The fluid should be sent for routine bacterial, fungal, and mycobacterial cultures; spinal fluid should also be sent for viral culture as enteroviruses (71%) may be cultured directly from this fluid.[35] Simultaneous viral cultures should be obtained from throat washings and stool specimens. The presence of eosinophils may suggest angiostrongylus and cysticercosis. Serologic confirmation from either CSF or blood is necessary to make the diagnosis.[39,40]

A spinal-fluid glucose should be compared with a simultaneously drawn blood glucose; levels in the CSF of 40 mg/dl or less than 50% of blood levels are suggestive of viral meningitis.[41] The protein is usually elevated; levels greater than 800 mg/L are suggestive of spinal-fluid block from either chronic infection or tumor (though it has been seen in chemical meningitis).

Other tests on spinal fluid to differentiate viral meningitis from pyogenic infections may be performed. These tests include lactate,[42,43] C-reactive protein,[44,45] amino acids,[46] and adenosine deaminase.[47] While alpha-inteferon alpha may be increased,[48,49] in most cases, the levels for these tests are lower in patients with viral meningitis as compared with other infectious etiologies.[50,51] However, these tests should not be relied on in a definitive way, but if negative, only considered corroborative in nature.

The peripheral white-blood-cell count is usually normal, or less than 5,000/mm^3; the differential is usually normal, though occasionally a left shift in the polymorphonuclear leukocytes series is observed. Eosinophilia has been noted in patients with drug- and serum-sickness[21] reactions. Blood cultures should be performed since bacterial agents such as *L monocytogenes, brucella,*[52,53] or typical pyogens (i.e., *Streptococcus pneumoniae , Neisseria meningitidis,* and *Hemophilus influenzae)* may present initially without a predominance of polymorphonuclear leukocytes in the spinal fluid.[54] Infectious endocarditis, from either bacteria or fungi, is usually considered in the appropriate clinical setting with positive blood cultures.

When fungal disease is suspected, serologic studies should be carried out on the peripheral blood for cryptococcal antigen, *H capsulatum,* and *C immitis;* complement fixation for *Mycoplasma pneumoniae* is warranted when a viral-like infection is suspected. In all cases in which the etiology is not clear, a VDRL should be determined on spinal fluid. A complement fixation test for *Rickettsia rickettsii* when Rocky Mountain spotted fever is suspected and a Lyme titer to look for evidence of infection with *B burgdorferi* should be performed. If rabies is suspected, an immunofluorescence test on conjunctival scrapings is the most accurate method of establishing the diagnosis.

A chest x-ray specifically looking for evidence of soft infiltrates, cavitary disease, or pleural or pericardial involvement can suggest either mycoplasmal, mycobacterial, or fungal infection. Evidence of a mass lesion suggests a carcinoma and the possibility of meningeal carcinomatosis. Serologic tests, including antinuclear antibody (ANA) to rule out lupus erythematosus, may be necessary, as well as other tests for autoimmune diseases. In the appropriate clinical setting and with the permission of the patient, HIV testing may be warranted. In patients with evidence of HSV-2 infections, serial serologic determinations three to four weeks apart should be carried out, though a fourfold rise is suggestive of HSV-2 but not diagnostic.

Focal involvement on neurologic examination requires a CT scan to seek evidence of an intracranial infection (i.e., brain, epidural/subdural abscess, or intracranial malignancy). Epidermoid tumors have presented with a clinical syndrome of recurrent meningitis mimicking Mollaret's meningitis, with macrophages noted in the spinal fluid.[22]

If vesicular skin lesions are present, immunofluorescent staining for HSV-1–2, and varicella zoster virus (VZV) can be performed, as can a viral culture; if syphilis is a consideration, though not with vesicular lesions, careful examination by dark field will reveal evidence of *T pallidum.* Petechial lesions can be Gram stained and cultured for bacteria and immunofluorescent staining for *R rickettsii* performed.

Treatment

At this time, the only treatments for viral infections of the central nervous system causing meningitis are AZT for HIV infections and intravenous acyclovir for HSV-1 infection causing encephalitis. Since early bacterial meningitis may present with spinal-fluid pleocytosis and a predominance of lymphocytes, it may be necessary to consider treatment with antibiotics even if the patient does not appear toxic; evidence or suspicion of bacterial infection coupled with sound clinical judgment is necessary. However, in patients with a predominance of polymorphonuclear leukocytes in whom a viral infection is suspected because of the clinical syndrome, some authors recommend that antibiotics be withheld and a spinal tap be repeated in 8–10 hours.[55,56] If there is a shift from polymorphonuclear leukocytes to mononuclear cells, then viral infection is more likely. However, others have not been able to confirm this finding.[57] In the rapidly deteriorating patient with a predominance of lymphocytes, it appears prudent to begin antibacterial treatment with agents such as ampicillin to cover *L monocytogenes* and third-generation cephalosporins (i.e., cefotaxime or ceftriaxone) to cover other bacterial causes; treatment of tuberculous meningitis also appears prudent if there are signs of CNS deterioration. While CSF glucose is usually normal in the aseptic meningitis syndrome, as is the CSF glucose/blood ratio,[58] patients with viral meningitis caused by herpes simplex, mumps, LCM, or polio may present with depressed CSF glucose.[58] A clinical judgment must then be made as to whether these patients should be treated with the above antibiotic regimens.

Infections secondary to *Mycobacteria tuberculosis* and fungi, including *Cryptococcus neoformans, Histoplasma* sp, and *Coccidiodes,* usually require therapy with specific agents (see other chapters). When bacterial endocarditis is suspected, antimicrobial therapy to cover either *Streptococcus viridans, Enterococcus faecalis,* or *Staphylococcus aureus* seems appropriate; in the intravenous-drug user, further coverage of gram-negative bacilli is warranted. In a patient with sinusitis with secondary infection of the CNS (i.e., a subdural or epidural abscess), surgical therapy and antimicrobial agents are usually necessary. With brain abscesses, the spinal fluid usually reveals no microorganisms unless there is a rupture into the ventricular space; this is usually associated with a catastrophic event. Therapy for brain abscess would include agents that penetrate the CNS and are effective against anaerobic bacteria; such therapies include penicillin V or a semisynthetic antistaphylococcal penicillin plus metronidazole.[59] Serial CT scans have revealed cures with antimicrobial agents given during a 3–6-week period.[60,61] If CNS syphilis is confirmed, therapy with intravenous penicillin for 10 to 14 days, 12–16 million units a day, is warranted; this may be better than 2.4 million units of benzathine penicillin given weekly for 3 weeks.[62] Penicillin has recently been shown to be beneficial for *Leptospira* infection, quickening the clinical response.[63] If evidence of *mycoplasma* infection is found, then therapy with either erythromycin [500 mg every 6 hours (Q6H)] or tetracycline (500 mg Q6H) (not in children or pregnant women) appears warranted; the effect on meningitis is not known. For Lyme disease with CNS involvement, therapy for two weeks with either intravenous penicillin (12–14 million units a day) or ceftriaxone (2–4 g/day)[64] appears to be effective.

When rickettsial infection is suspected on the basis of either the clinical setting or skin biopsy, therapy with tetracycline (500 mg Q6H), or in patients who are seriously ill and for whom meningococcal disease cannot be ruled out, with intravenous chloramphenicol (1 g Q6H), should be instituted. The latter drug will be effective against both *R rickettsii* and *N meningitidis*. The treatment of meningeal carcinomatosis is best left to an oncologist. With evidence of collagen vascular disease, or Bechet's syndrome, corticosteroids or immunosuppressive drugs may be warranted. When no infectious agent is found and the patient is taking certain of the above-mentioned drugs, their withdrawal may be beneficial. While most patients with varicella zoster meningitis recover completely without therapy, it is suggested from clinical trials that treatment with acyclovir may be beneficial in the immunocompromised[65,66] but is not necessary in the normal host.[67]

Viral Etiology of Aseptic Meningitis

The Centers for Disease Control reported 11,487 cases of aseptic meningitis in the year 1987, compared with 6,573 reported in 1978. The number of cases per 100,000 in the United States was 4.72 in 1987 versus 3.01 in 1978.[68]

Enteroviruses are the most common causes of aseptic meningitis, being responsible for up to 90% of all cases.[69,70] The enteroviruses consist of polio virus (3 types), group A Coxsackie virus (24 types), group B Coxsackie virus (6 types), ECHO virus (33 or 34 types), and enterovirus types 68–71 (new enteroviruses). Isolation of enterovirus is highest in June and decreases through December.[68] Most infections are endemic and caused by several types of enteroviruses, but single serotypes may be associated with outbreaks. While aseptic meningitis is the most common CNS manifestion of this disease, encephalitis, ataxia, peripheral neuritis, and paralysis have been noted. The enteroviruses have been, on occasion, associated with viremia and involvement of other organs. The incubation period is usually 1–5 days following initial contact. Meningeal involvement occurs 7–10 days thereafter, resulting in a biphasic illness. Most cases occur in children less than 5 years of age, with males predominating by 1.5 to 1. However, 14% of cases reported at the University of Texas Medical Branch[71] involved patients older than 5 years of age. The predominance of males has not been observed in the age group 20–35 years and a reversal in the sex ratio noted in children is seen in patients over 60 years of age. Previous disposition for meningeal invasion is believed to be a function of the viral inoculum, diet, and lower socioeconomic status where oral-fecal transmission is greater, and also with physical exertion.[72] In the University of Texas Medical Branch study, most patients presented with fever, rash, or other signs of viral infection of the respiratory or gastrointestinal tract; irritability and lethargy were often found. In adults, headache is a more prominent finding. In this study, the median peripheral blood count was 11,700/mm^3 with a range between 4,800 and 29,800/mm^3. In the CSF, a median range of 100 leukocytes/ml with 38% segmented neutrophils was observed. The median ranges for protein and glucose were within normal limits. In some cases, pleocytosis may not be present in the spinal fluid.[35–69,73] In patients with X-linked agammaglobulinemia, a severe form of enteroviral infection has been described.[74] In these patients, neurologic manifestations with altered mental status and seizures may be seen; severe cranial-nerve deficits and other neurologic problems have been associated with these syndromes.

Direct examination of the CSF by immunofluorescent microscopy has not proved useful clinically.[75,76] Since the isolation rate of enteroviruses from the CSF ranges between 40 and 77%, an attempt should be made to culture this virus. CSF fluid, throat, and rectal swabs should be collected in viral transport media and sent immediately to the laboratory or stored frozen. Blood culture for the detection of virus in mononuclear cells or in the serum for enterovirus has been productive. This subject has been extensively reviewed.[72] Growth from rectal swabs is faster than CSF, proportional to the inoculum in the feces; children excrete more virus than adults.[35] These viruses grow well in a variety of cell types, including primary monkey kidney cells and human diploid fibroblast cells such as WI-38 or MRC-5. The cytopathic effect (CPE) produced by enteroviruses is recognizable by the viral technician; this allows for at least a presumptive diagnosis within the first 4–5 days. It is difficult to grow Coxsackie group A viruses in cell cultures and specimens should be inoculated into either newborn mice or guinea-pig embryos.[77] Specific identification of any viral isolate depends on the use of virus-specific antiserum using neutralization antibody testing. For serologic diagnosis, a four fold rise in neutralizing antibody titer in the appropriate clinical setting is consistent with infection; approximately 3 weeks are necessary for a rise in either IgM or IgG. Since many serotypes of ECHO viruses exist, serology is impractical, except for public-health officials doing retrospective studies or to determine etiology during epidemics.

Under development are rapid diagnostic tests for enteroviral infections of the CNS. Immunofluorescence staining of white blood cells in the CSF looking for viral antigen has been reported.[76] However, the large numbers of antisera that are necessary and the low sensitivity of the test, especially in the absence of pleocytosis, are some disadvantages. Newer techniques using nucleic-acid hybridization are under development. Monoclonal antibodies directed against epitopes on the enterovirus are being investigated.[77,78] Enzyme-linked immunoadsorbant assays (ELISA) for the detection of Coxsackie viruses in stool show promise,[79] but virus may be detected in the stool of asymptomatic shedders and therefore is not proof of infection in the CNS. Enteroviral meningitis is more frequent in neonates, for whom severe sequelae may occur. These infants should be followed over the long term to note possible development of neurologic defects, including speech and language impairments.[32]

The second most common cause of aseptic meningitis is the mumps virus, which is most prevalent in the spring. While mumps is generally benign, hearing deficits have been reported.[80] CSF abnormalities occur in about 15% of patients.[81] The institution of a vaccine program has markedly decreased the number of cases in the United States. Since only 37–50% of patients have parotitis with the development of CNS symptoms[80] (i.e., headache, lethargy), this sign is not always suggestive of the diagnosis. Some observers note that the meningitis may precede by one week the development of parotitis,[80,82] but others have stated that meningitis takes place approximately 1 week after the development of parotitis, pancreatitis, otitis, and so on.[82] However other viral agents (i.e., CMV, LCM) may cause parotitis.[67]

Among other viruses that cause aseptic meningitis are togaviruses, bunyaviruses, and reoviruses. These agents are transmitted by insects, usually mosquitoes or ticks. Togaviruses include the families causing equine encephalitis (i.e., eastern, western, Venezuelian, and St. Louis encephalitis viruses); others in this group are Murray Valley fever, the Japanese encephalitis virus, and the tick-born encephalitis virus. Bunyaviruses include the LaCrosse virus. All of these agents may produce a meningitis, although clinically a picture of encephalitis is more common; up to 50% fatality rates with eastern equine encephalitis have been reported[83] and many patients are left with neurologic sequelae requiring hospitalization or institutionalization. St. Louis encephalitis is the most frequent virus infection; 60% of cases in children present with aseptic meningitis, although the disease is more common in adults. The fatality rate is 8%.[31–84] The case fatality rate for western equine encephalitis is 3%, and reoviruses and Venezuelan encephalitis less than 1%. California encephalitis virus is the most common cause of human infection, with a rate of 31.6/100,000 in 1978.[85] LaCrosse virus is the least severe; a recent paper reported no evidence of sequelae.[86] A reovirus produces Colorado tick fever, which is endemic in the mountainous areas of the western United States and Canada. Usually a self-limited disease with very low mortality, it generally exists in rodents and is transmitted by ticks. Since the virus enters red-cell precursors, it is often associated with prolonged viremia.

Herpes simplex viruses are responsible for severe neonatal and adult encephalitis, which require treatment with antiviral agents. On the other hand, aseptic meningitis from this virus represented 0.5–3% of reported cases.[87] Usually associated with HSV-2 infection, it is benign and requires no treatment. In some of these vesicular lesions on the lip, oral or vaginal mucosa suggest the diagnosis. A recurrent meningeal syndrome has been reported.[88]

The VZV is rarely associated with CNS involvement during primary infection, with a frequency of 0.1–0.8%[89] in chicken pox; the mortality is 5%.[90] A postinfectious meningoencephalitis or cerebritis, which is associated with seizures in 50% of patients, may occur.[91] Disseminated VZV is often seen in immunocompromised patients with underlying diseases. The CNS disease is not usually fatal, though neurologic sequellae may occur. Examination of the CNS usually reveals pleocytosis and hypoglycorrhachia in the absence of CNS infection in 30–40%.[92] Other herpes viruses associated with aseptic meningitis include the Epstein-Barr virus (EBV)[93,94] and CMV.[95] In patients with EBV infection, CSF abnormalities have been reported in from 0.37 to 26.5% of cases; atypical lymphocytes have been noted on direct examination of the spinal fluid.[93]

Measles encephalitis is reported in approximately 0.1% of measle cases,[96] although immunization has markedly decreased the incidence of clinical disease and encephalitis. CSF pleocytosis can be found in 12–30% of cases of uncomplicated cases in children.[97]

LCM is found in mice. Patients usually present with a prodromal fever, anorexia, headache, and nuchal rigidity; pneumonitis, coma, or death have rarely been reported.[98] Rabies classically presents with encephalitis.

HIV invades the CNS and may produce aseptic meningitis in 5–10% of cases, often early in the presentation.[99] A dementia-like picture with wasting syndrome has been reported in these patients.[100]

Further Diagnostic Methods

The incubation period for Venezuelan and western equine encephalitis is short, and blood culture may yield positive results within the first 3 to 5 days. However, diagnoses of the togaviruses, bunyaviruses, and reoviruses are best made by serologic testing: hemagglutination inhibition, complement fixation, and virus-neutralizing antibody tests. Cross-reactions have been noted in patients who have received the yellow-fever vaccine and hemagglutination inhibition and neutralization tests would be better suited to those patients.

Rocky Mountain spotted fever "sans" rash (spotless fever) is said to occur in approximately 15% of cases. In the absence of the rash, physicians often fail to consider this as a diagnosis and fatal outcomes have been reported.[101] In patients with petechial skin lesions, culture and immunofluorescence staining for *R rickettsii* may reveal this organism. It is more common to see Rocky Mountain spotted fever during the spring and summer months (i.e., April through September), but people who own dogs may be susceptible throughout the year. In a review of 262 cases,[102] 5% of patients had fever and meningismus. The Weil-Felix test is nonspecific and insensitive; other tests—latex agglutination, microagglutation, indirect hemagglutination assay, and complement fixation—are preferred. Most of these tests require 2 to 3 weeks to become positive. Inappropriate antidiuretic hormone has been reported with Rocky Mountain spotted fever and mycobacterial infections.[102]

Patient management can be directly affected by making a definitive diagnosis of a viral etiology for the aseptic meningitis syndrome. Most viral meningitides are benign in nature and require no therapy; however, the patient with HIV infection might benefit from early institution of antiviral therapy with AZT. While many patients may have antimicrobial therapy begun initially when the etiology is unclear, proof of viral diagnosis by either culture or some of the newly evolving rapid diagnostic tests allows the physician to stop antibiotics without worrying that a bacterial infection is being missed. This will enable patients to return to their usual environment, decrease hospital stays, and markedly decrease hospital costs, including per-day, nursing, and antibiotic costs. It behooves the physician, however, to search carefully for the treatable causes that have been described in this chapter.

References

1. Ellis SG, Verity MA: Central nervous system involvement in systemic lupus erythematosus: a review of neuropatholigic findings in 57 cases: 1955–1977. *Semin Arthritis Rheum* 1979;8:212-221.
2. Nadeau SE, Watson RT: Neurologic manifestations of vasculitis and collagen vascular syndromes, in Baker AB, Joynt, Robert J (eds): *Clinical Neurology,* Vol 4. Philadelphia, Harper & Rowe, 1984, chapt 59.
3. Delaney P: Neurological manifestations in sarcodisis: review of the literature with a report of 23 cases. *Ann Intern Med* 1977;87:336–345.
4. Nelson DA, Vates TS Jr., Thomas RD Jr: Complications from intrathecal steroid therapy in patients with multiple sclerosis. *Acta Neurol Scand* 1973; 49:176–188.
5. Vik-Mo M, Mauer H-J: Meningeal reactions following myelography: effects of detergent washing agent. *Acta Radiol (Diag)* 1975;16:39–42.
6. Weiss HD, Walker MD, Wiernick PH: Neurotoxicity of commonly used antineoplastic agents. *N Engl J Med* 1974;291:75–81.
7. Fischman RA: Cerebrospinal fluid, in *Diseases of the Nervous System*. Philadelphia, WB Saunders, 1980.
8. Becker WJ, Watters GV, de Chadarevian JP, et al: Recurrent aseptic meningitis secondary to intracranial epidermoids. *Can J Neurol Sci* 1984;11: 387–389.
9. Lawson JM, Grady MJ: Ibuprofen-induced aseptic meningitis in a previously healthy patient. *West J Med* 1985;143:386–387.
10. Hilton E, Stroh EM: Aseptic meningitis associated with administration of carbamazepine. *J Infect Dis* 1989;159:363–364.
11. Ballas ZK, Donta ST: Sulindac-induced aseptic meningitis. *Arch Intern Med* 1982;142:165–166.
12. Thordarson H, Talstad I: Acute meningitis and cerebral dysfunction complicating high-dose citosine arabinoside therapy. *Acta Med Scand* 1986;220: 493–495.
13. Carlson J, Wilholm BE: Trimethoprim associated aseptic meningitis. *Scand J. Infect Dis* 1987;19: 687–691.
14. Bouland DL, Specht NL, Hegstad DR: Ibuprofen and aseptic meningitis (letter). *Ann Intern Med* 1986;104:731.
15. Garagusi VF, Neefe LI, Mann O: Acute meningoencephalitis: association with isoniazid administration. *JAMA* 1976;235:1141–1142.
16. Haas, EJ: Trimethoprim-sulfamethoxazole: another cause of recurrent meningitis. *JAMA* 1984;252:346–347.
17. Hyman CB, Bogle JM, Brubaker CA, et al: Central nervous system involvement by leukemia in children. I: Relationship to systemic leukemia and description of clinical and laboratory manifestations. *Blood* 1965;25:1–12.
18. Sorenson SC, Eagan RT, Scott M: Meningeal carcinomatosis in patients with breast or lung cancer. *Mayo Clin Proc* 1984;59:91–94.
19. Wasserstrom WR, Glass JP, Posner JB: Diagnosis and treatment of leptomeningeal metastases from solid tumors: experience with 90 patients. *Cancer* 1982;49:759–772.
20. Park Am, Richardson JC: Cerebral complications of serum sickness. *Neurology* 1953;3:277–283.
21. Reik L. Jr: Disorders that mimic CNS infections. *Neurol Clin* 1986;4:223–248.
22. Mascia RA, Smith CW Jr: Mollert's meningitis: an unusual disease with a characteristic presentation. *Am J Med Sci* 1984;287:52–53.
23. Weiner LP, Fleming JO: Pathophysiology and epidemiology of acute viral infections, in Thompson RA, Green Jr (eds): *Infectious Diseases of the Central Nervous System,* vol. 6 PMA Publishing Corp., Chap 1, 1984.
24. Johnson RT, Mims CA: Pathogenesis of viral infections of the nervous system. *N Engl J Med* 1965;278:23–30
25. Johnson RT, Mims CA: Pathogenesis of viral infection of the nervous system. *N Engl J Med* 1965; 278:84–92.
26. Johnson KP: The pathogenesis of viral infections of the nervous system. *Neurol Clin* 1984;2:179–185.
27. Martin MA, Massanari RM, Nghiem DD, et al:

Nosocomial aseptic meningitis associated with administrations of OKT-3. *JAMA* 1988;259:2002–2005.
28. Vilaseca J, Tor J, Guardia J, et al: Periodic meningitis and familiar Mediterranean fever. *Arch Intern Med* 1982; 142:378–379.
29. Ellner JJ, Wilhelm C: Chronic meningitis. *Neurol Clin* 1986;4:115–142.
30. Pruitt AA, Rubin RH, Karchmer AW, et al: Neurologic complications of bacterial endocarditis. *Medicine* 1978;57:329–343.
31. Rennels MB. Arthropod-borne virus infections of the central nervous system. *Neurol Clin* 1984;2: 241–264.
32. Wilfert CM, Nusinoff Lehrman S, Katz SL: Enteroviruses and meningitis. *Pediatr Infect Dis* 1983; 2:333–341.
33. Wilfert GM: Mumps meningoencephalitis with low cerebrospinal fluid glucose, prolonged pleocytosis and elevation of protein. *N Engl J Med* 1969; 280:855–858.
34. Hevron JE: Herpes simplex virus type 2 meningitis. *Obstet Gynecol* 1976;49:622–624.
35. Wildin S, Chonmaitree T: The importance of the virology laboratory in the diagnosis and management of viral meningitis. *Am J Dis Child* 1987; 141:454–457.
36. Patrick BS, Smith RR, Bailey TO: Aseptic meningitis due to spontaneous rupture of craniopharyngioma cyst: case report. *J Neurosurg* 1974;41:387–390.
37. Laveter A, Laedom JM, Mathies AW, et al: Meningitis due to listeria monocytogenes. A review of 25 cases. *N Engl J Med* 1979;285:598–603.
38. Peters AC, Versteeg Gt, Bots AM, et al: Nervous system complications of herpes zoster: immunofluorescent demonstration of varicella-zoster antigen in CSF cells. *J. Neurol Neurosurg Psychiatry* 1979; 42:452–457.
39. Koo J, Pien F, Kliks MM: Angiostrongylus (Parastrongylus) eosinophilic meningitis. *Rev Infect Dis* 1988;10:1155–1162.
40. Earnest MP, Barth Reller L, Filley CM: Neurocysticercosis in the United States: 35 cases and a review. *Rev Infect Dis* 1987;9:961–979.
41. Singer JI, Mauer RP, Riley JP, et al: Management of central nervous system infections during an epidemic of enteroviral aseptic meningitis. *J Pediatr* 1980;96:559–563.
42. Nelson N, Eeg-Olofsson O, Larson L: The diagnostic and predictive value of cerebrospinal fluid lactate in children with meningitis. Its relation to current diagnostic methods. *Acta Paeditr Scand* 1986; 75:52–57.
43. Briem H: Comparison between cerebrospinal fluid concentrations of glucose, total protein, chloride, lactate and total amino acids for the differential diagnosis of patients with meningitis. *Scand J Infect Dis* 1983;15:277–284.
44. Peltola HO: C-reactive protein for rapid monitoring of infections of the central nervous system. *Lancet* 1982;980–983.
45. James Corrall C, Pepple JM, Moxon ER., et al: C-reactive protein in spinal fluid of children with meningitis. *J Pediatr* 1981;99:365–369.
46. Schott KJ, Meier D: Free amino acid pattern of cerebrospinal fluid in meningeal pathology. *Acta Neurol Scand* 1987;75:304–309.
47. Malan C, Donald PR, Golden M, et al: Adenosine deaminase levels in cerebrospinal fluid in the diagnosis of tuberculous meningitis. *J Trop Med Hyg* 1984;87:33–40.
48. Ho-Yen DO, Carrington D: Alpha interferon responses in cerebrospinal fluid of patients with suspected meningitis. *J Clin Pathol* 1987;40:83–86.
49. Abbott RJ, Bolderson I, Gruer PJ: Assessment of an immunoassay for interferon alpha in cerebrospinal fluid as a diagnostic aid in infections of the central nervous system. *J Infect Dis* 1987;15:153–160.
50. Donald PR, Malan C: Cerebrospinal fluid lactate and lactate dehydrogenase activity in the rapid diagnosis of bacterial meningitis. *S Afr Med J* 1986;69:39–42.
51. Jordan GW, Statland B, Halsted C: Cerebrospinal fluid lactate in diseases of the central nervous system. *Arch Intern Med* 1983;143:85–87.
52. Clinicopathologic Conference. Ludmerer KM, Kissane JM, eds: Chronic meningitis in a 68 year old man. *Am J Med* 1988;85:407–413.
53. Abramsky O: Neurologic features as presenting manifestations of brucellosis. *Eur Neurol* 1977; 15:281–284.
54. Karandanis D, Shulman JA: Recent survey of infectious meningitis in adults: review of laboratory findings in bacterial, tuberculous, and aseptic meningitis. *South Med J* 1976;69:449–457.
55. Feigin RD, Shackelford PG: Value of repeat lumbar puncture in the differential diagnosis of meningitis. *N Engl J Med* 1973;289:571–574.
56. Varki Ap, Puthuran P: Value of a second lumbar puncture in confirming a diagnosis of aseptic meningitis. *Arch Neurol* 1979;36:581–582.
57. Harrison SA, Risser WL: Repeat lumbar puncture in the differential diagnosis of meningitis. *Pediatr Inf Dis J* 1988;7:143–145.
58. Francke E. The many causes of meningitis. *Postgrad Med* 1987;82:175–188.
59. Ingham MR, Selkon JB, Roxby CM: Bacteriological study of otogenic cerebral abscesses: chemotherapeutic role of metronidazole. *Br Med J* 1977; 2:991–993.
60. Berg B, Franklin G, Cuneo R, et al: Nonsurgical cure of brain abscesses: early diagnosis and follow-

up with computerized tomography. *Ann Neurol* 1978;3:474–478.
61. Earsoum AH, Lewis MC, Cannillo PA: Non-operative treatment of multiple brain abscesses. *Surg Neurol* 1981;16:283–287.
62. 1985 STD Treatment Guidelines. Supplement, *MMWR* 1985;34(4S).
63. Watt G, Tuazon L, Santiago E, et al: Placebo-controlled trial of intravenous penicillin for severe and late leptospirosis. *Lancet* 1988;1:433–435.
64. Dattwyler RJ, Halperin JJ, Pass H, et al: Ceftriaxone as effective therapy in refractory Lyme disease. *J Infect Dis* 1987;155:1322–1327.
65. Peterson LR, Ferguson RM: Fatal central nervous system infection with varicella-zoster virus in renal transplant recipients. *Transplantation* 1984;37:366–368.
66. Steele RW, Keeney RE, Bradsher BW, et al: Treatment of varicella-zoster meningoencephalitis with acyclovir: demonstration of virus in cerebrospinal fluid by electron microscopy. *Am J Clin Pathol* 1983;80:57–60.
67. Ratzan KR: Viral meningitis. *Med Clin North Am* 1985;69:399–413.
68. Summary of Notifiable Diseases, United States, 1987. *MMWR* 1988;36(54).
69. Chonmaitree T, Menegus MA, Powell KR. The clinical relevance of CSF viral culture. A two-year experience with aseptic meningitis in Rochester, New York. *JAMA* 1982;247:1843–1847.
70. Centers for Disease Control. Aseptic meningitis surveillance, annual summary 1976. Atlanta, US Department of Health, Education and Welfare, Jan 1979.
71. Chonmaitree T, Baldwin CD, Lucia HL: Role of the virology laboratory in diagnosis and management of patients with central nervous system disease. *Clin Microbiol Rev* 1989;1–14.
72. Centers for Disease Control. Enteroviral disease in the United States, 1970–1979. *J Infect Dis* 1982; 146:103–108.
73. Krober MS, Bass JW, Powell JM, et al: Bacterial and viral pathogens causing fever in infants less than 3 months old. *Am J Dis Child* 1985;139:889–892.
74. Wilfert CM, Buckley RH, Mohanakumar T, et al: Persistent and fatal central nervous system echo virus infections in patients with agammaglobulinemia. *N Engl J Med* 1977;296:1485–1489.
75. Grandien M, Olding-Stenkvist E: Rapid diagnosis of viral infections in the central nervous system. *Scand J Infect Dis* 1984;16:1–8.
76. Taber LH, Mirkovic RR, Adam V, et al: Rapid diagnosis of enterovirus meningitis by immunofluorescent staining of CSF leukocytes. *Intervirology* 1973;1:127–134.
77. Yousef GE, Mann GF, Brown IN, et al: clinical and research application of an enterovirus group-reactive monoclonal antibody. *Intervirology* 1987;28:199–205.
78. Yousef GE, Mann GF, Smith DG, et al: Chronic enterovirus infection in patients with postviral fatigue syndrome. *Lancet* 1988;1:146–150.
79. Yolken RH, Torsch VM: Enzyme-linked immunosorbent assay for detection and identification of coxsackie virus A. *Infect Immun* 1981;31:742–750.
80. Johnstone JA, Ross CA, Dunn M: Meningitis and encephalitis associated with mumps infection. A 10 year survey. *J Dis Child* 1972;47:647–651.
81. Centers for Disease Control: Aseptic meningitis surveillance, annual summary 1976. Jan. 1979.
82. Jubelt B: Enterovirus and mumps virus infections of the nervous system. *Neurol Clin* 1984;2:187–213.
83. McGowan JE Jr., Bryan JA, Gregg MB: Surveillance of arboviral encephalitis in the United States, 1955–1971. *Am J Epidemiol* 1973;97:199–207.
84. Barrett FF, Yow MD, Phillips CA: St. Louis encephalitis in children during the 1964 epidemic. *JAMA* 1965;193:381–385.
85. Arboviral infections of the central nervous system—United States 1987. *MMWR* 1988;37:506–513.
86. Sikes RK, Calisher CH, Smith JD: Human infections with La Crosse virus in Georgia, 1982. *South Med J* 1984;77:972–974.
87. Olson LC, Buescher EL, Artenstein MS, et al: Herpes virus infections of the human central nervous system. *N Engl J Med* 1967;277:1271–1277.
88. Steel JG, Dix RD, Baringer JR: Isolation of herpes simplex virus type 1 in recurrent (Mollaret) meningitis. *Ann Neurol* 1982;11:17–21.
89. Applebaum E, Rachelson MH, Dolgopol VB: Varicella encephalitis. *Am J Med* 1953;15:223–230.
90. Barnes DW, Whitley RJ: CNS diseases associated with varicella zoster virus and herpes simplex virus infection: pathogenesis and current therapy. *Neurol Clin* 1986;4:265–283.
91. Johnson R, Milbourn PE: Central nervous system manifestations of chicken pox. *Can Med Assoc J* 1970;102:831–834.
92. Karp SJ: Meningitis and disseminated cutaneous zoster complicating herpes zoster infection. *J Neurol Neurosurg Psych* 1983;46:582–583.
93. Grose C, Henle W, Henle G, et al: Primary Epstein-Barr virus infections in acute neurologic diseases. *N Engl J Med* 1975;292:392–395.
94. Silverstein A, Steinberg G, Nathanson M: Nervous system involvement in infectious mononucleosis. *Arch Neurol* 1972;26:353–358.
95. Phillips CA, Fanning WL, Gump DW, et al: CMV encephalitis in immunologically normal adults: successful treatment with vidarabine. *JAMA* 1977; 238:2299–2300.

96. *Morbidity and Mortality Weekly Report.* 1981; 30:362–364.
97. Hanninen P, Arstila P, Lang M, et al: Involvement of the nervous system in acute, uncomplicated measles virus infection. *J Clin Microbiol* 21:610–613, 1980.
98. Peters CJ: In *Adenovirus Textbook of Human Virology,* Belshe RB, ed. 1985, ch 19, pp 513–545.
99. Gabuzda DH, Hirsch MS: Neurologic manifestations of infection with immunodeficiency virus. *Ann Intern Med* 1987;107:383–391.
100. Price RW, Navia BA, Eun-Sook CHO: AIDS encephalopathy. *Neurol Clin* 1986;4:285–301.
101. Westerman EL: Rocky Mountain spotless fever. A dilemma for the clinician. *Arch Intern Med* 1982;142:1106–1107.
102. Helmick CG, Bernard KW, D'Angelo LJ: Rocky Mountain spotted fever: clinical, laboratory and epidemiological features of 262 cases. *J Infect Dis* 1984;150:480–488.

4
Chronic Meningitis

TARVEZ TUCKER AND JERROLD J. ELLNER

Introduction

The clinical presentation of chronic meningitis is quite uniform, despite a diversity of etiologies. Patients describe a subacute onset of headache, most often associated with fever and stiff neck, and occasionally accompanied by encephalopathy (i.e., confusion, disorientation, or lethargy). Examination of the cerebrospinal fluid (CSF) reveals a lymphocytic pleocytosis in most cases with elevation of protein and, particularly with the fungal meningitides, lowered glucose. By definition, this constellation of signs and symptoms is generally present for four weeks before the label of chronic meningitis applies.[1,2] However, in practice, important therapeutic decisions need to be made well before this empiric deadline, particularly because a delay in diagnosis can result in irreversible neurologic deficits. In addition, correct diagnosis of a specific underlying cause is important, in that many of the drugs used to treat chronic meningitis have potentially serious toxicities, making empiric drug trials before diagnosis risky.

Rarely, clues in the history, physical examination, or CSF formula help distinguish the various causes of subacute or chronic meningitis. A cardinal example is the characteristic rash of Lyme disease, erythema chronicum migrans, preceding the clinical picture of meningitis. The presence of uveitis or granulomatous periphlebitis in a patient with meningitis suggests the diagnosis of sarcoid. Demographics can be helpful on occasion. For example, histoplasmosis would be uncommon in a patient from the rural plains states. A history of exposure to tuberculosis, or a miliary pattern of pulmonary tuberculosis on chest x-ray, might guide the diagnosis. In general, these situations are, however, exceptional. More often, the clinician is faced with a uniform clinical picture typical of chronic meningitis with no clue to the specific infectious agent from physical examination or history.

Therefore, an organized approach to the patient with chronic meningitis is useful. If features of encephalitis accompany the signs and symptoms of meningitis, specific infectious agents may be implicated. In particular, cysticercosis and toxoplasmosis frequently present with both cerebral and meningeal signs,—that is, a meningoencephalitis. Alteration of consciousness in the absence of hydrocephalus and increased intracranial pressure is much less common with specific fungal agents, such as histoplasma and cryptococcus. Similarly, until its late stages, Lyme disease usually does not depress consciousness. Infections that have a predilection for the basilar meninges may produce a characteristic neurologic picture consistent with raised intracranial pressure. Patients present with a change in mental status, ataxia, headache, nausea, and vomiting, in addition to meningeal signs. Fungal and granulomatous processes affect the basal meninges; therefore, cranial-nerve involvement may be evident early. In particular, ocular motor palsies or eighth-nerve dysfunction may herald the diagnosis of tuberculosis, sarcoidosis, fungal infection, or syphilis. On the other hand, although the racemose form of cysticercosis does produce clusters of cysts in the basal meninges, this parasitic infection rarely presents with cranial-nerve palsies. The specific cranial nerve involved can be useful diagnostically: syphilitic infections frequently involve cranial nerves VII, VIII, and II, whereas sarcoidosis has a predilection for cranial nerve VII. Unfortunately, however, certain cranial-nerve pareses, such as VIth-nerve palsies, can be nonlocalizing signals of raised intracranial pressure attributable to causes other than that of direct infection, such as hydrocephalus or parameningeal foci of infection.

Exposure history may be useful in identifying specific infectious agents. *Histoplasma capsulatum* and *Blastomyces dermatiditis* have high endemicity in the Mississippi and Ohio River valleys. *Coccidiodes immitis* is prevalent in the semiarid Southwest. Lyme disease has primarily been reported in the northeastern United States and has its peak prevalence in late summer and early fall, reflecting the activity of the tick vector. Cysticercosis in endemic in Mexico and South America, and in immigrants to the United States from those areas.

The physical examination is generally less helpful in identifying a diagnosis. The findings on general physical exam, however, may specify a biopsy site, which may lead to diagnosis. Depigmentary choroidal tubercles are present in both sarcoidosis and tuberculosis. Diseases associated with an inflammatory CSF, though not necessarily a specific infectious agent, such as Behcet's disease and Vogt-Koyanagi-Harada (VKH) syndrome, cause uveitis, and in VKH syndrome, also vitiligo and poliosis. Draining sinuses and ulcerative lesions are seen in blastomycosis; subcutaneous nodules and abscesses can be a source of diagnostic culture. An example of this are palatal lesions of the oral mucosa that are seen in histoplasmosis.

Laboratory data, particularly CSF parameters, may help organize the search for diagnosis in chronic meningitis. Most fungal meningitides present with a moderate lymphocytic pleocytosis of 50–100 white cells with a low glucose. Tuberculosis, syphilis, and parasitic and some viral infections also fall into this category. If the glucose is low but there is less of an inflammatory pleocytosis (usually less than 50 white cells), the diagnosis of carcinomatous meningitis, sarcoidosis, or subarachnoid hemorrhage should be considered.

A lymphocytosis in the presence of normal glucose changes the differential diagnosis somewhat. When the pleocytosis is modest (50–100 white cells), sarcoidosis, chronic-benign lymphocytic meningitis, vasculitis, intracranial mass lesions including abcesses, and multiple sclerosis are in the differential. When there is a brisk pleocytosis with normal glucose, fungal and parasitic infections must be considered, as well as chemical meningitis.

A unique CSF profile emerges in the category of "pleocytosis with neutrophilic predomiance."[3] In this case, certain bacteria (specifically, *Norcardia, Actinomyces,* and *Brucella),* as well as specific fungi (*Blastomyces, Coccidiodes, Aspergillus,* and *Zygomycetes),* may be implicated. Systemic lupus erythematosis and chemical meningitis that results from a discharge from epidermoid tumors or craniopharynhioma, for example, causes a neutrophilic CSF pleocytosis, as does the administration of contrast agents and intrathecal drugs.

When eosinophilia is present in the CSF, certain diseases must be considered. Hodgkin's disease, parasitic meningitis, tuberculosis, *Coccidiodes,* and chemical meningitis, particularly that caused by ibuprofen and related drugs, all cause an eosinophilic predominance.[3–6]

Lumbar puncture at times needs to be repeated periodically, both to assure adequate material for culture and cytology and to follow the course of meningeal inflammation. India-ink preparations can be quickly diagnostic, particularly in cryptococcal meningitis in immunosuppressed partients, especially those with the acquired immunodeficiency syndrome (AIDS). In these patients, the numbers of yeast may outnumber the white-cell response and the organisms are readily apparent on an India-ink slide as refractile yeast bodies surrounded by a large capsule, impermeable to the ink particles.

Multiple lumbar punctures are especially important when the diagnosis of meningeal carcinomatosis is a consideration. Cytologic examination may not be positive in the initial CSF exams. In addition, lymphocyte staining with monoclonal antibodies can help identify cells of lymphoma or leukemic origin.

CSF culture is, of course, the mainstay of the diagnosis of chronic meningitis. Because the likelihood of obtaining a positive culture increases with the passage of time, lumbar punctures may need to be repeated at regular intervals, if cultures at first are negative. All samples should be sent for bacteria and acid-fast bacilli, as well as fungi. Usually, three samples will be adequate for diagnosis of most bacteria and mycobacteria; more may be required for accurate fungal diagnosis. The yield from cultures containing few organisms may be improved by inoculating Sabaroud's agar with large volumes of CSF. Laboratories should be advised to observe cultures for at least four to six weeks because of the slow growth of some organisms.

Radiographic procedures can help to focus the diagnostic workup and, in many cases, should be performed before a lumbar puncture. Mass lesions, including brain abscess, may present with a clinical picture identical to that of chronic meningitis and need to be excluded before a needle enters the subarachnoid space. Contrast-enhanced computed tomography (CT) and, particularly, magnetic resonance imaging (MRI) scanning, are useful for visualizing the basilar enhancement seen in granulomatous and fungal meningitides. Effacement of the basilar cisterns may also occur from the inflammatory reaction. Hydrocephalus is detected well by both CT and MRI, as is cerebral infarction, which may occur with vasculitis or tuberculosis, for example, that affects vessels primarily at the base of the brain.

Algorithms for enigmatic cases involve decision making based on the CSF formula, the results of the physical examination and history, and specific laboratory tests. In many cases, the clinician is faced with deciding whether to perform an invasive diagnostic procedure such as meningeal biopsy or to attempt an empiric trial of therapy before a specific diagnosis has been made by culture or serology results.

If the CSF demonstrates a lymphocytic pleocytosis with 50–500 cells and depressed or normal glucose, an infectious disease is extremely likely. If the tuberculin skin test is positive, this picture makes empirical therapy for tuberculosis appropriate. If the skin test is negative, tuberculosis is still a possibility, and antituberculous drugs may be started empirically after cryptococcal polysaccharide antigen and other specific antibodies, such as FTA-ABS, in the serum and CSF are drawn. Because fungal meningitis may progress to irreversible disease in an unpredictable fashion, simply observing a patient for response to antituberculous therapy is risky unless invasive procedures such as biopsy are contraindicated. If vasculitis is a clinical diagnostic possibility, cerebral angiography may be helpful. Ventricular fluid can have a higher cultural yield than lumbar CSF in some settings, such as the fungal meningitis of histoplasmosis, blastomycosis, and sporothrix.

The algorithm changes if the lymphocytic pleocytosis is less brisk (less than 50 white cells). In this case, an infectious etiology is less likely and, even when no diagnosis is forthcoming, many of these patients spontaneously improve.[7] Early empiric corticosteroid therapy is usually not indicated because of its risk if the diagnosis is unsuspected tuberculous or fungal meningitis. It is difficult to recommend an empiric trial of antifungal therapy in any clinical situation because of its potential toxicity and the uncertainty as to the appropriate dose, duration, and route of administration without an identifiable infectious agent.

Specific Infectious Causes of Chronic Meningitis

Tuberculosis Meningitis

When a parameningeal (Rich) tuberculous focus ruptures into the subarachnoid space, meningitis due to *Mycobacterium* tuberculosis develops. Exudation of protein and cells into the CSF results, the equivalent of an in situ delayed type of hypersensitivity.

In populations in whom tuberculosis is common, meningeal involvement usually occurs in children three months to five years of age. Associated pulmonary involvement with hilar adenopathy is seen in 50–90% of cases. Because tuberculous infection in general is decreasing in prevalence in the United States, more cases of tuberculous meningitis are seen now in adults. The chest x-ray may be normal and, as stated above, the skin test may not be reactive.

An exudative basilar meningitis may spread into the parenchyma, also causing encephalitis, but the pathologic hallmark of tuberculosis is vasculitis. Small, medium, and large arteries are involved, as well as veins, causing cerebral infarctions resulting from vasculitis in approximately a third of patients. Hydrocephalus is a common finding, although it not infrequently resolves with medical therapy and does not require surgical shunting.

Clinically, tuberculous meningitis presents with a subacute onset of nonspecific symptoms of low-grade fever, mild confusion or encephalopathy, personality or behavioral changes, and lassitude.[8–13] After approximately two weeks, the next phase of the illness reflects the meningeal inflammatory process, with headache and stiff neck. Cranial-nerve palsies, particularly of nerve III, IV, VI, or I, are present in about one third of patients. Focal neurologic signs such as hemipareses, hemianopsias, and hemisensory deficits may occur due to stroke.

The CSF shows depressed glucose in 50–95%, of patients, with a mononuclear pleocytosis of 100–500 cells,[14,15] which intially may be neutrophilic. Elevations of protein and opening pressure are often seen, as is serum hyponatremia caused by inappropriate antidiuretic hormone secretion. The yield of acid-fast bacilli stains of the CSF is extremely variable (10–87%), but may be improved by sedimenting high volumes (10–20 ml) of CSF at high speeds. Yield of culture is also variable (47–87%).

Empiric therapy with isoniazid, rifampin, and Ethambutol may be necessary before cultures become positive in 4–6 weeks. Pyrazinamide may be used if drug resistance is suspected. The use of corticosteroids should be limited to patients with life-threatening progressive illness such as multiple strokes, a relentless increase in intracranial pressure, or coma.

Cryptococcal Meningitis

Even before the AIDS epidemic, cryptococcal meningitis was most common in chronically immunosuppressed patients. Because the organism is a common environmental saprophyte, exposure is widespread, although the disease itself is infrequent. The portal of entry is generally the lungs, though a pulmonary focus may not be demonstrable, presumably because of spontaneous regression. Patients present with a chronic febrile syndrome with headache,[16–20] or only with mild cognitive changes such as early dementia without specific meningeal symptoms. Forty percent of patients have demonstrated ocular abnormalities such as papilledema and cranial-nerve palsies. The CSF-cell counts range from 40 to 400, and rarely above 800. The protein is generally elevated and hypoglycorrhachia is present in 55% of patients. India-ink CSF preparations are positive in one third to one half of patients and may be diagnostic, particularly in the setting of immunosuppression. Serum cryptococcal polysaccharide antigens, as well as CSF antigens, are helpful in yielding the diagnosis early since cultures may not become positive for as long as two to six weeks. Current therapy for cryptococcal meningitis includes amphotericin B and flucytosine. Fluconazole is a drug that is proving effective for cryptococcal meningitis in the initial therapy as well as for maintenance therapy, particularly in patients with AIDS.

Other Fungal meningitides

Coccidiodes immitis is prevalent in California, New Mexico, and Texas, and infects through the respiratory route. *Histoplasma capsulatum* is another fungus more commonly found in the soil of the Ohio and Mississipppi river valleys. Both of these chronic meningitides present with mental-status changes and signs of encephalopathy, such as disorientation, lethargy, confusion, or memory loss. Large volumes of CSF may be necessary to culture the organism. *Blastomyces dermatitides* causes disease around the Mississippi River base and the Great Lakes, and in the Southeast. The meningitis associated with blastomycoses is often associated with other manifestations of disseminated disease.

Candida meningitis should be sought when chronic meningitis occurs in intravenous-drug abusers, patients who have indwelling venous catheters or who undergo abdominal surgery, and those receiving corticosteroid therapy. Unlike some of the other infectious chronic meningitides, fever is almost invariably part of the presentation. Otherwise, the clinical and laboratory picture is indistinguishable from that of other fungal meningitis.

Neurosyphilis

Despite the widespread availability of antibiotic treatment for early forms of syphilis, primary and secondary forms of syphilis have increased worldwide in the past decade. Some of this is due to the increased incidence of syphilitic infections in people who are positive for the human immunodeficiency virus (HIV). Because all the classical syndromes of neurosyphilis occur in the setting of active meningeal inflammation, abnormal CSF is the hallmark of the disease. The only exception to this rule is tabes dorsalis, which in the late stages may present with a normal spinal-fluid picture. Otherwise, a pleocytosis, positive CSF VDRL, or elevation of protein occurs in all patients with cerebrovascular syphilis or paretic neurosyphilis (dementia paralytica).

Treponemal involvement of the meninges may cause a clinical meningitis or may be asymptomatic. Infection localizing at the meninges of the base of the brain causes either hydrocephalus or cranial-nerve palsies. Obliterative endarteritis affects cerebral blood vessels, causing stroke. In syphilitic meningitis, a brisk lymphocytic pleocytosis with values greater than 500 is common, although there is a less vigorous lymphocytic response (50–200 white cells) in syphilitic vascular disease or general paresis. The CSF pleocytosis is probably the most sensitive indicator of the disease. The fluorescent treponemal antibody (FTA) tested serum is reactive in more than 95% of patients with late syphilis[21] and remains reactive despite therapy, unlike the nontreponemal flocculation test, the VDRL. However, the VDRL test is more useful as an indicator of active disease in the CSF.

Standard treatment regimens for neurosyphilis have recently been revised because of several reports of recurrence of persistence of infection following "adequate" penicillin therapy, and the original recommendations have been challenged.[22] Success of treatment is determined by resolution of CSF pleocytosis with repeat lumbar punctures at 6, 12, and 24 months. Because relapse occurs, changes of clinical status should prompt a repeat lumbar puncture.

Lyme Disease

The newly recognized spirochete *Borrellia burgdorferi* causes a unique syndrome of oligoarthritis and cardiac and neurologic involvement, often preceded by a localized skin rash at the site of the tick bite. Cases were originally described from Lyme, Conn., but endemic areas in the United States include central New Jersey, Long Island, and Cape Cod. Its characteristic seasonal occurence in late summer and early fall is helpful in making the diagnosis, particularly because the tick bite is recalled by only a small proportion of patients and the characteristic skin rash does not always appear.

The neurologic picture of Lyme meningitis includes cranial neuritis, particularly with facial palsies, and a lymphocytic meningitis that takes place early in the illness. Interestingly, the classic signs of meningeal irritation such as Kernig's and Brudzinski's signs, cervical pain, or stiffness of the neck are frequently absent. Headache, however, is a prominent symptom. In the latter stage of the disease, often associated with arthritis, less fulminant central-nervous-system (CNS) symptoms appear. such as memory difficulties and nonspecific cognitive changes.

All patients suspected of having Lyme disease should also have the fluorescent trepenemal antibody test because patients with syphilis may have false-positive serology to the species of borrelia that cause Lyme disease. The initial stage of illness is treated with oral tetracycline or penicillin. However, when neurologic manifestations develop, intravenous penicillin or ceftriaxone is now recommended.[23]

Cysticercosis

Although most cases in the United States are found in the southwestern part of the country, worldwide cysticercosis is the most common parasitic infection of the CNS, endemic to South and Central America, Mexico, Africa, India, Eastern Europe, China, and Indonesia.

Two distinct forms of cysticercosis occur—*Cysticercus cellulosae* primarily in brain parenchyma and *Cysticercus racemosus* in basilar cisterns, the ventricles, or the subarachnoid space as grapelike clusters.

Clinical manifestations are diverse, and include cognitive changes, seizures, and symptoms associated with increased intracranial pressure. When cysts are located in the ventricle, hydrocephalus may ensue. Cysts expanding within the subarachnoid space may cause meningitis, as well as hydrocephalus, and may obstruct CSF flow. Chronic meningitis may be subclinical over many years, not becoming apparent in some patients until ten to fifteen years after immigration to the United States.

An indirect hemagglutination (IHA) test performed by the Centers for Disease Control is positive in most patients with meningitis. Nonactive, calcified, cerebral lesions, however, may not yield diagnostic titers. Enzyme-linked immunosorbent assay (ELISA) of IgM antibodies against cysticercosis antigens has been found to be 87% sensitive in CSF samples in a recent study.[24]

Therapy varies according to the clinical presentation. Cysts producing seizures alone may need only anticonvulsant therapy. The calcified lesions are usually not progressive and, unless they cause hydrocephalus, usually do not require surgical resection. The clinical response to ventricular shunting procedures often depends on the activity and number, as well as location, of the basilar and intracerebral cysts. Larvicides such as praziquantel have been used as cysticerccidal agents.

Specific Causes of Noninfectious Chronic Meningitis

Sarcoidosis

Sarcoidosis afflicts the nervous system in 5% of patients. A chronic aseptic meningitis is seen at the time of neurologic presentation in some patients with sarcoidosis, and also as a recurrent syndrome, along with headache and meningeal signs. VIIth cranial-nerve palsies are frequent. The CSF shows a lymphocytic pleocytosis in the range of 6–200 cells, protein is usually elevated less than 200 mg/dL, and 20% of patients have hypoglycoracchia.[25]

Vasculitis and Collagen Vascular Disease

Rheumatologic and vasculitic diseases may cause an inflammatory meningitis, most often in the setting of systemic disease. On occasion, however, CNS involvement may be the presenting feature of an unrecognized systemic illness such as systemic lupus erythematous or rheumatoid arthritis.

Granulomatous angitis of the nervous system is a vasculitic process confined to cerebral vessels. Patients typically present with headache and encephalopathy, followed by a progression to stroke like syndromes with hemipareses and other focal signs. A change in mental status, elevated CSF protein, and cells in the spinal fluid should be present before the diagnosis is entertained. The erythrocyte sedimentation rate is variably elevated and cannot be counted on to confirm the diagnosis. Angiography may show irregularity or "beading" of vessels.

Other vasculitides, such as that associated with herpes zoster ophthalmicus or with Cogan's syndrome (vestibulo-auditory dysfunction with interstitial keratitis in young adults), can present a clinical and CSF picture consistent with chronic meningitis. The presence of herpetic lesions in the former and the specific cranial-nerve involvement in the latter help to guide the diagnosis.

Polyarteritis Nodosa

Polyarteritis nodosa may present with meningeal symptoms such as headache, fever, and leukocytosis, as well as a "toxic delirium" with confusion and disorientation. Neurasthenic symptoms such as weight loss, fatigue, anorexia, and generalized weakness may also be present at the time of diagnosis, as well as upper-respiratory symptoms such as sinusitis, mastoiditis, or otitis. The CSF may be entirely normal or may show a low-grade pleocytosis with minimally elevated protein.[26] Interpretation of the CSF formula may be complicated because some patients present with seizure, stroke, or subarachnoid hemorrhage, syndromes that similarly produce a mild pleocytosis in the CSF.

Systemic Lupus Erythematosus

Systemic lupus erythematosus is another collagen vascular disorder causing a chronic meningeal inflammation. CSF is abnormal in approximately a fourth of patients with nervous system dysfunction in lupus, commonly showing a slight elevation of protein and minimal pleocytosis. Although glucose is not often depressed, hypoglycoracchia can be seen with the transverse myelopathy associated with systemic lupus erythematosus

Sjogren's syndrome, Behcet's disease, and rheumatoid arthritis should also be included in the differential diagnosis of noninfectious chronic meningitis. The occurrence of Sicca syndrome in Sjogren's, recurrent oral and genital ulceration with ocular lesions in Behcet's, and the extraneural manifestations of rheumatoid arthritis help to distinguish these three rheumatologic disorders.

Chemical Meningitis

Chemical meningitis may occur when intrathecal injection of certain compounds causes an inflammatory reaction of the leptomeninges. Examples are contrast agents for radiographic studies, chemotherapeutic agents, antibiotics, and local anesthetics. The CSF may reflect a partial or complete spinal block with lowered opening pressure, lymphocytic pleocytosis, and elevated protein. The CSF abnormalities usually resolve within 1 to 2 weeks.

Chronic Meningitis Associated with Malignancies

The diagnosis of primary or metastatic cerebral tumors is generally made by CT and MRI scanning, rather than lumbar puncture, which carries a risk in a patient with a cerebral mass lesion. In the era preceding these radiographic studies, hallmarks of brain tumor were the presence of raised intracranial pressure and elevated CSF protein. Necrotic malignant gliomas, in particular, may be associated with very high CSF-cell counts.

The leptomeningeal spread of solid tumors may produce a CSF profile similar to that seen in chronic meningitis. Cell count and protein are elevated and, in particular, hypoglycoracchia may be a prominent finding. The definitive diagnosis is, of course, confirmed by cytologic examination of malignant cells in the CSF. It may take more than one lumbar puncture to yield positive cytology, and larger volumes are more likely to yield a diagnosis than will small aliquots.

In contrast to some of the other causes of noninfectious chronic meningitis that present a nonspecific clinical picture, the neurologic presentation of leptomeningeal carcinomatosis can be quite characteristic. Neurologic deficits appear at multiple levels of the neuroaxis simultaneously: cranial-nerve pareses, long-tract signs, and radiculopathies, in addition to deep tendon reflex changes, may occur simultaneously in the same patient, suggesting the diffuse nature of the pathological process.

Chronic Meningitis in Immune-Compromised Patients

Recognition that a patient is from a group at high risk for infection with HIV results in a paradigmatic shift in the clinician's differential diagnosis of chronic meningitis. Because of the AIDS epidemic, the numbers of immunosuppressed patients are increasing. In addition, the widespread use of immunosuppressive and radiation therapy for transplant recipients and cancer patients has altered the sanctity of the blood–brain barrier, changing the body's vulnerability to microbial agents.

A usually self-limited syndrome of acute meningitis may occur at the time of seroconversion in HIV infection. On rare occasions, this meningitis persists or recurs. Patients manifest headache and fever with a mild CSF pleocytosis periodically over months after the onset of symptoms.

More commonly, patients with HIV infection develop cryptococcal meningitis. Unlike patients with competent immune systems, AIDS patients may present with nonspecific symptoms such as headache or lethargy alone. Although fever is common, meningeal signs do not occur in most patients with cryptococcal meningitis, and papilledema and photophobia are usually absent. Similarly, the CSF profile is less likely to be abnormal in AIDS patients than in the immune-competent host. Modest cell-count elevations and protein increases may be seen, and the glucose is greater than 40 mg% in most cases.[27,28] Fortunately, however, specific cryptococcal antigen tests in CSF and serum are frequently positive in AIDS patients.

Although the initial response to amphotericin B is favorable in 58% of the cases, sustained clinical improvement is less prevalent and relapse rates and therapeutic failures on amphotericin B alone or in combination with flucytosine are, unfortunately, common. Recent experience with fluconazole shows promise of improving therapeutic results.

Toxoplasma meningoencephalitis is the most commonly encountered neurologic opportunistic infection in AIDS patients.[29] Although cerebral toxoplasmosis generally presents as a focal mass lesion in the brain, it may also present as a diffuse chronic meningitis with mental-status changes, lethargy, and cognitive decline indistinguishable from the AIDS dementia complex or other indolent causes of chronic meningitis in the immune-compromised host.

CSF protein usually is mildly elevated and there is a minimal mononuclear pleocytosis. Although negative IgG antibody titers to toxoplasmosis make the diagnosis less likely, neither positive nor negative blood or CSF serologies are diagnostic. Specific IgG may be undetectable in the CSF in patients with biopsy or autopsy-proved CNS toxoplasmosis.

Because of the high prevalence of toxoplasmosis, many physicians begin an empiric trial of therapy for patients suspected of having CNS lesions or meningoencephalitis attributable to toxoplasmosis. Pyrimethamine and sulfadiazine evoke an initial response in up to 90% of patients.[28] Lifelong maintenance therapy is recommended.

AIDS patients also suffer chronic meningitis caused by other organisms, such as *Candida albicans, Mycobacterium* tuberculosis, *Aspergillus fumigatus, H capsulatum,* and *C immitis*. Once again, there are few clinical indicators for these fungal infections, and diagnosis of necessity is made by CSF culture or serologies as discussed above. *Mycobacterium avium intracellulare* is commonly found in nervous tissue at autopsy but is not felt to be pathogenic. Tuberculous meningitis usually responds to drug therapy.

Neurosyphilis may take a clinically agressive course in HIV-positive persons[31] and there have been several reports of patients who go on to develop neurosyphilis even after recommended therapy for early syphilis with benzathine penicillin.[32,33] Higher doses of antibiotics for longer periods thus may be necessary. Repeat CSF examinations with serologies are helpful in gauging response to therapy. Whether *Treponema pallidum* is acting as an opportunistic infection in patients also afflicted with HIV, or whether the natural clinical course of syphilis is altered by the profound immune defects caused by the AIDS virus, is still speculative.

References

1. Wilhelm C, Ellner JJ. Chronic meningitis. *Neurol. Clin* 1986;4:115–141.
2. Ellner JJ, Bennett JE. Chronic meningitis. *Medicine* 1976; 55:341–369.
3. Peacock JE Jr, McGinnis MR, Cohen MS. Persistent neutropholic meningitis: report of four cases and review of the literature. *Medicine* 1984;63:379–395.
4. Hyslop NE Jr, Swartz MN. Bacterial meningitis. *Postgrad Med* 1975;58(3):120–128.
5. Koo J, Pieu F, Kliks MM. Angiostrongylus (parastrongylus) esinophilic meningitis. *Rev Infect Dis* 1988;10:1155–1162.
6. Kuberski T. Eosinophils in the cerebrospinal fluid. *Ann Intern Med* 1979;91:70–75.
7. Hopkins AP, Harvey PKP. Chronic benign lymphocytic meningitis. *J. Neurol Sci* 1973;18:443.
8. Molavi A, LeFrock JL. Tuberculous meningitis. *Med Clin North Am* 1985;69:315–331.
9. Lepper M H, Spies HW. The present status of the treatment of tuberculosis of the central nervous system. *Ann NY Acad Sci* 1963;106:106.
10. Weiss W, Flippin HF. The changing incidence and prognosis of tuberculous meningitis. *Am J Med Sci* 1965;50:46.
11. Barrett-Conner EB. Tuberculous meningitis in adults. *South Med J* 1967;60:1061.
12. Kennedy DH, Fallon FJ. Tuberculous meningitis. *JAMA* 1979;241:264–268.
13. Johnson J, Ellner JJ. Tuberculous meningitis, in Evans RW, Baskin DS, Yatsu FM (eds). *Prognosis in Neurological Disease*. Cambridge, England, Oxford University Press, 1990, in press.
14. Merritt HH, Fremont-Smith F. Cerebrospinal fluid in tuberculous meningitis. *Arch Neurol Psychol* 1935; 33:516.
15. Jeren T, Beus L. Characteristics of cerebrospinal fluid in tuberculous meningitis. *Acta Cytol* 1982; 26:678.
16. Stocksill MT, Kauffman CA. Comparison of cryptococcal and tuberculous meningitis. *Arch Neurol* 1983;40:81–85.
17. Spickard A, Butler WT, Andriole V, et al. The improved prognosis of cryptococcal meningitis with amphotericin B therapy. *Ann Intern Med* 1963;58:66.
18. Butler WT, Alling DW, Spickard A, et al. Diagnostic and prognostic value of clinical and laboratory findings in cryptococcal meningitis. A follow-up study of forty patients. *N Eng J Med* 1964;270:59.
19. Littman ML, Walter JE. Cryptococcosis: current status. *Am J Med* 1968;45:922.
20. Diamond RD, Bennett JE. Prognostic factors in cryptococcal meningitis. A study of 111 cases. *Ann Intern Med* 1974;80:176.
21. Simon RP. Neurosyphilis. *Arch Neurol* 1981;42: 606–613.
22. Willcox RR. Treatment of syphilis. *Bull WHO* 1981;59:655–663.
23. Abramowicz, M (ed). Treatment of Lyme disease. *Med Lett Drugs Therapeut* 1989;31.
24. Rosas N, Sotelo J, Nieto D. ELISA in the diagnosis of neurocysticercosis. *Arch Neurol* 1986;43:353–356.
25. Gaines JD, Eckman PM, Remington JS. Low CSF glucose level in sarcoidosis involving the central nervous system. *Arch Intern Med* 1970;125:333–336.
26. Scully RE, Mark EJ, McNeely BU. Case 43-1986. *Case Rec Mass Gen Hosp* 1986;315:1143–1154.
27. Kovacs JA, Kovacs AA, Polis M, et al. Cryptococcosis in the acquired immunodeficiency syndrome. *Ann Intern Med* 1985;103:533–538.
28. Dismukes W E. Cryptococcal meningitis in patients with AIDS. *J Infect Dis* 1988;157:624–628.
29. Levy RM, Bredesen DE, Rosenblum ML. Neurological manifestations of the acquired immunodeficiency syndrome (AIDS): experience at UCSF and review of the literature. *J. Neurosurg* 1985;62:475–495.
30. McArthur JC. Neurologic manifestations of AIDS. *Medicine* 1987;66:407–437.
31. Johns DR, Tierney M, Felsenstein D. Alterations in the natural history of neurosyphilis by concurrent infection with the human immunodeficiency virus. *N Engl J Med* 1987;316:1569–1602.
32. Emskitter TH, Jenzevski H, Pulz M, Spehn J. Neurosyphilis in HIV infection—persistence after high-dose penicillin therapy. *Neuroimmunol* 1988; 20:153–166.
33. Berry CD, Hooton TM, Collier AC, Lukehart SA. Neurologic relapse after benzathine penicillin therapy for secondary syphilis in a patient with HIV infection. *N Engl J Med* 1987;316:1587–1589.

5
Posttraumatic Meningitis

REBECCA A. CLARK AND NEWTON E. HYSLOP, JR.

The central nervous system (CNS) is normally protected from pathogenic organisms by mechanical barriers and the host's natural defense system. The two primary routes of access for infecting organisms are hematogenous spread or direct advancement from a parameningeal focus.

Infection is facilitated in the presence of a cerebrospinal-fluid (CSF) fistula that occurs when the natural physical barriers are disrupted. Acute trauma, either accidental or surgical, is often the cause of CSF leaks. If trauma acutely disrupts the dura or causes it to erode over time, the thin arachnoid membrane is generally not able to contain the CSF and there is subsequent leakage.

The generally accepted classification for CSF leaks is based on etiology. As proposed by Ommaya in 1976, the principal distinction is between traumatic and nontraumatic causes. Traumatic causes may be accidental or iatrogenic. Onset of leak is either acute or delayed.[1] Nontraumatic leaks are rare and more apt to be insidious in onset. CSF leaks are important because they predispose patients to bacterial CNS infection A significant proportion, up to 17%, of patients presenting with first episode bacterial meningitis will have had a history of head trauma.[2] Onset of meningitis may occur immediately after trauma or years later. When CSF leaks are asymptomatic, meningitis may be the initial presenting sign.

Any patient with recurrent bacterial meningitis should be evaluated for the possible presence of a CSF leak. The association between recurrent bacterial meningitis and CSF leak is stressed by the observation that 11–21% of patients with posttraumatic meningitis will have recurrent episodes.[2,3] This chapter reviews posttraumatic meningitis, particularly focusing on its etiology, diagnosis, and treatment. Although bacterial meningitis is a well-known complication of head trauma, there continues to be limited information and therefore controversy in management of some aspects. The role of prophylactic antibiotics for acute CSF leak and optimal surgical management of various fistulas require more data for unequivocal recommendations.

Signs and Symptoms

Posttraumatic CSF leak is either accidental or due to surgical trauma. Accidental leaks follow mid-face trauma and fractures of the base of the skull, which contains the pneumatized temporal, sphenoid, ethmoid, and frontal bones. Both types of trauma may be complicated by acute or delayed onset of meningitis. Clear or bloody rhinorrhea, otorrhea, otorhinorrhia, and pneumocephalus are diagnostic of a CSF leak. Other suggestive signs include hemotympanum, Battle's sign, bilateral periorbital ecchymoses, and specific cranial-nerve deficits.

Rhinorrhea

Rhinorrhea is the term for CSF leaking from the nose. The most common site of skull fracture associated with rhinorrhea is either lateral frontal, resulting from a blow to the side of the head, or central, in which the blow is taken head on.[4] The onset is variable, taking place anywhere from 24 hours to years later, but generally rhinorrhea is apparent within the first few days. In a series of 81 patients, Westmore and Whittam[3] noted that 61 (75%) had rhinorrhea within the first month and 46 (57%) within 48 hours, but presentation was delayed for as long as 35 years. Rhinorrhea complicates basilar skull fractures 6.5%[5] to 26%[6], transphenoidal hypophysectomies 7%[7] to 8%,[8] and middle third facial fractures in 43%.[2]

Otorrhea

Otorrhea is defined as CSF present in the external auditory canal and is usually secondary to temporal bone fractures that may be longitudinal or transverse. The frequency of otorrhea complicating traumatic skull fractures varies from 9%[5] to 59.5%.[6] Postoperative otorrhea complicates removal of acoustic neurominas in up to 18%.[11]

Longitudinal fractures of the temporal bone are the most common cause of otorrhea, accounting for 70–80% of the cases.[9] They characteristically follow a blow to the temporal and parietal region in which the forces tear apart the base of the skull in an anterior–posterior direction, resulting in a fracture passing through the external auditory canal, middle ear, and mastoid. The petrous bone is split longitudinally along the weaker eustacian tube, and there may be a fracture of the auditory ossicles that results in a conductive hearing loss. If the dura in the tegmen tympani is lacerated, CSF leaks into the middle ear. However, otorrhea will only occur if the tympanic membrane is lacerated; otherwise, CSF will drain from the nose (paradoxical rhinorrhea or otorhinorrhea). The incidence of otorhinorrea is very low.[9]

Transverse fractures account for 20% of cases of otorrhea. They result from an occipital blow and begin in the region of the foramen magnum. The fracture traverses the internal auditory meatus and labyrinth or the internal cochlea and may terminate in the middle cranial fossa. There is often a total sensorineural hearing loss on the side of the lesion. Since this type of fracture involves the otic capsule, which contains endochrondral bone that heals by fibroplastic proliferation rather than by osteogenesis, a persistent CSF fistula is more likely in this type of fracture.

CSF Leakage into Tissue: Subgalleal and Orbital Collections

CSF can leak from the skull fracture unobtrusively into subgalleal and other sites and be missed on physical exam. Unusual examples have been a few cases of frontoethmoidal fracture where CSF tracked laterally from the ethmoidal region into the orbital tissues to give rise to a fluctuant mass above and medial to the globe.[12] Postoperative subgalleal CSF collections also often complicate posterior-fossa craniotomies.

Hemotympanum

Hemotympanum refers to bleeding behind the tympanic membrane which is generally obvious on exam. If the tympanum ruptures, blood is then visible in the external canal. Hemotympanum following head trauma generally indicates a temporal bone fracture involving the inner or middle ear and consequently is suggestive of a CSF leak. It occurs in 27%[13] to 81%[14] of cases of basilar skull fractures.

Battle's Sign

Battle's sign refers to ecchymosis over the mastoid area. In traumatic skull fracture, Battle's sign occurs in 12%[14] to 13%.[13] Its appearance, which may be delayed 1–2 days after trauma, is a sign of basal skull fracture. Periorbital ecchymoses ("raccoon eyes") is another sign of basilar skull fracture.[13,14]

Cranial-Nerve Palsies

Specific cranial nerves may be compromised by skull fracture, depending on the location of the injury. The olfactory canals traverse the cribriform plate, and it is clear that a fracture involving the cribriform plate area may result in olfactory-nerve deficit or anosmia. In a series of 1,000 cases of consecutive closed-head injuries, anosmia developed in 50 (5%). The incidence was higher in frontal injuries.[4]

The facial nerve is injured in about 15% of longitudinal temporal-bone fractures, usually at the geniculate ganglion or above the oval window. If there is a transverse temporal-bone fracture, the facial nerve is injured medial to the geniculate ganglion in approximately 45%.[15] The eighth nerve can be injured in a transverse temporal-bone fracture, as previously described.

Settings Predisposing to CSF Fistula

Surgical Trauma

Any pericranial or perispinal surgery with the potential to disrupt the dura or intracranial procedures where watertight dural closures are difficult can produce a CSF leak.

Ophthalmological Surgery: Global Enucleation

Enucleation even in the presence of endophthalmitis does not increase the risk of postoperative meningitis, provided that perioperative intensive and appropriate antibiotic therapy is used. Formerly, this operation posed a serious risk for extension of infection.[16]

Nasal Surgery

Transnasal ethmoidectomy is the most common otolaryngologic procedure causing CSF rhinorrhea, principally due to the surgeon's inability to visualize the outer limits of the sinus during this approach. Fistulae may develop acutely or be delayed in onset.[15]

Elective nasal surgery, such as submucous resection of the nasal septum for nasal deviation or rhinoplasty for cosmetic purposes, rarely will have subsequent intracranial complications, due to the contiguous relationship between the bony portion of the ala nasae and the cribriform plate area. Patients undergoing septum surgery whose deviation is due to previous nasal trauma may be predisposed to fistula formation because previously damaged anterior cranial fossa floor is more easily fractured during manipulation of the bony ala nasae.

Otologic Surgery

Mastoidectomies[19] and stapendectomies[10] infrequently produce dural tears, but removal of acoustic neuromas carries a higher risk, especially when accessed by the suboccipital approach.

The incidence of otorrhea or rhinorrhea following suboccipital approach to the cerebellarpontine angle and internal auditory meatus, approaches 20%.[11] Highly pneumatized temporal bones, where air cells extend along the posterior wall of the internal auditory meatus, may predispose to CSF fistulization following suboccipital craniotomy.[20] Temporal bone pneumatization, which begins in fetal life and progresses during infancy, varies considerably among individuals. Approximately 20% of temporal bone pneumatization progresses to the posterior wall of the internal auditory meatus, leaving a thinner table of calvarium. While any operation which requires removing bone from the posterior wall of the internal auditory meatus carries the risk of CSF leak, hyperpneumatized temporal bones carry a greater risk.[20]

Extracranial Hypophysectomies

Hypophysectomies can be complicated by CSF leaks, and occasionally meningitis, if the dural defect in the sella turcica is not adequately sealed. A dural defect may occur following any of the three extracranial approaches: transethmoid, transphenoid, or transnasal. With present techniques, the incidence of CSF leak following hypophysectomy is 7%[7] to 8%[8] and the rate of postoperative meningitis is 6%[7] to 10%.[8]

Accidental Trauma

Basilar Skull Fractures

Accidental cranial trauma is an important predisposing factor for CSF leaks. Trauma that fractures portions of the cranium containing pericranial air sinuses, aerated bone, or middle ear carry high risk of CSF fistulization. Furthermore dura is most apt to rupture with a fracture of the cranial bone to which it adheres.[5]

Fractures involving the basilar skull especially predispose to CSF leak, in part because adhesion between inner table bone and dura is most pronounced at the base of the skull. The frequent localization of CSF fistula in frontal, ethmoid, and sphenoid sinuses following trauma is attributable to the thin bony inner table being especially susceptible to fracture plus dural adherence. While the cribriform plate itself is quite thick, the immediately adjacent bony areas forming the floor of the anterior cranial fossa and the roof of the ethmoid complex are very fragile and easily fractured with midface forces. The frontal fossa is therefore the area from which most traumatic leaks arise in adults.[22,23]

Middle cranial fossa leaks may result from temporal bone fractures where the only barrier between endolymph and middle ear is the stapes foot plate and membrane of the oval window. Posterior fossa leaks are very rare but may also occur as a consequence of a fracture of the petrous bone.[22]

Temporary self-limiting CSF fistula formation occurs in 16%[14] to 24%[13] of adults and 3.5% of children experiencing basilar skull fracture.[5] The overall risk of developing meningitis following basilar skull fracture is increased if there is clinical evidence of CSF leak, such as rhinorrhea, otorrhea, or pneumocephalus. In the presence of an obvious leak, the incidence of meningitis ranges from 7%[6] to 35%.[3] For basilar skull fracture without rhinorrhea or otorrhea, the incidence of meningitis varies from 0[25] to 2%.[13] The high prevalence of CSF leak complicating basilar skull fractures in adults is especially relevant to the advantages and dangers posed by use of antibiotics in such patients, especially for prophylaxis against meningitis.

Facial Bone Fractures

The prevalence of a dural tear after fracture of the middle third of the facial skeleton is greater than after a direct skull injury. The zygomatic arch transfers midface forces to periorbital and paranasal structures, causing secondary pericranial trauma and dural laceration. Characteristic groupings of findings have been defined by Le Fort.

The prevalence of dural tear increases with the anatomic height and increasing severity of the fracture. In a review of 247 patients with fracture of the middle third of the facial skeleton, 107 had CSF leaks (43%). Dura tears occurred in 49% (72/148) of Le Fort II and 73% (19/26) of Le Fort III fractures. Remarkably, the incidence of subsequent meningitis was only 2% (2/107).[2] Of 98 patients who had rhinorrhea, 91% experienced cessation within two weeks of fracture reduction. Persistent CSF leak (>2 weeks) occurred in 6% of those with Le Fort II and 18% of those with Le Fort III fractures.[2]

Characteristics of Posttraumatic Meningitis

The signs and symptoms of posttraumatic meningitis are similar to those of any patient presenting with meningitis. Common complaints include headache, confusion, recent upper-respiratory infection, chills, myalgia, meningismis, nausea, vomiting, and seizures. The most frequent findings are fever, confusion, nuchal rigidity, and cranial-nerve deficits.[24]

Posttraumatic meningitis does differ by having a relatively good prognosis if appropriately treated.[24] The mortality in treated posttraumatic meningitis remains about 6%.[2,24] Patients with posttraumatic meningitis tend to do well, probably because they are younger and have less underlying disease.

Bacteriology

Posttraumatic Meningitis

Streptococcus pneumoniae has traditionally been the predominant pathogen in posttraumatic meningitis. In 1970, Hand and colleagues[24] published a large series of 16 patients with 32 episodes of posttraumatic meningitis. *S pneumoniae* was found to be the etiologic agent in 17 of 24 (71%) definitely and was implicated in three more cases. Other organisms isolated included a *Hemophilus* species and probable *Nersseria meningitidis*. The remainder of the cultures were unknown or sterile.

Over the past 10 years, meningitis following accidental trauma is still primarily due to *S pneumoniae,* but there is a trend toward an increasing percentage caused by Gram-negative bacilli. In 1984, a second large series showed *S pneumoniae* was again the main pathogen, being implicated in 70% (21/30) of episodes of posttraumatic meningitis.[2] In six other large series published since 1978 that reviewed posttraumatic meningitis, a total of 50 patients had the causative organism known. Bacteria isolated included *S pneumoniae* in 56%, aerobic Gram-negative bacilli in 26% (including *Enterobacter aerogenes, Serratia marcesens, Escherichia coli, Pseudomomas aeruginosa, Proteus mirabilis, Klebsiella* sp), *Hemophilus influenzae* in 8%, streptococcus other than *S pneumoniae* in 6%, *N meningitidis* in 2%, and *Staphylococcus aureus* in 2%. Note that CSF cultures were sterile in 30% of cases even when biochemical parameters were consistent with bacterial meningitis.[3,6,13,14,23,44] Anaerobes have been isolated in some postoperative cases and may be more frequent than is generally recognized in traumatic cases. Unusual organisms have been cultured from the CSF in patients who developed meningitis after head injuries, including *Pasteurella multocida*[26] and *Brucella melitensis*.[27]

Postoperative Meningitis

Meningitis as a complication of neurosurgery, such as transphenoidal hypophysectomy, is less likely to be due to *S pneumoniae*. Gram-negative bacillis, anaerobes, and staphylococcus are more prominent, and sometimes more than one organism is isolated. Combining the results from Gansden[8] and Romanowski's[7] series, a total of 15 organisms were isolated from the CSF (lumbar) of 17 patients following transphenoidal hypophysectomy. Five patients had sterile cultures. Aerobic Gram-negative bacilli [*E coli* (4), *P mirabilis* (1), *Proteus vulgaris* (1), *P aeruginosa* (1)] were prominent, accounting for 46% of the cases. Other bacteria included streptococcus species in 13%, anaerobes in 13%, *Staphylococcus epidermidis* in 7%, *S aureus* in 7%, *Hemophilus parainfluenza* in 7%, and diptheroids in 5%.

Antibiotics

Neurologic and Otologic Surgical Prophylaxis

The most significant factor in the development of a postoperative infection is bacterial contamination during surgery. This contamination can be caused either by inoculation of organisms spreading from an adjacent previously infected area or by airborne bacteria. The latter can be better controlled by shortening operating time and using special techniques, such as laminar air-flow units, in the operating room.

The need for prophylaxis is influenced by the nature of the surgery (clean versus contaminated) and potential of a coexisting infection. Prophylaxis should begin immediately preoperatively and not be continued for longer than 12–48 hours. It is not the same as treatment.[28,29]

Otologic Surgery

In clean surgery with low risk of CSF fistula formation or wound hematoma, such as stapendectomy, the incidence of infection is rare and prophylaxis is not felt to be warranted. However, if operating in the presence of purulent otorrhea and a probably infected operative site, prophylactic antibiotics would be prudent, especially if dural disruption is anticipated. Since the bacteriology of suppurative otitis media includes a combination of anaerobes, particularly Bacteroides and Peptococci, aerobic Gram-negative bacilli, *S aureus,* and streptococci,[28] broad-spectrum coverage should be chosen.

Because of the inherent risk of contamination of subdural tissues, prophylaxis has been used in resection of an acoustic neuroma. Until recently, there were no studies available to critically determine the benefits and drawbacks. In 1988, Kartush and coworkers[30] reported on a prospective study of 236 patients undergoing translabyrinth resection of an acoustic neuroma or retrolabyrinth vestibular-nerve section. Patients were divided into four groups: (1) no antibiotics, (2) intravenous cephalosporin only, (3) topical bacitracin irrigation intraoperatively, and (4) both bacitracin irrigation and intravenous cephalosporin. There was no difference in the incidence of meningitis among any of the groups, but patients treated with topical bacitracin irrigation intraoperatively with or without intravenous antibiotics had both a lower incidence of wound infection (2% versus 9%) and CSF leak (5% versus 12%). In addition, in the bacitracin-treated groups with CSF leak, fewer sutures were needed for subsequent closure of the wound. Note that the benefits of bacitracin were cited as early as 1950 by Teng and colleagues.[31]

From these studies, the following conclusions can be made:

1. Intravenous antimicrobial prophylaxis in clean otologic surgery does not appear to lower the incidence of postoperative meningitis.
2. Bacitracin-irrigation solution appears to play an important role in intraoperative prophylaxis, particularly in the removal of acoustic neuromas, and mainly in lowering the risk of postoperative leak and local wound infection.

Neurosurgery

Routine antimicrobial prophylaxis for any neurosurgical procedure is now common but still controversial. Shapiro and co-workers[32] addressed this issue by performing a large prospective, double-blind, placebo-controlled randomized clinical trial in an institution where there was a baseline neurosurgical postoperative wound-infection rate of 6%. A total of 148 patients undergoing any neurosurgical procedure were divided into two groups; one group received one to two doses of intravenous vancomycin and gentamicin immediately preoperatively and one group received intravenous placebo. The wound irrigant in the antibiotic group also had streptomycin added to the saline. The overall infection rates of the antibiotic and placebo groups were 2.8% and 11.7%, respectively. None of the operations following trauma were complicated by infection. This study suggested that the general incidence of neurosurgical postoperative infections may be lessened by prophylactic intravenous vancomycin, gentamicin, and streptomycin irrigant. However, prophylactic antimicrobial use in specific neurologic procedures was not analyzed separately and efficacy was confined to preventing wound infection rather than targetted only at preventing meningitis.

Recently, two retrospective studies looked specifically at the risk of acquiring meningitis during hypophysectomies. Romanowski and colleagues[7] studied 98 patients who underwent a transphenoidal hypophysectomy. Of these, 64 received prophylaxis and 5 developed meningitis. Of the 34 patients not treated, 1 developed meningitis. Rhinorrhea and diabetes mellitus were both found to be significant risk factors for the postoperative development of meningitis. The relative risk of meningitis was 22 times greater for those with rhinorrhea than for those without, and 36.8 times greater for those with diabetes than for those without. Rhinorrhea occurred in three of the patients with meningitis and in four of the other 92 patients. Five of the six patients with meningitis had diabetes mellitus.[47]

In the second study, Gransden and others[8] described 114 patients who underwent a transsphenoidal removal of pituitary tumor using a combined transethmoidosphenoidal and transnasal route. All but two patients received systemic prophylaxis with either intravenous chloramphenicol alone or chloramphenicol plus sulfamethoxazole. Four patients were receiving prophylaxis at the onset of meningitis, and in three of these patients, the organism isolated from CSF was sensitive to at least one antibiotic. Organisms resistant to the prophylactic antibiotics were isolated from four patients and included a chloramphenicol-resistant *P mirabilis*.

The data from these studies imply the following:

1. Intraoperative intravenous vancomycin, gentamicin, and topical antibiotic irrigant can lower the risk of neurosurgical postoperative wound infections in institutions that may have a relatively high infection rate (6%). Other regimens may be equally effective, providing they recognize prevailing nosocomial antibiotic resistance patterns.
2. The routine administration of prophylactic antibiotics in transsphenoidal hypophysectomies does not appear to be necessary and may predispose patients to meningitis with resistant organisms. However, patients with diabetes mellitus appear to be especially prone to postoperative meningitis, and in these patients prophylaxis should be considered.
3. The presence of rhinorrhea following transsphenoidal surgery carries an increased risk of postoperative meningitis, and broad spectrum antibiotics plus possible surgical correction should be considered if leakage is persistent.

The recognition that intraoperative antibiotic administration will reduce wound infection for all clean surgical procedures makes any kind of placebo-controlled study in neurosurgical procedures essentially passé. When surgery is expected to carry a risk of CSF leak into a mucosal-lined surface, choice of narrow spectrum prophylaxis, such as vancomycin, may reduce the selection of highly resistant Gram-negative rods.

Accidental-Head-Trauma Prophylaxis

Basilar Skull Fractures

Knowing the hazard of meningitis following head trauma, physicians often administer "prophylactic" antimicrobial treatment if there appears to be any evidence suggestive of a CSF leak. "Empiric treatment for subclinical meningitis" is better terminology, because the antibiotics are started after the head trauma occurs and generally are continued for several days. Routine administration of antibiotics has been controversial as there can be obvious drawbacks, and the benefits are at times questionable. To find a better answer to this question, several studies have analyzed the efficacy of prophylactic antibiotics in basilar skull fractures independent of whether or not a persistent CSF leak was present.

Ignelzi and colleagues[25] prospectively studied 75 patients with basilar skull fractures, observing 50 and treating the remainder with intravenous antibiotics. They also retrospectively reviewed 54 patients with basilar skull fractures treated with various antibiotics. Results of combining both groups showed that in the untreated patients, there were no CNS infectious complications, whereas in the treated group, there was one fatal case of meningitis, and another patient had a brain abscess.[3]

Frazee and co-workers[13] retrospectively studied 347 patients with basilar skull fractures, of whom 251 (72%) were treated prophylactically and 96 (28%) were observed. Fifty-one percent of the treated group had a leak as compared with 10.5% of the observed group. A total of six patients, two with a CSF leak, developed meningitis. There was no significant difference between the two groups (1.6% incidence in the treated group versus 2% incidence in the observed group).[19] These two studies reveal that the incidence of meningitis in patients with basilar skull fractures was not decreased by antimicrobial prophylaxis.

Moreover, there are important potential detrimental side effects to antibiotic prophylaxis. The primary danger is change in normal flora, which predisposes the patient to acquire a resistant, usually Gram-negative-bacillus meningitis. For example, the normal nasopharyngeal flora, composed of mainly alpha-hemolytic streptococci on routine cultures, is replaced by enteric organisms, particularly *P aeruginosa* in patients receiving systemic antibiotics (Sprunt and others[33]). Serial cultures taken on neurosurgical patients with CSF leaks confirm antibiotic-induced changes in respiratory flora. Ignelzi[25] prospectively randomized ten patients with traumatic CSF leaks so that five received prophylactic intravenous ampicillin and cephalothin and five none. Cultures of the posterior nasopharynx were taken on days 1, 5, and 10. None of the patients developed meningitis, but four of the five prophylaxed had significant changes in their posterior pharyngeal flora, shifting to a Gram-negative-bacillus predominance.

The addition of antibiotics not only increases the risk that a CNS infection will be caused by resistant organisms, but may predispose patients to non-CNS superinfections. Zrebeet and Huang[6] studied 42 patients with basilar skull fractures of whom 28 received prophylactic antibiotics. There was no significant difference in incidence of meningitis (two in the treated group and one in the untreated group), but there was a tendency toward an increased incidence of non-CNS infections in the treated patients (14% versus 21%). These included four pulmonary infections, two urinary-tract infections, one otitis media, and one wound infection in 28 treated patients. In 14 untreated patients, no non-CNS infections developed.

Mid-Facial Fracture

Major middle face fractures commonly are complicated by dural tears and accompanying CSF rhinorrhea. Pressure ventilation with a face mask is avoided to prevent forced intracranial entry of secretions. Closed reduction of facial bone fractures is undertaken within the first few days. No studies of antibiotic prophylaxis in this group of patients has been undertaken; they routinely receive parenteral antibiotics.[2]

Indications for Prophylaxis

Ideally, antibiotics should be reserved for patients who are particularly susceptible to CNS infections. The risk of posttraumatic meningitis does appear to be related to specific parameters such as size, location, and duration of the leak, since most small leaks are transient and self-sealing.

The presence of air in the subarachnoid space (pneumocephalus) is an objective sign of dural fistula and is usually a consequence of a relatively large defect in the dural envelope, generally as a result of trauma. Such defects are less apt to heal spontaneously and therefore place the patient at high risk for the invasion of organisms into the subarachnoid space. The patient, upon straining, coughing, or sneezing, transports air and secretions from the nose, the paranasal sinuses, and even the pharynx into the subarachnoid space. In one series of 13 patients with pneumocephalus, not surprisingly, seven (54%) developed meningitis.[23] Delayed onset rhinorrhea also has a higher incidence of meningitis of up to 56%, possibly because of increased length of exposure.[23]

Patients with posttraumatic rhinorrhea after a basilar skull fracture had a decreased incidence of meningitis when treated prophylactically in at least one series. Of 18 patients with active rhinorrhea, 13 were treated with antibiotics on presentation and none developed meningitis. Of the five untreated patients, two (40%) progressed to meningitis, one with a beta-hemolytic streptococcus and one with *S pneumoniae*.[14] However, while the difference between the treated and untreated groups in this nonrandomized retrospective study was noteworthy, it was not statistically significant.

Although antimicrobial administration continues to be controversial in the setting of potential CSF leak complicating head trauma without evidence of meningitis, some conclusions can be derived from the available data.

1. The overall incidence of meningitis in basilar skull fractures is not lessened by prophylactic antibiotics; thus routine administration is not warranted.
2. The several potential detrimental side effects of antibiotics should be taken into consideration before initiating prophylaxis, except under the following circumstances: (a) certain subpopulations of patients with mid-facial and basilar skull fractures appear to have an increased risk of meningitis and should be considered for

both early surgical intervention and antimicrobial prophylaxis; (b) those with large dural defects who present with pneumocephalus; and (c) those who present with profuse rhinorrhea, acute or delayed. However, there is no clear data supporting the efficacy of antibiotics in these settings.

Treatment

The essential ingredient for optimal outcome in patients with CSF leak and bacterial meningitis is rapid clearing of the CSF. Early treatment is not only essential for preventing CNS complications but also to promote spontaneous healing of the fistula if it is acute. Antibiotics recommended for the treatment of meningitis depend on the organism isolated and are the same regardless of their route of access to CSF. If cultures remain sterile, the setting must be taken into consideration.

The treatment of choice for pneumococcal meningitis continues to be high-dose intravenous penicillin in most areas of the world, although relative resistance is prevalent in some places and increasing everywhere. Vancomycin is effective against these strains.

Gram-negative meningitis remains notoriously difficult to treat although third-generation cephalosporins have excellent CNS penetration and some patients respond well. Gilbert and colleagues[34] evaluated the use of intrathecal amikacin in such patients. They reasoned that large doses were needed because much of the drug could be lost in the leaking CSF. They treated six patients who had CSF leaks and Gram-negative meningitis *(P aeruginosa, S marcescens, Enterobacter aerogenes)* with large doses of intrathecal amikacin (20–40 mg) and systemic antibiotics. Five of the patients had no bactericidal activity in the CSF with systemic antibiotics alone or with low-dose intrathecal amikacin. With higher doses of intrathecal amikacin, bactericidal levels in the CSF improved to 1:8 to 1:32 in five patients. All six patients were cured, and three of four patients had cessation of CSF leaks within 72 hours.

Identification of CSF Leak

Identifying the leak can be extremely difficult. Basic characteristics of a CSF leak include the tendency to be intermittent and often to be positional. Fluid may drain down the throat and can produce hoarseness, coughing, or a sweet or salty taste. In otorrhea, there may be hearing difficulties or intermittent dizziness. A loss of the sense of smell may indicate a cribriform fracture.[35]

Analysis of Fluid

Unless contaminated with blood by acute trauma, the CSF is clear and colorless, with a low specific gravity (1.006), and contains a low amount of protein (<50 mg%), a modest amount of glucose (50–70 mg%), and a chloride content higher than blood or serum (about 120 mM). Lacrimal and nasal mucous secretions both have a low glucose. The easiest bedside test to do is to measure the nasal drainage for glucose. If Dextrostix is used, the result may be inaccurate.[35]

A second diagnostic chemical study is the identification of an extra band of transferrin in the beta-2 fraction in the protein electrophoresis of the spinal fluid. There are two electrophorectically distinct transferrins in the CSF fluid, which differ in their amounts of neuraminic acid. The transferrin is pathognomonic for CSF, not being present in the serum, nasal secretions, saliva, tears, perilymph, or endolymph.[36]

Localization of Otorrhea by Fluorescein Dye in CSF

Fluid in the tympanomastoid compartment of adults demands a diligent diagnostic search to determine whether it is actually CSF, since disorders other than CSF fistulas may present in a similar manner. Both serous otitis media in vacuo (SOV) and adult serous effusion (ASE) should be differentiated from otorrhea. In all three diagnoses, the usual complaint is unilateral hearing loss and the main finding is a unilateral fluid-filled tympanomastoid compartment. After performing the chemical tests discussed, specific diagnostic maneuvers can be helpful.[37]

In SOV, placement of a pressure-equalizing tympanostomy tube will result in resolution of the SOV as long as the tube remains patent because SOV is the result of blockage of the eustacian tube. ASE is characterized by the active secretion of serous fluid from mucous membrane lining the tympanomastoid compartment. Unlike ASE, otorrhea will increase when the patient increases intracranial pressure with a Valsalva maneuver.[37]

The fluorescein-dye test can be used both to identify CSF otorrhea and to help identify the source of the leak. The fluorescein should be injected about 4 to 24 hours prior to surgery to take full advantage of the stain as an aid in locating the site. A mixture of 9.5 cc CSF removed by lumbar puncture (LP) and 0.5 cc of 10% fluorescein is then reinjected very slowly (over 5 minutes) into the CSF via the lumbar spinal needle. Two hours later, the fluid is removed from the middle ear and examined. The presence or absence of fluorescein will determine whether the fluid is secondary to ASE or a CSF leak.[37]

If a patient subsequently proceeds to surgery, it is preferable first to enter the mastoid through a postauricular approach and to explore the dural surfaces of the middle and posterior fossas for CSF leaks, looking specifically for the fluorescein stain. If no dural defect is identified, the surgical exploration proceeds to the middle ear via a transcanal approach. The three principal sites for a CSF fistula in the middle ear, in order of frequency, are the oval window, the round window, and Hyrtl's fissure.[37]

Radiographic Studies

Although skull roentgenograms are usually routinely performed, the sensitivity for revealing a CSF leak is low. In a series of 51 patients with CSF rhinorrhea, plain roentgenograms of the head and tomography of the skull base demonstrated findings consistent with a source for the leak in 21% (8/89) and 53% (18/34), respectively.[38]

Computed tomography (CT) scanning is helpful in revealing possible cranial-bone anomalies and evaluating other potential coexistent pathology, such as hydrocephalus or tumor. High-resolution computed tomography can localize the approximate site of the CSF fistula before a metrizimide study is performed.

Radioactive tracers have been used to identify and locate a CSF leak. Indium (In-111 DTPA) has become the most frequently used cisternography radioisotope. It is very sensitive, but specificity is a problem since it frequently produces overly positive scans. As it has a long half-life, it may be effective in detecting arachnoid cysts by imaging beyond 12 hours.[23] Radioactive indium can be injected by either cisternal tap or LP. Tagged, numbered pledgets placed at the ostia of the sinuses and in the meatus of the nose may help localize the region of the leak.[38] If this is performed, simultaneous use of fluorescein in CSF provides a visible marker.

Radionuclide tracer can also be injected through two skull drill holes under local anesthesia. The dura matter is pierced and radionuclide material is injected into the subarachnoid space. In one series, CSF leaks were confirmed in 221 of 269 patients (82%). Certain locations were clearly better visualized by this method. Ninety-seven percent of the fistulas in the anterior or middle part of the ethmoid were satisfactorily seen, but precise localization of posterior ethmoidal, or sphenoidal fistulas could not be obtained in 21%.[39]

Metrizamide CT cisternography is now probably the most widely used and most useful diagnostic test for active fistulas. Metrizamide is a water-soluble contrast agent used to study the intracranial subarachnoid spaces. Side effects frequently include headache, nausea, and vomiting, and, rarely, short-lived perceptual aberrations.[40] The metrizamide is injected into the lumbar or cervical subarachnoid space with the patient in a prone position. After removal of the spinal needle, the fluoroscopy table is tilted into a negative 70-degree position (with the neck in gentle flexion) to bring the contrast material into the basal subarachnoid space, and then the patient is returned to a 5- to 10-degree position and transported to CT. The combination of metrizamide with high-resolution 5-mm coronal and axial cuts in head CT has proved extremely useful in locating leaks. The anatomic site and extent of the fistula can be demonstrated precisely by observing metrizamide passing through the bony defect.[45] When necessary, 1.5 mm thick cuts in the area of interest are necessary to demonstrate the fistula. Valsalva maneuver or cough may be required to provoke leakage during the procedure.

However, metrizamide CT-cisternographs appear to work best in patients with active rhinorrhea.[41] Patients with slower, or intermittent CSF leaks, may not have the leak identified initially. If unsuccessful, Spetzler and Wilson[42] have recommended that the intracranial pressure can be elevated briefly electively for radionuclide cisternography. Naturally, patients with signs of elevated intracranial pressure or expanding intracranial masses, and those in early stages after head injury, should not be studied by this technique.[42] There are no large series reporting on the success of this hyperbaric method for metrizamide CT cisternography.[41] Some surgeons use lumbar drains during surgery to infuse saline or dye to visualize the leak and then postoperatively to provide decompression.[35]

Surgery

The decision to perform surgery is influenced by the etiology, severity, and location of the CSF leak. The majority, approximately 70%, of CSF fistulas tend to cease leaking spontaneously within the first several weeks.[35] General recommendations include bed rest with the head up, and caution against nose blowing or sniffing.[35] Laxatives are given to minimize increased intra-abdominal and intrathoracic pressures during bowel movements.[23] For CSF leak following middle third facial fractures, immobilization of the fractures is also required.

Under certain circumstances, decreasing the intracranial CSF pressure by the repeated removal of CSF fluid, either by repeat lumbar taps or by an indwelling lumbar subarachnoid catheter, has been recommended,[43] although with large CSF leaks, pressures are already low. Continuous external lumbar subarachnoid drainage of CSF has been used to treat both postoperative and posttraumatic fistulas. The hazards of secondary infection may outweigh the advantages of this procedure.[43]

Note that temporary increases in CSF pressure may occur after head injury or during meningitis, which can cause persistent CSF leakage. If hydrocephalus develops, then shunting is the appropriate first step to try to reverse continuing CSF leak.[35]

For most patients, if the leakage is gradually decreasing, surgical intervention can be delayed for four to six weeks. If the leakage does not decrease after two weeks, or the leak persists longer than six weeks, surgical intervention should be strongly considered because of the increased risk of meningitis.[1,15]

Certain populations of patients should be considered for immediate cranial exploration and repair; these include patients with open dural wounds, closed head injuries with intracranial complications such as hemorrhage, or the presence of pneumocephalus, implying a more extensive dural tear. There is an increased predisposition to meningitis and frequent failure to close spontaneously in these patients.[23] Spontaneous repair of CSF fistula complicating mid-facial trauma is unlikely to occur when there is gross damage to the anterior cranial fossa, significant associated frontal bone fracture, or aerocele.[2]

Fat, muscle, and fascia are the preferred tissues that should be used for repair. It is better to use natural tissue than prosthetic or foreign material because of the higher risk of infection with the latter.[35] The second cardinal principle of reconstructive surgery refers to the manner of using tissue transfer to span gaps. Flaps are always superior to a graft.[46]

Approaches

Surgical management of CSF rhinorrhea can be undertaken through either an intracranial or an extracranial approach. The intracranial approach has the advantages of having direct visualization of the dural tear and adjacent cortex, and theoretically a better opportunity to tamponade a leak in the face of increased intracranial pressure. The disadvantage is probable prolonged operative time with associated increased morbidity. Although extracranial approaches generally have less morbidity, the cortex cannot be examined for coexistent cerebral damage in severe head trauma.[23]

Besides less morbidity extracranial approaches provide superior exposure of sphenoid, parasellar and posterior ethmoid areas. Also, good visualization of leaks in the posterior wall of the frontal sinuses, cribriform plate, and fovea ethmoidalis regions is a major advantage. For CSF rhinorrhea, extracranial rhinological repair is the most appropriate surgical approach, assuming that any intracranial hypertension has first been reversed,[23] and that other indications for an intracranial approach are absent.[2] The patient should always be forewarned that the risk of relapse may approach 20% even in the most experienced hands.[35]

Anterior Fossa

Anterior fossa leaks can be difficult to repair adequately because of the many possible leakage sites through the sinuses. The extracranial approach is favored when the leakage site can be properly visualized and reached.[35]

If the fistula cannot be readily visualized and approached extracranially, then an intracranial approach should be considered.[35] However, extracranial approaches are much less hazardous. The most commonly used intracranial technique for mid-face fracture tears is via a frontal craniotomy with an intradural approach and placement of the graft to cover the defect.[2]

Frontal Sinus

An extracranial approach is preferred for frontal sinus repairs. The incision should be made through the brow or bicoronal with care so as not to preclude an intracranial approach.[35] Both frontal sinuses are exposed by reflecting the osteoplastic flap anteriorly and inferiorly. The mucous membranes of both sinuses and the interfrontal septum are removed, and defects in the posterior wall of the frontal sinus can be identified. If the dural defect cannot be sutured, repair can be done with either the temporalis or frontalis muscle fascia or frontal pericranium. The tissue is then tucked between the posterior wall of the frontal sinus and dura around the periphery of the bony defect. Before obliterating the sinus defect with adipose tissue, the entire cortical lining of the frontal sinus must be removed with a rotating cutting burr. This procedure ensures complete removal of the mucosal lining of the sinus and adequate blood supply for the adipose implant. Subcutaneous adipose tissue obtained from the abdominal wall is trimmed and implanted so as to fill completely the frontal sinus complex. If the adipose tissue is obtained atraumatically and immediately prior to its implantation, revascularization of adipose tissue from ingrowth of blood vessels from the bone will take place during the first few days following implantation. The osteoplastic flap is replaced in its anatomic position and sutured with multiple periosteal sutures.[11,15]

Ethmoid Sinus

Leaks through the ethmoidal sinus may be approached transnasally through the lateral rhinotomy exposure or through an external Chiari incision. When a leak is found in the ethmoidal region, an ethmoidectomy is usually performed.[22] The gap from the transnasal or external ethmoidectomy is patched by either free fascia and muscle graft or by a septal or turbinate mucosal flap.[15] The tissue is then maintained in position by medicated-gauze nasal packing for at least seven days.[15] If the leak is in the posterior ethmoid/sphenoid region, there tends to be a higher recurrence rate with repairs by an extracranial approach.[3]

Cribriform-Plate Area

The cribriform-plate region or roof of the ethmoid is the site most commonly involved in CSF leaks. To repair a defect in this area, an external ethmoidectomy is done and the middle turbinate removed. The dural defect is exposed, and then the septal mucosal nasal septal flap is rotated approximately 90 degrees to cover the leakage points and adjacent dura of the olfactory bulb and roof of the ethmoid regions.[15]

Middle Cranial Fossa

Middle fossa leaks generally take place through the temporal bone. Leakage may be classified as closed or open. In the closed leak, the eardrum is intact and CSF flows through the middle ear and out the eustachian tube. In the open leak, either the tympanic membrane may be perforated or the external canal lacerated.[35] Immediate surgery is needed if there is evidence of otitis.[15]

It is essential to support the middle fossa floor because if a dural tear is present, there is the hazard of potential cerebral herniation.

Sphenoid Sinus

A transseptal sphenoidotomy can be accomplished through a sublabial approach. If the ethmoid sinus is involved, an external or transnasal ethmoidectomy route can also be used. The anterior sphenoid sinus wall is opened and the mucosal lining completely stripped. It is generally necessary to remove the intersphenoid septum and a small portion of the posterior wall of the nasal septum in order to expose the sphenoid sinus complex adequately. The fascial graft is placed as an external patch and can be made relatively watertight by tissue adhesive. The sinus cavity is packed with a free muscle graft and the nasal cavities with a medicated-ointment-impregnated gauze for seven days.[15]

Otic Region

A CSF leak of otic origin following accidental or surgical trauma can almost always be prevented by obliterating the mastoid translabyrinth route to the internal auditory canal and cerebellopontine angle with adipose tissue. The first piece of subcutaneous adipose tissue is placed in the labyrinthine defect to seal the communication between the mastoid and cerebellopontine angle. The second piece is placed in the mastoid antrum and the remainder of the mastoidectomy defect is closed by a third piece of adipose tissue. The wound is closed without drainage and the sutures remain in place for two weeks.[11]

If otorrhea is found to emanate from the mastoid area, there are several surgical methods that can be used for correction. The defect can be repaired intracranially or extracranially. If an extracranial approach is chosen, either a mastoidectomy can be done with an obliteration procedure or tissue can be placed over the defect. If the cellular development of the mastoid cavity is not extensive, an inferiorly based pedicle-tissue flap can be placed over the leak. Otherwise, the mastoid area can be packed with abdominal fat, and fascia from the temporalis muscle can be used as a graft by laying the fascia on top of the tegmen and under the dural defect for support.[19]

Posterior Fossa

CSF leaks through the posterior fossa generally are a result of surgery, particularly the removal of acoustic neuromas, and may present in the oropharynx following trauma. Posterior fossa leaks can be corrected through a suboccipital approach, laying fascia over the defects and plugging small crevices, or through a translabyrinthine approach using fat.[35] Craniotomies and mastoidectomies are less effective for controlling rhinorrhea originating from fistulas in the middle and posterior fossas.[42]

Complications of Surgical Repair of CSF Fistulas

Reoccurrence rates of up to 20% are common after extracranial repair.[3] One of the highest reported rates of recurrence was in patients who had a transethmoid repair using fascia lata and hammered muscle, particularly in the posterior ethmoid sphenoid area.[3]

Intracranial approaches to anterior fossa leaks may require sacrifice of cranial nerves (especially olfaction).[15] Also patients with midfacial fractures and subsequent intracranial dural repair have had many unfortunate sequelae described: in 31 patients with LeFort I, II, or III fracture, anosmia occurred in 19 of 31 (61%); two of 31 (7%) sustained frontal paresthesia and one (3%) had significant memory loss postoperatively.[2]

Role of Surgery

Surgery is indicated in the following instances.

1. If leakage is profuse and not decreasing after two weeks or has not ceased after six weeks following trauma;
2. In recurrent CSF leaks;
3. If pneumocephalus or a large leak is demonstrated.
4. If meningitis developed with a demonstrable CSF leak.
5. If CSF leak is associated with ear infections.

Summary

Posttraumatic meningitis may complicate CSF leakage into pneumatized bones of the base of the skull following (1) mid-face trauma, (2) basilar skull fracture, and (3) certain surgical procedures, especially extracranial approaches to the pituitary and posterior fossa lesions. Disruption of bone and attached dura brings arachnoid membrane into direct contact with either mucosa-lined air sinuses (frontal, ethmoid, sphenoid), middle ear, or mastoid.

CSF leakage is suggested by clear or blood-stained fluid exiting from the nose (rhinorrhea) or external auditory canal (otorrhea). Delay in onset of recognizable leakage is common and may be due to temporary blockage of the fistula by early tissue edema or herniated brain, or time required to erode arachnoid membrane. Clinical findings suggestive of CSF leak also include hemotympanum and ecchymoses over the mastoid (Battle's sign) and periorbitally (raccoon sign). Pneumocephalus on x-ray is diagnostic but infrequent.

Self-sealing of CSF fistula is a common feature of basilar fractures but somewhat less frequent with mid-face fractures, even after appropriate immobilization. Postoperative leaks represent a failure of the initial repair of the surgical defect required for the procedure and rarely close spontaneously.

The preoperative location of CSF fistula is most efficiently identified by high-resolution CT metrizamide cisternography. Intraoperative use of fluorescein dye appropriately diluted in CSF and hydrostatic control of CSF pressure help identify the leak in extracranial approaches.

The role of antibiotics in preventing meningitis in the presence of suspected or documented CSF leak remains controversial. Most patients with mid-face injuries receive antibiotics for other reasons, and it is common practice to give antibiotics to patients with basilar skull fractures. However, the few studies of prophylaxis do not support their efficacy and suggest that selection of resistant organisms may promote Gram-negative rod meningitis instead of infection with common respiratory flora *(S pneumoniae, H influenza, N meningitidis).*

Indications for repair of acute CSF leaks include: pneumocephalus, large leaks, leaks through infected bone, postoperative leaks and meningitis. Otherwise, leaks should be given adequate time to resolve spontaneously before considering repair.

Extracranial approaches to repair of anterior, middle, and posterior fossa leaks are safer and more effective than intracranial approaches. Postoperative recurrence remains a problem in up to 20% of cases complicating accidental trauma, even when concomitant intracranial hypertension and hydrocephalus have been ruled out.

References

1. Ommaya AK: Spinal fluid fistulae. *Clin Neurosurg* 1979;23:363–392.
2. O'Brien MD, Reade PC: The management of dural tear resulting from mid-facial fracture. *Head Neck Surg* 1984;6:810–818.
3. Westmore GA, Whittam DE: Cerebrospinal fluid rhinorrhoea and its management. *Br J Surg* 1982; 69:489–492.
4. Lewin W: Cerebrospinal fluid rhinorrhoea in closed head injuries. *Br J Surg* 1954;17:1–18.
5. Einhorn A, Mizrahi EM: Basilar skull fractures in children. *Am J Dis Child* 1978;132:1121–1124.
6. Zrebeet HA, Huang PS: Prophylactic antibiotics in the treatment of fractures at the base of the skull. *Del Med J* 1986;58:741–748.
7. Romanowski B, Tyrrell DL, Weir BKA, Goldsand G: Meningitis complicating transsphenoidal hypophysectomy. *Can Med Assoc J* 1981; 124:1172–1175.
8. Gransden WR, Wickstead M, Eykyn SJ: Meningitis after transsphenoidal excision of pituitary tumours. *J Laryngol Otol* 1988;102:33–36.
9. Henry RC, Taylor PH: Cerebrospinal fluid otorrhoea and otorhinorrheoea following closed head injury. *J Laryngol Otol* 1978;92:743–756.
10. Gunderson T, Haye R: Cerebrospinal otorrhea. *Arch Otolaryngol* 1970;91:19–23.
11. Montgomery WW: Common complications following removal of vestibular schwannoma. *Adv Otorhinolaryngol* 1983;31:228–239.
12. Lewin W: Cerebrospinal fluid rhinorrhea in nonmissile head injuries. *Clin Neurosurg* 1964;12:237–252.
13. Frazee RC, Mucha P, Farnell MB, Ebersold MJ: Meningitis after basilar skull fracture. *Postgrad Med* 1988;83:267–274.
14. Dagi RD, Meyer RB, Poletti CA: The incidence and prevention of meningitis after basilar skull fracture. *Am J Emerg Med* 1983;3:295–298.
15. Hyslop, NE Jr, Montgomery WW: Diagnosis and management of meningitis associated with cerebrospinal fluid leaks. In: Remington JM, Swartz MN, eds. *Current Concepts in Infectious Diseases*. Vol 3. Philadelphia: McGraw-Hill, 1982:254–285.
16. Afran SI, Budenz DL, Albert DN: Does enucleation in the presence of endophthalmitis increase the risk of post-operative meningitis? *J Opthalmol* 1987;94: 235–237.
17. Marshall DR, Slattery PG: Intracranial complications of rhinoplasty. *Br J Plast Surg* 1983;36:342–344.
18. Haddad FS, Hybballa J, Zaytoun G, Haddad GF: Intracranial complications of submucous resection of the nasal septum. *Am J Otolaryngol* 1985;6:443–447.
19. Moore GF, Nisson AJ, Yonkers AJ: Potential complication of unrecognized cerebrospinal fluid leaks secondary to mastoid surgery. *Am J Otol* 1984;5:317–323.
20. Allam AF: Pneumatization of the temporal bone. *Ann Otol* 1969;78:49–64.
21. Gordon DS, Kerr AG: Cerebrospinal fluid rhinorrhea following surgery for acoustic neurinoma. *J Neurosurg* 1986;64:676–678.
22. Briant TDR, Snell D: Diagnosis of cerebro-spinal rhinorrhea and the rhinologic approach to its repair. *Laryngoscope* 1967;77:1390–1409.
23. Park JI, Strelzow VV, Friedman WH. Current management of cerebrospinal fluid rhinorrhea. *Laryngoscope* 1983;93:1294–1300.
24. Hand WL, Sanford JP: Posttraumatic bacterial meningitis. *Ann Intern Med* 1970;72:869–874.
25. Ignelzi RJ, VanderArk GD: Analysis of the treatment of basilar skull fractures with and without antibiotics. *J Neurosurg* 1975;43:721–726.
26. Roberts SR, Esther JW, Brewer JH: Posttraumatic Pasteurella multocida meningitis. *South Med J* 1988; 81:675–676.
27. Michowiz SD, Wald U, Shapiro M: Brucella melitensis meningits following head trauma. *Southern Med J* 1988;8:675–676.
28. Fitzgerald DC: Use of prophylactic antibiotics in otologic and neuro-otologic surgery. *Am J Otol* 1985;6:121–125.
29. Voth D: Perioperative prevention of infection in neurosurgery. *Antibiot Chemother* 1985;33:165–183.
30. Kartush JM, Cannon SC, Bojrab DI, et al: Use of bacitracin for neurotologic surgery. *Laryngoscope* 1988;98:1050–1054.
31. Teng P, Cohen I, Meleney FL: Bacitracin in neurosurgical infections. *Surg Gynecol Obstet* 1951;92:53–63.
32. Shapiro M, Wald U, Simchen E, et al: Randomized clinical trial of intra-operative antimicrobial prophylaxis of infection after neurosurgical procedures. *J Hosp Infect* 1986;8:283–295.
33. Sprunt K, Redman W: Evidence suggesting importance of role of interbacterial inhibition in maintaining balance of normal flora. *Ann Intern Med* 1968;68:579–590.

34. Gilbert VE, Beals JD, Natelson SE, Tyler WA: Treatment of cerebrospinal fluid leaks and gram-negative bacillary meningitis with large doses of intrathecal amikacin and systemic antibiotics. *Neurosurgery* 1986;18:402–406.
35. Myers DL, Sataloff RT: Spinal fluid leakage after skull base surgical procedures. *Otolaryngol Clin North Am* 1984;17:601–611.
36. Meurman OH, Irjala K, Suonpaa J, Laurent B: A new method for the identification of cerebrospinal fluid leakage. *Acta Otolaryngol* 1979;87:366–369.
37. Schuknecht HF, Zaytoun GM, Moon CN: Adult-onset fluid in the tympanomastoid compartment. *Arch Otolaryngol* 1982;108:759–765.
38. Lant EJ, Forbes GS, Brown ML, Laws ER: Radiology of cerebrospinal fluid rhinorrhea. *Am J Roentgenol* 1980;135:1023–1030.
39. Mamo L, Cophignon J, Rey A, Thurel C: A new radionuclide method for the diagnosis of posttraumatic cerebrospinal fistulas. *J Neurosurg* 1982;57:92–98.
40. Drayer BP, Wilkins RH, Boehnke M, et al: Cerebrospinal fluid rhinorrhea demonstrated by metrizmide CT cisternography. *Am J Roentgenol* 1977; 129:149–151.
41. Prere J, Puech JL, Deroover N, et al: Rhinorrhea and meningitis due to post-traumatic osteo-meningeal defects in the anterior cranial fossa. *J Neuroradiol* 1986;13:278–285.
42. Spetzler RF, Wilson CB: Management of recurrent CSF rhinorrhea of the middle and posterior fossa. *J Neurosurg* 1978;49:393–397.
43. Swanson SE, Kocan M, Chandler WF: Flow-regulated continuous spinal drainage: technical note with case report. *Neurosurgery* 1981;9:163–165.
44. Lau YL, Kenna AP: Post-traumatic meningitis in children. Injury. *Br J Acc Surg* 1986;17:407–409.
45. Ahmadi J, Weiss MH, Segall HD, et al: Evaluation of cerebrospinal fluid rhinorrhea by metrizamide computed tomographic cisternography. *Neurosurgery* 1985;16:54–59.
46. McCabe BF: The osteo-mucoperiosteal flap in repair of cerebrospinal fluid rhinorrhea. *Laryngoscope* 1976;86:537–539.

6

Infections of Central-Nervous-System Shunts

JANARA J. YOUNGER AND FRED F. BARRETT

Hydrocephalus has been recognized throughout the ages as a condition in which excess fluid accumulates within the cranium. Hippocrates is credited with the first efforts to drain the dilated ventricles.[1] During the 1700–1800s, treatment of hydrocephalus was limited to bleeding, purges, and diuretics. Head wrapping, radiation therapy, and thyroid extract were also transiently believed to be efficacious. Some of the earliest surgical efforts at control of this condition involved removal of the choroid plexus, tying the common carotid arteries, and intermittent puncture of the lateral ventricles.[1,2]

The first successful internal cerebrospinal-fluid (CSF) diversion system was placed by Miculicz in 1893. Subsequently, gold, silver, glass, platinum, and rubber tubes were used with variable success to divert CSF from the ventricles to the subdural and subarachnoid spaces. The first operations to channel CSF into more distand body cavities took place in the early 1900s.[1,2] Since then, many different materials and surgical techniques have been tried to shunt CSF into other speaces such as the pleural space, ureters, fallopian tubes, gallbladder, cisterna magna, right atrium and peritoneum. Ventriculoperitoneal (V-P) and ventriculoatrial (V-A) shunts have been the most successful. Long-term survival and improved quality of life in hydrocephalic patients have resulted from these shunting techniques. Unfortunately, excessive complication rates remain a problem. The most frequent and serious complications are shunt malfunction and shunt infection.

Shunt infection occurs at a rate of 10–15%. Infection is associated with significant morbidity and mortality and has been shown to be directly associated with reduced intelligence in hydrocephalic children.[3,4] There is an extensive literature dealing with shunt infection. In this chapter, we will attempt to summarize the current knowledge on this subject.

Incidence

Reported rates of infection following CSF-shunt procedures vary from 1.5% to 30%.[5–13] Rates from different institutions are difficult to evaluate because of varying methods of calculation. In order to compare shunt-infection rates, the following variables must be known: (1) definition of shunt infection; (2) type of infections included in the numerator, that is, wound infection, ventriculitis, positive shunt-tubing cultures, hematogenously spread meningitis, and so on; (3) duration of postoperative follow-up; and (4) patient population and/or neurosurgical procedures included in the denominator.

Including only shunt infections occurring within six weeks of surgery can reduce the infection rate by 30% or more.[10] Similarly, including in the denominator shunt revisions, as well as new shunt procedures, significantly changes the infection rate. Thus, operation-related CSF-shunt-infection rates need to be accompanied by completed numerator and denominator definitions to allow valid interpretation.

Factors Associated with Shunt Infections

Host Factors

Patient-related factors found to correlate with the incidence of postoperative shunt infections include age, abnormal skin conditions, peripheral sites of infection, and presence of meningomyelocele.[5–7,11–16] The influence of meningomyelocele is controversial, and many authors maintain that there is no correlation between the etiology of hydrocephalus and the risk of infection.

Although most studies report an increased incidence of infection in young infants, the age at which this risk is reported to decline varies from one week to three years. Ammirati and Raimondi[13] reported an infection rate of 48% for infants with meningomyelocele operated on prior to one week of age versus a rate of 24% after one week of age, and a further decline in infection rate after two months of age was observed. Renier and colleagues[14] noted shunt infection to occur 2.6 times more frequently during the first six months of life than after one year of age. Nelson[11] reported an incidence of 13% in patients younger than one year and 8% for older children.

Dermatitis, decubiti, and other skin conditions were reported by both Renier and colleagues[14] and Spanu and colleagues[15] to increase the infection rate from to 3% to 15%. These same authors reported significant increases in infection rates in patients with preceding infection of the urinary tract, ears, chest, or other sites, even if appropriately treated prior to surgery.

Patient factors that have *not* been associated with an increased risk for shunt infection include sex, degree of hydrocephalus, number of preceding neurosurgical procedures, and CSF glucose level and leukocyte count.

Neurosurgical Technique

There are conflicting data regarding the influence of the neurosurgeon's expertise on shunt-infection rates. In one recent study, no correlation between the infection rate and the neurosurgeon was identified,[14] but most authors feel that the surgeon is one of the most significant factors and quote surgeon-specific rates ranging from 1.8% to 50%.[10–12,16] Yogev[12] described an increased rate of shunt infection at his institution yearly between July and September, which correlated with the arrival of new neurosurgery residents.

Forrest and co-workers[17] found that prolonged operating time is associated with higher infection rates. Techniques aimed at reducing airborne intraoperative transmissions of bacteria, such as reducing operating-room traffic and using a surgical isolator, have been reported to reduce infection rates.[18]

Shunt Factors

There are no firm data indicating that either the V-A or V-P shunt is more prone to postoperative infection. The consequences of infection in a V-A shunt, however, are more serious since the patients is bacteremic and frequently develops immune-complex-mediated disease.

Significant differences in the rate of infection have been described depending on whether the surgery was for primary placement of a shunt or for shunt revision.[7,11] In addition, ventricular catheter revisions are associated with a higher incidence of infection than distal revisions (7.7% versus 2.6%), as reported by Renier. Renier[14] also reported an infection rate of 8.4% after primary insertions.

In general, there as been no correlation of value or shunt types with infection, but Raimondi and colleagues[2] reported a decrease in infection rate from 17% to 7% with the use of a simpler one-piece shunt.

Pathogenesis

Operative Causes

Most operatively related shunt infections are due to microorganisms that are introduced at the time of surgery. This hypothesis is supported by the perioperative clustering of infections and the predominance of etiologic agents that are components of the normal skin flora. Bayston and Lari[19] were able to show that, in most cases, the organism found in the colonized shunt originated from the patient's skin flora. Most shunt infections are caused by skin commensals, organisms generally associated with low virulence. The presence of the foreign body, in this case the CSF shunt, enables these organisms to become pathogenic. Bayston and Penny[20] reported that coagulase-negative staphylococci isolated from CSF shunts produced a viscous, extracellular "mucoid" material that bound the organism to the surface of the shunt. This mucoid material is now referred to as "slime" and appears to be a virulence factor for the organism in the setting of foreign-body infections.[21–26] Coagulase-negative staphylococci isolated from infected prosthetic devices are significantly more likely to produce slime than isolates considered to be contaminants.[25,26] Additionally, infections caused by slime-producing strains of coagulase-negative staphylococci are more difficult to eradicate with antibiotics alone and frequently require removal of the prosthetic device.[22,25,26] In vitro data suggest that slime also interferes with the function of lymphocytes and neutrophils.[27]

In addition to the organism-protective factor of slime, shunt materials themselves may predispose to infection by interfering with host defenses. Borges[28] has shown in vitro that neutrophils and monocytes have difficulty adhering to shunt catheters and valves. Bacteria on the surface of inoculated catheters were not phagocytized after several hours of incubation with white-cell suspensions. Borges also noted that neutrophils released myeloperoxidase, a major component of the intracellular killing system, into the extracellular environment when in contact with shunt tubing or value material, thus further diminishing the cell's bactericidal capacity.

Nonoperative Factors

Nonoperative events by which shunt infection can develop include hematogenous dissemination and retrograde contamination. Central-nervous-system (CNS) infection attributable to the usual meningitis pathogens (*Hemophilus influenzae, Streptococcus pneumoniae,* and *Neisseria meningitidis*) is acquired via the hematogenous route, and occurs in children with CSF shunts at the same or greater rate than in normal children.[5,29] These infections are usually cured without shunt removal, using standard antimicrobial therapy for meningitis.[5,12,29]

Gram-negative enteric CSF-shunt infection occurring remotely from the time of surgery is hypothesized to arise via perforation of the bowel wall by the shunt tubing and subsequently ascending infection.[30] This complication was relatively common when the ureter was used as the site of placement for the distal catheter as a result of the reflux of urinary-tract pathogens into the system.

Etiologic Agents

Coagulase-negative staphylococci account for more than 50% of all CSF-shunt infections. *Staphylococcus aureus* is the second most common pathogen involved, and these two organisms together are causative in 75% of cases.[5–12,31–35]

Enter gram-negative organisms are isolated in 5–20% of shunt infections and when acute are somewhat more commonly seen in infants.[5,7,12,30,32] Infections with these organisms may develop remotely from surgery and are often associated with such abdominal complications as bowel perforation by the shunt and peritonitis.

Other organisms occasionally isolated from CSF shunts include *Pseudomonas* sps, *Streptococcus* sps (including group D enterococcus, nonenterococcal group D streptococci, *Streptococcus viridans,* and *Streptococcus pyogenes), Propionibacterium acnes,* other diphtheroides, and *Candidae*.[5,6,15,16,31,32,34,35]

Shunt infection can be caused by *H influenzae, S pneumoniae, N meningitidis,* and *Listeria monocytogenes* in the setting of bacteremia.[5,29,30]

Clinical Features

Except for cases in which there is associated cellulitis or wound infection, there are usually no clinical features that are diagnostic of shunt infection. Fever is the most common symptom and is present in 42–100% of cases.[5,9,32] Irritability and changes in sensorium are also frequently seen with shunt malfunction found in 20–80% of cases.[7,32] Twenty percent of cases with V-P shunt infection will have evidence of peritoneal irritation with abdominal pain, vomiting, or diarrhea.[7] Only one third of patients will manifest meningeal symptoms.[5]

The majority of shunt infections are diagnosed within the first two months after surgery; however, in 25% of cases, the presentation is delayed for months or, rarely, years after surgery.[5,6,7,9,10,16] These late infections invariably are due to coagulase-negative staphylococci or other organisms of low pathogenic potential, such as diphtheroides, which can cause indolent shunt colonization without clinical symptoms. These patients frequently present with shunt malfunction and the diagnosis is established unexpectedly when cultures of the removed shunt or CSF samples are positive.[32]

An unusual presentation of shunt infection that needs to be kept in mind is distal V-P shunt infection that presents with acute or recurrent/chronic abdominal pain.[37–41] These patients do not have CNS symptomatology or shunt malfunction, and cultures of the ventricular CSF are frequently sterile. Diagnosis is established by exteriorizing the peritoneal end of the V-P shunt and obtaining Gram strains and cultures of distal CSF and shunt tubing. This procedure not only is diagnostic, but also results in rapid improvement of symptoms. Patients have undergone unnecessary abdominal explorations because of the failure to consider the diagnosis of distal-shunt infection. Laparotomy should be reserved for patients with negative distal CSF studies whose abdominal symptoms do not improve within a few hours after shunt exteriorization.

Laboratory Diagnosis

The laboratory findings very depending on whether the patient has a V-A or V-P shunt. With infected V-A shunts, bacteremia is the rule, and thus blood cultures are usually diagnostic. These patients may have other laboratory abnormalities if the infection is chronic, such as anemia, thrombocytopenia, sterile pyuria, hematuria, and abnormal renal function secondary to immune-complex-mediated glomerulonephritis.[5] Bacteremia is rarely seen with V-P shunt infection unless would infection or severe peritonitis is present. The peripheral white-blood-cell count is too variable to be helpful. Twenty-five percent of patients with active infection have white counts of less than 10,000 and only one third of patients manifest leukocytosis of 20,000 or greater.[5]

Diagnosis of shunt infection depends almost entirely on obtaining CSF samples from the shunt reservoir for Gram-stained smears and cultures. Cultures of CSF obtained via lumbar puncture are not reliable.[34] The diagnosis is confirmed when two or more individual cultures of the shunt-reservoir fluid or shunt hardware yield the same bacterial species, or if the Gram stain of CSF reveals an organism that is morphologically compatible with the bacterium isolated via culture. Surgical-wound infections with erythema along the shunt tract or wound dehiscence can be bacteriologically diagnosed by needle aspiration and wound cultures. In these cases, CSF from the shunt reservoir still needs to be obtained in order to establish the presence or absence of ventriculitis.

Most of the pathogens infecting CNS shunts are readily cultured by routine laboratory techniques. The exceptions are anaerobic organisms such as *P acnes* and diphtheroides.[36] These bacteria may require seven to ten days to grow, and repeated CSF sampling is occasionally necessary. The microbiology laboratory should hold CSF obtained from shunts and shunt-tubing cultures a minimum of ten days before reporting them as negative.

CSF parameters such as leukocytosis and levels of glucose and protein vary widely in shunt infections.[34] In general, the CSF inflammatory response is mild with a median leukocyte count of 156 cells per cubic millimeter (range 0–2,623 cells per cubic millimeter), median glucose concentration of 25 mg/dl (range 4–42 mg/dl), and median protein concentration of 136 mg/dl (range 40–1,375 mg/dl).[7] In comparison, children with shunt malfunction, but without infection, have median CSF leukocyte counts of 18 cells per cubic millimeter and average CSF glucose and protein concentrations of 42 mg/dl and 40 mg/dl respectively.[7]

There is often considerable reluctance to "invade" the shunt for the purpose of obtaining CSF for culture and Gram stains in patients who do not present with strong clinical evidence of shunt infection. This argument is not supported by data. Noetzel and Baker[42] have reported an 18-month follow-up of 91 patients who had undergone 209 diagnostic "shunt taps," in whom no complications—mechanical or infectious—were noted either acutely or long term. Since CSF-shunt cultures often become negative within 24–48 hourts of beginning antibiotics, CSF should be obtained for culture before initiating antimicrobial therapy in any shunted patient in whom another definate focus of infection is not identified.

Treatment

When acute wound infection or cellulitis is present, all investigators agree that shunt removal combined with antimicrobial therapy is the only curative approach.[7,12] There is, however, no agreement on the optimum therapy of the more common presentation of infected shunts. In general, there are three different approaches to the problem, and each has its advocates.

1. Administration of prolonged systemic antibiotic therapy, usually in conjunction with intraventricular antibiotics via the shunt reservoir, without any surgical intervention.
2. Complete removal of the shunt, with either immediate or delayed replacement in the same or new location, combined with systemic and occasionally intraventricular antibiotics.
3. Establishment of external ventricular drainage, usually by exteriorizing the distal shunt, with administration of systemic and intraventricular antibiotics, followed by either complete or partial shunt replacement.

The appeal of the antibiotics-only approach is that patients are spared the risks and trauma of surgery. This approach can only be attempted in patients with well-functioning shunts. Overall, the success rates reported with this therapy are dismal, particularly if intraventricular antibiotics are not used. Reported cure rates vary from 9% to 16%.[31–33] The addition of intraventricular antibiotics improves the outlook somewhat, with published cure rates of 9–80%.[31,43–46]

Although occasional cures do occur without surgical intervention, the mortality rates with this form of shunt-infection treatment are 10–36%, and most patients relapse and ultimately require some surgical manipulation of the shunt.[31–33,43–46]

There are many variations of the second type of treatment. Removal of the shunt with immediate replacement in the same location without antibiotics is associated with persistent infection in 20% and so is seldom used.[17] In patients without overt ventriculitis, Forrest and co-workers[17] reported no relapses in 12 patients treated by having the shunt removed and immediately replaced in a new site without the use of antibiotics. Cure rates in excess of 90% are found in almost all reported series using any of the following combinations: (1) antibiotics initially with a delayed single surgical removal and replacement of the entire shunt; (2) immediate removal of the shunt, followed by a period of antibiotics prior to replacement of the shunt; (3) immediate removal and replacement of the shunt followed by two weeks of intraventricular and systemic antibiotics.[5,7,12,34,35,45]

The third therapeutic approach includes antibiotics and external ventricular drainage (EVD) for a variable period of time followed by complete or partial shunt replacement. There are several ways in which EVD can be established, the least invasive of which is to externalize the distal shunt at the neck or upper chest and connect it to a closed drainage system. This form of exteriorization can usually be accomplished using local anesthesia. Another method is to remove the existing shunt completely and place an EVD device either in the old shunt tract or via a new burr hole. EVD allows uninterrupted CSF drainage and an access through which antibiotics can be administered intraventricularly and CSF samples obtained for culture and antibiotic levels. The patient is treated with systemic plus intraventricular antibiotics followed by either complete shunt replacement or replacement of the distal components. The main disadvantages of this therapy are the possibility of secondary infection and the loss of fluid and electrolytes (which occasionally can be excessive). Cure rates are approximately 90% and are comparable to those achieved with any form of therapy that includes shunt removal.[7,12,47,48]

Antibiotic Therapy

The choice of antimicrobial agents is guided by knowledge of the causative organism, its susceptibility pattern, CSF penetration of the antibiotic, and potential antimicrobial toxicities. Because of the low CSF levels achieved with most antibiotics in the absence of meningeal inflammation, intraventricular antibiotics are commonly used in conjunction with either orally or parenterally administered systemic antibiotics in the therapy of CSF shunt infections.

Staphylococcal Infection

Shunt infection by *S aureus* in which the organism is methicillin sensitive is usually managed by a combination of parenteral nafcillin at a dose of 12 g/day or 200 mg/kg/day and intraventricular vancomycin.[12,46] Intraventricular methicillin, nafcillin, and cephalothin have also been used successfully by some investigators.[31,45,56]

Coagulase-negative staphylococci are usually resistant to the antistaphylococcal penicillins and cephalosporins. They are best treated with vancomycin, both parenterally at 2 g/day or 40 mg/kg/day and intraventricularly.[49,50,51] Because of the variable metabolism in children, vancomycin levels should be monitored. Rifampin is often added as adjunctive therapy.[44,49,52]

Vancomycin penetrates the blood–brain barrier poorly in the absence of inflamed meninges. Odio and colleagues[53] found CSF levels of only 0.2–1.0 μg/ml in pediatric patients who received two 15-mg/kg doses of vancomycin intravenously for shunt-surgery prophylaxis. Since most coagulase-negative staphylococci have minimum inhibitory concentrations (MICs) to vancomycin of 1–2 μg/ml, these levels would be unlikely to achieve sterilization of a foreign body. Accordingly, many centers are now using daily intraventricular injections of vancomycin to achieve CSF bactericidal activity.[26,47,50] Doses of 2–25 mg per day have been utilized. McLaurin and Frame [47] recommend that the dose be adjusted to achieve CSF trough levels of 20 φg/ml, which is 10 to 20 times the MIC of most coagulase-negative staphylococci. No adverse effects have been reported with the use of intraventricular vancomycin.

Rifampin is very active against staphylococci, however, it cannot be used alone owing to the rapid development of resistance. It has been used successfully in combination with vancomycin, nafcillin, and trimethoprim/sulfamethoxazole in the treatment of shunt infection, even where shunt removal followed by appropriate antibiotics had failed.[44,47,49] Rifampin crosses the blood–brain barrier well, achieving CSF concentrations of 0.5–4 μg/ml, which exceeds the MIC for staphylococci by 1,000-fold.[52]

Frame and McLaurin[44] are now recommending intraventricular vancomycin plus a combination of oral rifampin and trimethoprim/sulfamethoxazole in cases of staphylococcal shunt infection. Both components of the trimethoprim/sulfamethoxazole combination penetrate the CSF well. Use of these antibiotics avoids intravenous therapy with its possible complications. The dosage of trimethoprim/sulfamethoxazole used in their regimen is 10–20 mg/kg/day of the trimethoprim component and 50–100 mg/kg/day of sulfamethoxazole. The dosage is adjusted to achieve serum sulfamethoxazole levels of 75–150 μg/ml. Rifampin is given in daily doses of 15–20 mg/kg/day.

Infections Caused by Other Organisms

Most nonstaphylococcal gram-positive infections, as well as anaerobic infections such as *P acnes* and diphtheroides, can be effectively treated with a combination of intraventricular vancomycin and parenteral penicillin or ampicillin. Shunt infections caused by *Pseudomonas* or enteric gram-negative organisms have been treated with a variety of antimicrobial agents. The advent of third-generation cephalosporins with their ability to achieve excellent CSF levels may allow some of these infections to be treated with parenteral therapy alone. In the past, such infections were treated with parenteral ampicillin, aminoglycosides or chloramphenicol, and intraventricular gentamicin at doses of 1–4 mg per day.[7,30,54] However, intraventricular gentamicin may cause toxicity.[8,54,55] An autopsied patient who had received intraventricular gentamicin for *Pseudomonas aeruginosa* meningitis had neuropathic changes similar to those seen in animals given large doses of the agent experimentally.[34] Other studies have reported no side effects from this treatment. The mortality rate in one published series of gram-negative CSF-shunt infections using earlier therapies was 35%, with significant morbidity in the survivors.[30] No deaths occurred in two small referenced series of patients treated with ceftriaxone alone for gram-negative shunt infections; however, some of these patients were infected with *H influenzae*, and this organism is more readily eradicated than are the enteric gram-negative pathogens.[34,56]

Treatment of Hematogenously Acquired Shunt Infection

Therapy of shunt infections with *H influenzae, N meningitidis*, and *S pneumoniae* can be successfully accomplished using the standard treatment for meningitis attributable to these pathogens. In general, neither shunt removal nor intraventricular antibiotics is required.[5,29,34] Parenteral therapy with a third-generation cephalosporin such as cefotaxime or ceftriaxone and therapy with a combination of ampicillin and chloramphenicol are equally effective in treating *H influenzae* infections. High-dose penicillin is used for infections with *N meningitidis* and *S pneumoniae*.

Prophylactic Antibiotics

The efficacy of prophylactic antibiotics given at the time of shunt surgery in reducing the infection rate remains extremely controversial. Ideally, a blinded, randomized controlled trial needs to be performed; however, as discussed by Odio and colleagues[53] and by Walters and co-workers,[57] large numbers of patients (692–1,100) would be required to achieve a significance level of 0.05. The published randomized controlled trials all suffer the bias induced by small sample size. Odio and colleagues[53] found no difference in the infection rates with two perioperative doses of intravenous vancomycin (four of 17 control patients infected compared with three of 18 prophylaxed patients). This particular study was discontinued because of multiple adverse reactions to the vancomycin. Wang and colleagues[58] found a similar incidence of shunt infection in patients who were given three doses of intravenous trimethoprim/sulfamethoxazole (four of 55) and in a control group (five of 65). In a double-blind, randomized trial, Haines and Taylor[59] were unable to document a significant difference in the incidence of shunt infection using 72 hours of methicillin as the prophylactic antibiotic. Bayston[60] also found no effectiveness of antibiotic prophylaxis using either cloxacillin or gentamicin. In contrast, two randomized controlled trials using oxacillin and trimethoprim/sulfamethoxazole showed reduced infection rates in the prophylaxis group.[61,62] One recent *case-control* study indicated a threefold reduction in the shunt-infection rate with the use of various antibiotics.[57]

The rest of the published prophylaxis studies are either retrospective and sequential, uncontrolled, and nonrandomized, or compare retrospective controlled group with prospective prophylaxis groups.[63–67] The flaws inherent in these studies preclude any definitive conclusions regarding the efficacy of prophylactic antibiotics.

Future Research

Use of antibiotic-impregnated shunt materials has shown some promise in animal models, but human trials have not yet been published.[68] Other potential areas of investigation include changes in shunt materials[69] that would prevent or induce microbial adherence and further efforts at prophylaxis. In view of the large number of CNS shunts placed each year in this country, information on the usefulness of any new treatment showed be rapidly generated; however, such dissemination of data would require cooperation among the centers that perform shunt surgery.

References

1. Davidoff LM: Treatment of hydrocephalus. *Arch Surg* 1929;18:1737–1762.
2. Raimondi AJ, Robinson JS, Kuwamura K: Complications of ventriculo-peritoneal shunting and a critical comparison of the three-piece and one-piece systems. *Childs Brain* 1977;3:321–342.
3. McLone DG, Czyzewski D, Raimondi AJ, et al: Central nervous system infections as a limiting factor in the intelligence of children with myelomeningocele. *Pediatrics* 1982;70:338–342.
4. Shurtleff DB, Foltz EL, Loeser JD: Hydrocephalus. *Am J. Dis Child* 1973;125:688–693.
5. Schoenbaum SC, Gardner P, Shillito J: Infections of cerebrospinal fluid shunts: epidemiology, clinical manifestations, and therapy. *J Infect Dis* 1975;131: 543–552.
6. Meirovitch J, Kitai-Cohen Y, Keren G, et al: Cerebrospinal fluid shunt infections in children. *Pediatr Infect Dis J* 1987;6:921–924.
7. Odio C, McCracken GH, Nelson JD: CSF shunt infections in pediatrics. *Am J Dis Child* 1984; 138:1103–1108.
8. Venes JL: Control of shunt infection. *J Neurosurg* 1976;45:311–314.
9. Gardner BP, Gordon DS: Postoperative infection in shunts for hydrocephalus: are prophylactic antibiotics necessary? *Br Med J* 1982;284:1914–1915.
10. Younger JJ, Simmons CH, Barrett FF: Operative related infection rates for ventriculoperitoneal shunt procedures in a children's hospital. *Infec Cont* 1987;8:67–70.
11. Nelson JD: Cerebrospinal fluid shunt infections. *Pediatr Infect Dis* 1984;3:S30–S31.
12. Yogev R: Cerebrospinal fluid shunt infections: a personal view. *Pediatr Infect Dis* 1985;4:113–118.
13. Ammirati M, Raimondi AJ: Cerebrospinal fluid shunt infections in children. *Childs Nerv Syst* 1987;3:106–109.
14. Renier D, Lacombe J, Pierre-Kahn A, et al: Factors causing acute shunt infection. *J Neurosurg* 1984; 61:1072–1078.
15. Spanu G, Karussos G, Adinolfi D, et al: An analysis of cerebrospinal fluid shunt infections in adults. A clinical experience of twelve years. *Acta Neurochir* 1986;80:79–82.
16. George R, Leibrock L, Epstein M: Long-term analysis of cerebrospinal fluid shunt infections. *J Neurosurg* 1979;51:804–811.
17. Forrest DM, Tabara ZB, Towu E, et al: Management of the colonised shunt. *Z Kinderchir* 1987;42:21–22.
18. Hirsch JF, Renier D, Pierre-Kahn A: Influence of the use of a surgical isolator on the rate of infection in the treatment of hydrocephalus. *Childs Brain* 1978;4: 137–150.
19. Bayston R, Lari J: A study of the sources of infection in colonised shunts. *Dev Med Child Neur* 1974; 16(suppl. 32):16–21.
20. Bayston R, Penny SR: Excessive production of mucoid substance in staphylococcus SIIA: a possible factor in colonization of Holter shunts. *Dev Med Child Neurol* 1972;14(suppl. 27):25–28.
21. Christensen GD, Simpson WA, Bisno AL, et al: Adherence of slime-producing strains of *Staphylococcus epidermidis* to smooth surfaces. *Infect Immun* 1982;37:318–326.
22. Diaz-Mitoma F, Harding GKM, Hoban DJ, et al: Clinical significance of a test for slime production in ventriculoperitoneal shunt infections caused by coagulase-negative staphylococci. *J Infect Dis* 1987; 156:555–560.
23. Christensen GD, Simpson WA, Bisno AL, et al. Experimental Foreign Body Infections in Mice Challenged with Slime-Producing *Staphylococcus epidermidis*. *Infec Immun* 1983;40:407–410.
24. Christensen GD, Simpson WA, Younger JJ, et al: Adherence of coagulase-negative staphylococci to plastic tissue culture plates: a quantitative model for the adherence of staphylocci to medical devices. *J Clin Microbiol* 1985;22:996–1006.

25. Davenport DS, Massanari RM, Pfaller MA, et al: Usefulness of a test for slime production as a marker for clinically significant infections with coagulase-negative staphylococci. *J Infect Dis* 1986;153:332–338.
26. Younger JJ, Christensen GD, Bartley DL, et al: Coagulase-negative staphylococci isolated from cerebrospinal fluid shunts: Importance of slime production, species identification, and shunt removal to clinical outcome. *J Infect Dis* 1987;156:548–554.
27. Sugarman B: Infections and prosthetic devices. *Am J Med* 1986;81(suppl 1A):78–84.
28. Borges LF: Cerebrospinal fluid shunts interfere with host defenses. *Neurosurgery* 1982;10:55–60.
29. Leggiadro RJ, Atluru VL, Katz SP, et al: Meningococcal meningitis associated with cerebrospinal fluid shunts. *Brief Reports* 1984;3:489–490.
30. Sells CJ, Shurtleff DB, Leoser JD: Gram-negative cerebrospinal fluid shunt-associated infections. *Pediatrics* 1977;59:614–618.
31. James HE, Walsh JW, Wilson HD, et al: The management of cerebrospinal fluid shunt infections. A clinical experience. *Acta Neurochir* 1981;59:157–165.
32. Walters BC, Hoffman HJ, Hendric EB, et al: Cerebrospinal fluid shunt infection. *J Neurosurg* 1984; 60:1014–1021.
33. Connolly B, Guiney EJ, Fitzgerald RJ: CSF/shunt infections—the bane of our lives. *Z Kinderchir* 1987;42:13–14.
34. Fan-Havard P, Nahata MC: Treatment and prevention of infections of cerebrospinal fluid shunts. *Clin Pharmacol* 1987;6:866–880.
35. Gardner P, Leipzig T, Phillips P: Infections of central nervous system shunts. *Med Clin North Am* 1985; 69:297–314.
36. Beeler BA, Crowder JG, Smith JW, et al: *Propionibacterium acnes:* pathogen in central nervous system shunt infection. *Am J Med* 1976;61:935–938.
37. Younger JJ, Simmons JCH, Barrett FF: Occult distal ventriculoperitoneal shunt infections. *Pediatr Infect Dis* 1985;4:557–-558.
38. Rekate HL, Yonas H, White RJ, et al: The acute abdomen in patients with ventriculoperitoneal shunts. *Surg Neurol* 1979; 11:442–445.
39. Tchirkow G, Verhagen AD: Bacterial peritonitis in patients with ventriculoperitoneal shunt. *J Pediatr Surg* 1979; 14:182–184.
40. Hutschmann OR, Countee RW: Acute abdomen in children with infected ventriculoperitoneal shunts. *Arch Surg* 1980;115:305–307.
41. Reynolds M, Sherman JO, Mclone DG: Ventriculoperitoneal shunt infection masquerading as an acute surgical abdomen. *J Pediatr Surg* 1983;18:951–953.
42. Noetzel MJ, Baker RP: Shunt fluid examination: risks and benefits in the evaluation of shunt malfunction and infection. *J Neurosurg* 1984;61:328–332.
43. McLaurin RL: Treatment of infected ventricular shunts. *Childs Brain* 1975;1:306–310.
44. Frame PT, McLaurin RL: Treatment of CSF shunt infections with intrashunt plus oral antibiotic therapy. *J Neurosurg* 1984;60:354–360.
45. Shurtleff DB, Foltz EL, Weeks RD, et al: Therapy of *Staphylococcus epidermidis:* infections associated with cerebrospinal fluid shunts. *Pediatrics* 1974; 53:55–61.
46. Wald SL, McLaurin RL: Cerebrospinal fluid antibiotic levels during treatment of shunt infections. *J Neurosurg* 1980;52:41–46.
47. McLaurin RL, Frame PT: Treatment of infections of cerebrospinal fluid shunts. *Rev Infect Dis* 1987; 9:595–602.
48. Mori K, Raimondi AJ: An analysis of external ventricular drainage as a treatment for infected shunts. *Childs Brain* 1975;1:243–250.
49. Gombert ME, Landesman SH, Corrado ML, et al: Vancomycin and rifampin therapy for *Staphylococcus epidermidis* meningitis associated with CSF shunts. *J Neurosurg* 1981;55:633–636.
50. Bayson R, Barnicoat M, Cudmore RE, et al: The use of intraventricular vancomycin in the treatment of CSF shunt-associated ventriculitis. *Z Kinderchir* 1984;39:111–113.
51. Bayston R: Intraventricular vancomycin for treatment of shunt-associated ventriculitis. *J Antimicrob Chemothe* 1987;20:283.
52. Ring JC, Cates KL, Belani KK, et al: Rifampin for CSF shunt infections caused by coagulase-negative staphylococci. *J Pediatr* 1979;95:317–319.
53. Odio C, Mohs E, Sklar FH, et al: Adverse reactions to vancomycin used as prophylaxis for CSF shunt procedures. *Am J Dis Child* 1984;138:17–19.
54. Frenkel LD, Patno K, Rayport M: Safety and effectiveness of intraventricular gentamicin in CNS infections. *Inf Surg* 1986;March:163–170.
55. McCracken G, Mize S: Intraventricular gentamicin treatment in gram-negative bacillary meningitis of infancy. *Lancet* 1980;1:787–791.
56. Steele RW: Ceftriaxone: increasing the half-life and activity of third generation cephalosporins. *Pediatr Infect Dis* 1985;4:188–191.
57. Walters BC, Hoffman HJ, Hendrick EB, et al: Decreased risk of infection in cerebrospinal fluid shunt surgery using prophylactic antibiotics: a case-control study. *Z Kinderchir* 1985;40:15–18.
58. Wang EEL, Prober CG, Hendrick BE, et al: Prophylactic sulfamethoxazole and trimethoprim in ventriculoperitoneal shunt surgery. *JAMA* 1984;251: 1174–1177.
59. Haines SJ, Taylor F: Prophylactic methicillin for shunt operations: effects on incidence of shunt

malfunction and infection. *Childs Brain* 1982;9:10–22.

60. Bayston R: Antibiotic prophylaxis in shunt infection. *Dev Med Child Neurol* 1975;17(suppl 35):99–103.
61. Djindjian M, Fevrier MJ, Otterbein G, et al: Oxacillin prophylaxis in cerebrospinal fluid shunt procedures: results of a randomized open study in 60 hydrocephalic patients. *Surg Neurol* 1986;25:178–180.
62. Blomstedt GC: Results of trimethoprim-sulfamethoxazole prophylaxis in ventriculostomy and shunting procedures. *J Neurosurg* 1985;62:694–697.
63. McCullough DC, Kane JG, Presper JH, et al: Antibiotic prophylaxis in ventricular shunt surgery. I. Reduction of operative infection rates with methicillin. *Childs Brain* 1980;7:182–189.
64. McCullough DC, Kane JG, Harleman G, et al: Antibiotic prophylaxis in ventricular shunt surgery. II. Antibiotic concentrations in cerebrospinal fluid. *Childs Brain* 1980;7:190–194.
65. Ajir F, Levin AB, Duff TA: Effect of prophylactic methicillin on cerebrospinal fluid shunt infections in children. *Neurosurgery* 1981;9:6–8.
66. Younger JJ, Simmons JC, Barrett FF: Failure of single dose intraventricular vancomycin for cerebrospinal fluid shunt surgery. *Pediatr Infect Dis* 1987;6:212–213.
67. Slight PH, Gundling K, Plotkin SA, et al: A trial of vancomycin for prophylaxis of infections after neurosurgical shunts. *N Engl J Med* 1985;312:921.
68. Bayston R, Milner RDG: Antimicrobial activity of silicone rubber used in hydrocephalus shunts, after impregnation with antimicrobial substances. *J Clin Pathol* 1981;134:1057–1062.
69. Guevara JA, Torre JL, Denoya C, et al: Microscopic studies in shunts for hydrocephalus. *Childs Brain* 1981;8:284–293.

7
Noninfectious Causes of Acute CNS Inflammation

LOUIS REIK, JR. AND MORVEN C. BARWICK

A variety of noninfectious, inflammatory diseases of the central nervous system (CNS) can mimic CNS infection, both acute and chronic. The focus of this chapter is on those that mimic acute CNS infection: allergic and hypersensitivity reactions, vasculitis and the collagen vascular diseases, Behcet's disease, the uveomeningitic syndromes, Mollaret's meningitis, sarcoidosis, and chemical meningitis. The para- and postinfectious encephalitides and the causes of chronic meningitis are discussed elsewhere in this volume.

Allergic and Hypersensitivity Reactions

Drug-Induced Meningitis

Drug-induced meningitis is an acute, febrile meningitis or meningoencephalitis that has been reported following the administration of nonsteroidal anti-inflammatory drugs (ibuprofen,[1–8] naproxen,[9] sulindac,[10,11] tolmetin sodium[12]), sulfamethizole,[13] trimethoprim alone[14,15] and in combination with sulfamethoxazole,[14–18] isoniazid,[19] phenazopyridine,[20] azathioprine,[21,22] and cytosine arabinoside.[23] Affected patients, particularly those reacting to nonsteroidal anti-inflammatory drugs, often have an underlying collagen vascular disease, usually systemic lupus erythematosus (SLE) or mixed connective-tissue disease. But apparently healthy individuals have been affected also.

The pathology is not known. New Zealand mice, susceptible to a spontaneous SLE-like illness, do develop a massive lymphocytic and mononuclear infiltration of the meninges and choroid plexus when fed ibuprofen chronically,[24] but earlier, more acute changes have not been described.

Circumstantial evidence suggests that an immediate hypersensitivity reaction is involved.[15] The interval between drug ingestion and the onset of symptoms is brief and becomes briefer with repeated exposure, while the symptoms become more intense, allergic features accompany the onset, and recovery is prompt when the drug is discontinued. The meningeal deposition of circulating immune complexes seems a less likely mechanism: in at least two cases, no circulating complexes were detectable when sought,[8,11] and in a third, complexes were present in serum but not cerebrospinal fluid (CSF).[15]

Symptoms may begin less than an hour after ingestion of a drug to which the patient is already sensitized and usually within weeks of the start of treatment with a new drug, although the onset of meningitis after two years of therapy has been reported.[25] The onset is typically explosive with fever up to 40.7°C, chills, headache, nausea, vomiting, neck stiffness, and photophobia. Accompanying systemic signs and symptoms include pruritis,[10,13,14] rash,[3,4,6] conjunctivitis,[4,6,12–14,16] facial swelling,[12] myalgias and arthralgias,[4,14,16,19] and lymphadenopathy.[12] Lethargy, irritability, confusion, and delirium are common,[1,8,11,14,19,20] and papilledema,[4,9,19] coma,[2–4,15] seizures,[3,15] and residual hearing loss[3,4] have been reported. Signs and symptoms persist until the responsible drug is discontinued, and then resolve over 24–72 hours.

Most routine laboratory tests are normal, although leukocytosis of up to 29,000 cells/mm^3, mainly polymorphonuclear (PMN), is common,[5–7,10–13,15,19] and eosinophilia (26%) has been reported.[16] The CSF is always abnormal. The pressure may be increased (up to 400 mm CSF),[4,5,12,15,19] and pleocytosis (44–19,000 cells/mm^3, usually greater than 90% PMN) and increased protein (54–522 mg/dl) are always present.[1–23] Exceptionally, CSF lymphocytes may predominate,[4] and CSF eosinophilia has been reported.[7] Hypoglycorrhachia has been present in at least three cases.[7,8,10] CSF changes, like the clinical abnormalities, resolve within days once the offending drug is stopped. The electroencephalogram (EEG) in two cases has shown nonspecific slowing,[14,15] whereas computerized tomography (CT) scans have been consistently normal,[4,14,15,18,23]

Drug-induced meningitis most resembles acute bacterial meningitis, and empiric antibiotic therapy may be necessary until the distinction can be made. The results of CSF cultures and Gram stain and the prompt resolution of symptoms after the responsible drug is stopped all aid in the distinction. Recurrent meningitis results when the drug is taken episodically at long intervals.[2–4,14–16,19,20] Then a careful drug history should establish the correct diagnosis. Only symptomatic treatment is necessary. Symptoms and signs resolve within a day or two once the responsible drug is discontinued.

Serum Sickness

Serum sickness is an acute, monophasic, multisystem inflammatory disease that was formerly a common reaction to the injection of horse-serum antitoxins used in the treatment of bacterial infections. Routine vaccination and effective antibiotic therapy have made the use of antitoxins largely obsolete for this purpose,[26] and serum sickness is less common today. However, heterologous serum still is used in the prophylaxis and treatment of botulism, gas gangrene, diphtheria, venomous-snake bites, and bites of the black-widow spider, and it can cause serum sickness, as do other injected foreign proteins—hymenoptera venoms, streptokinase, and antilymphocyte globulin.[26,27] But drug reactions are not the most common cause of the illness.[26–28] A number of commonly prescribed medications have been implicated: penicillin, cephalosporins, streptomycin, sulfonamides, para-aminosalicylic acid, thiouracils, hydantoins, captopril, hydralazine, methyl dopa, propranolol, procainamide, quinidine, phenylbutazone, naproxen, and sulindac, among others.[26,27]

Serum sickness results when immune complexes formed in response to foreign antigens precipitate in blood-vessel walls. Complement is fixed and consumed, and inflammatory vascular lesions develop that range from PMN infiltration and fibrinoid necrosis to noninflammatory degeneration, depending on the amount of antigen–antibody interaction.[29] Such multifocal vascular lesions are present throughout the nervous systems of laboratory animals with experimental serum sickness: in choroid plexus, leptomeninges, cerebral cortex, subcortical and subependymal white matter, and peripheral nerves (where they are accompanied by perivascular demyelination).[30] Less is known about the nervous-system pathology of human serum sickness, but the abnormalities reported from the few fatal cases include vascular congestion, hyalinization, and endothelial swelling; perivascular edema, demyelination, hemorrhage, and round-cell infiltration; and focal areas of necrosis in the brain and spinal cord.[31,32]

The illness begins acutely, usually 7 to 10 days after the injection of a foreign protein or the start of treatment with a new drug, but the onset may be as late as 3 weeks, or as early as 1 to 4 days if the patient has been previously sensitized. Typical systemic manifestations are fever, urticaria, abdominal pain, arthralgias or arthritis, lymphadenopathy, and immune-complex nephritis.[26,27,29]

Neurologic abnormalities are also common, especially in serum cases. They usually appear on the first or second day of systemic illness but sometimes occur alone. A mild meningoencephalitis is most frequent. Headache, nausea, and vomiting are common at onset, 50% of patients have lymphocytic pleocytosis,[31] and drowiness and mild encephalopathy are almost always present.[33] More overt parenchymal involvement also occurs. Peripheral-nervous-system (PNS) abnormalities are most frequent, typically brachial neuritis, radial-nerve palsy, or ascending polyneuritis.[34] However, about 10% of those with overt parenchymal involvement have severe CNS disease[34]; papilledema, aphasia, hemiplegia, hemianopia, coma, convulsions, chorea, cerebellar ataxia, cranial neuropathies, and transverse myelitis have all been reported.[31,33]

Typical laboratory abnormalities are an increased erythrocyte sedimentation rate (ESR), mild anemia, leukocytosis, occasional eosinophilia (with drug reactions), proteinuria, microscopic hematuria and red-cell casts, hypergammaglobulinemia, depressed serum-complement levels, and elevated levels of circulating immune complexes.[26–28,35] The electrocardiogram (ECG) may show conduction block. The CSF pressure may be increased, and a lymphocytic pleocytosis is usual (10–30 cells/mm^3, occasionally up to 500). CSF protein is only occasionally increased (up to 290 mg/dl); the glucose is normal.[31,33,36] The EEG is often slowed in patients with cerebral symptoms.[33]

CNS involvement in serum sickness can mimic acute infectious meningoencephalitis. When CNS signs and symptoms follow heterologous serum injection or are accompanied by the typical systemic manifestations of serum sickness, the diagnosis should be straightforward. When CNS involvement develops in isolation, the simultaneous development of peripheral neuropathy is one clue, and the typical laboratory abnormalities of serum sickness another.

Serum sickness resolves spontaneously and completely within 2 weeks in most cases, but recovery may take longer after large doses of serum or reactions to slowly metabolized drugs. Treatment with antihistamines may block the further deposition of immune complexes, thereby shortening the course and lessening the severity of the illness. Prednisone, 40–60 mg daily for two weeks, is usually recommended for severe cases,[28] but even higher doses of corticosteroids given preventively did not stop the development of serum sickness in a group of patients treated with horse antithymocyte globulin.[35] Plasma ultrafiltration, on the other hand, was effective in preventing renal deposition of immune complexes in rabbits with acute serum sickness,[37] suggesting that plasmapheresis could be of value in severe human cases.

Vasculitis and Collagen Vascular Disease

Neurologic dysfunction that mimics acute CNS infection is common in the vasculitides and collagen vascular disorders, usually developing in the setting of established disease. Neurologic abnormalities suggesting infection can be the initial manifestation, but even then the diagnosis usually can be made on the basis of associated clinical findings of systemic involvement. Confusion occurs when symptoms and signs of CNS infection are the only manifestation. This situation arises most often in primary angiitis of the CNS, SLE, lymphomatoid granulomatosis, and Behcet's disease.[28,38–40]

Primary Angiitis of the CNS

Primary angiitis of the central nervous system (PACNS), also known as granulomatous angiitis of the nervous system, is a rare disease of unknown etiology that affects all ages and is seen in men slightly more often than in women. Five percent of reported cases have involved patients with lymphoma, particularly Hodgkin's disease.[28,39,41–44]

The characteristic pathologic change in the CNS is a segmental granulomatous inflammation and fibrinoid necrosis of small arteries and arterioles (less than 200–500 μm) in the leptomeninges and parenchyma, with vascular narrowing and occlusion resulting in tissue ischemia and infarction.[40,42–45] Capillaries, veins, and venules are less often and less severely affected.[28,40] Larger arteries can be affected, often with disruption of the internal elastic lamina.[40] The vasculitic process may rarely involve the spinal cord and temporal arteries.[39,40] Microscopic evidence of systemic involvement, usually in the lung and kidney, has been reported, but clinically significant manifestations do not occur.[28,39–41]

The cause of PACNS is unknown. Proposed mechanisms include infectious agents (varicella-zoster and herpes-simplex viruses or Mycoplasma)[39–41] and defects in immune regulation as suggested by its association with malignant lymphoma.[41,46] To date, direct evidence of viral infection, circulating immune complexes, or defective lymphocyte function has not been reported.[41]

The usual clinical presentation is that of an acute or subacute diffuse or diffuse and multifocal encephalopathy with headache, confusion, altered mentation, nausea, and vomiting, frequently progressing to stupor and coma. Constitutional symptoms such as fever and weight loss are present in 25% of patients. Focal and multifocal signs ultimately appear in 60–80%, including seizures, hemiparesis, dysphasia, papilledema, visual loss, and cranial neuropathies (nerve III, VI, or VII.)[28,38–41,47]

Routine laboratory tests are generally normal, although the ESR is increased in 70% of reported cases.[40,41] The CSF is almost always abnormal. Opening pressure may be elevated. Increased protein, usually less than 500 mg/dl (range, 75–825 mg/dl), and lymphocytic pleocytosis, usually less than 200/mm^3 (range, 40–500/mm^3), are reported in 95% of published cases.[28,39–41,45] Red cells (up to 800/mm^3) are sometimes seen. A low CSF glucose has been reported in several cases.[39,40] Abnormal EEGs with diffuse and sometimes superimposed focal slowing have been documented in 82% of cases studied.[40] Neuroimaging techniques useful in identifying CNS disease include, in ascending order, radionuclide brain scans, CT, magnetic-resonance imaging (MRI), and cerebral angiography.[40] CT may demonstrate multiple low-density, non-contrast-enhancing areas.[339,41] MRI is more sensitive (but not specific) in detecting vasculitic brain lesions, whether clinically apparent or silent, and should prove useful in screening patients for subsequent angiography and in assessing response to treatment.[40,48] Cerebral angiography has been abnormal in 60–80% of patients studied, revealing segmental narrowing and ectasia (beading), vessel irregularities, and, on occasion, avascular mass lesions.[28,39–41,49]

The diagnosis of PACNS is difficult to establish. Its onset may mimic acute or subacute infectious meningoencephalitis, even to the presence of hypoglycorrhachia. Serologies and CSF stains and cultures are negative. Cerebral angiography may be abnormal, but the characteristic vascular changes are not specific for PACNS. Similar changes have been reported in association with infections, emboli, drugs, neoplasia, and atherosclerosis.[47] Furthermore, a normal angiogram does not exclude the diagnosis. [28,39,41,47] Histologic confirmation of suspected PACNS by leptomeningeal and parenchymal biopsy is recommended, but may fail to establish the diagnosis owing to the patchy, segmental nature of the process.[39,41,47]

In the past, PACNS usually was fatal, with death occurring within days to three or four years from the time of onset.[45,47] Recent studies suggest that prolonged remissions may be induced by treatment with a combination of prednisone (1 mg/kg/day) and cyclophosphamide (2mg/kg/day).[41,45,50] When clinical assessment and neuroimaging suggest PACNS, diagnostic confirmation should be sought by leptomeningeal and parenchymal biopsy before starting therapy. If clinical suspicion is strong, and infectious causes have been excluded, a negative biopsy need not prevent an empiric trial of corticosteroids alone or in combination with cyclophosphamide.

Systemic Lupus Erythematosus

A chronic remitting and relapsing autoimmune inflammatory disorder, SLE is characterized by multiple-organ-system involvement and a predilection for young and middle-aged adults, especially women.[28,51]

The primary pathologic lesion is a bland vasculopathy marked by fibrinoid necrosis and endothelial swelling of small arteries, arterioles, and capillaries, presumably the result of immune-complex deposition. True systemic vasculitis, with inflammatory cell infiltration of vessel walls, is seen less frequently, either in the form of hypersensitivity angiitis or as a polyarteritis nodosa (PAN)-like necrotizing process involving muscular arteries.[28] Within the CNS, true vasculities has been found in less than 10% of patients in autopsy series.[28,52,53] The microvasculopathy common to all organ systems is accompanied by organ-specific responses to immune-complex deposition, and possibily to antibody-mediated cytotoxic reactions. These are expressed pathologically as glomerulonephritis, verrucous endocarditis (Libman-Sacks), myocarditis and pericarditis, interstitial pneumonitis, oninon-peel hypertrophy of splenic vessels, focal lymph-node necrosis, and vasculitis.[28,54]

Within the CNS, microvasculopathy is prominent with intimal swelling and proliferation, hyaline necrosis of vessel walls, and perivascular lymphocytic and microglial infiltrates.[28,52,54,55] Microinfarcts, larger infarcts, and hemorrhages (sometimes subarachnoid) are common. While microvascular lesions can account for clinical findings in some SLE patients, there is often a remarkable lack of clinicopathologic correlation.[52,55]

SLE is an immunologically mediated disorder whose etiology is multifactorial, including genetic predisposition and environmental triggers.[56] Numerous immune abnormalities have been described, of which B-cell abnormalities are the most important.[28,56] B-cell hyperactivity is manifested by hypergammaglobulinemia, increased numbers of circulating antibody-producing cells, and overproduction of autoantibodies directed against cell membranes and cytoplasmic and nuclear proteins (especially DNA). These autoantibodies, in combination with their respective antigens, are responsible for cell lysis and immune-complex formation. The former leads, for example, to Coombs' positive hemolytic anemia. The latter, in the presence of complement, results in glomerulonephritis and systemic vasculitis and may contribute to CNS disease.[28,39,55–57] A variety of T-cell abnormalities have been reported during active disease, including reduced helper and suppressor T-cell activity. How these relate to B-cell hyperfunction is not clear.[56]

Indirect evidence suggests that the pathogenesis of CNS disease in SLE is a function of two mechanisms operating independently or in concert—immune-complex vasculopathy and autoantibodies directed against brain tissue.[28,52,55] Antibody to DNA and DNA/anti-DNA complexes have been demonstrated in the CSF of patients with lupus meningitis.[58] The fourth component of complement (C_4) is reduced in the CSF of some patients with acute CNS lupus.[59] Immunoglobulin and immune-complex deposition in choroid plexus take place in patients both with and without symptomatic CNS disease.[52] Cell-mediated nervous-system damage may also play a role. Antineuronal IgG antibodies in CSF correlate highly with diffuse CNS disease, particularly dementia and seizures.[52] Whether such antibodies enter the CNS via an immune-complex-damaged blood–brain barrier in cerebral vessels or choroid plexus or are synthesized intrathecally is not known.[51,52]

Initial clinical manifestations usually include skin lesions, arthralgia, and arthritis, variably followed by any or all of the following: constitutional symptoms (fever, weight loss, anorexia, malaise, fatigue, nausea, and vomiting), lymphadenopathy, pleuritis, pericarditis, renal disease including nephrotic syndrome, Raynaud's phenomenon, splenomegaly, and vasculitis.[28,39]

Neuropsychiatric abnormalities are frequent, occurring in up to 75% of patients.[51,54] They arise early in the course prior to the diagnosis of SLE or within the first year after diagnosis in 63% of cases. Neurologic manifestations are associated with active disease in 85%. The most common CNS abnormalities are dementia, psychosis, and seizures.[28,39,52,60] Various other diffuse and focal manifestations have been reported, including delirium, coma, pseudotumor cerebri, aseptic meningitis, hemiplegia, cerebellar ataxia, myelitis, cranial neuropathies (usually supranuclear), chorea, migraine headache, and peripheral neuropathies (Guillain-Barre syndrome, mononeuritis multiplex).[28,39,52,60] CNS involvement can be the initial indication of disease, particularly in the form of seizures, myelitis, chorea, and, rarely, meningitis.[28,39]

Among common laboratory abnormalities are anemia, leukopenia, thrombocytopenia, increased ESR, hyperglobulinemia, proteinuria, and microscopic hematuria. Serologic findings include a positive antinuclear antibody (ANA), anti-n DNA antibodies, and false-positive VDRL. In addition, the LE cell test may be positive, circulating immune complexes and cryoglobulins can be demonstrated, and serum complement may be decreased. Skin biopsy can reveal immunofluorescent staining of immune complexes at the dermal–epidermal junction (lupus band test).[28,39]

CSF abnormalities are present in one third of patients.[28,39] They include increased protein (usually less than 200 mg/dl) and lymphocytic pleocytosis (usually less than 100 cells/mm^3, but occasionally higher counts with PMN predominance). CSF glucose of less than 30 mg/dl has been reported in both myelitis and aseptic meningitis.[39] Elevated IgG and oligoclonal bands can be present in patients with diffuse CNS disease.[51] Nonspecific diffuse or focal EEG abnormalities occur in 80% of patients with cerebral disease.[28,39] CT identifies cerebral atrophy in patients with diffuse disease (as well as in a subset of steroid-treated patients without CNS disease),[51,52] and is also useful in the differentiation of large infarcts and hemorrhage. MRI is more sensitive, but not more specific, detecting lesions in twice as many patients. It may prove useful in monitoring disease activity and response to therapy.[52,61] Cerebral angiography is normal in the presence of lupus microvasculopathy but can detect the PAN-type vasculitis sometimes seen.[39,52]

Acute infectious meningitis and meningoencephalitis are common complications of SLE, particularly in steroid-treated patients. CNS lupus, which can mimic acute CNS infection, usually occurs in established SLE during periods of active systemic disease. The diagnosis can be suspected when diffuse and multifocal CNS and PNS involvement is seen in this setting, but infection must be excluded by appropriate serologies, CSF stains, and cultures.[39] When CNS abnormalities suggestive of acute infection occur alone as the initial manifestation of SLE, appropriate CSF studies must first rule out infection. Then clinical and laboratory evidence of multisystem disease can be sought.[39]

Treatment of CNS lupus remains controversial in the absence of controlled trials. Prednisone is usually prescribed in doses of 50–100 mg daily when CNS disease manifests and then is tapered as rapidly as disease activity permits. Recently, there has been a trend toward the use of high-dose intravenous corticosteroids (pulse therapy) in the management of severe exacerbations of SLE, including neuropsychiatric lupus (NP-SLE). Several studies have reported rapid improvement in NP-SLE following such therapy.[51] Immunosuppressants have not been shown to be superior to steroids in the therapy of cerebral lupus, but do have a steroid-sparing effect.[28,39,51,52]

Lymphomatoid Granulomatosis

Lymphomatoid granulomatosis (LYG) is a rare, often fatal, systemic disease with prominent pulmonary, cutaneous, and nervous-system involvement. Progression to lymphoma is common. All ages are affected, as well as both sexes, although males are affected twice as often as females. It is distinct from Wegener's granulomatosis with which it shares certain clinical, radiologic, and histologic features.[28,39,62–64]

Pathologically, LYG is an angiocentric and angiodestructive granulomatous and lymphoreticular proliferative process. Small and medium-sized muscular arteries are particularly vulnerable. Any organ system may be invaded by an infiltrating polymorphocellular mass of lymphocytes, plasma cells, histiocytes, and atypical lymphoreticular cells.[28,62,63] In the CNS, this process leads to formation of multiple necrotizing inflammatory parenchymal mass lesions or areas of tissue ischemia and infarction secondary to vessel narrowing, occlusion, and necrosis. Extensive infiltration of meninges and cranial and peripheral nerves is common.[28,39,62] Progression to lymphoma resembling immunoblastic sarcoma occurs in 12–47% of reported cases.[62–64]

The etiology of LYG remains obscure, but it may represent a lymphoproliferative disorder arising in a setting of disordered or impaired immunity.[28,39,69]

Clinically, the most common presenting symptoms are constitutional (fever, 58%; weight loss and malaise, each 35%) and pulmonary (cough, 56%; dyspnea, 29%). Skin lesions, often ressembling erythema nodosum, occur in 40%. Other organ systems can be involved, including the kidney, heart, adrenal glands, liver, pancreas, bowel, and prostate.[28,39,63]

Neurologic manifestations occur in 20–30% of reported cases. They are frequently among the presenting symptoms, can antedate other features of the illness by as much as five years, and may be the only clinical expression of disease.[62,63,65–68] CNS findings are protean, including headache, raised intracranial pressure, confusion, coma, seizures, and focal deficits such as hemiparesis and aphasia. Cranial neuropathies and peripheral neuropathy (mononeuritis multiplex) are common; myelopathy is less commonly found.[28,63]

There are no consistent laboratory abnormalities. Chest radiography is almost invariably (97%) abnormal with characteristic multiple rounded densities in both lower lung fields.[63]

CSF abnormalities include pressure elevations, lymphocytic pleocytosis, increased total protein (up to 250 mg/dl) and IgG (one case), and abnormal nondiagnostic cytology.[28,39] Parenchymal mass lesions, sometimes ring enhancing, are seen on CT. Cerebral angiograms are usually normal, but may show fusiform vessel narrowing.[28,62]

Definitive diagnosis depends on tissue biopsy, usually of lung. When neurologic abnormalities occur exclusively, or are accompanied only by constitutional systems, LYG may be confused with acute or subacute CNS infections, whether meningitis, meningoencephalitis, or brain abscess. Serology and CSF stains, cultures, and glucose determination can aid in the distinction, but leptomeningeal and parenchymal biopsy may be necessary.[39,66,68]

The overall mortality of patients with LYG is 63%, with 94% of deaths occurring within three years of onset. Neurologic involvement is associated with a poor prognosis; mortality rates range from 83 to 94% in this setting.[63] CNS disease may progress even as pulmonary involvement responds to therapy.[39,62,63,69] Early initiation of combined therapy with steroids and cyclophosphamide can induce complete remission and prevent progression to lymphoma.[28,64] Isolated CNS disease diagnosed by brain biopsy appeared to carry a better prognosis in two reported cases.[66] Cranial radiation may be indicated if CNS disease fails to repond to combined therapy.[28,69] More aggressive chemotherapy is indicated should lymphoma develop.[28]

Behcet's Disease

Behcet's disease is a multisystem disorder of unknown cause featuring recurrent oral and genital ulcerations, relapsing uveitis, and skin eruptions. It affects all ages, but particularly young adults.[70–72] It is found most frequently among Asian and Eurasians (especially the Japanese and Turks) living between latitudes 30° and 45° north, but is being increasingly recognized worldwide.[72]

Pathologically, the characteristic lesion is a perivascular lymphocytic infiltrate affecting small arteries (including vasa vasorum) and veins. Endothelial proliferation and occasional fibrinoid necrosis occur. Small-vessel vasculopathy underlies the mucocutaneous, ocular, pulmonary, and gastrointestinal manifestations.[70–72] Occlusive disease of large veins and arteries is attributed to involvement of the vasa vasorum.[70,72] Within the nervous system, perivascular (often perivenular) and meningeal lymphocytic infiltrates are prominent, together with scattered foci of gray- and white-matter necrosis and occasional demyelination. These findings are most prominent in the brain stem, basal ganglia, and internal capsule. Frank vasculitis with inflammatory cell invasion of vessel walls has been reported infrequently.[40,71,73,74]

The cause remains unknown, but immunologic abnormalities abound. These include autoantibodies against oral mucosa, tissue-damaging serum factors such as skin necrotizing factor, and lymphokine-induced PMN hyperactivity. There is a decrease in the $T_4:T_8$ ratio, and an increase in natural killer T-cells. In the serum, IgG, IgM, and IgD are elevated during an attack, as is serum complement. Immunoglobulin (IgG, IgM, and BIA globulin) deposition in vessel walls (especially venules) has been demonstrated[72,75,78,79] in non-CNS tissues, and circulating immune complexes have been reported in up to one third of patients.[75] An increased incidence of HLA-B5 is reported in patients with Behcet's disease.[72,75] In neuro-Behcet's syndrome, elevations of C_3, alpha$_2$-macroglobulin, and IgA in CSF have been correlated with active disease.[72] Accumulating evidence points to immune-complex-induced vasculitis triggered by as yet unknown factors (possibly viral or toxic) as the basis for disease.[40,72]

The most common clinical abnormalities in Behcet's disease are oral aphthous ulcers, genital ulcers, skin eruptions (especially erythema nodosum), ocular symptoms, and arthritis. Ocular involvement includes episcleritis, iridocyclitis with hypopyon, Keratitis, retinal-vein thrombosis, and retinal or vitreous hemorrhages.[72,80] Progression to permanent loss of vision is likely, being reported in 50–80% of Japanese patients.[72] Gastrointestinal ulcers (ileocecal) and epididymitis can occur. Vascular involvement develops later in the course in 8–10% of cases. This takes the form of arterial occlusions or aneurysms and venous occulusions or varices and carries a poor prognosis.[72]

Neurologic manifestations are seen in 5–28% of cases, usually in the setting of established disease, but may be the initial feature in 5% of patients.[70–73,81,82] The subclassification of neuro-Behcet's is applied when neurologic features predominate.[72] Involvement of the CNS raises the mortality of a fairly benign disease from 4% to approximately 40%.[70,72,79] The onset of CNS disease is frequently associated with fever, headache, and meningeal signs. Neurologic abnormalities include aseptic meningitis, meningoencephalitis, dementia, seizures, limb paresis, bulbar and pseudobulbar palsy, cerebellar ataxia, intracranial hypertension with or without sagittal sinus thrombosis, cranial neuropathies, and myelopathy.[40,71–74,81,82] Peripheral neuropathies are rare. The clinical course is usually remitting and relapsing, but may be progressive with chronic deficits.

There are no diagnostic laboratory findings in blood or urine. An acute attack may be accompanied by a high ESR; a positive test for C-reactive protein; increased fibrinolysis; elevated prostaglandins E and F2; increased concentrations of IgG, IgM, and IgD; and the presence of circulating immune complexes. These abnormalities disappear during remissions.[72,75] Lymphocytic pleocytosis and elevated CSF protein are common.[40,71,73] The EEG demonstrates focal or diffuse slowing.[40] A CT scan shows hypodense areas that frequently enhance with contrast, typically in the brain stem, basal ganglia, internal capsule, and hemispheric white matter. Contrast enhancement may correlate with active disease.[80] The use of MRI has been reported in several cases of neuro-Behect's disease and has been shown to be more sensitive than CT in detecting lesions.[48,83] Cerebral angiography is usually normal, but occasionally has shown vessel occlusion or displacement.[73]

Diagnosis of Behcet's disease in complete form depends on the appearance of all four major criteria—recurrent oral and genital ulcers and skin and ocular lesions—during the clinical course. The diagnosis can also be made when recurrent aphthous stomatitis is associated with at least one other major criterion and one minor criterion (neurologic, vascular, arthritic, or gastrointestinal).[72,73,79] Diagnostic confusion is likely when neurologic abnormalities are the initial manifestation of disease. Acute meningeal involvement can be confused with acute infectious meningoencephalitis. Serologies and CSF analysis, stains, and cultures should exclude an infectious process, but a definitive diagnosis of Behect's disease may have to await the development of more specific clinical features.

The prognosis for patients with Behcet's disease varies, and spontaneous remissions can occur. Ocular involvement is a major cause of morbidity; vascular and neurologic disease contribute significantly to morbidity and mortality. Early institution of therapy with high-dose prednisone (60 mg/day) can control both neurologic and systemic manifestations. The addition of azathioprine or chlorambucil may prove beneficial.[71,72,75] Colchicine and cyclosporine-A are reported to suppress ocular lesions, but not CNS disease.[75–78]

Vogt-Koyanagi-Harada Syndrome

The Vogt-Koyanagi-Harada (VKH) syndrome, also known as the uveomeningoencephalitic syndrome, is a rare disease of unknown cause that affects both sexes and all ages, particularly adults between the ages of 20 and 40.[84–86] Orientals may be more susceptible.[86,87] The symptom complex includes bilateral anterior and posterior uveitis with exudative retinal detachment; integumentary changes (poliosis, canities, and alopecia); auditory dysfunction (dysacousis and tinnitus); and neurologic, particularly CNS, involvement in up to 60% of cases.[84,86]

The characteristic ocular pathology consists of diffuse granulomatous uveitis with an infiltrate of plasma cells, lymphocytes, and macrophages, and marked retinal pigment epithelial disturbance.[87,89] Neuropathologically, adhesive arachnoiditis (with a mononuclear meningeal infiltrate) has been found at craniotomy.[84,88]

The etiopathogenesis remains obscure. A viral origin has been suspected but not substantiated.[86,89,90] Accumulating evidence points to an autoimmune process directed primarily against melanocytes in eye, skin, and meninges. Cellular hypersensitivity to uveal pigment and lymphocyte-mediated cytotoxicity to melanocyte antigen have been demonstrated. Humoral immunity may also be involved, suggested by antipigment antibodies in the sera of patients with the VKH syndrome, by the elevations of serum IgD, and by the accumulation of plasma cells and B-cells in the eye. An immunogenetic predisposition is suggested by the increased incidence of certain human-lymphocyte-antigen haplotypes, especially DRW53, in these patients.[79,87,89]

Clinically, the disease frequently evolves through three stages: (1) meningeal, (2) ophthalmic, and (3) convalescent, characterized by subsiding uveitis and the appearance of auditory and dermatologic manifestations. However, this pattern is variable, and the ear and skin abnormalities may be lacking.[86]

The meningeal phase is characterized by fever, headache, photophobia, and meningeal signs. These can develop simultaneously with eye symptoms, but in more than half of the patients with CNS involvement, meningeal symptoms and signs will precede or follow the uveitis by as much as ten days.[3] Other reported neurologic abnormalities include diffuse or focal encephalopathy with confusion, delirium, coma, seizures, psychosis, diabetes insipidus, raised intracranial pressure, hemiparesis, and aphasia; cranial neuropathies (especially nerves II, sensory, V, VI, VII, and VIII); myelopathy with paraparesis and sphincter disturbance; peripheral neuropathy; and myopathy.[79,84–86] The CSF may be under increased pressure. Lymphocytic pleocytosis and mildly elevated protein are usually present. EEG abnormalities occur in association with encephalopathy.

The ophthalmic phase is marked by the appearance of acute uveitis affecting both eyes simultaneously in 70% of patients. The ultimate deficit in visual acuity does not correlate with the presence or absence of CNS, dematologic, or auditory involvement.[86]

The convalescent phase is characterized by the development of auditory dysfunction and patchy depigmentation of skin and hair. Fluctuating or persistent neurologic deficits such as cranial neuropathies (especially nerve VI) or hemiparesis or paraparesis, are variably present.[84]

Diagnosis is straighforward when bilateral panuveitis occurs in association with symptoms and signs of meningitis or meningoencephalitis. But when neurologic symptoms and signs precede ocular involvement, the VKH syndrome may mimic acute or subacute CNS infection. Serologies and CSF glucose determination, stains, and cultures should aid in exclusion of an acute infectious process.

The disease is usually self-limited, becoming inactive within one year.[84,86] The acute meningeal and ophthalmic phases, which may coincide or overlap, generally run a course measured in weeks. Skin and auditory manifestations begin to appear one or two months after disease onset, together with fluctuating or persistent neurologic deficits.[84,87] Topical and high-dose systemic corticosteroids are utilized in therapy, but no controlled trials have been carried out. Early systemic administration of steroids appears to increase the likelihood of recovery of visual acuity, to shorten the duration of the disease, and to prevent the development of ear and skin lesions.[86] Whether steroid therapy prevents permanent neurologic deficits is unclear. Recently, an encouraging response to cyclosporine-A has been reported in patients with uveoretinitis who failed steroid therapy.[89]

Mollaret's Meningitis

Mollaret's meningitis is an uncommon disease of unknown etiology characterized by recurrent attacks of fever and meningeal inflammation, lasting days, and separated by symptom-free intervals of weeks to months.[91–95]

Neither its pathology nor its pathogenesis is known. Infection has been suspected often but seldom confirmed; an infectious agent has been isolated in only two cases—herpes-simplex virus type I in one[96] and an unidentified virus in another.[95] More recently, a relation to recurrent hereditary polyserositis (RHP) has been suspected instead, based on several lines of evidence: (1) accompanying splenomegaly in one case,[97] (2) the development of renal amyloidosis in another case,[98] (3) the precipitation by metaraminol infusion of an attack of Mollaret's meningitis in a case of typical RHP,[99] and (4) a favorable response to colchicine in several cases of Mollaret's meningitis without other features of RHP.[100–103]

Mollaret's meningitis can begin at almost any age (5 to 88 years),[92,94,104] and it affects men and women equally. The first attack begins without prodromal symptoms in a previously healthy individual. Headache and neck stiffness begin suddenly and became maximum in hours, often in less than 1 hour.[92,95] There is usually accompanying fever (up to 40°C), generalized malaise, nausea, vomiting, muscle and joint pain, and generalized hyperesthesia.[91–95] Exceptionally, fever is absent,[105] and in a few cases, there has been an urticarial rash.[97,100] Kernig's and Brudzinskis' signs are regularly present, and transient parenchymal nervous-system signs and symptoms may accompany the attack in as many as 50% of cases. Seizures, hallucinations, confusion, coma, dysphasia, diplopia, facial weakness, anisocoria, vertigo hypoactive, and hyperactive reflexes, Babinski signs, hemiparesis, and monoparesis have all been reported.[91–95,100,101,104,105] Symptoms and signs persist for days (usually 1 to 3), and then disappear rapidly, only to recur in attacks identical to the first after intervals of weeks to months. In most cases, the disease remits spontaneously after three to 5 years and an average of five attacks[92]; but in one case, the illness lasted 28 years,[106] and some patients have experienced dozens of attacks.

Routine laboratory tests are usually normal, although both leukocytosis[91,93,99,100,102,103,105,106] and leukopenia[94,95,97] have been reported, the ESR is somtimes increased,[91,93,98,100,101,106] and a few patients have had eosinophilia.[94,95,100]

The CSF is always abnormal during attacks.[91–95] The pressure is often moderately increased (usually less than 350 mm CSF), and there is invariably a mixed pleocytosis of up to several thousand cells/mm^3 during the first 12–24 hours. At first, the pleocytosis consists mainly in PMNs plus up to 66% "endothelial" or Mollaret's cells—large mononuclear cells with irregular nuclear and cytoplasmic membranes that rapidly lyse in the counting chamber to form ghosts. However, Mollaret cells are not always present—and even when they are, they usually disappear by the end of 24 hours. Shortly afterwards, the PMNs disappear in turn, to be replaced by lymphocytes. By the end of 3 or 4 days, only a few lymphocytes remain. Moderate increases in CSF protein are also common during attacks (usually 70–100 mg/dl, occasionally up to 250 mg/dl),[100] and increases in CSF gamma globulin and IgG and oligoclonal bands of IgG have been reported.[91–93,96,103,107] The CSF glucose is usually normal, but values as low as 30 mg/dl have been recorded.[91,94] Between attacks, the CSF is usually normal.

Most other investigations are normal, including the radionuclide brain scan, CT, cerebral angiography, and EEG.[94,96–98,100,101,105] Occasionally, the EEG has shown nonspecific slowing during attacks.[100,105]

During the initial attack, Mollaret's meningitis can be confused with acute bacterial or viral meningitis or meningoencephalitis, and then it may be necessary to prescribe antibiotics until cultures prove sterile. If present, Mollaret cells are a clue to the correct diagnosis, but they are not pathognomonic: apparently, identical cells have been seen in cases of herpes-simplex encephalitis,[106] parasellar tumor,[91] and posterior fossa epidermoid cyst.[108] Once the typical pattern of recurrence is established, Mollaret's meningitis must be differentiated from other causes of recurrent aseptic meningitis,[94] including recurrent viral meningitis, sarcoidasis, Behcet's syndrome, the uveomeningitic syndromes, hydatid cyst, and dermoid and epidermoid tumors; but the resemblance in most causes is only superficial. Repeated episodes of drug-induced meningitis should also be considered but can be ruled out by a careful history.

The best treatment for Mollaret's meningitis is not known, but the use of colchicine 0.5 mg two or three times daily as in RHP seems promising. At least four patients with Mollaret's meningitis and no other evidence of RHP have responded to colchocine therapy with fewer and less severe attacks,[109–103] as did one patient with associated renal amyloidosis.[98] Corticosteroids and antihistamines, on the other hand, appear to be ineffective.[97,102,104,107]

Sarcoidosis

Sarcoidosis is a chronic multisystem granulomatous disease of unknown etiology that most commonly affects young adults, particularly women and especially blacks.[109]

The characteristic pathologic change is the sarcoid granuloma, a noncaseating epithelioid-cell granuloma containing Langhans'-type giant cells and occasional central areas of fibrinoid necrosis. The organ systems most often affected are the lymph nodes, lungs, skin, and eyes. Less often involved are the liver, spleen, mucous membranes, salivary glands, bones, muscle, heart, and central and peripheral nervous systems.[109]

CNS involvement is found at autopsy in up to 14% of case[110]; granulomatous meningitis is the most common pathologic change.[111] Fibrosis, thickening, nodularity, and opacification of the meninges, particularly at the base of the brain, are typical, often enveloping the optic chiasm, cranial nerves, and spinal roots. Typical granulomas are present in the thickened meninges, are frequently perivascular, and can infiltrate the walls of pial and spinal arteries, causing infarction.[111–117] Granulomas are also present, either scattered or coalesced into nodules, in the parenchyma, particularly in the pituitary, hypothalamus, and floor of the third ventricle, but also in the cerebral cortex, cerebellum, brain stem, spinal cord, and nerve roots.[112,113,115–120] Hydrocephalus is common and results from granulomatous infiltration of the choroid and ependyma, brainstem or cerebellar lesions, or subarachnoid block from basal meningitis.[111,113,116,117,119–126] Less commonly, the granulomas coalesce to form large circumscribed mass lesions, either solitary or associated with meningeal or ependymal diseases elsewhere, and usually supratentorial in the cerebral hemispheres, but also in the pineal, brain system, cerebellum, ventricles, and spinal cord.[111,115,116,121,122,125,127,128] Similar coalescence of granulomas in the meninges results in the formation of large subdural plaques or either intradural extramedullary or extradural spinal lesions.[117,118] Finally, identical granulomas are also found in the PNS embedded along the nerve trunks.[111]

The clinical picture in sarcoidosis ranges from incidental asymptomatic radiographic abnormalities to severe disability, or even death, depending on the degree and site of tissue involvement. The onset may be acute or indolent. The lungs and intrathoracic lymph nodes are most commonly involved, sometimes without symptoms, but often causing chest discomfort, cough, dyspnea, and even respiratory failure and cor pulmonale. Other common signs and symptoms at onset are fever, iritis, erythema nodosum, and other skin lesions. Less common are hepatomegaly, splenomegaly, hypersplenism, lymphadenopathy, renal calculi, cardiac abnormalities, salivary-gland enlargement, muscle pain and weakness, and polyarthritis.[109]

Neurologic dysfunction occurs in 5% of cases[122,129] and is the presenting complaint in up to two thirds of these patients.[111,116,117,125,126,128,130] Most, but not all, of those who present with neurologic abnormalities will have other stigmata of sarcoid, usually hilar adenopathy or uveitis.[111,116,117,126,130] CNS abnormalities usually occur early in the course of the illness.[111] The most common abnormality is an acute or subacute meningoencephalitis which multiple cranial neuropathies and, less often, spinal-root abnormalities.[111,117,125,126,128,130–132]

Common CNS signs and symptoms include headache, confusion, mental and personality change, seizures, papilledema, focal motor weakness, spinal-cord syndromes, and ataxia. Cranial-nerve palsies are the most common abnormality—usually nerves II, VII (often bilateral), sensory V, and the acoustic portion of VIII, but any of the cranial nerves may be affected, often in multiples. Spinal meningeal involvement causes neck stiffness and root involvement mainly causes sensory symptoms. Coalescence of granulomas in the hypothalamus and pituitary causes abnormal thirst, diabetes insipidus, inappropriate secretion of antidiuretic hormone, and endocrine deficiencies. Large intracranial granulomas present as mass lesions.[127] Pure PNS abnormalities arise later, either as a mononeuritis multiplex or as a polyneuropathy.[111]

Typical laboratory abnormalities in sarcoidosis are mild anemia, leukopenia, elevated ESR, hypergammaglobulinemia, hypercalciuria and hypercalcemia, hyperuricemia, elevated serum levels of angiotensin-converting enzyme (ACE) and lysozyme, and skin-test hyporeactivity.[109] Chest radiographs show bilateral hilar adenopathy or parenchymal change, or both, in about 90% of cases, while pulmonary-function tests may be abnormal even if the chest x-ray is negative.[109] Since sarcoid granulomas avidly take up gallium, gallium scans may show accumulation of radiotracer in the lungs, and in other sites of active disease as well.[109,133]

The CSF is abnormal in up to 75% of neurologic cases.[111,114,115,117,125,126,130,131,134] The pressure is increased in 20%; as many as 70% have pleocytosis (up to 300 cells/mm^3, mainly lymphocytes); 70% have increased protein (usually less than 100 mg/dl, occasionally up to 2 g/dl); and 20% have hypoglycorrhachia (glucose as low as 15 mg/dl). Additional CSF abnormalities include increased gamma globulin, an elevated IgG index, and increased levels of ACE in the CSF.[135] The EEG is often nonspecifically abnormal because of generalized or focal slowing or spike and wave discharges.[117,126,128,130] Isotope brain scans are usually normal,[116,126] but a radionuclide scan in one case showed diffuse breakdown of the blood–brain barrier and uptake, suggesting ventriculitis.[123] CT–scan abnormalities are more common and include hydrocephalus; hypodense areas in the periventricular white matter, sometimes with contrast enhancement; diffuse contrast enhancement of the cerebral hemispheres; noncalcified hyperdense intraparenchymal mass lesions with homogeneous postcontrast enhancement; mass lesions with uneven enhancement and marked white-matter edema; and dense symmetric enhancement in the basal meninges.[113,116–118,122,–127,136] In cases of large intraparenchymal granuloma, angiograms show an avascular mass. [116–118,121,125,127,128] In a few patients with meningoencephalitis, angiography has shown multiple short segments of narrowing alternating with dilated segments, suggesting vasculopathy.[120,125] MRI seems most sensitive: in one series, abnormalities were detected in all 14 patients studied.[122] These abnormalities were usually hyperintense on T_2-weighted images and were basilar, periventricular, periaqueductal, convexity (meningeal), and hemispheric. Myelography in cases of spinal-cord involvement has shown arachnoiditis with or without partial subarachnoid block, intradural extramedullary mass lesions, and cord swelling.[111,116,118] Peripheral-nerve involvement is reflected in slowed nerve-conduction velocity and denervation potentials.[128] Endocrine abnormalities and renal concentrating defects may be demonstrated when the pituitary and hypothalamus are infiltrated.

Aseptic meningitis in sarcoidosis can begin acutely and then mimic viral and other acute lymphocytic meningitides. Sarcoid meningoencephalitis is more often subacute or chronic and then mimics tuberculosus and fungal meningitis, syphilis, and Lyme disease, among others. When neurologic abnormalities appear in the course of known sarcoidosis, the diagnosis is straightforward, but superimposed opportunistic infection should still be ruled out as the incidence of both cryptococcosis and tuberculosis is increased in sarcoidosis.[131] In other cases, neurologic abnormalities are the presenting feature but are accompanied by symptoms from other organ systems. These symptoms, plus typical laboratory and radiographic abnormalities of sarcoidosis, are clues to the diagnosis. Those tests particularly useful in identifying disease outside the nervous system are the chest x-ray, eye and skin examinations, nerve-conduction studies, endocrine-function tests, and gallium scan. When disease is confined to the nervous system, a presumptive diagnosis is made by exclusion; the demonstration of meningeal granulomas by biopsy is not specific.[131] In such cases, hypothalamic or pituitary dysfunction and simultaneous CNS and PNS disease are clues. Definite diagnosis, however, requires clinical or radiographic evidence of the involvement of more than one organ system plus histologic evidence of widespread granulomas. Lymph nodes, skin lesions, minor salivary glands, liver, lung, and muscle are all appropriate sites for biopsy,[109] and a gallium scan may help to pinpoint those most suitable. Biopsy at the site of injected Kveim antigen has also been used to diagnose CNS sarcoidosis.[116,117,126]

The course of nervous-system sarcoidosis is often benign, with spontaneous remission in many cases, particularly in those with cranial or peripheral-nerve involvement and in those with the acute monophasic form of neurologic disease.[126] The outcome in cases with CNS involvement and in those that are chronically progressive or remitting and relapsing is less good, and persisting abnormalities are common.[126] Corticosteroids are felt to be the treatment of choice in sarcoidosis,[111,117,126–128,130,132] although their use has not been subjected to a controlled trial, and spontaneous improvement does take place. Moderate doses (30–40 mg prednisone daily) should be prescribed initially and tapered as disease activity permits. Treatment should be continued for at least six to 12 months. Surgery should be considered in patients with hydrocephalus and those with large solitary intracranial granulomas unresponsive to steroids.[118,128]

Chemical Meningitis

Chemical meningitis is an acute, sterile meningeal inflammation that has been reported following both spinal[137–140] and epidural[141] anesthesia, lumbar puncture,[142] pneumoencephalography,[143] isotope cisternography,[144–146] myelography with both lipid and water-soluble contrast agents,[147–154] intracranial surgery (especially posterior fossa surgery in children),[155,156] and the intrathecal injection of cytosine arabinoside,[157] methotrexate,[158,159] and methylprednisolone acetate.[157,160–162]

In contrast to chronic adhesive arachnoiditis, which may follow many of the same antecedents,[163] acute chemical meningitis is self-limited and its pathology is not known. In some cases, the injected material itself or its diluent[157,160] is at fault. In others, contaminants are probably responsible: detergents and disinfectants on inadequately rinsed glass syringes,[137,138,140,153] bacterial endotoxins in radioisotopes,[146] and starch powder from surgical gloves.[156]

Symptoms begin acutely, usually four to 24 hours after intrathecal injection or operation, with fever up to 40.2°C, headache, nausea, vomiting, photophobia, neck stiffness, and, occasionally, leg pain.[137,162] In some cases, there is accompanying irritability, confusion, disorientation, lethargy, delirium, obtundation, and even seizures and coma.[142,144,148,150,151,158,161] Both Kernig's and Brudzinski's signs may be present, but there are seldom other physical signs aside from neck stiffness and fever. The symptoms and signs resolve spontaneously within 2 to 4 days, although occasional cases are more protracted,[145,156,161] and fever may persist for days to weeks in children after posterior fossa surgery.[155]

Leukocytosis of up to 17,800 cells/mm^3 has been reported,[137,142,144,148,154] but other routine laboratory tests are usually normal. The CSF pressure may be increased (up to 275 mm CSF),[144,154] and there is always a pleocytosis.[137–162] PMNs predominate, and cell counts often reach several thousand/mm^3 (range, 150–50,000; usually 1,000–3,000). The CSF protein is increased to 100–800 mg/dl, and hypoglycorrhacia is common (glucose as low as 4 mg/dl).[137,144,151,153–155,162] Like the clinical findings, the CSF abnormalities resolve spontaneously: the CSF usually returns to normal within 3 to 7 days.

Acute chemical meningitis must be differentiated from acute bacterial meningitis caused by contamination of the CSF at the time of lumbar puncture or surgery. Symptoms of nosocomial bacterial meningitis often begin later, 24–96 hours after intraspinal procedures.[151] But neither the timing of symptoms nor the results of a CSF Gram stain (positive in only 60% of cases of postmyelographic bacterial meningitis)[164] are adequate to rule out infection, and broad-spectrum antibiotics should be prescribed until the results of CSF cultures are known. No other treatment is usually necessary, although corticosteroids may suppress symptoms in postsurgical cases.[155]

Cyst Rupture

Another, less common variety of chemical meningitis results from the spontaneous, posttraumatic, or intraoperative rupture and spillage of the contents of certain cystic CNS tumors into the CSF: craniopharyngiomas, dermoids, and epidermoids.[108,165–173] All three originate from embryonic rests of epithelial cells within the nervous system, and all three contain desquamated epithelial cells, keratin, fatty material, and cholesterol.[168,169] Among these, keratin is probably most responsible for the meningeal inflammation.[166,168]

Pathologic changes range from mild leptomeningitis to widespread granulomatous inflammation throughout the meninges, ependyma, and subarachnoid space infiltrating cranial- and spinal-nerve roots and around blood vessels, and causing secondary cerebellar degeneration and dorsal-column demyelination.[168,173]

The onset is acute, with fever, headache, nausea, vomiting, photophobia, neck stiffness, and sometimes lethargy, confusion, or convulsions.[108,165–172] Kernig's and Brudzinski's signs may be present, as may a dermal sinus or focal signs of an intracranial or intraspinal mass. The meningeal symptoms and signs typically resolve over days to three weeks, but the attacks may be recurrent,[108,166,170,171] hydrocephalus may develop,[171] and chronic dementia and amyotrophy with parkinsonian features have been reported.[173]

Routine laboratory tests are normal. The CSF pressure may be increased to over 300 mm CSF,[169] and pleocytosis (up to 24,000 cells/mm^3, mainly PMNs) and increased protein (up to 850 mg/dl) are always present.[108,166–172] Hypoglycorrhachia is common and sometimes profound (as low as 6 mg/dl).[108,168–171] Fat droplets may be visible in the CSF,[169] and birefringent keratin may be identified by polarized microscopy.[168]

Confusion with acute bacterial meningitis is likely. However, chemical meningitis from cyst rupture can be suspected when a CT scan shows an intracranial cyst or when signs of cauda equina or conus dysfunction are present, suggesting an intraspinal cyst. Once suspected on clinical or radiologic grounds, the diagnosis can be confirmed by polarized microscopy of the CSF.[166] Nonetheless, antibiotics may still be necessary until cultures prove negative, particularly in postoperative cases and in those in which the presence of a dermal sinus suggests a portal of entry for bacteria. Recurrent cases may suggest Mollaret's meningitis among others, but CT should again suggest the correct diagnosis, as it should in the rare chronic case, and yet the cyst may remain undetected for years.[108]

The meningitis usually resolves spontaneously in days to weeks, although corticosteroids may speed recovery.[166,168,169] Successful removal of the cyst is curative.

References

1. Bernstein RF: Ibuprofen-related meningitis in mixed connective tissue disease. *Ann Intern Med* 1980; 92:206–207.
2. Bouland DL, Specht, NL, Hegstad DR: Ibuprofen and aseptic meningitis. *Ann Intern Med* 1986; 104:731.
3. Durback MA, Freeman J, Schumacher HR: Recurrent ibuprofen-induced aseptic meningitis: third episode after only 200mg of generic ibuprofen. *Arthritis Rheum* 1988;31:813–815.
4. Jensen S, Glud TK, Bacher T, et al: Ibuprofen-induced meningitis in a male with systemic lupus erythematosus. *Acta Med Scand* 1987;221:509–511.
5. Katona BG, Wigley FM, Walters JK, et al: Aseptic meningitis from over-the-counter ibuprofen. *Lancet* 1988;1:59.
6. Lawson JM, Grady MJ: Ibuprofen-induced aseptic meningitis in a previously healthy patient. *West J Med* 1985;143:386–387.
7. Quinn JP, Weinstein RA, Caplan LR: Eosinophilic meningitis and ibuprofen therapy. *Neurology* 1984; 34:108–109.
8. Widener HL, Littman BH: Ibuprofen-induced meningitis in systemic lupus erythematosus. *JAMA* 1978;239:1062–1064.
9. Sylvia LM, Forlenza SW, Brocavich JM: Aseptic meningitis associated with naproxen. *Drug Intell Clin Pharmacol* 1988;22:399–401.
10. Ballas ZK, Donta ST: Sulindac-induced aseptic meningitis *Arch Intern Med* 1982;142:165–166.
11. Von Reyn CF: Recurrent aseptic meningitis due to sulindac. *Ann Intern Med* 1983;99:343–344.
12. Ruppert GB, Barth WF: Tolmetin-induced aseptic meningitis. *JAMA* 1981;245:67–68.
13. Barrett PVD, Thier SO: Meningitis and pancreatitis associated with sulfamethizole. *N Engl J Med* 1963;268:36–37.
14. Carlson J, Wiholm B-E: Trimethoprim associated aseptic meningitis. *Scand J Infect Dis* 1987;19:687–691.
15. Derbes SJ: Trimethoprim-induced aseptic meningitis. *JAMA* 1984;252:2865–2866.
16. Haas EJ: Trimethoprim-sulfamethoxazole: another cause of recurrent meningitis. *JAMA* 1984;252:346.
17. Kremer I, Ritz R, Brunner F. Aseptic meningitis as an adverse effect of co-trimoxazole. *N Engl J Med* 1983;308:1481.
18. Streiffer RH, Hudson JG: Aseptic meningitis and trimethoprim-sulfamethoxazole. *J Fam Pract* 1986; 23:314.
19. Garagusi VF, Neefe LI, Mann O: Acute meningoencephalitis: association with isoniazid administration. *JAMA* 1976:235:1141–1142.
20. Herlihy TE: Phenazopyridine and aseptic meningitis. *Ann Intern Med* 1987;106:172–173.
21. Sergent JS, Lockshin MD, Klempner MS, et al: Central nervous system disease in systemic lupus erythematosus: therapy and prognosis. *Am J Med* 1975;58:644–654.
22. Sergent JS, Lockshin M. Azathioprine-induced meningitis in systemic lupus erythematosus. *JAMA* 1978;240:529.
23. Thordarson H, Talstad I: Acute meningitis and cerebellar dysfunction complicating high-dose cytosine arabinoside therapy. *Acta Med Scand* 1986;220: 493–495
24. Berliner S. Weinberger A, Shoenfeld Y, et al: Ibuprofen may induce meningitis in (NZB× NZW) F2 mice. *Arthritis Rheum* 1985;28:104–107.
25. Mandell BF, Raps EC: Severe systemic hypersensitivity reaction to ibuprofen occurring after prolonged therapy. *Am J Med* 1987;82:817–820.
26. Naguwa SM, Nelson BL: Human serum sickness. *Clin Rev Allergy* 1985;3:117–126.
27. Erffmeyer JE: Serum sickness. *Ann Allergy* 1986; 56:105–109.
28. Nadeau SE, Watson RE: Neurologic manifestations of vasculitis and collagen vascular syndromes, in Joynt RJ, (ed.). *Clinical Neurology*, vol 4. Philadelphia, Harper & Row, 1988, ch 59.
29. Cochrane CG, Dixon FJ: Immune complex injury, in Samter M (ed): *Immunological Diseases*. vol 1. ed 3. Boston, Little Brown & Co., 1978, pp. 210–229.
30. Krajewski S, Szablowska-Krajewski M. Disseminated vasculomyelinopathy in the peripheral nervous system mediated by immune complexes (ICs). *J. Neurol Sci* 1986;72:131–145.
31. Kraus WM, Chaney L: Serum disease of the nervous system. *Arch Neurol Psychiatry* 1937;37:1035–1047.
32. Miller HG: Clinical manifestations of tissue reactions in the nervous system, in Williams D (ed): *Modern Trends in Neurology* (2nd series). London, Butterworth, 1957; pp. 164–176.

33. Park AM, Richardson JC: Cerebral complications of serum sickness. *Neurology* 1953;3:277–283.
34. Iqbal A, Arnason BGW: Neuropathy of serum sickness, in Dyck PJ, Thomas PK, Lambert EH, et al (eds): *Peripheral Neuropathy,* vol 2., ed 2. Philadelphia, Saunders, 1984, pp 2044–2049.
35. Lawley TM, Bielory L, Gascon P, et al: A prospective clinical and immunological analysis of patients with serum sickness. *N Engl J Med* 1984;311:1407–1413.
36. Delavergne V, Abel E: Des modifications de liquide cephalorachidienne au cours des reactions seriques. *Bull Soc Med Paris* 1926;50:488–490.
37. Kilpatrick JM, Pitt A, Allen S, et al: Treatment of acute serum sickness by plasma ultrafiltration. *Am J Med Sci* 1987;293:75–84.
38. Moore PM, Cupps TR: Neurological complications of vasculitis. *Ann Neurol* 1983;14:155–167.
39. Reik L: Disorders that mimic CNS infections. *Neurol Clin* 1986;4:223–248.
40. Sigal LH: The neurologic presentation of vasculitic and rheumatologic syndromes: a review. *Medicine* 1987;66:157–180.
41. Calabrese LH, Mallek JA: Primary angiitis of the central nervous system: report of 8 new cases, review of the literature, and proposal for diagnostic criteria. *Medicine* 1987;67:20–39.
42. Hughes JT, Brownell B: Granulomatous giant-celled angiitis of the central nervous system. *Neurology* 1966;16:293–298.
43. Kolodny EH, Rebeiz JJ, Caviness VS, et al: Granulomatous angiitis of the central nervous system. *Arch Neurol* 1968;19:510–524.
44. Harrison PE: Granulomatous angiitis of the central nervous system. *J. Neurol Sci* 1976;29:335–341.
45. Case records of the Massachusetts General Hospital. *N Engl J Med* 1989;320:514–525.
46. Reik L: Granulomatous angiitis presenting as chronic meningitis and ventriculitis. *Neurology* 1983;33:1609–1612.
47. Moore PM: Diagnosis and management of isolated angiitis of the central nervous system. *Neurology* 1989;39:167–173.
48. Miller DH, Ormerod IEC, Gibson A: MR brain scanning in patients with vasculitis: differentiation from multiple sclerosis. *Neuroradiology* 1987;29: 226–231.
49. Younger DS, Hays AP, Booss JCM, et al: Granulomatous angiitis of the brain: an inflammatory reaction of diverse etiology. *Arch Neurol* 1988;45:514–518.
50. Cupps TR, Moore PM, Fauci AS: Isolated angiitis of the central nervous system. *Am J Med* 1983; 74:97–106.
51. Adelman DC, Saltiel E, Klienberg JR: Neuropsychiatric manifestations of systemic lupus erythematosus: an overview. *Semin Arthritis Rheum* 1986; 15:185–199.
52. McCune WJ, Bolbus J: Neuropsychiatric lupus. *Rheum Dis Clin North Am* 1988;14(1):149–168.
53. Devinsky O, Petits CK, Alonso DR: Clinical and neuropathological findings in system lupus erythematosus: the role of vasculitis, heart emboli, and thrombocytopenic purpura. *Ann Neurol* 1988;23: 380–384.
54. Johnson RT, Richardson EP: The neurological manifestations of systemic lupus erythematosus: a clinico-pathological study of 24 cases and review of the literature. *Medicine (Baltimore)* 1968;47:337–369.
55. Ellis SG, Veirty MA: Central nervous system involvement in systemic lupus erythematosus: a review of neuropathologic findings in 57 cases. *Semin Arthritis Rheum* 1979;8:212–221.
56. Steinberg AD, Klinman DM: Pathogenesis of systemic lupus erythematosus. *Rheum Dis Clin North Am* 1988;14(1):25–42.
57. Zuailfler NJ, Bluestein HG: The pathogenesis of central nervous system manifestations of systemic lupus erythematosus. *Arthritis Rheum* 1982;25:861–866.
58. Keefe EB, Bardana EJ, Hanbeck RJ, et al: Lupus meningitis. *Ann Intern Med* 1974;80:58–60.
59. Hadler NM, Gerwin RD, Frank MM, et al: The fourth component of complement in the cerebrospinal fluid in systemic lupus erythematosus. *Arthritis Rheum* 1973;16:507–521.
60. Feinglass EJ, Arnett FC, Dorsch CA, et al: Neuropsychiatric manifestations of systemic lupus erythematosus: diagnosis, clinical spectrum, and relationship to other features of the disease. *Medicine (Baltimore)* 1976;55:323–339.
61. Vermess M, Bernstein RM, Bydder GM, et al: Nuclear magnetic imaging (NMR) of the brain in systemic lupus erythematosus. *J Comput Assist Tomogr* 1983;7:461–467.
62. Liebow AA, Carrington CRB, Friedman PJ: Lymphomatoid granulomatosis. *Hum Pathol* 1972;3: 457–558.
63. Katzenstein AL, Carrington CB, Liebow AA: Lymphomatoid granulomatosis: a clinicopathologic study of 152 cases. *Cancer* 1979;43:360–373.
64. Fauci AS, Haynes BF, Costa J, et al: Lymphomatoid granulomatosis: prospective clinical and therapeutic experience over 10 years. *N Engl J Med* 1982;306:68–74.
65. Patton WF, Lynch JP: Lymphomatoid granulomatosis: clinicopathologic study of four cases and literature review. *Medicine (Baltimore)* 1982;61:1–11.
66. Schmidt BJ, Meagher-Villemure K, Del Carpio J. Lymphomatoid granulomatosis with isolated involvement of brain. *Ann Neurol* 1984;15:478–481.
67. Kokman E, Billman JK, Abell MR: Lymphomatoid

granulomatosis clinically confined to CNS. *Arch Neurol* 1977;34:782–784.
68. DeRemae RA, Weiland LH, McDonald TJ. Polymorphic reticulosis and lymphomatoid granulomatosis: two diseases or one? *Mayo Clin Proc* 1978;53:634–640.
69. Bone RC, Vernon M, Sobonya R, et al: Lymphomatoid granulomatosis: report of a case and review of the literature. *Am J Med* 1978;65:709–715.
70. Chajek T, Fainaro M. Behcet's disease: report of 41 cases and a review of the literature. *Medicine (Baltimore)* 1975;54:179–195.
71. O'Duffy JD, Goldstein NP: Neurologic involvement in seven patients with Behcet's disease. *Am J Med* 1976; 61:170–178.
72. Shimuza T, Ekolich GE, Inaba G, et al: Behcet disease (Behcet syndrome). *Semin Arthritis Rheum* 1979;8:223–260.
73. Wolff SM, Schotland DL, Phillips LL: Involvement of nervous system in Behcet's syndrome. *Arch Neurol* 1965;12:315–324.
74. McMenemey WH, Lawrence BJ: Encephalomyelopathy in Behcet's disease: report of necropsy findings in two cases. *Lancet* 1957;2:353–358.
75. James DG: "Silk route disease" (Behcet's disease). *West J Med* 1988;148:433–437.
76. Lee S, Kim DH, Bang D, et al: Immunological aspects of the four types of Behcet's syndrome, in Lehner T, Barnes CG (eds): *Recent Advances in Behcet's Disease*. Royal Society of Medicine Services International Congress and Symposium Series no. 103. London, Royal Society of Medicine Services Ltd, 1986; pp 47–50.
77. Mizuskima Y: Recent research into Behcet's disease in Japan. *Int J Tissue React* 1988;10:59–65.
78. Gramble CN, Weigner KB, Shapiro RE: The immune complex pathogenesis of glomerulonephritis and pulmonary vasculitis in Behcet disease. *Am J Med* 1979;66:1031–1039.
79. Wilhelm C, Ellner JJ: Chronic meningitis. *Neurol Clin* 1986;4:115–141.
80. Herskowitz S, Lipton RB, Lantos G: Neuro-Behcet's disease: CT and clinical correlates. *Neurology* 1988;38:1714–1720.
81. Pamir MN, Kansu T, Erbengi A, et al: Papilledema in Behcet's syndrome. *Arch Neurol* 1981;38:643–645.
82. Serdaroglu P, Yaziei H. Ozdemir C, et al: Neurologic involvement in Behcet's syndrome: a prospective study. *Arch Neurol* 1989;46:265–269.
83. Willeit J, Schmutzhand F, Aichner U, et al: CT and MR imaging in neuro-Behcet disease: case report. *J Comput Assist Tomogr* 1986;10:313–315.
84. Pattison EM: Uveomeningoencephalitis syndrome (Vogt-Koyanagi-Harada). *Arch Neurol* 1965;12: 197–205.
85. Rield JL, Andrews J: The uveomeningoencephalitis syndrome. *Neurology* 1966;16:603–609.
86. Ohno S, Char DH, Kimura SJ, et al: Vogt-Koyanagi-Harada syndrome. *Am J Ophthalmol* 1977;83:735–740.
87. Sugiura S: Vogt-Koyanagi-Harada disease. *Jpn J Opthalmol* 1978;22:9–35.
88. Reed H, Lindsay A, Silversides JL, et al: The uveoencephalitic syndrome or Vogt-Koyanagi-Harada disease. *Can Med Assoc J* 1958;79:451–459.
89. Chan C: Relationship between sympathetic ophthalmia, phacoanaphylactic endophthalmitis, and Vogt-Koyanagi-Harada disease. *Ophthalmology* 1988; 95:619–624.
90. Ohoro S: Vogt-Koyanagi-Harada's disease, in Saari KM (ed): *Uveitis Update*, Proceedings of the First International Symposium on Uveitis, Hanasaari, Espoo Finland, May 16–19, 1984. Amsterdam, Excerpta Medica, 1984, pp. 401–405.
91. Bruyn GW, Straathof LJA: La meningite endothelio-leucocytaire multirecurrente benigne de Mollaret. *Presse Med* 1961;69:1741–1743.
92. Fredericks JAM, Bruyn KW: Mollaret's meningitis, in Vinken PJ, Bruyn GW (eds): *Handbook of Clinical Neurology*, vol 34. Amsterdam, North-Holland Publishing Co., 1978, pp 545–52.
93. Galdi AP: Benign recurrent aseptic meningitis (Mollaret's meningitis). *Arch Neurol* 1979;36:657–658.
94. Hermans PE, Goldstein NP, Wellman WE: Mollaret's meningitis and differential diagnosis of recurrent meningitis: report of a case and review of the literature. *Am J Med* 1972;52:128–140.
95. Mollaret P: Benign recurrent pleocytic meningitis and its presumed causative virus. *J. Nerv Ment Dis* 1952;116:1072–1080.
96. Steel JG, Dix RD, Baringer JR: Isolation of herpes simplex virus type I in recurrent (Mollaret) meningitis. *Ann Neurol* 1982;11:17–21.
97. George RB, Westfall RE: Periodic meningitis: an unusual manifestation of periodic disease. *Ann Intern Med* 1965;62:778–785.
98. Vilaseca J, Tor J, Guardia J, et al: Periodic meningitis and familial Mediterranean fever. *Arch Intern Med* 1982;142:378–379.
99. Barakat MH, Mustafa HT, Shakir RA: Mollaret's meningitis: a variant of recurrent hereditary polyserositis, both provoked by metaraminol. *Arch Neurol* 1988;45:926–927.
100. Swithinbank IM, Rake MO: A case of Mollaret's meningitis associated with a lymphoma. *Postgrad Med J* 1978;54:682–685.
101. Mascia RA, Smith CW Jr: Mollaret's meningitis: an unusual disease with a characteristic presentation. *Am J Med Sci* 1984;287:52–53.
102. Gledhill RF, Lewis PD, Marsden CD, et al: Is Mol-

laret's meningitis another periodic disorder responsive to colchicine? *Lancet* 1975;2:415.

103. Mora JS, Gimeno A: Mollaret meningitis: report of a case with recovery after colchicine. *Ann Neurol* 1980;8:631–633.
104. Haynes BF, Wright R, McCracken JP. Mollaret meningitis: a report of three cases. *JAMA* 1976; 236:1967–1969.
105. Iivanainen M: Benign recurrent aseptic meningitis of unknown etiology (Mollaret's meningitis). *Acta Neurol Scand* 1973;49:133–138.
106. Tyler KL, Adler D: Twenty-eight years of benign recurring Mollaret's meningitis. *Arch Neurol* 1983; 40:42–43.
107. Kinnman J, Kam-Hansen S, Link H, et al: Studies on the humoral and cell-mediated immune response in a patient with Mollaret's meningitis. *J Neurol Sci* 1979;43:265–275.
108. Chadarevian JP, Becker WJ: Mollaret's recurrent aseptic meningitis: relationship to epidermoid cysts. *J. Neuropathol Exp Neurol* 1980;39:661–669.
109. Winterbauer RH: Sarcoidosis, in Petersdorf RG, Adams RD, Braunwald E, et al (eds): *Harrison's Principles of Internal Medicine,* ed 10. New York, McGraw-Hill Book Co., 1983, pp 1248–1253.
110. Richer W, Clark M: Sarcoidosis: a clinicopathologic review of 300 cases, including 22 autopsies. *Am J Clin Pathol* 1949;19:725–749.
111. Delaney P: Neurological manifestations in sarcoidosis: review of the literature with a report of 23 cases. *Ann Intern Med* 1977;87:336–345.
112. Camp WA, Frierson JG: Sarcoidosis of the central nervous system: a case with postmortem studies. *Arch Neurol* 1962;7:432–441.
113. Cordingley G, Navarro C, Brust JCM, et al: Sarcoidosis presenting as senile dementia. *Neurology* 1981;31:1148–1151.
114. Douglas AC, Maloney AFJ: Sarcoidosis of the central nervous system. *J Neurol Neurosurg Psychiatry* 1973;36:1024–1033.
115. Gaines JD, Eckman PB, Remington JS: Low CSF glucose level in sarcoidosis involving the central nervous system. *Arch Intern Med* 1970;125:333–336.
116. Kendall BE, Tatler GLV: Radiological findings in neurosarcoidosis. *Br J Radiol* 1978;51:81–92.
117. Stern BJ, Krumholz A, Jones C, et al: Sarcoidosis and its neurological manifestations. *Arch Neurol* 1985;42:909–814.
118. Cahill DW, Salcman M: Neurosarcoidosis: a review of the rarer manifestations. *Surg Neurol* 1981;15: 204–211.
119. Dickinson ES: Sarcoid meningoencephalitis: diagnostic difficulties encountered in two cases. *Dis Nerv Syst* 1971;32:118–124.
120. Lawrence WP, El Gammal T, Pool WH Jr., et al: Radiological manifestations of neurosarcoidosis: report of three cases and review of literature. *Clin Radiol* 1974;25:343–348.
121. Bahr AL, Krumholz A, Kristt D, et al: Neuroradiological manifestations of intracranial sarcoidosis. *Radiology* 1978;127:713–717.
122. Hayes WS, Sherman JL, Stern BJ, et al: MR and CT evaluation of intracranial sarcoidosis. *AJR* 1987; 149:1043–1049.
123. Ho SU, Berenberg RA, Kim KS, et al: Sarcoid encephalopathy with diffuse inflammation and focal hydrocephalus shown by sequential CT. *Neurology* 1979;29:1161–1165.
124. Morehouse H, Danziger A: CT findings in intracranial neurosarcoid. *Comput Tomogr* 1980;4: 267–370.
125. Oksanen V: Neurosarcoidosis: clinical presentations and course in 50 patients. *Acta Neurol Scand* 1986;73:283–290.
126. Pentland B, Mitchell JD, Cull RE, et al: Central nervous system sarcoidosis. *Q J Med* 1985;56:457–465.
127. Powers WJ, Miller EM: Sarcoidosis mimicking glioma: case report and review of intracranial sarcoid mass lesions. *Neurology* 1981;31:907–910.
128. Silverstein A, Feuer MM, Siltzbach LE: Neurologic sarcoidosis: study of 18 cases. *Arch Neurol* 1965; 12:1–11.
129. Siltzbach LE, James DG, Neville E, et al: Course and prognosis of sarcoidosis around the world. *Am J Med* 1974;57:847–852.
130. Wiederholt WC, Siekert RG: Neurological manifestations of sarcoidosis. *Neurology* 15:1147–1154.
131. Ellner JJ, Bennett JE: Chronic meningitis. *Medicine* 1976;55:341–369.
132. Matthews WB: Sarcoidosis of the nervous system. *J Neurol Neurosurg Psychiatry* 1965;28:23–29.
133. Gupta RG, Bekerman C, Sicilian L, et al: Gallium 67 citrate scanning and serum angiotensin converting enzyme levels in sarcoidosis. *Radiology* 1982; 144:895–899.
134. Colover J: Sarcoidosis with involvement of the nervous system. *Brain* 1948;71:451–475.
135. Oksanen V, Grönhagen-Riska C, Fyhrquist F, et al: Systemic manifestations and enzyme studies in sarcoidosis with neurologic involvement. *Acta Med Scand* 1985;218:123–127.
136. Weisberg LA, Jacobs L: Clinical and computed tomography findings in intracranial sarcoidosis involving the juxtasellar region. *Comput Radiol* 1984;8:107–111.
137. Austin DA, Sokolowski JW: Postlumbar puncture chemical meningitis. *NY State J Med* 1968;68:2444–2446.
138. Bert AA, Laasberg LH: Aseptic meningitis following spinal anesthesia—a complication of the past? *Anesthesiology* 1985;62:674–677.
139. Backer-Gröndahl N: Recherches sur les alterations

dans le liquide rachidien apres rachianesthesie. *Acta Chir Scand* 1934;73:485–499.
140. Winkelman NW: Neurologic symptoms following accidental intraspinal detergent injection. *Neurology* 1952;2:284–291.
141. Jenicek JA: Aseptic meningitis following lumbar epidural block: case report. *Anesthesiology* 1955; 16:464–472.
142. Reynolds KE, Wilson G: Aseptic meningitis following diagnostic lumbar puncture. *JAMA* 1934; 102:1460–1462.
143. Bickerstaff ER: Changes in the cerebrospinal fluid after pneumoencephalography. *Lancet* 1951;1: 1209–1210.
144. Barnes B, Fish M: Chemical meningitis as a complication of isotope cisternography. *Neurology* 1972;22:83–91.
145. Nicol C: A second case of aseptic meningitis following isotope cisternography using I^{131} human serum albumin. *Neurology* 1967;17:199–200.
146. Rhodes BA, Kamanetz GS, Wagner HN Jr: The use of Limulus testing to reduce the incidence of adverse reactions to cisternographic agents. *Neurology* 1974;24:810–812.
147. Broadbridge AT, Bayliss SG, Brayshaw CI: The effect of intrathecal iohexol on visual evoked response latency: a comparison including incidence of headache with iopamidol and metrizamide in myeloradiculography. *Clin Radiol* 1987;38:71–74.
148. DiMario FJ: Aseptic meningitis secondary to metrizamide lumbar myelography in a 4½-month-old infant. *Pediatrics* 1985;76:259–262.
149. Gelmers HJ: Adverse side effects of metrizamide in myelography. *Neuroradiology* 1979;18:119–123.
150. Gelmers HJ: Exacerbation of systemic lupus erythematosus, aseptic meningitis and acute mental symptoms, following metrizamide lumbar myelography. *Neuroradiology* 1984;26:65–66.
151. Sand T, Anda S, Hellum K, et al: Chemical meningitis in metrizamide myelography: a report of seven cases. *Neuroradiology* 1986;28:69–71.
152. Tarlov IM: Pantopaque meningitis disclosed at operation. *JAMA* 1945;129:1014–1016.
153. Vik-Mo H, Maurer H-J: Meningeal reactions following myelography: effects of detergent washing agents. *Acta Radiol (Diag)* 1975;16:39–42.
154. White WB: Metrizamide meningitis. *South Med J* 1984;77:88–89.
155. Carmel PW, Fraser RAR, Stein BM: Aseptic meningitis following posterior fossa surgery in children. *J. Neurosurg* 1974;41:44–48.
156. Dunkley B, Lewis TT: Meningeal reaction to starch powder in the cerebrospinal fluid. *Br Med J* 1977;2:1391–1392.
157. Band PR, Holland JF, Bernard J, et al: Treatment of central nervous system leukemia with intrathecal cytosine arabinoside. *Cancer* 1973;32:744–748.
158. Mott Mg, Stevenson P, Wood CBS: Methotrexate meningitis. *Lancet* 1972;2:656.
159. Weiss HD, Walker MD, Wiernik PH: Neurotoxicity of commonly used antineoplastic agents. *N Engl J Med* 1974;291:75–81.
160. Nelson DA: Dangers from methyeprednisolone acetate therapy by intraspinal injection. *Arch Neurol* 1988;45:804–806.
161. Nelson DA, Vates TS Jr., Thomas RB Jr: Complications from intrathecal steroid therapy in patients with multiple sclerosis. *Acta Neurol Scand* 1973; 49:176–188.
162. Plumb VJ, Dismukes WE: Chemical meningitis related to intrathecal corticosteroid therapy. *South Med J* 1977;70:1241–1243.
163. Whisler WW: Chronic spinal arachnoiditis, in Vinken PJ, Bruyn GW (eds): *Handbook of Neurology*, vol 33. Amsterdam, North-Holland, 1978, pp 263–274.
164. Schelkun SR, Wagner KF, Blanks JA, et al: Bacterial meningitis following pantopaque myelography: a case report and literature review. *Orthopedics* 1985;8:73–76.
165. Arseni C, Nash F: Epidermoid tumors of the brain. *Confin Neurol* 1959;19:442–453.
166. Cantu RC, Wright RL: Aseptic meningitic syndrome with cauda equina epidermoid tumor. *J. Pediatr* 1986;73:114–116.
167. Decker RE, Gross SW: Intraspinal dermoid tumor presenting as chemical meningitis: report of a case without dermal sinus. *J. Neurosurg* 1967;27:60–62.
168. De Klerk OJJ, Spence J: Chemical meningitis with intracranial tumors. *S Afr Med J* 1974;48:131–135.
169. Patrick BS, Smith RR, Bailey TO: Aseptic meningitis due to spontaneous rupture of craniopharyngioma cyst: case report. *J Neurosurg* 1974;41:387–390.
170. Roberts AP: A case of intracranial dermoid cyst associated with Klippel-Feil deformity and recurrent meningitis. *Arch Dis Child* 1958;33:222–225.
171. Schwartz JF, Balentine JD: Recurrent meningitis due to an intracranial dermoid. *Neurology* 1978; 28:124–129.
172. Schwartz MN, Dodge PR: Bacterial meningitis—a review of selected aspects. I. General clinical features, special problems and unusual meningeal reactions mimicking bacterial meningitis. *N Engl J Med* 1965;272:898–902.
173. Tomlinson BE, Walton JN: Granulomatous meningitis and diffuse parenchymatous degeneration of the nervous system due to an intracranial epidermoid cyst. *J Neurol Neurosurg Psychiatry* 1967;30:341–348.

Part II
Brain—Diffuse and Focal Processes

8
Brain Abscess and Related Focal Intracranial Suppuration

Richard T. Sokolov, Jr. and Richard D. Meyer

Brain Abscess

Abscesses may form in brain parenchyma as a result either of metastatic spread from infection elsewhere in the body or of contiguous spread from structures in close proximity, such as the paranasal sinuses, ears, and nose. Trauma and surgical procedures may introduce infectious agents to vulnerable cerebral tissue. Since brain abscess is a curable condition, prompt recognition of predisposing factors and knowledge of the varied clinical presentations, as well as of the diagnostic and therapeutic approaches, are essential for cure.

Abscesses in the brain substance are frequently sequelae of disease elsewhere in the body. Organisms may be directly implanted in brain parenchyma as a result of trauma, by spread of pyogenic infections in the head and neck, or by hematogenous spread from distant sites such as the heart, lungs, or distal bones.[1,2] Bacterial endocarditis may give rise to cerebral emboli, but usually does so in a "miliary" pattern of multiple abscesses as opposed to single, large space-occupying lesions.[2] History and physical examination may indicate the etiology of intracranial infection in the majority of patients.[1] Early institution of appropriate therapy is a critical determinant of outcome.

Incidence

An understanding of the incidence of brain abscess and the patients at risk requires an appreciation of the predisposing conditions. Harrison[1] described in a retrospective review a male predominance, especially in the third decade of life, with a definite predisposing condition in approximately 15% of patients. Others found intracranial abscesses three times as common in males as in females and estimated an incidence of about four abscesses annually per million population.[3] Many estimates of incidence may, however, be lower than the true incidence owing to the fact that patients may die without accurate diagnosis. In the review by Chun and colleagues,[4] a peak incidence in the winter months was noted, perhaps correlating with the frequent occurence of parameningeal respiratory infections during these months. The large number of infants and young children affected in other series may be attributed to the greater prevalence of otic infections in this group.[4] Patients with cyanotic congenital heart disease represent a group at risk for brain abscess, for example, for abscesses located in the cerebellum.[5]

Source of Infection

Knowledge of the predisposing conditions that give rise to brain abscesses is essential in order to recognize the various clinical presentations and to choose an empiric therapy. Brain abscesses commonly arise from primary infections in the paranasal sinuses and middle ear and from intrathoracic foci of infections such as lung abscesses.[6] Head and neck suppurative processes can seed the brain parenchyma by contiguous spread, whereas hematogenous spread probably accounts for brain abscesses secondary to empyema thoracis, lung abscesses, and bronchiectasis. The risk for brain abscess in cyanotic congenital heart disease is due in part to loss of pulmonary filtration of the cardiac output, as occurs in patients with right-to-left shunts.[7] Loss of structural barriers to brain parenchyma increases the vulnerability to suppurative disease, such as with neurosurgical procedures complicated by abscess formation.[8] Beller and co-workers[9] found that primary ear and nose infections preceded 38% of the cerebral abscesses in a study of 89 cases. Carey and colleagues,[2] in a review of 86 patients, attributed 20 cases to right-to-left cardiac shunts in predisposed individuals and 25 to preceding sinus infection, and found eight cases secondary to skull trauma or osteomyelitis. Others note that a wide variety of systemic infections, such as those in skin, the oral cavity, and throat, can precede brain abscesses.[1] Such studies clearly illustrate that patients with chronic infections of the middle ear, sinuses, or thoracic cavity, and those with cyanotic congenital heart disease and head trauma will account for the majority of patients with brain abscess. The origin of infection is not apparent on presentation in some cases or after initial diagnostic tests, suggesting that the disease may occur in patients without obvious predisposition.

Site of Suppuration

McClelland and co-workers[3] reviewed 172 cases of brain abscess over a 30-year period and found 29% of lesions localized to the temporal lobes, 10% to the frontal lobes, 3% to the occipital lobes, and 20% involving multiple sites of suppuration. There is a strong correlation between the location of intracranial suppuration and the predisposing cause of infection. De Louvois and colleagues[10] found strong correlation between temporal-lobe abscesses and otitis and between frontal-lobe abscesses and sinusitis. Multiple brain abscesses usually result from metastatic spread of infection from distant primary sites, whereas single abscesses more frequently result from continguous spread of head and neck infection or from trauma.[4] This strong relationship between the site of brain-abscess formation and the predisposing condition can be helpful in seeking an etiologic agent in patients with documented brain abscess. Conversely, the existence of an infection known to give rise to brain abscess would heighten the clinical suspicion of this diagnosis. Brain abscesses from hematogenous sources commonly involve the middle-cerebral-artery distribution.

Sinusitis is frequently associated with frontal- and temporal-lobe abscesses, while otogenic infections are frequently associated with temporal-lobe and, occasionally, cerebellar abscesses.[4] Studies in which the vast majority of ear and sinus infections caused intracranial suppuration ipsilateral or adjacent to primary foci of infection support the notion that contiguous spread is the means by which most head and neck infections cause brain abscesses.[9]

Bacteriology

Medical therapy of the patient with suspected brain abscess usually precedes the definitive identification of involved microorganisms. Knowledge of the bacteria involved in predisposing conditions allows for rational empiric therapy. De Louvois and colleagues[10] studied pus samples from 46 patients with brain abscesses and found predominantly streptococci with *Streptococcus milleri* (Lancefield group F) in 36 of their patients. In this study, streptococci were isolated from multiple sites and from abscesses resulting from a variety of preceding sites of infection, while staphylococci assumed importance in abscesses following trauma and surgery.[10] Anaerobic Gram-negative bacteria, including *Bacteroides fragilis* and *Bacteroides melaninogenicus,* were invariably associated with preceding sinus, otogenic, or pleuropulmonary infection.[3,4,10] In their study of 18 cases of brain abscess or cerebritis, Mathisen and colleagues[11] occasionally found anaerobes isolated as sole pathogens, but more frequently found anaerobes in mixed culture with faculative bacteria. This group found fusobacteria to be the most common isolates in abscesses secondary to prior pulmonary infection.[11]

In a study of brain abscesses associated exclusively with preceding otogenic infection, obligate anaerobic bacteria were isolated from all patients studied, strengthening the belief that these organisms are extremely important in brain abscess secondary to otogenic disease, and in particular with chronic infection of the middle ear.[12] Other studies demonstrate anaerobic bacteria as major pathogens causing chronic sinusitis.[13] Frontal-lobe abscesses resulting from disease of the frontal sinuses usually involve anaerobes, both streptococci and *Bacteroides* sp.[14] Gas-containing brain abscesses are associated with wounds, especially with puncture wounds of the brain substance,[15] but an air shadow may be seen with other sources and conditions, as in frontal sinusitis and spread of infection.

Aerobic gram-negative bacilli are found in 20–40% of brain abscesses and assume great clinical importance in abscesses related to preceding otogenic infections.[4] *Proteus* species are the most common isolates, but *Escherichia coli, Klebsiella* sp, *Pseudomonas* sp, and *Enterobacter* sp have also frequently been isolated in mixed culture.[4] The enterobacteriaceae, especially *E coli* and *Proteus* sp, are often found in mixed cultures of abscesses following surgery and trauma, while streptococci are rarely identified in abscesses following neurosurgery.[10] *Hemophilus* species have been found in 5–10% of pediatric cases, while *Nocardia* sp and the *Actinomyces* group emerge in the immunocompromised and in patients with prior pulmonary or odontogenic infection respectively.[4] Fungal brain abscesses and infarcts are rare in the general population, but assume importance in the immunocompromised patient. Toxoplasmosis may involve the central nervous system (CNS), particularly in patients with the acquired immunodeficiency syndrome, causing brain abscess and encephalitis. Ring-enhancing lesions are frequently seen on contrast-enhanced computerized axial tomographic (CT) scans of such patients, particularly in the basal ganglia. Organisms that are associated with bacterial meningitis are rarely isolated from cerebritis or brain abscesses. Thus, isolation of an organism unlikely to cause bacterial meningitis should raise suspicion of the possibility of brain abscess with rupture into the ventricles.[4,16] Of note are *Listeria monocytogenes,* which can cause either meningitis or cerebritis,[17] and *Citrobacter diverusus,* which in infants causes meningitis with concomitant brain abscess in a high percentage of cases.[18]

Clinical Features

The possibility of brain abscess must be considered in any patient with or without a predisposing condition who presents with any feature suggesting intracranial disease, such as headache, focal neurologic defect, or signs or symptoms related to intracranial hypertension. Focal neurologic defects or overt signs of intracranial hypertension such as papilledema ordinarily do not occur early in the course of pyogenic meningitis, and their presence suggests the possibility of brain abscess or other mass lesion.[19] Headache is a fairly constant feature of brain abscess, and by itself in a patient with or without focal neurologic deficits who has concomitant extracranial suppurative disease would be enough to prompt a thorough search for brain abscess. Fever is a fairly frequent but by no means reliable accompaniment of brain abscess. In one neurosurgical review of 86 patients with brain abscess, 40 patients were febrile, 13 patients were hypothermic, and five of six patients with temperatures greater than 101.5°F had concurrent meningitis.[2] In another series of 18 cases studied at a Veterans Administration hospital, fever was seen in two thirds of the patients.[11] Other reviews note that as many as 60% of patients with brain abscess do not mount fevers, stressing the point that the absence of fever should not deter the consideration of brain abscess in predisposed patients.[4]

The presentation of brain abscesses derives many features from the effects of an expanding intercranial mass, rather than from an acute suppurative process. Focal neurologic defects, like the presence of fever, are frequent though not constant features of brain abscesses. Thus, the finding of fever and headache, even without neurologic deficit, would be enough to justify the consideration of brain abscess in predisposed patients. In one series of patients with brain abscess, 17 of 20 of the patients presented with focal neurologic deficit,[20] while others have found the incidence of focal neurologic deficit to range from 67 to 90%.[1,9] In Harrison's[1] review of 67 surgically proved cases of brain abscess, focal findings were evident in 75% of cases on initial examination, followed in frequency by depressed sensorium, nuchal rigidity, and fever. Others found nuchal rigidity a presenting feature in roughly half the cases.[4] Nausea and vomiting occur in roughly 50% of patients,[21] and seizures in about a quarter to a third of patients.[21,22] Series done before the widespread use of CT scanning are likely to emphasize more severe signs and symptóms. The tempo of presentation can be rapid and fulminant if one is dealing with an expanding mass lesion, or somewhat indolent if one sees the patient with only smaller areas of cerebritis prior to frank encapsulation. Clues to extracranial foci of infection are frequently present with acute disease and may be absent or subtle in more chronic disease states. Suspicion and recognition of brain abscess are made possible by appreciation of the varied modes of presentation. The type of focal deficit present can be expected to correlate with the location of the mass lesion. Patients with cerebellar abscesses invariably present with headache, nausea, and vomiting.[5] Signs and symptoms referable to disease in the posterior fossa, notably ataxia and nystagmus, also are frequently present, while coma and papilledema are seen with extensive crebellar lesions.[5]

Pathology

The pathogenesis of brain abscesses proceeds in predictable fashion, usually beginning with establishment in a vulnerable cerebral focus; this focus is seeded by bacteria and then cerebritis, followed by encapsulation, ensues. Initial bacterial seeding of vulnerable brain parenchyma can be accomplished by hematogenous spread or by contiguous spread from head and neck foci. This sequence of events has therapeutic implications, and influences diagnostic test results, particularly imaging studies. The importance of recognizing cerebritis, prior to encapsulation, rests on the finding that cerebritis alone may respond to antimicrobial therapy without neurosurgical intervention.[8] Hypoxia and reduction in cerebral perfusion render brain parenchyma vulnerable to infection.[23] Nonetheless, abscesses do occur in previously normal individuals. Most abscesses begin with cellulitis and inflammation, followed by implantation of organisms, edema, subsequent necrosis, and finally encapsulation by collagen fibers. Gates and colleagues,[24] in their review of metastatic brain abscesses, delineate the pathogenesis and suggest time courses of disease. They describe an early stage of "local suppurative encephalitis" that spanned the seven days after cerebral implantation of bacteria, followed by a second stage of frank abscess formation without encapsulation around 8–10 days after implantation.[24] The time to complete encapsulation may vary from 17 days to 6 weeks after the onset of cerebral infection.[24] The firmness and speed of encapsulation may be influenced by the pathogenicity of the bacteria involved and by the intensity of the patient's immune response.[7] The lesion prior to encapsulation has been referred to as cerebritis, while the final encapsulated mass containing necrotic tissues constitutes the abscess cavity.[7] Some authors have suggested that cerebritis may represent a "reversible presuppurative stage of disease."[25]

Diagnostic Tests

Most series on brain abscess advise caution in the performance of lumbar puncture in patients with suspected mass lesions. The yield of examination of cerebrospinal fluid (CSF) in patients with brain abscess is frequently low and it seems prudent to consider performing lumbar punture only after examinations, including imaging studies, confidently exclude the possibility of intracranial hypertension and risk of herniation. The study of spinal fluid, while not diagnostic, may at times be helpful. Most studies show the majority of CSF examinations in cases of documented abscesses to exhibit moderate pleocytosis.[1,4,20] In a review of 400 cases of brain abscesses in China, the CSF pressure was normal in one third of the cases, while the CSF white-blood-cell count was less than 10/mm^3 in roughly 20% of cases.[26] The spinal fluid is sterile unless the abscess cavity ruptures into the subarachnoid space or ventricles.[4,25] The finding of an extremely high white-blood-cell count and/or multiple bacterial isolates may suggest a leaking or ruptured abscess. Depressed spinal-fluid glucose concentrations occur in 15–30% of patients, and increased protein concentrations in 60–85% of patients.[4] Overall, however, results of CSF examination are usually of such a nonspecific nature that they are not useful in the diagnosis of brain abscess.

The peripheral white-blood-cell count provides little discrimiation from other infectious processes, but may have a limited use in distinguishing brain abscess from noninfectious diseases. One series found 75% of patients with brain abscess had a significant leukocytosis, whereas patients with brain tumors had peripheral leukocytosis in 25% of cases.[1] Others have found white-blood-cell counts less helpful, with 20–40% of affected patients having normal counts.[2,22] An elevation of the erythrocyte sedimentation rate is consistent with focal brain infection, but the rate is also elevated in other infections, as well as in many inflammatory and neoplastic processes.

Imaging Studies

The introduction of CT scanning has had a significant impact on the morbidity and mortality associated with brain abscesses. CT scanning allows for earlier diagnosis than in the past and for anatomic localization, which is vital for diagnosis, therapy, follow-up, and particularly neurosurgical intervention. CT scanning provides a noninvasive technique for the detection of brain edema and allows for the safe performance of lumbar puncture, when indicated, by excluding dangerous intracranial hypertension and involvement of a site at risk for supratentorial herniation. Much has been written comparing the sensitivity and specificity of CT scans in the detection of brain abscesses with electroencephalography (EEG) and radionuclide brain scanning. In one series of ten patients found to have discrete CT-defined abscesses, only seven patients had EEG abnormalities corresponding to the CT-defined lesions.[20] The same series showed that of ten patients with CT scans demonstrating brain abscess, only five had a positive radionuclide brain scan.[20] Other series have noted greater sensitivity with radionuclide brain scanning,[19,27] but most series suggest that CT scanning is overall the best method. Radionuclide imaging sometimes, however, may be more sensitive than contrast-CT scanning, particularly in cases of extensive inflammation or in lesions that are not as yet well organized.[28]

The distinction between cerebritis and encapsulated abscess has important therapeutic and prognostic implications. In view of reports of successful therapy with antimicrobials alone in the cerebritis stage, it is clear that the ability of an imaging procedure to delineate the pathologic stage of a brain abscess is important. Although CT scans reliably demonstrate ring enhancement when used with contrast agents, this feature may be absent or incomplete in the early cerebritis stage.[1] The ring of enhancement seen on CT scans may represent contrast material released into areas where vascular permeability has been altered by inflammation, representing a preencapsulation stage.[7] Inhomogenous enhancement may correlate with cerebritis while homogenous enhancement may represent encapsulation.[7,29] Corticosteroid administration can affect the results of imaging procedures. Some studies have found that in patients given steroids, presumably to counteract the edema accompanying brain abscess, there may be a reduction in enhancement in the late cerebritis stage, conceivably causing understaging of the process.[30] Moreover, such a response may be falsely ascribed to antimicrobial therapy concomitantly given with corticosteroids. Others note increased ring enhancement after corticosteroid therapy was discontinued, making follow-up CT scans appear to worsen in the face of otherwise effective therapy.[20]

Magnetic-resonance imaging (MRI) appears to be more sensitive than CT scanning in the early detection of cerebritis, but this observation may be moot since virtually all patients already have abnormalities on CT scans by the time of clinical presentation.[31] MRI is also useful in excluding other focal lesions, but may not be more helpful than contrast-CT scanning in distinguishing metastatic tumor from abscess. Also, MRI has been reported to be superior to CT scanning in distinguishing necrosis from cerebritis.[32] Gadolinium diethylenetriamine pentaacetic acid (DTPA) enhances the MRI image of brain abscesses in a manner similar to that obtained with contrast-CT scanning, and gadolinium MRI scanning can also elucidate components of a mature abscess, namely, the core, the rim of collagen, and surrounding edema.[32]

Differential Diagnosis

Early diagnosis is important in brain abscess because early institution of therapy has a major effect on patient outcome. Because of varied presentations and similarities to other disease entities, brain abscesses are difficult to diagnose in the earlier stages. Any disease process causing intracranial mass lesions can simulate a brain abscess. Although symptoms referable to a mass lesion are present in most patients with a brain abscess, clinical presentation will not invariably include focal neurologic features. The most frequent presenting symptoms include headache in more than 80% of patients, lethargy in 50–65%, nausea and vomiting in about 50%, and seizure activity in 25–33%.[21,22] Primary and metastatic tumors, pituitary abscess, cerebrovascular disease, and subdural, epidural, or intracerebral hematoma can all produce a clinical picture similar to that of brain abscess.[1,33] Of note, the hemiparesis resulting from brain abscess may be mild as compared with the severe deficits seen in patients with cerebral hemorrhage.[1] Meningitis is a consideration in any patient with fever and neurologic signs or symptoms.[34] Headache and fever may be prominent symptoms in viral encephalitis, as may a prodrome of malaise, fever, and gastrointestinal or respiratory symptoms typical of certain viral illness.[34] Focal neurologic defects and seizures may also be prominent features in patients with herpes simplex virus encephalitis;[35] seizures occur in certain other viral encephalitides and in cases of bacterial meningitis, as with some caused by *Hemophilus influenzae*. Signs and symptoms referable to an extracranial infection known to predispose to brain abscess can be helpful in sorting through diagnostic possibilities.

Imaging studies may not convincingly delineate brain abscess from other entities. Gliomas, metastatic tumors, and cerebral infarcts may appear as enhancing lesions on contrast-CT studies, although ependymal enhancement argues in favor of an abscess as the cause of ring enhancement.[20] The "doughnut" lesion revealed on technetium brain scanning is seen in well-encapsulated abscesses, but has also been described in patients with subdural hematoma, tumor, and cerebral infarction.[19]

Therapy

In most cases of brain abscess, antimicrobial therapy and surgical drainage are utilized. Since the cerebritis stage may respond to antimicrobial therapy alone, the therapeutic goal is to reach a diagnosis prior to encapsulation, thus possibly avoiding neurosurgical intervention. However, some type of surgery is required in any tightly encapsulated abscess. In view of the relationship between the bacteriology of brain abscesses and the predisposing condition, knowledge of the bacteriology of paranasal sinuses, otogenic sources, and intrathoracic infections allows for the selection of appropriate empiric therapy in the absence of specific results of cultures and susceptibility-test results. Staphylococci are frequently encountered pathogens following surgery and trauma, streptococci are found in almost all abscesses, and *Bacterioides* sp and *Fusobacterium* sp are important in patients with chronic paranasal sinus disease.[10,13] *Nocardia asteroides* would be a consideration in an immunocompromised patient, especially with prior pulmonary disease, but it also occurs in previously healthy individuals.[36] *Candida* sp may cause single or multiple abscesses, usually as part of widely disseminated disease in immunocompromised patients.

In the past, the standard recommended regimen for empiric antibiotic therapy of brain abscess was penicillin G and chloramphenicol. Although penicillin G is bactericidal against streptococci, recent studies show problems with it as monotherapy for brain abscess, particularly those involving *Bacteroides* sp.[37] *B melaninogenicus* may produce beta-lactamases, which can cause penicillin hydrolysis.[11] With meningeal inflammation, penicillin G penetration into the spinal fluid is increased, and doses of 20 million units daily lead to levels of 0.2 μg/ml.[38] Chloramphenicol readily penetrates the blood–brain barrier[39] and is bactericidal against pneumococci, *H influenzae*, and many anaerobes, but has unreliable activity against enterobacteriaceae.[4,40] There has been a suggestion that antagonism exists between concomitantly administered penicillin and chloramphenicol, potentially reducing the efficacy of each agent.[41] Corticosteroid therapy has not been shown to affect chloramphenicol penetration across the blood–brain barrier.[42]

Metronidazole has assumed an important role in the therapy of brain abscesses. Obligate anaerobic bacteria are important pathogens in brain abscesses secondary to chronic paranasal sinus or chronic middle-ear infections.[12] It has excellent activity against anaerobic bacteria, with 99% of *B fragilis* inhibited by <8 μg/ml of the drug, although activity against anaerobic cocci is not nearly this good.[43] Metronidazole has excellent penetration into intracerebral abscesses and rapid bactericidal activity against anaerobes.[44] Thus, with its excellent activity in the CNS, it is extremely valuable in treating brain abscesses in patients with prior otogenic and sinus infection;[12] penicillin G or ampicillin is almost always given concomitantly for adequate treatment of streptococci. The combination of penicillin G or ampicillin with metronidazole is generally preferred, but it has never been compared in a clinical trial with penicillin G or ampicillin with chloramphenicol. A summary of the more commonly used agents is presented in Table 8.1 and recommendations for empiric use in Table 8.2.

Gram-negative bacilli assume importance in brain abscesses secondary to otogenic disease.[4] Effective therapeutic agents need to have adequate activity against Gram-negative bacilli at levels achieved in the CNS; aminoglycosides do not meet these requirements.[45] Some of the newer cephalosporins (e.g., cefotaxime and ceftizoxime) have excellent penetration into the spinal fluid and attain levels of 10–12 μg/ml in the presence of inflammation.[46] Cefotaxime also has reasonable activity against gram-positive cocci (except for staphylococci), but should not be considered for therapy of *Pseudomonas aeruginosa* infection in the CNS. Ceftazidime has an even wider spectrum of activity against gram-negative bacilli that include *P aeruginosa,* and it

Table 8.1. Summary of selected antimicrobial agents useful in therapy of brain abscess.

Antimicrobial agent	Usual total daily dose*	Usual interval between doses
Penicillin G	20–24 million units	Every 2–4 hr
Ampicillin	12 g	Every 4 hr
Oxacillin	12 g	Every 4–6 hr
Mezlocillin	16–18 g	Every 4–6 hr
Piperacillin	16–18 g	Every 4–6 hr
Cefotaxime	9–12 g	Every 4 hr
Ceftazidime	8–12 g	Every 8 hr
Metronidazole	2 g	Every 6 hr
Chloramphenicol	4–6 g	Every 6 hr

*Adults with normal renal, hepatic, and hematologic function.

Table 8.2. Suggested regiments for empiric use.

Site of infection	Common suspected pathogens	Suggested empiric therapy
Otogenic	Anaerobic gram-negative bacilli Aerobic gram-negative bacilli	Metronidazole with penicillin G and cefotaxime
Sinusitis	Peptostreptococci Other anaerobic gram-positive cocci *Bacteroides* sp Aerobic gram-negative bacilli	Penicillin G with metronidazole, ± cefotaxime
Wounds—traumatic	*S aureus* Gas-containing abscess Secondary to puncture wounds: *Clostridia* sp	Oxacillin or nafcillin or vancomycin with penicillin G
Postoperative neurosurgery	Enterobacteriaceae *S aureus*	Cefotaxime* or a ueidopenicillin ± oxacillin or nafcillin or vancomycin
Immunocompromised patients	*N asteroides*	Sulfadiazine or trimethoprim/sulfamethoxazole
	L monocytogenes	Ampicillin or trimethoprim/sulfamethoxazole

*Another third-generation cephalosporin such as ceftazidime or ceftizoxime may be substituted.

appears to enter the spinal fluid readily, although data are not complete for this agent in terms of spinal-fluid penetration.[46]

The extended-spectrum penicillins, notably mezlocillin and piperacillin, possess excellent activity against many enterobacteriaceae, but data on penetration into cerebral abscesses are incomplete for these agents as compared with the "third-generation" cephalosporins.[4] Aztreonam, a monobactam, has proved to be effective therapy in experimental models of cerebritis.[47] The choice for therapy for staphylococcal brain abscesses remains either nafcillin, oxacillin, or methicillin; vancomycin therapy is reserved for methicillin-resistant strains.[48] One study of antibiotic penetration of brain abscesses found that methicillin attained therapeutic concentrations in abscess tissue, while nafcillin failed to penetrate cerebral abscesses adequately.[49] Preliminary data suggest that of the fluoroquinolones, ciprofloxacin and perfloxacin penetrate into the CSF in patients with inflamed meninges.

Sulfadiazine alone or sulfamethoxazole combined with trimethoprim is used to treat nocardial brain abscess; no agent is a definite alternative in the patient intolerant of sulfonamides but the following may be of benefit: minocycline, cycloserine, or high-dose cefotaxime. Amphotericin B, alone or with flucytosine, is the current treatment of choice for candidal brain abscess.

Boom and Tuazon[50] studied patients with multiple abscesses who were treated solely with antibiotics. The shortest course of successful therapy in their study was 14 weeks, although therapy and follow-up in some patients may require up to two years.[50] The duration of antimicrobial therapy will vary with each patient, but in most instances it will be a total of 6 weeks of therapy with 2–3 weeks of this therapy given intravenously.[50] Others require longer therapy. Authoritative authors suggest intravenous therapy for 4–6 weeks followed by oral therapy for 2–6 months.[31]

The majority of brain abscesses will require some form of surgical drainage. Much has been written in the neurosurgical literature regarding the best surgical techniques for cerebral abscesses. Whether drainage, aspiration, or excision is used, the priority remains to employ a procedure to reduce life-threatening intracranial pressure before the onset of irreversible cerebral-tissue destruction, and to operate early in the face of deteriorating neurologic or cognitive status.[2] The type of procedure employed will depend on the type, number, and location of the lesion(s) and the results of imaging studies.[4] Large series suggest that excision may be the procedure of choice based on comparisons of postoperative seizures, frequency of relapse, and overall mortality.[4] The advantages of primary excision over repeated aspiration may include expeditious decompression, visualization of the involved site for additional foci, the ability to remove encapsulated abscesses, and a shorter stay in the hospital.[51]

CT scanning is very useful in following patients treated for brain abscesses. Patients who show clinical improvement will generally have decreased ring enhancement and reductions in edema and mass effect on interval scans.[20] During the initial treatment phase, CT examinations are recommended at 3–4-day intervals.[52]

Prognosis

The outlook for the patient with a brain abscess has improved for many reasons, but principally relates to improved understanding of bacteriology, more effective use of antimicrobials, and, importantly, better imaging procedures. The source of infection may have prognostic value, with high mortality associated with abscesses secondary to distant primary foci and lower overall mortality in cases resulting from surgery or trauma.[8] Some have not found age to correlate with overall mortality,[9] whereas others suggest higher mortality in the very young or very old.[4] The patient's level of consciousness at the time of presentation has great prognostic value. Most authors note a poorer prognosis in patients with a depressed sensorium at presentation as shown by a study done nearly 20 years ago. Others note a correlation between outcome and abscess location, with temporal-lobe lesions being the most likely ultimately to cause herniation, while a comparable frontal-lobe lesion might be better tolerated.[3]

Subdural Empyema

Many similarities exist between brain abscesses and subdural empyema, particularly with regard to presentation, therapy, bacteriology, and predisposing conditions. Subdural empyema most often results from preexisting otogenic and paranasal sinus disease, although cases may also occur after surgery, placement of a ventriculoperitoneal shunt, or trauma.[53] Distant infectious processes may seed the subdural space hematogenously.[54] Infection of the paranasal sinuses may reach the subdural space by contiguous spread through bone or by communicating veins.[54] The suppurative process acutely involves the subdural space, causing intense inflammation on the surface of the cortex.[55] By and large, most cases of subdural empyema occur in patients with prior sinusitis or middle-ear infections.[56] The typical presentation is one of headache and fever, followed by changes in cognitive function, and finally the appearance of focal neurologic signs or seizures.[57] Clinical suspicion of subdural empyema should be high in the patient with advancing focal deficits superimposed on prior paranasal sinus or middle-ear infection. Signs and symptoms are related to this intense cortical reaction. The clinical picture of cerebral dysfunction and meningeal irritation could also be seen with brain abscesses, meningitis, subdural hematoma, and certain brain tumors.[56]

The bacteriology of subdural empyema relates to predisposing conditions. Some authors have stressed the consistent involvement of anaerobic bacteria,[58] while others note frequent involvement by streptococci and staphylococci, or even gram-negative bacilli.[59] Gram staining of material recovered at the time of drainage is crucial in selecting antimicrobial therapy. The spinal fluid in cases of true subdural empyema is sterile and shows mild pleocytosis, moderate protein elevation, and moderate decreases in glucose concentration.[55] Successful therapy consists of early drainage and parenteral antimicrobial therapy, the choice of which is influenced by the predisposing condition and by bacteriologic results.[54]

Intracranial Epidural Abscess

Intracranial epidural abscess is a rare condition that virtually always originates from frontal sinusitis, mastoiditis, or craniotomies. Persistent headache and fever are usually ascribed to the underlying infectious process. Severe and progressive neurologic deficits ensue unless therapy and operative drainage are introduced promptly. Radiographic evidence of frontal sinusitis or skull osteomyelitis frequently accompanies the condition.[60]

Successful management of subdural and epidural empyemas requires early diagnosis and urgent surgery to evacuate pus. Unfortunately, CT scanning may miss some of these lesions, and MRI scanning appears to be a more sensitive diagnostic modality in all stages of subdural and epidural empyemas. The superior sensitivity of MRI is attributable in part to its better detection of superficial lesions due to the absence of bone artifact and its ability to distinguish true empyemas from sterile effusions and chronic hematomas.[61] MRI may demonstrate a "hypointense medial rim" in epidural empyemas that result from dural inflammation.[61] The absence of this feature in subdural empyemas can be used to distinguish these two lesions.[61]

Dural Sinus Syndromes

Septic thromboses of the intracranial venous sinuses are being less commonly seen in the antimicrobial era than they were previously. Nonetheless, the serious neurologic consequences of the spread of infection along these related venous channels, as well as the continued occurrences of septic thromboses, dictate their consideration.[62]

Cavernous sinus thrombosis represents a true infectious-disease emergency, requiring prompt and aggressive intervention the moment the diagnosis is seriously considered. As soon as a patient's clinical presentation suggests this diagnosis, empiric antimicrobial therapy should be instituted, followed by consideration of an alternative diagnosis and performance of diagnostic tests.[63] Understanding the basic anatomy is essential for recognition of this entity and appreciation of its etiology, pathogenesis, and presentation. The cavernous sinuses are bilateral structures lying between the inner and outer layers of dura matter. They serve to collect venous drainage from multiple sources, principally the superior and inferior ophthalmic veins, some cerebral veins, and the middle third of the face (periorbital and nasal areas).[63,64] They are interconnected by circular sinuses, explaining the frequent bilaterality of the signs of this disease.[64] Many important structures transit the cavernous sinuses and explain many clinical features of thrombosis. The oculomotor, trochlear, and ophthalmic divisions of the trigeminal nerve lie within the lateral wall of the cavernous sinus. The abducens nerve lies within the sinus in close proximity to the internal carotid artery. The anatomic arrangement explains the frequent ophthalmic and neurovascular complications of this disease.

Pathogenesis begins with a bacterial infection involving the upper part of the face, periorbital or paranasal sinuses, which, by virtue of drainage systems, allows the process to reach the cavernous sinus.[65] Sphenoid sinusitis was the most frequent predisposing condition in a large modern series.[62] Thrombophlebitis of the cavernous sinus may ensue and quickly become a bilateral process owing to circular sinuses. The dural sinuses contain septa that are felt to make these structures vulnerable to thromboembolic phenomena.[63] Headache precedes fever and periorbital edema.[61] The patient with cavernous sinus thrombosis is acutely ill, with early complaints of neck pain and stiffness, eye pain, headache, and fever. On examination, chemosis, proptosis, edema, and injection of the upper facial structures may be prominent.[65] A number of pupillary abnormalities may occur owing to the involvement of the oculomotor nerve, internal carotid artery, and associated sympathetic plexus.[64] Changes in sensorium and papilledema are late events.[57,65] Some patients show a slower or attenuated pace.[62]

The bacteriology of this syndrome is somewhat predictable, considering the predisposing roles of skin infection and other deep oculonasal disease. Staphylococci and streptococci are frequent pathogens in preceding skin and soft-tissue infections, while gram-negative bacilli and anaerobes are frequent with prior otogenic and paranasal sinus disease. *H influenzae* and *Streptococcus pneumoniae* are always considerations in younger patients and in those with ethmoid or maxillary sinusitis.[62,64]

Important differential diagnostic considerations include orbital tumors, orbital cellulitis, acute ethmoid sinus infection, mucormycosis in uncontrolled diabetic patients, meningiomas, and arteriovenous aneurysms.[57,63,65] The orbital apex syndrome—consisting or proptosis, lid edema, forehead and orbital pain, and restriction in the mobility of the globe—is also a diagnostic consideration. Cavernous sinus thrombosis may be distinguished from these entities by its bilateral signs and symptoms, meningeal signs, and rapid progression to coma and the late appearance of papilledema without early intervention. Leukocytosis is a common feature.[65] Examination of the CSF is usually normal. Contrast-CT scanning combined with angiography allows for precise diagnosis of venous sinus thrombosis.[66] Orbital venography is considered to be the definitive method of diagnosis.[62]

Therapy includes administration of high doses of parenteral antimicrobials, which play an unquestioned role in management whereas controversy continues regarding the utility of anticoagulation.[62-65] The selection of antimicrobials is based to some extent on predisposing conditions. An antistaphylococcal penicillin is part of all regimens where skin and soft-tissue infections are involved. Metronidazole and the extended-spectrum cephalosporins are important considerations when, respectively, anaerobes and gram-negative bacilli are suspected. All antimicrobial regimens are administered in high doses until there is clinical resolution of all parameters of the syndrome.[64]

Lateral sinus thrombophlebitis is a complication of otitis media and mastoiditis in most cases, and is a disease of young or otherwise healthy patients. Early symptoms include ear pain or sinus tenderness, which can progress to fever, headache, nausea, emesis, and signs and symptoms attributable to increased intracranial pressure. Fever in the face of apparently appropriate antimicrobial therapy is a relatively constant feature.[62] Focal neurologic defects are uncommon, but Gradenigo's syndrome, consisting of abducens-nerve paralysis and trigeminal-nerve inflammation, is seen with involvement of the inferior petrosal sinus and is very suggestive of lateral sinus thrombophlebitis.[67] Bacteriologic results resemble those seen in chronic sinus and otogenic disease, involving principally *Proteus* sp, *E coli, Staphylococcus aureus,* and anaerobes.[62,67]

Septic thrombosis of the superior sagittal sinus most commonly results from meningitis and can also spread from nearby paranasal sinus disease, cavernous or lateral sinus disease, osteomyelitis, or extradural infection.[62,67] Clinical features include headache associated with increased intracranial pressure, grand mal seizures, and focal neurologic deficits, such as quadriplegia or hemiplegia.[62,67] An increased tendency to thrombosis, as is seen with pregnancy, hemodynamic instability, and in patients receiving oral contraceptives, is felt to play an etiologic role.[68] *S pneumoniae* is a common pathogen, but other streptococci, *S. aureus,* anaerobes, and gram-negative bacilli may also be involved.[62,68] Thereapy of lateral-sinus and superior-sagittal-sinus disease includes early institution of high-dose parenteral antimicrobials and drainage of involved paranasal sinuses.[67]

Summary

Advances in noninvasive diagnostic techniques in the past 10 years have led to better management, less morbidity, and lower mortality rates in brain abscesses.

A better understanding of the microbiology in different cases, as well as knowledge of risk factors and predisposing conditions, will lead to earlier diagnostic consideration of this entity. Although some cases, if discovered early enough, may be amenable to antimicrobial therapy alone, many will require combined neurosurgical and medical management. Successfully managed patients need long-term antimicrobial therapy and follow-up, including clinical evaluation and serial CT scanning. Timely diagnosis of other focal intracranial infections and septic thromboses also requires a high index of suspicion and prompt management.

Acknowledgment. The authors acknowledge the assistance of Glenn E. Mathisen, M.D., in reviewing the manuscript.

References

1. Harrison MJG: The clinical presentation of intracranial abscesses. *Q J Med* 1982;204:461–468.
2. Carey ME, Chou SN, French LA: Experience with brain abscesses. *J Neurosurg* 1972;36:1–9.
3. McClelland CJ, Craig BF, Crockard HA: Brain abscesses in Northern Ireland: a 30 year community review. *J Neurol Neurosurg Psychiatry* 1978;41: 1043–1047.
4. Chun CH, Johnson JD, Hofstetter M, Raff MJ: Brain abscess. A study of 45 consecutive cases. *Medicine (Baltimore)* 1986;65:415–431.
5. Morgan H, Wood MW: Cerebellar abscesses: a review of seventeen cases. *Surg Neurol* 1975;3:93–95.
6. Durack DT: Prevention of central nervous system infections in patients at risk. *Am J Med* 1984;76:231–237.
7. Garvey G: Current conepts of bacterial infections of the central nervous system. Bacterial meningitis and bacterial brain abscess. *J Neurosurg* 1983;59:735–744.
8. Karandanis D, Shulman JA: Factors associated with mortality in brain abscess. *Arch Intern Med* 1975; 135:1145–1148.
9. Beller AJ, Sahar A, Praiss I: Brain abscess. Review of 89 cases over a period of 30 years. *J Neurol Neurosurg Psychiatry* 1973;36:757–768.
10. De Louvois J, Gortvai P, Hurley R: Bacteriology of abscesses of the central nervous system: a multicentre prospective study. *Br Med J* 1977;2:981–984.
11. Mathisen GE, Meyer RD, George WL, et al: Brain abscess and cerebritis. *Rev Infect Dis* 1984;6(suppl. 1):S101–S106.
12. Ingham HR, Selkon JB, Roxby CM: Bacteriological study of otogenic cerebral abscesses: chemotherapeutic role of metronidazole. *Br Med J* 1977;2:991–993.
13. Frederick J, Braude AI: Anaerobic infection of the paranasal sinuses. *N Engl J Med* 1974;290:135–137.
14. Heineman HS, Braude AI: Anaerobic infection of the brain. *Am J Med* 1963;35:682–697.
15. Norrell H, Howieson J: Gas-containing brain abscesses. *Am J Roentgenol Rad Nuclear Med* 1970; 109:273–276.
16. De Louvois J: Bacteriological examination of pus from abscesses of the central nervous system. *J Clin Pathol* 1980;33:66–71.
17. Pollock SS, Pollock TM, Harrison MJG: Infection of the central nervous system by *Listeria monocytogenes:* a review of 54 adult and juvenile cases. *Q J Med* 1984;211:331–340.
18. Graham, DR, Band JD: *Citrobacter diversus* brain abscess and meningitis in neonates. *JAMA* 1981; 245:1923–1925.
19. Crocker EF, McLaughlin AF, Morris JG, et al: Technetium brain scanning in the diagnosis and manage-

ment of cerebral abscess. *Am J Med* 1974;56:192–200.
20. Whelan MA, Hilal SK: Computed tomography as a guide in the diagnosis and follow-up of brain abscesses. *Radiology* 1980;135:663–671.
21. Samson DS, Clark K: A current review of brain abscess. *Am J Med* 1973;54:201–210.
22. Morgan H, Wood MW, Murphey F: Experience with 88 consecutive cases of brain abscess. *J Neurosurg* 1973;38:698–704.
23. Fischbein CA, Rosenthal A, Fischer EG, et al: Risk factors for brain abscess in patients with congenital heart disease. *Am J Cardiol* 1974;34:97–102.
24. Gates EM, Kernohan JW, Craig WMcK: Metastatic brain abscess. *Medicine* 1950;29:71–96.
25. Heineman HS, Braude AI, Osterholm JL: Intracranial suppurative disease. Early presumptive diagnosis and successful treatment without surgery. *JAMA* 1971; 218:1542–1547.
26. Yang SY: Brain abscess: a review of 400 cases. *J Neurosurg* 1981;55:794–799.
27. Brewer NS, MacCarty CS, Wellman WE: Brain abscess: a review of recent experience. *Ann Intern Med* 1975;82:571–576.
28. Kim EE, DeLand FH, Montebello J: Sensitivity of radionuclide brain scan and computed tomography in early detection of viral meningoencephalitis. *Radiology* 1979;132:425–429.
29. New PFJ, Davis KR: The role of CT scanning in diagnosis of infections of the central nervous system, in Remington, Swartz (eds): *Current Clinical Topics in Infectious Diseases No. 1*. New York, McGraw-Hill, 1980, pp 1–12.
30. Enzmann DR, Britt RH, Placone RC, et al: The effect of short-term corticosteroid treatment on the CT appearance of experimental brain abscesses. *Radiology* 1982;145:79–84.
31. Wispelwey B, Scheld WM: Brain abscess. *Clin Neuropharmacol* 1987;10:483–510.
32. Sze G: Infections and inflammatory diseases, in Stark DD, Bradley WG (eds): *Magnetic Resonance Imaging*. St. Louis, C. V. Mosby Co, 1988, pp 316–343.
33. Domingue JN, Wilson CB: Pituitary abscesses: report of seven cases and review of the literature. *J Neurosurg* 1977;46:601–608.
34. Van Voris LP, Roberts NJ Jr: Central nervous system infections, in Reese RE, Douglas RG Jr. (eds): *A Practical Approach to Infectious Diseases*. Boston, Little, Brown & Co., 1986, pp 123–143.
35. Griffith JF, Ch'ien LT: Herpes simplex virus encephalitis. Diagnostic and treatment considerations. *Med Clin N Am* 1983;67:991–1006.
36. Young LS, Armstrong D, Blevins A, et al: *Nocardia asteroides* infection complicating neoplastic disease. *Am J Med* 1971;50:356–367.
37. Hackman AS, Wilkins TD: Influence of penicillinase production by strains of *Bacteroides melaninogenicus* and *Bacteroides oralis* on penicillin therapy of an experimental mixed anaerobic infection in mice. *Arch Oral Biol* 1976;21:385–389.
38. Jawetz E, Melnick JL, Adelberg EA: Antimicrobial chemotherapy, in Jawetz E, Melnick JL, Adelberg EA (eds): *Review of Medical Microbiology*. Norwalk, Conn, Appleton & Lange, 1987, pp 130–159.
39. AMA Division of Drugs: Amphenicols. *AMA Drug Evaluations*. Philadelphia, W. B. Saunders Co, 1983, pp 1643–1650.
40. Rahal JJ, Simberkoff MS: Bactericidal and bacteriostatic action of chloramphenicol against meningeal pathogens. *Antimicrob Agents Chemother* 1979; 16:13–18.
41. Haley EC, Costello GT, Rodeheaver GT, et al: Treatment of experimental brain abscess with penicillin and chloramphenicol. *J Infect Dis* 1983;148:737–744.
42. Kramer PW, Griffith RS, Campbell RL: Antibiotic penetration of the brain. A comparative study. *J Neurosurg* 1969;31:295–302.
43. Jones RN, Thornsberry C: Cefotaxime: a review of in vitro antimicrobial properties and spectrum of activity. *Rev Infect Dis* 1982;4(suppl):S300–S312.
44. Bartlett JG: Recent developments in the management of anaerobic infections. *Rev Infect Dis* 1983;5:235–242.
45. Berk SL, McCabe WR: Meningitis caused by gram-negative bacilli. *Ann Intern Med* 1980;93:253–260.
46. Neu HC: The new beta-lactamase-stable cephalosporins. *Ann Intern Med* 1982;97:408–419.
47. Scheld WM, Brodeur JP, Gratz JC, et al: Evaluation of aztreonam in experimental bacterial meningitis and cerebritis. *Antimicrob Agents Chemother* 1983;24: 682–688.
48. Scheld WM, Winn HR: Brain abscess, in Mandell GL, Douglas RG, Bennett JE (eds): *Principles and Practices of Infectious Diseases*, 2nd ed. New York, Wiley, 1985, pp 585–592.
49. Black P, Graybill JR, Charache P: Penetration of brain abscess by systemically administered antibiotics. *J Neurosurg* 1973;38:705–709.
50. Boom WH, Tuazon CU: Successful treatment of multiple brain abscesses with antibiotics alone. *Rev Infect Dis* 1985;7:189–199.
51. Choudhury AR, Taylor JC, Whitaker R: Primary excision of brain abscess. *Br Med J* 1977;2:1119–1121.
52. Holtas S, Tornquist C, Cornqvist S: Diagnostic difficulties in computed tomography of brain abscesses. *J Comp Assist Tomogr* 1982;6:683–688.
53. Tahmouresie A: Subdural empyema secondary to vetriculoperitoneal shunt. *NY State J Med* 1979;79:375–376.
54. Coonrod JD, Dans PE: Subdural empyema. *Am J Med* 1972;53:85–92.
55. Luken MG III, Whelan MA: Recent diagnostic expe-

rience with subdural empyema. *J Neurosurg* 1980:52:764–771.
56. Farmer TW, Wise GR: Subdural empyema in infants, children and adults. *Neurology* 1973;23:254–261.
57. Harter DH, Petersdorf RG: Pyogenic infections of the central nervous system, in Braunwald E, Isselbacher KJ, Petersdorf RG, et al (eds): *Principles of Internal Medicine*. New York, McGraw-Hill. 1987, pp 1980–1987.
58. Yoshikawa TT, Chow AW, Guze LB: Role of anaerobic bacteria in subdural empyema. Report of four cases and review of 327 cases from the English literature. *Am J Med* 1975;58:99–104.
59. Vetrovec GW. Warner JF: Infected subdural hematoma: three case reports involving gram-negative organisms. *Am J Med Sci* 1975;269:113–115.
60. Handel SF, Klein WC, Kim YW: Intracranial epidural abscess. *Radiology* 1974;111:117–120.
61. Weingarten K, Zimmerman RD, Becker RD, et al: Subdural and epidural empyemas: MR imaging. *AJNR* 1989;10:81–87.
62. Southwick FS, Richardson EP, Swartz MN: Septic thrombosis of the dural venous sinuses. *Medicine (Baltimore)* 1986;65:82–106.
63. Yarington CT: The orbit in relation to rhinology. *Proc Roy Soc Med* 1977;70:456–459.
64. Zahller M, Spector RH, Skoglund RR, et al: Cavernous sinus thrombosis. *West J Med* 1980; 133:44–48.
65. Harter DH: Parameningeal infections, in Wyngaarden JB, Smith LH (eds): *Textbook of Medicine*. Philadelphia, W. B. Saunders Co, 1988, pp 2181–2187.
66. Rao KCVG, Knipp HC, Wagner EJ: Computed tomographic findings in cerebral sinus and venous thrombosis. *Radiology* 1981;140:391–398.
67. Anonymous: Infections of the dural venous sinuses (editorial). *Lancet* 1987;1:201–202.
68. Gettelfinger DM, Kokmen E: Superior sagittal sinus thrombosis. *Arch Neurol* 1988;34:2–6.

9
Acute Viral Encephalitis

MIGUEL MATEOS-MORA AND KENNETH R. RATZAN

In the simplest of terms, encephalitis is defined as inflammation of the brain. It can be caused by many etiologic agents, including viruses, bacteria, parasites, and fungi. Viral encephalitis may be caused either by direct viral infection of neuronal tissue with neuronal destruction and the inflammation that accompanies that destruction or by an immunologic process whereby demyelination of white matter and perivenular inflammation occur, a hallmark of postinfectious encephalitis. In either case, the clinical picture is characterized by an acute or subacute onset of neurologic symptoms, such as impairment of mental function, seizures, focal neurologic findings, coma, and abnormalities evidenced by such diagnostic procedures as the electroencephalogram, (EEG) nuclide brain scan, computed tomography (CT) scan, and magnetic-resonance imaging (MRI) of the brain. More often than not, an inflammatory response is present in the cerebrospinal fluid (CSF). In such cases, meningoencephalitis may be a more appropriate term. [1–4] There is very little about the clinical syndrome of viral encephalitis that discriminates among the various etiologic agents. To be sure, Herpes simplex virus (HSV) encephalitis typically causes focal symptoms, rabies virus usually causes hydrophobia, and the postinfectious encephalitis of varicella often produces cerebellar dysfunction. Yet there is so much overlap in the clinical presentation of encephalitis caused by viruses that one cannot rely on the clinical setting alone to make an etiologic diagnosis. Thus, once bacteria, fungi, parasites, and other etiologies are excluded (Table 9-1), the identification of the specific virus causing the encephalitis will depend on viral isolation from the brain or CSF, histologic demonstration of virus by electron microscopy, identification of viral antigen or specific antiviral antibody in spinal fluid, or demonstration of a fourfold change in antibody levels in serum. Despite all these tests, for 60–85% of patients with encephalitis described in large series in the literature, no etiology is determined. [3,5–14]

The number of viral agents reported to be responsible for encephalitis are legion (Table 9-2). We will limit our discussion to the most frequently identified causes of viral encephalitis in the United States, including HSV, western equine encephalitis (WEE), eastern equine ecephalitis (EEE), St. Louis encephalitis (SLE), the group of California encephalitis viruses (CE), Venezuelan equine encephalitis (VEE), rabies, enteroviruses, mumps, measles, rubella, varicella-zoster virus, and Epstein-Barr virus (EBV). We will describe those viral encephalitides in which the virus causes a primary infection of the central nervous system (CNS) with neuronal destruction, not those attributable to immunologic events such as postinfectious demyelinating disease. That entity is covered elsewhere in this book, as is encephalitis caused by infection with the human immunodeficiency virus (HIV).

Encephalitis is a reportable disease in the United States. From 1968 to 1987 an average of 1,587, cases were reported to the Centers for Disease Control (CDC) each year, [13] and it is estimated that each year only 18–60% of the actual cases of encephalitis that occur are reported to public-health authorities, [14] thus, the number of cases reported to the CDC at best represents a bare minimum of those that actually arise across the United States. Moreover, of all cases reported to the CDC, approximately 75% are given no etiology. [13] Although encephalitis is seen throughout the year, cases seen in the summertime tend to be due to infections with enteroviruses and arboviruses, reflecting the known occurrence of

Table 9.1. Nonviral conditions causing or simulating encephalitis.

Infections	
Bacterial	Brain abscess Infective endocarditis Tuberculosis, syphilis, *Mycoplasma pneumoniae*
Fungal	Cryptococcosis, coccidioidomycosis, histoplasmosis, candidiasis, nocardiosis, blastomycosis
Rickettsial	Rocky Mountain spotted fever
Parasitic	Amebic meningoencephalitis, malaria, toxoplasmosis, cysticercosis, trichinosis
Toxins	Heavy metals, salicylates, barbiturates, phencyclidine
Metabolic diseases	Electrolyte imbalances, hyperglycemia, hypoglycemia, acute porphyria, pheochromocytoma
Systemic diseases	Sarcoidosis, collagen diseases, neoplasms
Others	Subdural empyema, subdural hematoma, cerebral infarction, progressive multifocal leukoencephalopathy, demyelinating diseases, acute psychosis

Table 9.2. Causes of acute viral encephalitis.

Herpes simplex types 1 and 2 (HSV)
Arboviruses (in the United States: western equine, eastern equine, St. Louis, California group, Venezuelan equine, Powassan, Colorado tick fever)
Mumps virus
Measles virus
Rubella virus
Enteroviruses (coxsackie, echo, polio)
Epstein-Barr virus (EBV)
Varicella-zoster virus (VZV)
Human immunodeficiency virus (HIV)
Rabies virus
Cytomegalovirus (CMV)
Adenoviruses
Variola virus
Reoviruses
Influenza A and B
Lymphocytic choriomeningitis (LCM)
Hepatitis B virus

epidemics caused by enteroviruses and the increase in the mosquito population during this time of year. HSV infections occur all year as does encephalitis associated with EBV infection. Cases caused by measles and mumps usually follow epidemics, but since immunization against these viruses is widespread in the United States, viral encephalitis attributable to these organisms has become exceedingly uncommon.

Herpes Simplex Virus Encephalitis

HSV encephalitis (HSVE) is the most common cause of fatal sporadic encephalitis in the United States. It is estimated to affect approximately 1 in 250,000–500,000 persons per year.[15] HSVs have a worldwide distribution and encephalitis caused by these agents is found throughout the year in all age groups. In various series, HSVE accounted for 5–20% of the encephalitides with known etiology.[2–4,6,8,16–18] While 1941 marked the first reported case of HSVE, [19] interest in the problem has increased significantly during the past decade because of the efficacy of acyclovir in treating such infections.[18,20–22] Prompt diagnosis and treatment are essential since the infection rapidly progresses to serious morbidity, and even mortality.

Most cases of HSVE are caused by HSV 1. Encephalitis attributable to HSV type 2 is found in neonates during the course of a disseminated herpes infection, [15,23,24] where the virus causes a devastating CNS, illness with a high frequency of morbid sequelae despite the use of acyclovir.[15,23,24] Approximately 32% of babies infected with HSV 2 develop encephalitis.[15] Risk factors for the development of neonatal HSV 2 infections include a history of genital herpes in the mother and maternal exposure to a sexual partner with presumed HSV lesions.[23] Maternal infection can be asymptomatic in 70% of women at the time of delivery, [23] which makes the diagnosis a difficult one. The overall mortality rate for neonatal HSV 2 infections is 19%.[15]

Encephalitis attributable to HSV 1 is a disease of older children and adults. In 30% of patients with HSVE, the infection is a primary one, whereas 70% have had a prior infection with HSV on the basis of a history of labial infection or the presence of serum antibodies to HSV.[25] Nonetheless, not all patients with concurrent labial infection and encephalitis are infected simultaneously with the same strain of HSV. Whitley and colleagues, [26] using endonuclease-restriction analysis, have shown that, in some instances, the viral isolate from the brain is a different strain from that in the vesicle on the lip.

Clinical Presentation

Unfortunately, the clinical picture of HSVE is nonspecific. The disease may follow a brief influenza-like illness or begin abruptly. The most prominent symptoms are fever, headache, personality changes, altered consciousness, malaise, irritability, and lethargy. Occasionally, olfactory hallucinations occur. Meningeal signs are not common, but focal neurologic signs such as seizures, localized cranial-nerve dysfunction, and autonomic disorders are typical for HSVE.[16,25] Unusual presentations of HSVE include brain-stem encephalitis, [27,28] chronic encephalitis, [29], and psychosis.[30,31] Untreated, the disease progresses relentlessly and quickly and is rapidly followed by neurologic deterioration, coma, and then death. These changes may also be associated with uncontrollable seizures. Death usually is caused by herniation. Mortality in untreated patients ranges from 60 to 80%.[4,15,16,18,25,32,33]

Pathology and Pathogenesis

Typical of HSVE is localization of disease to the orbitofrontal and temporal lobes.[34–26] While cerebral disease may be bilateral, in cases that come to postmortem examination early in the course of the illness, findings are usually unilateral and are typically localized to the temporal lobes. Microscopically, one sees neuronal necrosis, hemorrhage, increased numbers of polymorphonuclear leukocytes and macrophages in severely involved areas, and typical eosinophilic Cowdry type A intranuclear inclusions in neurons and glial cells (Figure 9-1).[16,25,35,37] In one study in patients with biopsy-proved HSVE, typical Cowdry type A intranuclear inclusions were found in only 56%. Moreover, histologic findings in 13 specimens were normal.[37] An explanation for the localization of HSVE to the temporal and orbital frontal lobes still is a matter of debate. Intranasal inoculation of HSV 1 into newborn mice is followed by spread of the virus through the cribiform plate and along nerve fibers extending into the olfactory bulbs.[38] On the basis of these findings, it is postulated that during a primary infection in humans, HSV 1 might enter along the olfactory pathways and spread along the base of the brain.[39] However, this hypothesis does not explain all cases since olfactory-bulb necrosis is not a uniform finding in patients dying of HSVE.

Another hypothesis holds that the virus may spread in a retrograde fashion from its latent position in the trigeminal ganglion.[34] HSV has been cultured from trigeminal-nerve ganglia harvested from routine autopsies.[40] Moreover, fibers from the trigeminal ganglion innervate the basal meninges of the anterior and middle fossae. Thus, if virus can spread centrifugally from the trigeminal ganglion along axons to the oropharynx and mucocutaneous borders of the lips, one can envision that virus can spread in a retrograde fashion along fibers from the trigeminal ganglion to the anterior and middle fossae via tentorial nerves. In this way, virus would be deposited in the orbitofrontal and temporal lobes and would explain the location of neuronal destruction seen in HSVE.

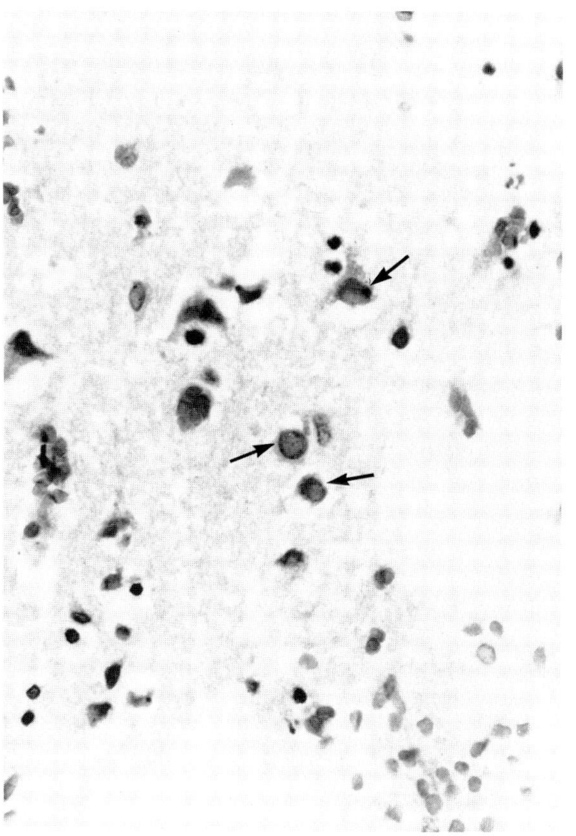

Figure 9.1. Eosinophilic Cowdry type A inclusions in herpes simplex encephalitis. Slide provided by the Dade County Medical Examiner Department. Micrograph by Dr. Jeffrey Morgan.

Diagnosis

Since HSVE is the only treatable viral infection of the CNS and the efficacy of therapy is directly related to the rapidity of treatment and the extent of the disease at the time of treatment, a rapid diagnosis of HSVE is essential.[15,17,18,20–22,37] While the disease tends to be localized to the orbitofrontal and temporal lobes and focal findings are typical of HSVE, any of the other viruses that invade the brain can cause focal lesions and involve the same anatomic areas as does HSV. Moreover, the differential diagnosis of HSVE includes not only other viral agents that can invade the CNS, but also tuberculosis, pyogenic brain abscess, subdural empyema, subdural hematoma, cerebral infarction, progressive multifocal leukoencephalopathy, disseminated cryptococcosis, acute demyelination, and subacute encephalitis, to name a few (Tables 9-1 and 9-2). The rapidity of the progression of neurologic damage is impressive. The replication cycle time for HSV 1 is 18 hours, so that a delay of only one day in establishing a diagnosis and initiating therapy can result in a potentially nonsalvagable state.[41]

Just as the clinical picture of HSVE is not pathognomonic, neither is any of the laboratory abnormalities. The CSF is usually abnormal, containing a pleocytosis of 50–1,000 cells/mm^3. Early on, the cells may be polymorphonuclear, but they soon change to a lymphocyte predominance typical of viral infections. In 75–85% of patients, red cells are seen in the spinal fluid, [42] which probably reflects the hemorrhagic necrosis caused by infection with HSV. CSF protein levels are usually slightly elevated, but may also be normal. CSF glucose is usually normal, but occasionally may be low.[42]. A normal spinal fluid should not exclude HSVE. A review of the literature revealed that 16 of 189 patients with culture-proven HSVE had a normal spinal fluid on initial lumbar puncture.[43] Isolation of the virus from the spinal fluid is rare, and this has been a major obstruction to the rapid noninvasive diagnosis of HSVE.[37] Much effort has been directed toward utilization of spinal fluid to measure specific HSV 1 antibodies, to detect the viral genome, and to find virus specific antigen in patients suspected of having HSVE. Each of these tests has its drawbacks, mainly because positive results do not develop early enough in the course of the disease to influence intervention with specific therapy. For example, the simultaneous measurement of antibodies to the virus in the CSF and serum provides information that can only be used to make a retrospective diagnosis.[37,44–46] A serum/CSF ratio of antibody to HSV 1 of less than 20 with either a passive hemagglutinating or immune adherence hemagglutinating antibody test occurred in every patient with HSVE.[46] However, diagnostic ratios were found in only three patients before brain biopsy and in four patients by the tenth day of disease. Ten days is too long to wait to begin specific therapy. When HSV 1 antigen was assayed in spinal fluid by means of an immunoblot assay, 24 of 26, or 92%, of patients were positive, with a specificity of 82%. While specificity and sensitivity improve with duration of disease, early in its course when a specific diagnosis is most important, these tests too often are negative.[47] These same limitations apply to attempts to find specific HSV 1 DNA in CSF.[48–50] The availability of more sensitive methods, such as passive hemagglutination, immunofluorescence, and enzyme-linked immunosorbent assay (ELISA), has not significantly improved the early diagnosis of HSVE.[37,51–53] The novel technique of polymerase chain reaction, also known as enzymatic gene amplification, may be helpful in the future for the early detection of HSV in spinal fluid. However, no data have been reported to date with this technique.[54]

One of the more sensitive tests for identifying and localizing infection in the brain is the EEG.[16,17,25,42,51,55–57] In 80–90% of patients, the initial EEG is abnormal and localizing[42,51,57]; the finding of bilateral abnormalities is a poor prognostic sign.[55] An abnormal EEG showing focal findings was the most sensitive neurodiagnostic test in patients with biopsy-proved HSVE. It was positive in 81% of patients, while technitium brain scanning was positive in 50% and CT in only 59%.[42]

It was hoped that CT would be exquisitely sensitive in detecting encephalitis resulting from HSV. Indeed, CT scanning may show low-density, contrast-enhancing areas, primarily in the temporal lobes. Also, there may be evidence of mass effect and brain edema [45,58,59]. However, CT scanning has been disappointing since only 59–64% of patients with biopsy-proven HSVE have an abnormal CT scan.[42,58] In fact, some studies have shown that CT scans may be normal when performed in the early stages of the infection, [42,59] which suggests that an abnormal CT scan may be associated with more advanced disease.

MRI may eventually prove to be the most sensitive radiologic test because of its high sensitivity to changes in brain-water content and excellent multiplanar imaging of the base of the skull. Moreover, this test may be abnormal early in the course of HSVE. Indeed, Schroth and co-workers[60] reported four cases of HSVE diagnosed by antibody to HSV in the CSF in which MRI scans demonstrated earlier and more diffuse changes than did CT scans.

The gold-standard test for diagnosing HSVE is the brain biopsy.[25,33,37,61,62] In experienced hands, the brain biopsy results in a morbidity of as low as 2%.[22,41] Brain biopsy should only be done at centers where a complete evaluation of brain tissue can be performed. This includes:

1. Histopathologic examination to look for eosinophilic Cowdry type A intranuclear inclusions. This technique has a sensitivity of only 56% but an 86% specificity.[37]
2. Identification of HSV antigens in brain tissue with electron microscopy. This procedure may be positive only 45% of the time, but it has a specificity of 98%[37]
3. The use of indirect immunofluorescence to detect HSV antigen. Although this test may be positive only 70% of the time, it has a specificity of 91%.[37]
4. Viral culture. This technique has a 90–95% sensitivity with 100% specificity.

On occasion, brain biopsy may yield false-negative results. In one study, 3 of 79 patients, or 4%, had negative biopsies, yet their autopsies revealed the presence of HSV 1 in the brain. The biopsies performed antemortem in these patients were from the wrong site.[22] The EEG, CT scan, and MRI can all help direct the site for biopsy. In the absence of focality, the best place to biopsy is the anterior portion of the inferior temporal gyrus.[37,41] While culture results may not be positive for 24–72 hours, immunofluorescent stains can be available within two to three hours, and electron-microscopy results in 24 hours. With negative-stain techniques, electron-microscopy results may be available in one to two hours.[25]

Brain biopsy not only can establish a specific diagnosis of HSVE and allow specific therapy, but it can also detect diseases that require other forms of therapy and would otherwise be missed. Several studies have analyzed the results of brain biopsy in patients suspected of having HSVE. In only 33–56% of these patients was that diagnosis proved by brain biopsy.[18,20,22,41,42] Other diagnoses were established in 46% of the patients negative for HSV, and in 20 of them, the biopsy led to appropriate management, with complete recovery in 13 instances.[18,22] These diagnoses included cryptococcal infection, tuberculosis, subdural hematoma, and brain abscess.

Treatment and Prognosis

As with any other of the viral encephalitides, general supportive treatment such as cardiorespiratory monitoring, intravenous fluids, adequate nutrition, control of the fever, treatment of increased intracranial pressure if present, and adequate management of seizures is of great importance in patient outcome. Fortunately, there is specific therapy for HSVE. The results of controlled trials performed since 1973 by the collaborative antiviral study group from the National Institute of Allergy and Infectious Disease (NIAD) show that the use of vidarabine decreased the rate of mortality from 70% to 28% one month after disease onset and to 44% six months later.[18] Patients under the age of 30 and with more normal levels of consciousness (lethargy as opposed to coma) were more likely to return to normal function than older, comatose patients.[22] In a comparative study involving 208 patients who underwent brain biopsy for presumptive HSVE and were randomly assigned to receive either vidarabine (15 mg/kg/day) or acyclovir (30 mg/kg/day) for 10 days, among 69 biopsy-proved patients, acyclovir was superior to vidarabine in decreasing both mortality and morbidity.[20] Mortality was directly related to level of consciousness at the onset of therapy, as well as age under 30 years. The deeper the level of coma at the onset of therapy, the poorer was the prognosis, no matter which drug was used. Patients under 30 without coma had the best prognosis. Indeed, 8 of 13 such patients treated with acyclovir fully recovered[20]. Skoldenberg and colleagues[21] reported similar results in a trial comparing acyclovir and vidarabine for HSVE. Disease duration of less than four days was associated with the best outcomes in each study; the mortality rate was 7% for acyclovir recipients. If the disease lasted more than 4 days, the mortality rate increased to 25%.[20] Thus, early specific antiviral treatment with acyclovir is currently the therapy of choice for HSVE.

Since time is of the essence in diagnosing and treating HSVE, a logical approach to a patient with suspected HSVE should be as follows: (1) Acyclovir should be started empirically and a brain biopsy scheduled as soon as possible. (2) Brain tissue should be processed as described above, and if the presence of HSV is demonstrated histologically or by means of immunofluorescence or electron microscopy, acyclovir should be continue for a full 10 to 14 days. (3) If these studies are negative, acyclovir should be continued for at least 5 days until culture results are reported. (4) If the cultures are negative, acyclovir can be discontinued. (5) If brain biopsy establishes a definitive diagnosis of a disease other than HSVE, acyclovir can be stopped and the appropriate alternative therapy instituted.

Arboviral Encephalitides

Currently, the term "arbovirus" no longer is officially in use. The more than 450 RNA viruses transmitted by arthropods are now grouped into five families: *Reoviridae, Togaviridae, Rhabdorividae, Filoviridae,* and *Bunyaviridae*. Most of the viruses causing encephalitis belong to the family *Togaviridae,* which is subdivided into two major groups, *Alpha virus* (formerly arbovirus group A) and *Flavivirus* (formerly arbovirus group B).[11,12,63] The *Alphavirus* encephalitides are all mosquito-borne and are restricted in distribution to the Americas, while those caused by flaviviruses are either mosquito-borne, tick-borne, or have an unknown vector and are distributed throughout numerous parts of the world.[63,64] In the United States, the four most common arthropod-borne viruses causing encephalitis belong to two families: (1) the *Togaviridae* family—WEE virus, EEE virus, and SLE virus; and (2) the *Bunyaviridae* family—California encephalitis (CE) viruses. Occasionally, VEE, Powassan, Tensaw, and Colorado tick fever viruses cause disease in the United States.[2,11,12,63,64]

Encephalitis caused by arthropod-borne viruses usually accounts for about 10% of all cases reported annually, but this figure can be as high as 50% during an epidemic year.[2] For example, cases of arboviral encephalitis reported to the CDC usually average around 100–150 per year, but in 1975 2,113 cases of arboviral encephalitis were reported because of a large epidemic of SLE during that year (Figure 9-2).[7]

The incidence of the most frequent arboviral encephalitides reported to the CDC from 1975 to 1987 can be appreciated from Figures 9.2 through 9.4.[13]

Mosquitoes are the arthropod vectors for the major arboviral encephalitides in the United States. The female mosquito acquires the virus from feeding on a viremic animal, usually a wild bird. For the mosquito to become infected, there must exist a high

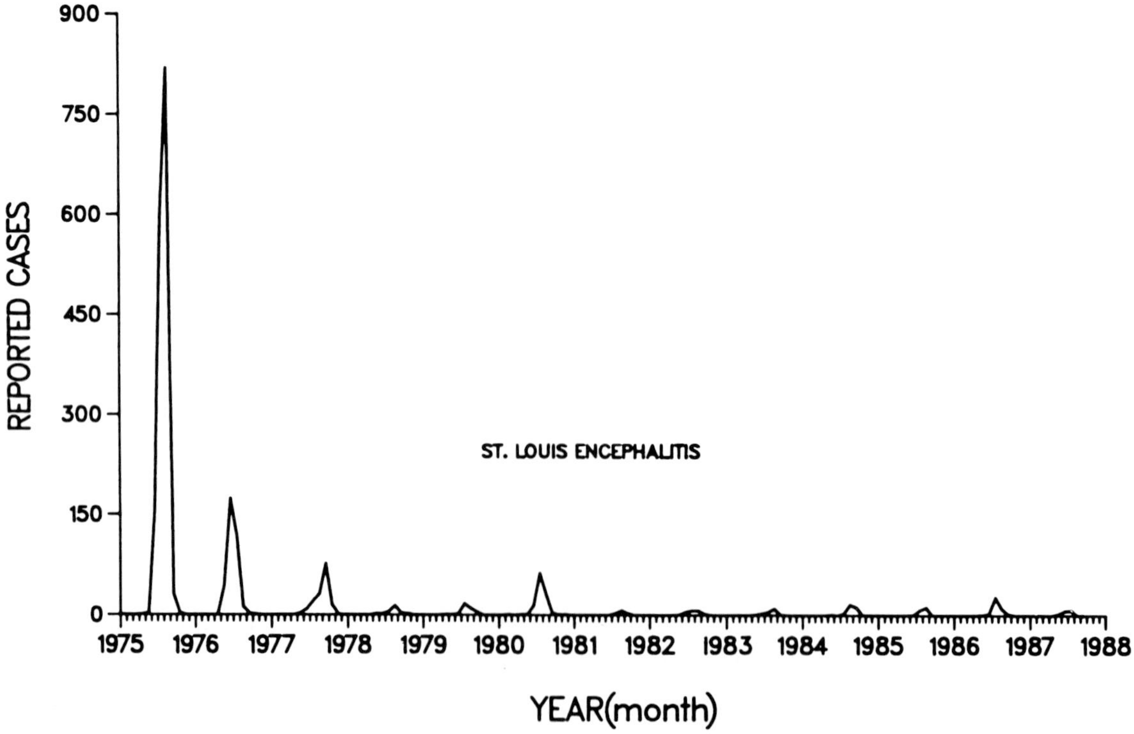

Figure 9.2. Arboviral infections of the central nervous system. Reproduced from Centers for Disease Control: Encephalitis Surveillance, 1978. CDC Annual Summary, May 1981.

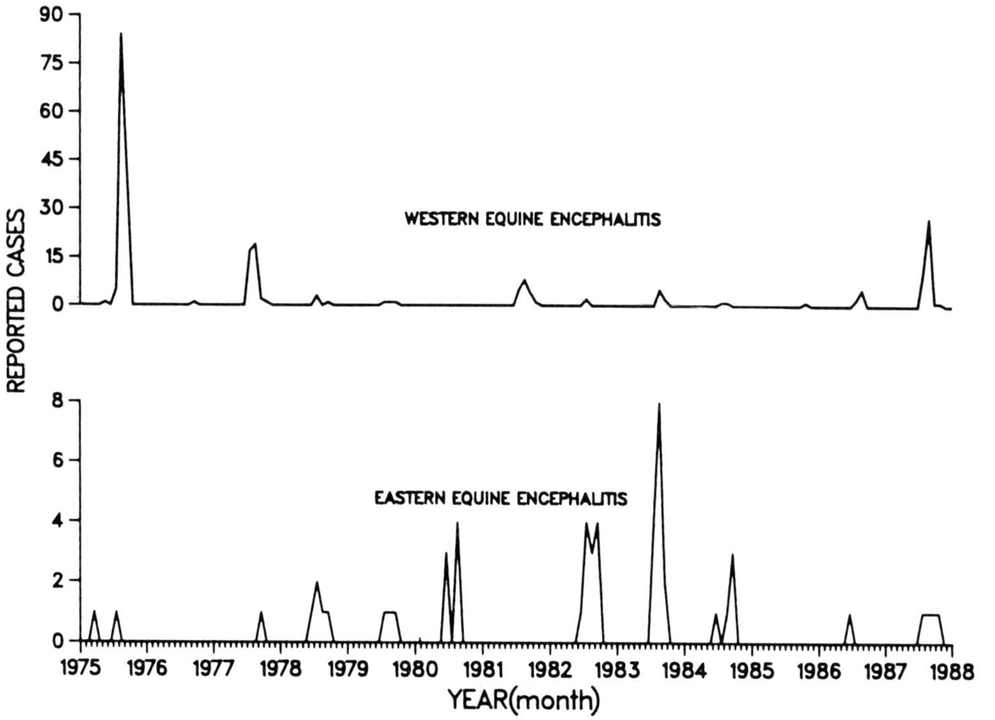

Figure 9.3. Arboviral infections of the central nervous system. Reproduced from: Centers for Disease Control: Summary of Notifiable Disease, United States, 1987. MMWR. 1988;3–11,18–19,53–59.

enough level of viremia in the host. Once the mosquito vector becomes infected, there is a one- to two-week period during which the virus multiplies in the salivary glands. The mosquito can then infect new hosts during feeding. Transmission is usually to birds of a specific species, which differs for each virus. Occasionally, in epidemic situations, the virus may be transmitted to horses, quails, and, rarely, to humans. However, these hosts are "incidental" since they do not develop sufficient vire-

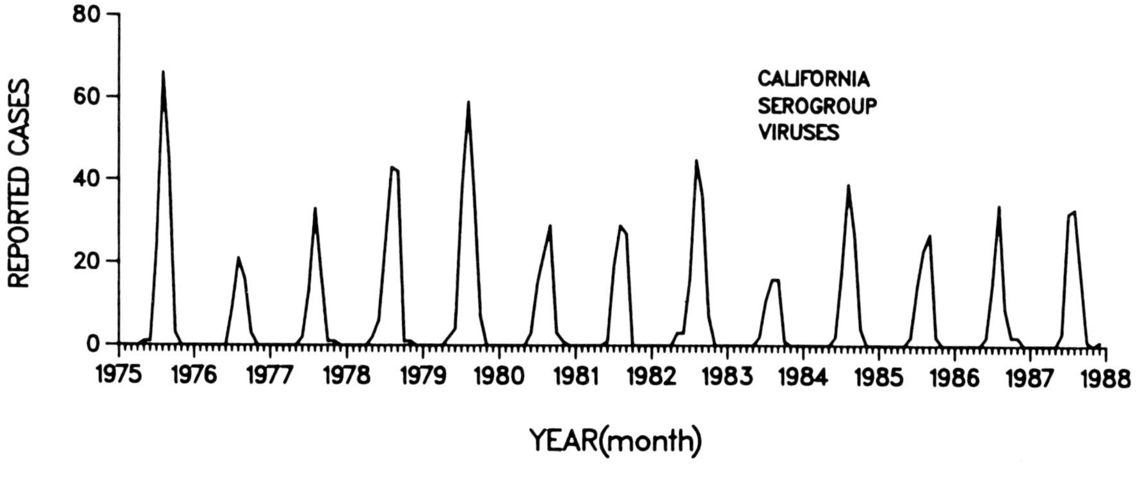

Figure 9.4. Arboviral Infections of the central nervous system. Reproduced from: Centers for Disease Control: Summary of Notifiable Disease, United States, 1987. MMWR. 1988;3–11,18–19,53–59.

mia to transmit the virus to uninfected mosquitoes.[63,64] Arboviruses are prevalent in the summer months when mosquito populations are at their highest. Cases begin to appear in June, peak in the summer and early fall, and usually cease by November. Epidemics of arboviral encephalitis, particularly SLE, WEE, and EEE, typically follow weather conditions that encourage large mosquito populations. How arboviruses are maintained in nature during the winter and how they reemerge each spring have not been fully determined, despite many theories of transovarian transmission among mosquitoes and persistence of the virus in the various infected hosts.[5,9,12,63–66]

Once there has been inoculation of the virus, local viral replication occurs, followed by viremia with dissemination of the virus to several organs, especially the lymphoid system. The virus can be demonstrated in brain tissue only after viremia and infection in other viscera are established, which suggests a hematogenous spread to the CNS.[64]

While infection with an arbovirus may produce a fulminating encephalitis or an aseptic meningitis, infection usually is not apparent. Clinical to subclinical ratios vary among the viruses and are age dependent. Neither the clinical picture nor the laboratory abnormalities distinguish one arboviral infection from another. There is typically a low-grade lymphocytosis in the CSF, a mildly elevated protein, and a normal glucose. Occasionally, the initial spinal fluid may have no cells or even a predominance of polymorphonuclear leukocytes. In fact, this clinical syndrome does not differentiate arboviral encephalitis from any of the other causes of encephalitis. Arboviral infections usually occur during the summer months, but so do enteroviral infections of the CNS. Therefore, seasonal distribution is not a discriminating feature of arboviral infections. Outbreaks of WEE and EEE are typically preceded by morbidity and mortality among horses in the geographical area, and this can predict potential disease among humans. Indeed, prior to an

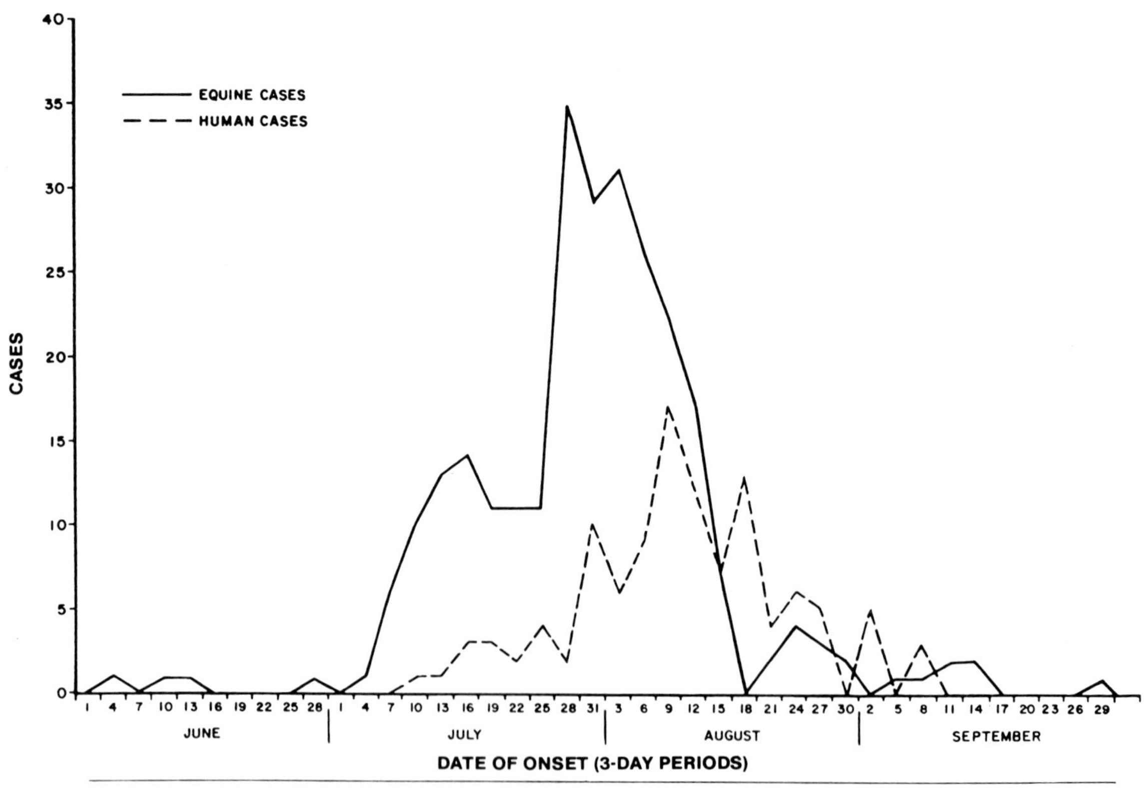

Figure 9.5. Encephalomyelitis in horses and human beings, northern Red River Valley, June to September, 1975. Reproduced with permission from: JAVMA. 1977;170:1396–1399 (Ref. 67).

epidemic of WEE in the northern Red River Valley of North Dakota and Minnesota in 1975, a sharp increase of WEE in horses preceded a similar epidemic in humans (Figure 9.5).[67]

The diagnosis of arboviral infections is made serologically. Hemagglutinating inhibition (HI) and neutralizing (NT) antibodies appear early in the illness and may be elevated when the patient first presents. Occasionally, they may rise so quickly that the demonstration of a fourfold increase in titer is not always possible; their titers remain detectable for several years after the infection. Complement-fixation (CF) antibodies, however, rise later in the course of illness and a fourfold change in titer may be more readily demonstrable with this test; these antibodies are shortlived and an elevated titer is, therefore, indicative of a recent infection.[63,64]

Pathologic findings in the brain are nonspecific for arboviral infections. The inflammatory process resembles that seen in other viral encephalitides. There is meningeal and perivascular inflammation, neuronal degeneration, glial nodules, and small hemorrhages. Lesions occur primarily in gray matter and are widely distributed throughout the brain, frequently with severe involvement of the basal ganglia.[63,64]

There is no specific antiviral therapy for arboviral infections. Careful attention to fluid and electrolyte management, antiseizure medications if necessary, and surveillance of the patient in a critical-care area are of utmost importance for patient survival.

Although experimental vaccines against some of the arboviruses are available, vaccination of the general public is not reasonable since the attack rate in endemic areas is so low and epidemics are so unpredictable. However, laboratory workers at high risk of infection might be candidates for vaccination. Mosquito-control programs provide an important deterrent for spread of infection. Surveillance of encephalitis and mortality among horses can be useful in predicting subsequent disease in humans. Hence, when there is a combination of increased morbidity among horses and a high density of mosquitoes, mosquito-control programs can be instituted to try to prevent the spread to humans.[10–12,63,64]

Western Equine Encephalitis

WEE is the third most common cause of arbovirus encephalitis in humans in the United States. It also causes severe epizootics in horses. WEE is caused by an *Alphavirus* (group A arbovirus) and is transmitted principally by *Culex tarsalis,* a mosquito vector that maintains the virus in nature through an enzootic cycle involving wild birds and other vertebrate hosts. *C tarsalis* predominates in flooded and irrigated areas, and cases occur in rural localities in the western two thirds of the United States and adjacent areas in Canada.[11,12,63,64] Rarely, WEE is found in the East. Approximately 36 cases of WEE are reported annually to the CDC, and small epidemics of WEE occasionally are noted in the United States following a wet winter or spring when conditions are favorable for the breeding of large numbers of *C tarsalis.* The largest single outbreak of WEE reported took place in 1941 and affected more than 3,400 humans in Minnesota, North and South Dakota, Nebraska, and Montana, and in Alberta, Manitoba, and Saskatchewan in Canada; equine cases were estimated to be in the hundreds of thousands.[64] Cases begin to appear in June, reach a peak in July and August, and decline in September (Figure 9-3). Horses play no role, however, in the transmission cycle.[11,12,63,64,67] In 1975, a WEE outbreak in the Red River Valley of North Dakota and Minnesota resulted in 281 equine and 133 human cases.[67] In 1987, 41 cases of WEE were reported to the CDC with 1 fatality, an elderly man.[68]

The WEE virus was isolated in 1930 and was the first arbovirus grown in the United States.[69] In 1938, it was isolated from the brain of a child who died of the disease.[70] Most infections with WEE are subclinical. There is a wide range of clinical: subclinical infection; it has been reported to be 1:58 in children one to four years of age and 1:1,150 in adults.[9,11,63,64,71] Attack rates have varied from 1 per 100,000 to 128 per 100,000[71]. The highest attack rates are usually in young children[11,64,71] and disease is more frequent in males, which can only be partially explained by occupational exposure.[64,72]

Clinical Manifestations

The presenting signs and symptoms of WEE are similar to and indistinguishable from those for the other viral encephalitides. The incubation period is five to ten days and the onset of the illness is typically abrupt, with the sudden appearance of fever, headache, malaise, chills, nausea, and vomiting. Signs of CNS infection become evident several days later, with dizziness, drowsiness, increased headache, stiff neck, and disorientation that can progress to coma. Seizures occur in 75–80% of infants less than 3 months old during the acute illness.[9,11,12,63,64]

Physical examination may reveal a normal neurologic status or, in acutely ill patients, a depressed sensorium, agitation, and restlessness may be present. Gravely ill patients may be comatose. The neurologic examination usually fails to reveal any localizing findings. In infants, the fontanelle is bulging, and spastic paraparesis and frequent generalized convulsions typify the course of the illness. Indeed, the disease may produce devastating neurologic damage in infants. Recovery usually begins gradually after a few days to 1 week, with progressive improvement in sensorium. Full recovery may follow after several weeks. Most adults recover completely. However, in 13% of patients there are major neurologic sequelae such as quadriplegia, hemiplegia, and spasticity. In children developmental delay, retardation, and convulsions may occur. The risk of serious neurologic sequelae in infants is three times that of other age groups and 30% of affected patients under 1 year of age may develop serious neurologic impairment.[12,63,64] Parkinson's syndrome has been reported in several adults surviving WEE.[64,73] The case fatality rate in outbreaks in the central United States and Canada in 1941, 1975, and 1981 ranged from 7 to 9%. Age-specific fatality rates were highest in the elderly.[64] Laboratory tests are nonspecific. CSF obtained at an early stage will show a normal glucose, increased protein, and a leukocyte count ranging from 10 to 300 cells/mm^3. Usually, mononuclear cells predominate but polymorphonuclear leukocytes may be present on the initial tap.

Pathology

At postmortem, the brain may appear normal or be congested and swollen. Microscopic changes affect both gray and white matter diffusely; however, the basal ganglia are often severely involved. Disseminated small focal abscesses infiltrated with neutrophils are a distinctive feature. Cuffs of both mononuclear and polymorphonuclear cells surround small veins and arteries, and there may be vasculitis and endarteritis with obstruction of the vascular lumen.[63,64] Extensive patchy areas of demyelination may be found throughout the brain. Neuronal degeneration may occur in areas with demyelination, hemorrhage, or inflammation.[63,64]

Diagnosis

The specific diagnosis of WEE rests primarily on serologic tests. Recovery of the virus from the spinal fluid is distinctly unusual. HI and NT antibodies increase in the first week, and by the second week, a diagnostic fourfold increase in these titers may occur. CF antibodies are slower to rise (3–5 weeks) and an elevated titer correlates with a recent infection. NT and HI antibody titers are long lasting and may be present, with minimal decay, for up to 30 months after acute illness.[63,64] An indirect immunofluorescent (IF) antibody test is highly sensitive. It can detect IgM immunoglobulin by means of an antibody-capture enzyme immunossay as early as 24 hours after the onset of illness[73] and may turn out to be the procedure of choice for the rapid diagnosis of human infections caused by the WEE virus.

Eastern Equine Encephalitis

The EEE virus is an antigenically distinct member of the *Alphavirus* genus in the *Togaviridae*. The virus was first isolated from a postmortem brain-tissue specimen from a horse in 1933 during an outbreak of equine encephalitis.[12,63,64,75] EEE was described as the etiologic agent of a human epidemic of encephalitis in Boston in 1938.[76]

EEE causes an acute encephalitis in horses and humans, especially children, in whom high case fatality and low subclinical : clinical infection ratios are described. It is the most severe of the arboviral encephalitides in the United States where equine cases occur each summer along the Gulf and Atlantic coasts, and occasionally inland in the eastern half of the country.[11,12,63,64,75,76] Major epidemics have been seen in the past in New Jersey and Massachusetts and the virus can be isolated from its natural transmission cycle virtually every summer.[12,63,64,75,77]

Epidemiology

EEE is a disease of low incidence, with less than 20 cases occurring in most years in the United States. The states with the highest rates of infection show an average annual incidence of 0.012 (New Jersey and Massachusetts) to 0.020–0.026 per 100,000 (Florida, Delaware).[64,75,77] Viral transmission among horses usually is seen from May to September, although in Florida it can occur sporadically all year. Human cases usually are found from June to August in Florida and in the Northeast from August to September, with occasional cases noted late in October.[11,64,75,77]

Although rates of infection seem to be equal for the different age groups, clinically apparent disease occurs mainly at the extremes of life. Serologic studies during the 1959 epidemic in New Jersey showed that infection took place with equal frequency in all age groups, but the ratio of subclinical to clinical infections was highest in patients in the middle years of life (29:1) and lowest in children under 4 years of age (8:1). The overall attack rate in the outbreak was 101 per 100,000 population.[75]

The main vector in the enzootic cycle is *Culiseta melanura,* a mosquito that breeds in freshwater swamps and feeds on birds. Infection and viremia occur almost exclusively in birds. Sparrows and various exotic birds, such as ringnecked pheasants, Peking ducks, and Chukar partridges, may become ill and die from infection. *C melanura* mosquitoes usually do not feed on humans or horses, and it is necessary for the virus to become established in *Aedes* spp mosquitoes before human and equine cases arise.[12,63,64,75]

Pathology

Pathologic changes in the brain include gross evidence of edema and multiple punctuate hemorrhages. Microscopically, there are neutrophilic infiltrates in the meninges and perivascular cuffs around small blood vessels in the cortex and cerebral nuclei. Extensive areas of necrosis of the brain may also be seen. There may be inflammation of the vessel walls, with intravascular thromboses.[63,64,75]

Clinical Manifestations

The clinical course of EEE is the most fulminant of the arboviral encephalitides.[2,11,12,63,64,75] In young children and infants, the onset of illness is usually rapid, with high fever, headache, irritability, vomiting, and stiff neck, closely followed by lethargy, confusion, seizures, and, in most patients, coma. In adults and older children, there may be a brief prodrome with some nonspecific symptoms such as headache, fever, and dizziness, followed by lethargy and coma. Paralyses are common during the acute phase, and EEE seems to produce a greater disturbance in autonomic function than do the other togaviruses. These abnormalities include impairment of respiratory function, which can lead to severe hypoxemia, and excessive salivation, which may cause airway obstruction in comatose patients. The entire course of illness is usually less than 10 days.[63,64,75]

The case fatality rate for EEE is the highest among all of the arboviral encephalitides in North America, and in survivors, EEE is associated with severe sequelae. The mortality in sporadic cases was 50% during a 20-year period in the United States. In outbreaks, fatality rates as high as 74% have been reported.[64] In the 1938 outbreak in Massachusetts, it was 67%, and in New Jersey in 1959, it was 68%.[64,75] Age-specific mortality is high in children 5 to 20 years of age (38–62%), with adults over 60 having the highest mortality (78%).[63,64,75,77] Up to 30% of patients surviving the acute infection, mostly young children, will develop neurologic sequelae that may range in severity from minimal brain dysfunction, unilateral spasticity, and seizure disorder to severe mental retardation and quadriplegia.[2,11,12,63,64] Specific therapy is not available.

Diagnosis

The laboratory diagnosis of EEE is usually made serologically. Isolation of virus from the CSF is unusual. Culture of virus from brain biopsies is possible, as is identification of viral particles by immunofluorescence. Serologic testing by IF, NT, HI, and CF is used to establish the diagnosis.[63,64,75]

NT and HI antibodies appear 3 to 4 days after the onset of illness and are long lived. CF antibody appears 11 days after onset, peaks in the third week, and then declines rapidly. More recently, the detection of IgM antibodies by capture enzyme immunoassay has been used to diagnose EEE and WEE as early as 1 or 2 days after the onset of illness with good sensitivity and specificity.[74] Because of the low prevalence of this disease, the presence of antibodies in an acute serum sample from a patient with encephalitis is suggestive of EEE.

Prevention

Control of the vector mosquitoes is an important but difficult task to perform. The use of mosquito repellents and the avoidance of outdoor activity one to two hours after sunset when the feeding activity of mosquitoes is high are prudent measures to take during epidemic periods.

St. Louis Encephalitis

SLE is the most frequent and geographically the most widespread mosquito-borne encephalitis of humans in the United States. The SLE virus is a member of the newly formed family *Flaviviridae* (group B arboviruses), which are RNA viruses that are smaller than the *Alphaviruses*. Other members of the *Flaviviridae* include the yellow-fever virus, the dengue virus, and the Japanese encephalitis virus. SLE occurs in endemic and epidemic form throughout the Americas.[2,10–12,63,64,77]

Epidemiology

Because of its potential to cause major epidemics involving thousands of cases, SLE is the most important arboviral encephalitis in the United States. It was first recognized in 1933 when an outbreak involving 1,095 cases occurred in the St. Louis area. More recently, outbreaks have been reported in diverse epidemiologic settings and from an extensive geographic distribution.[2,10–12,63,64,77–79]

Cases are reported yearly but their numbers vary widely depending on whether large epidemics occur. Between 1955 and 1982, 4,999 cases were reported to the CDC, and over one third of those cases (1,815) were reported during 1975 (Figure 9.2); 30 different states reported cases in that year.[10,11] On the other hand, in 1987 only 17 of the 148 (11.4%) reported cases of arboviral encephalitis were due to SLE.[68]

In western states, annual WEE- and SLE-virus activity leads to sporadic endemic infection, although epidemics can take place. In the east-central United States, sporadic transmission of SLE virus is minimal, and major outbreaks are intermittent. Because of the intermittent activity of the virus, there is a large susceptible population, and when epidemics do occur, they tend to be extensive. The attack rate in outbreaks depends on the size of the population at risk.[10,63,64,71] The level of immunity is directly related to the length of residence in an endemic area. Thus, adults have a lower susceptibility to the virus than do children.[63,64,71]

Most cases of SLE are seen in mid- to late summer, but in Florida where *Culex nigripalpus* is active until the beginning of winter, cases have been seen through mid-December.[64,71]

In most SLE epidemics, the age of the infected person is the most important determinant of the development and severity of illness. Case-fatality rates increase sharply after the age of 60, with rates as high as 35–38% reported.[2,10–12,63,64,71,77]

There are at least four vectors for SLE in the United States: *C tarsalis* in the western and central states, *Culex pipiens* and *Culex quinquefasciatus* in the east-central and Atlantic states, and *C nigripalpus* in Florida.[12,63,64,71,78]

In the western United States, *C tarsalis*, which is also a vector for WEE, serves as both an enzootic and epizootic vector. It feeds mainly on birds early in the summer and on mammalian hosts in midsummer.[10,64,71]

Wild birds, primarily of the passerine species, are the amplifier for SLE virus during the spring, summer, and fall. They are the only animals known to develop a viremia of sufficient magnitude to be able to infect mosquitoes.[10,63,64,71]

The *C pipiens* complex breeds in polluted water. Following hot, dry periods, rivers and streams become stagnant, their organic content increases, and mosquitoes multiply to large numbers. Outbreaks of the disease then may take place among urban–suburban populations living along these waters.[10–12,64,71]

Pathology

The neuropathology of fatal SLE is characterized by involvement of the midbrain, thalamus, brain stem, cerebral cortex, and cerebellum. The leptomeninges show mononuclear cell infiltrates, edema, and small hemorrhages. Perivascular and parenchymal inflammation with lymphocytic infiltrates and microglial cells is prevalent in the gray-matter nuclei, especially the substantia nigra and the thalamic nuclei, but the infection may also involve the white matter of the brain stem and spinal cord[63,64]

Clinical Manifestations

The incubation period after the bite of an infected mosquito varies from 5 to 21 days. The clinical expressions of SLE range from inapparent infections to fulminant encephalitis and death.[2,10–12,63,64,78,79] The subclinical:clinical ratio of SLE has ranged from 19:1 to 470:1. An inverse correlation exists between age and the severity of infection. Children are much more likely to have inapparent infection than are the elderly.[10,63,64] Among persons that become symptomatic, three different syndromes have been observed: febrile headache, aseptic meningitis, and encephalitis. Encephalitis is the most frequent presentation and accounts for approximately 58 to 78% of symtomatic cases. Although children as a group exhibit milder symptoms than do adults, more than half of confirmed and presumptive cases among children involve encephalitis.[11,63,64]

There are no characteristic clinical findings that will help differentiate SLE from other viral encephalitides. Onset may be abrupt or gradual with fever, headache, nausea, vomiting, photophobia, and malaise as prodromal symptoms. Manifestations of CNS involvement are characterized by disorientation, lethargy, stupor, coma, confusion, or delirium follow. Other neurologic disorders include cranial-nerve palsies, dysarthria, abnormal reflexes, paralysis, paresis, rigidity, and tremor. Convulsions are seen in less than 10% of the patients, mostly in children.[10,12,63,64,79]

Other symptoms that have been observed include intense muscle aching, urinary frequency, and dysuria.[12,63,64,79] Inappropriate secretion of antidiuretic hormone has been seen in up to 25% of the cases.[80] In most cases, fever resolves in 4 to 7 days after onset, and clinical improvement begins early in the second week of illness.

Mortality rates are strictly age related. In cases reported to the CDC from 1955 to 1971, 8% of the patients died, but the age-specific mortality rate in persons 60 years of age and older was 19.5%. Mortality in children ranges from 2 to 5%, with those under 5 years of age at the highest risk.[11,64] Recovery from SLE is usually complete or associated with few sequelae, such as emotional disturbances, dizziness, headache, memory impairment, and tremor. Children may have a higher frequency of sequelae.[64]

White-blood-cell counts range from 5,000 to 15,000 cells/mm^3, with an increase in neutrophils. Normal or decreased leukocyte counts are occasionally seen. Urinalysis may show pyuria, proteinuria, or microscopic hematuria. Elevation of the blood urea nitrogen (BUN) and serum creatinine occurs in one third to one half of patients.[11,12,63,64,79] Abnormal electromyograms and increased levels of serum aldolase were documented by Southern and co-workers.[79] CSF examination shows a mononuclear pleocytosis, generally in the range of 5–500 cells/mm^3. If the CSF is obtained early in the illness, there may be a predominance of polymorphonuclear cells. CSF glucose is generally normal and protein is elevated in approximately half of the patients.[10,12,63,64,78,79] EEG is usually abnormal, with diffuse generalized slowing the most common finding.[64]

Diagnosis

Isolation of the SLE virus from blood or CSF has been unrewarding; it may be isolated from postmortem brain tissue with more success.[81] As with the other arboviral encephalitides, serologic studies provide the means to diagnose SLE. Measuring HI, CF, and NT antibodies has been the usual way to make a diagnosis when a fourfold rise or fall is detected.[10,12,63,64,78] More recently, an IgM capture enzyme immunoassay has been recommended as the procedure of choice because of its sensitivity in measuring IgM antibody, which indicates a primary infection.[82] Indirect immunofluorescence is also a sensitive test, but interpretation may be subjective.[81,83]

As with the other arboviruses, no specific treatment exists, and supportive therapy is of utmost importance.

Prevention

Surveillance of viral activity is the foundation of preventive public-health efforts to decrease the incidence of SLE. This can be accomplished by performing serologic studies periodically on captured wild birds and sentinel chickens. Rising seroprevalence rates, associated with viral amplification, may precede the appearance of human cases by several weeks.[10,11] Mosquito-control programs with elimination of breeding sites, plus the use of larvicides and insecticides during appropriate seasons, would prevent urban SLE epidemics.[10] The recognition that SLE epidemics follow periods of drought that may or may not have been preceded by spring floods or heavy rain may alert some state health departments to the need to intensify mosquito control.[10]

California Encephalitis

The CE virus serogroup belongs to the *Bunyaviridae* family. Prototype California virus, La Crosse (LAC), snowshoe hare (SSH), Jamestown Canyon (JC), and trivittatus (TVT) viruses are all members of the serogroup known to cause human disease in North America. Most recognized bunyavirid viral infections are undifferentiated, febrile diseases. Humans are not known to be a natural amplifier or reservoir for any of these viruses. One is infected when entering the ecologic niche of the vector, so the epidemiology of human infection is determined by the prevalence of infected vectors and their habits.[63,64]

The California viruses are found in tropical, temperate, and arctic regions where they are closely associated with their mosquito vectors, generally of the genus *Aedes*. CE was first isolated in 1943 in California after 150 patients with apparent viral infection of the CNS were hospitalized. Their clinical course was different from that of patients with WEE or SLE.[84] A few years later, CE was serologically implicated as a cause of human encephalitis in several cases.[85] In 1964, a strain of the virus was isolated from brain tissue of a 4-year-old girl who died of fatal meningoencephalitis in a La Crosse, Wis., hospital in September 1960.[86] This virus, known as La Crosse, is the most frequent causative agent of CE.[11,12,64,87]

Because of cross-reactivity in serologic tests, encephalitis due to the California group of viruses has usually been reported under the rubric "California encephalitis." More specific testing and viral isolation studies have led to the inference that La Crosse virus infection is responsible for most CE, particularly in the Midwest.[11,12,64,87]

Epidemiology

California virus (La Crosse) encephalitis is the principal cause of endemic arboviral CNS infection in the United States, which is found mainly among children. Among reported cases in the United States from 1972 to 1981, 75% of cases involved children under ten years of age and only 3% persons older than 20 years. The male-to-female ratio during that period was 1.8:1, but it was related to a higher exposure rate secondary to occupation rather than to a true biologic difference.[64,75,87–89] During 1987, La Crosse virus caused 87 of the 148 (59%) arboviral encephalitides reported to the CDC in that year.[68]

LaCrosse infections are endemic in the United States (Figure 9.4), with sporadic infections occurring annually from July to September, mainly in rural areas of the east-central states. Patterns of disease are better understood in relation to mosquito exposure.[12,64,87,88] Inapparent infections may be frequent, which accounts for the increasing immunity with age.[64,87,88]

Aedes triseriatus is both the reservoir of the virus in nature and the vector for the transmission of infection to humans. It is a woodland species that breeds preferentially in tree holes and small artificial containers capable of catching rainwater, such as discarded bottles, cans, and tires.[11,12,64,87,88] Geographically, the mosquito is found principally in eastern hardwood forests. Watts and colleagues[65] established that infected adult female *A triseriatus* could transmit the infection to their ova, which, in turn, would be the means of virus survival over the winter season. They also showed that there is venereal transmission of the virus from transovarially infected males to their uninfected female partners during mating.[65,66] These mechanisms allow the virus to survive, at least partially, independently of a natural animal reservoir, and they may explain why there is constant, predictable yearly disease in endemic areas. The principal amplifying hosts of *A triseriatus* are small mammals, especially squirrels and chipmunks. Other vertebrates, such as foxes and woodchucks, may also contribute to the amplification cycle.[11,12,64,87,88]

Pathology

Pathologic examination of the few fatal cases of La Crosse encephalitis revealed cerebral edema, neuronal degeneration, perivascular cuffing of capillaries and venules, and glial nodules in the brain. Inclusion bodies were not seen. These findings do not distinguish infection with CE from that of the other arboviruses.[86]

Clinical Manifestations

The incubation period of CE has been estimated to be 3–7 days.[64,87,89] Clinical patterns of La Crosse infection are age dependent and likely to result in a spectrum of disease ranging from inapparent or mild febrile illness as the predominant presentation in adults to aseptic meningitis and severe encephalitis in children.[11,12,64,87] Children usually have a two- to three-day prodrome consisting of fever, malaise, headache, and gastrointestinal symptoms. The illness evolves with clouding of the sensorium and lethargy. Those with milder cases develop meningeal signs and disorientation and usually recover within a week. In more severe cases with greater alteration of consciousness, patients often develop seizures during the first or second days of the illness.[64,87] In a study by Balfour and colleagues,[89] an analysis of 66 cases of La Crosse infection showed that the highest incidence was among children 5–9 years of age (22.4%); also, two distinct clinical presentations were seen—a "mild" form characterized by fever, lethargy, nausea, and vomiting lasting approximately 1 week, and a "severe" form characterized by fever, headache, seizures, and coma lasting approximately 12 days. In the severe form, focal and generalized seizures occurred in 42–62% of the patients,[64,89] and up to 25% exhibited focal neurologic findings such as paresis, aphasia, and abnormal reflexes.

La Crosse encephalitis has a very low case-fatality rate. Up to 37% of the patients with the severe form of the infection may develop sequelae after discharge from the hospital, mainly seizure disorders.[89] The same study showed residual sequelae in 15% of the patients 1 to 5 years after diagnosis.[89]

Laboratory results are nonspecific. CSF exam is usually abnormal with mononuclear pleocytosis of 100 cells/mm^3, elevated protein in about one third of cases, and normal glucose. One series showed abnormal CT scans in 12 of 51 patients with CE (23%), and 4 of those had definite focal abnormalities.[64] Focal findings were demonstrated in 4 of 10 Tc-99mm pertechnetate brain scans performed in patients proved to have La Crosse encephalitis.[89] EEG abnormalities are seen in more than 90% of CE patients during the acute phase; findings consist of generalized or symmetric slow waves, with focal findings in up to 40% of the patients.[64,89]

Diagnosis

As with the other arboviral encephalitides, the diagnosis is based on serologic studies. Recovery of La Crosse virus from the brain in fatal cases is possible.[86] Diagnosis rests on a fourfold rise or fall in HI, NT, or CF antibodies. In CE, the HI and CF tests are relatively insensitive,[64] while NT is highly sensitive.[64,87] Among the most sensitive tests is the determination of IgM by an enzyme-linked immunosorbent assay (ELISA) or IF. These tests are quite sensitive.[64] Because of the frequency of focal findings (approximately 20%) reported in CE,[64,87,89] HSV encephalitis should be a diagnostic consideration in such patients.

Treatment is symptomatic and supportive.

Prevention

Public-health prevention has focused on elimination of breeding sites of *A triseriatus*. The sealing of tree holes with cement and the removal of discarded tires and other containers that provide breeding sites for the vector have played a role in controlling the mosquito population. Additional control relies on the use of repellents and insecticides.[11,64,87]

Venezuelan Equine Encephalitis

VEE is the most important arboviral disease in tropical America.[11,90] Since 1935, numerous outbreaks, many of considerable magnitude, have occurred in Venezuela, Colombia, Ecuador, and Peru, as well as in Central America, Mexico, and Texas.[90] The virus was first isolated from the brain of a dead horse in Venezuela in 1938.[90]

VEE is a togavirus belonging to the *Alphavirus* genus. There are at least six subtypes (1–6) of VEE virus; subtype 1 has been divided into at least six variants, 1A to 1F. Only subtypes 1A, 1B, and 1C have been associated with epidemics among humans and equines.[11,90] Subtype 2 is the Everglades virus (EVE), which is restricted in its geographic distribution to the state of Florida.[11,63]

Epidemiology

From 1962 through 1964 in Venezuela, there were 23,283 human cases, including 960 with neurologic syndromes and 156 deaths.[90] In the United States, EVE has caused sporadic cases of undifferentiated febrile illness and meningitis in southern Florida, first recognized in 1968.[11] In 1977, a German tourist visiting the Everglades National Park acquired the disease and virus was isolated from his blood.[11] An additional four cases have since been reported.[63]

Serosurveys have shown an antibody prevalence as high as 27% for EVE among residents of South Florida.[63] Infection rates are similar for all age groups, whereas the incidence of neurologic disease is highest among children.[90] Outbreaks occur during the rainy months and are more intense in tropical coastal regions. Epizootics in horses precede the development of human disease, and horses are the principal amplifying host for the virus. The virus is transmitted by a wide variety of mosquito vectors, principally belonging to the many species of the genera *Aedes, Mansonia,* and *Psorophora*.[11,90]

Pathologic findings are similar to those for the other arboviral encephalitides, and they are most prominent in the basal ganglia and substantia nigra.[90]

Clinical Manifestations

Inapparent infections are rare; most, if not all, persons infected with the epizootic strains appear to develop an overt febrile influenza-like illness. Encephalitis occurs in only about 4% of infected persons under the age of 15 years and is observed even more infrequently in adults.[9,11,90] CNS symptoms and CSF findings are not different from those of other arboviral encephalitides.

The overall fatality rate of encephalitic infections is approximately 20%, with the highest rates in children younger than 5 years of age.[11,90] A prolonged convalescence may ensue, with asthenia, recurrent headaches, and decreased memory, and can last up to 4 weeks after recovery.[9,90] Neurologic sequela may arise after the encephalitis.[90]

Treatment is based on supportive care of the patient to prevent complications and sustain life.

VEE outbreaks in horses and humans may be prevented by mass vaccination of equines, which reduces or eliminates the susceptible primary vertebrate host population.

Rabies Encephalitis

Rabies is one of the oldest and most feared of human diseases. It is of unique interest among human virologic diseases because it is universally fatal once the characteristic clinical symptoms appear. Rabies has been recognized as a dramatic disease throughout recorded history. The disease was recognized by the Babylonians in 2300 BC. Hippocrates was probably referring to rabies when he described the combined thirst and fear of water in patients who had been bitten by "mad" dogs. In 100 AD, Celsus was the first to display an accurate understanding of the disease by attributing infection to a "virus" (i.e., a poison) in the saliva. He advocated cauterization of wounds produced by rabid animals. Galen, writing a century later, advised surgical resection as the method of choice for preventing rabies.[91–95] Human cases and epidemics of animal rabies were recognized throughout Europe and in the Americas in the 1700s and 1800s. Animal-control measures eliminated rabies from Scandinavia in 1826.

Louis Pasteur began his work with rabies in 1880, and it was in early 1882 that he first experimentally transmitted rabies by inoculating spinal material of a rabid dog into the brain of another dog. Through serial passages of the "infectious" agent in brains of rabbits, he produced a preparation that he called "fixed virus." On July 6, 1885, Joseph Miester, a 9-year-old boy who had been bitten numerous times by a rabid dog, was treated by Pasteur with 12 injections of rabid spinal-cord vaccine and he survived. By October 1886, of 726 persons similarly treated by Pasteur, only 10 had succumbed to the disease, for a mortality rate of 1.3%.[91–95]

In 1903, Negri described the pathologic changes observed in rabies encephalitis, including the cytoplasmic inclusion bodies that now bear his name. Vaccines derived from the original of Pasteur emerged, with the duck-embryo-derived vaccine released in 1948. The use of passive immunization with rabies immune serum was added to the treatment of rabies in 1954. In 1973, the human-diploid-cell vaccine (HDCV) was experimentally introduced, but it did not become available for general use in the United States until 1980.[91–95]

The rabies virus is a member of the *Rhabdoviridae* family, which includes pathogens for a wide variety of mammals, fish, birds, and plants. It has a bullet-shaped, cylindrical morphology, rounded at one end and flat at the other.[91–95] The *Rhabdoviridae* viruses are RNA-containing viruses, and they are divided into two genera based on distinct antigenic and biologic characteristics, *Lyssavirus* and *Vesiculovirus*. Rabies virus belongs to the *Lyssavirus* genus.[92–95] The virus is inactivated by formalin, phenol, bichloride of mercury, trypsin, beta-propiolactone, and disinfectants. Drying, sunlight, x-irradiation, and heat will also destroy the infectivity of the virus.

Virus replication and disease can be caused in

numerous laboratory animals: mice, rabbits, hamsters, rats, and guinea pigs. Tissue-culture systems that have proved useful for virus cultivation include human diploid cells, chick-embryo cells, and hamster kidney cells. WI-38 and MRC-5 are the two human diploid cell lines currently used for production of killed vaccine in the United States and Europe respectively.[92–94]

Epidemiology

Rabies is another example of a zoonotic infection. The natural cycle of infection involves animals; human disease results from accidential exposure to infected animals and is not required to complete the cycle of the infection.[92,93]

In areas where domestic-animal rabies has not been adequately controlled, dog or cat bites account for 90% or more of the reported human cases. In contrast, in areas where domestic-animal rabies is well controlled, such as the United States, Canada, and many western European countries, most human rabies results from wild-animal bites or is imported from other countries.[91–97] The most common wild animals that transmit rabies are skunks, raccoons, bats, and foxes. The control of canine rabies has resulted in the virtual elimination of indigenously acquired human rabies in the United States. Since 1978, only 17 such cases have been reported, compared with 428 cases reported from 1938 to 1947.[13,96] Worldwide, the situation is different. According to the World Health Organization (WHO), there were 20,482 human deaths resulting from rabies in 1981.[91]

In the United States, the number of cases of rabies dropped off abruptly in the early and mid-1950s. This was attributed to a parallel decrease in the number of cases among dogs as a result of the development of domestic-animal-control programs.[93] Wild-animal cases have exceeded domestic cases each year since 1960. In the 1970s, there was a large increase in the number of rabid skunks in the Midwest, and in the late 1970s, surveillance detected the emergence and spread of a rabies epizootic in racoons in Virginia and West Virginia.[96,97] In 1987, 4,729 cases of rabies were reported to the CDC,[96] of which 4,169 involved wild animals and 559 involved domestic animals, with one human case reported from California.[98] Eleven of the 50 cases (22%) among humans reported to the CDC since 1960 had no history of animal exposure.[96,97]

The incidence of rabies appears to be higher in males (70–80% of the cases) than in females, and the greatest number of cases is in persons younger than 20 years.[93–99] People with outdoor occupations constitute mroe than half of reported cases.

Pathogenesis and Pathology

Knowledge of the pathogenesis of rabies is largely derived from the work of Pasteur, who inoculated the virus intravenously and detccted it again in the CNS and spinal cord.[94] Although the usual mode of transmission involves the inoculation of the virus into the subcutaneous tissue or muscles after an animal bite, other modes of transmission have been described, such as inhalation in caves heavily infested with bats, transplantation of corneal tissue containing the virus, and mucous-membrane inoculation.[92–94] The development of rabies following exposure to a potentially rabid animal is not a certainty, and it depends on the type and severity of exposure, the animal involved, the stage of disease in the biting animal, and the preexposure and postexposure treatment given.[92–95]

Rabies infections are generally established by virus inoculation into peripheral tissues. The virus reaches the spinal cord by centripetal ascent via afferent peripheral nerves. Thereafter, the virus travels very rapidly to the brain and ultimately infects neurons. The virus subsequently descends via peripheral nerves to other sites, including the salivary glands. Virus is excreted in saliva, which may, in turn, infect another host and complete the cycle of infection.[92–95] Sensory-nerve endings in head and neck skin and corneal epithelium contain virus antigen, which can be detected by immunofluorescent techniques. Such techniques can be used to make an antemortem diagnosis of rabies.[92] Viremia is apparently an inconstant occurrence of little importance in the dissemination of infection.

The incubation period after inoculation of the virus is variable. It may be as short as 9 days or as long as several years, but it usually ranges from 3 weeks to 3 months. It is related to the distance between the site of inoculation and the brain and to the severity of the exposure. Head, neck, and hand lesions have the shortest incubation periods.[92–95]

Once the virus reaches the brain, widespread infection occurs and nearly all neurons in many different regions may be infected. The most severely involved areas appear to be the hippocampus, brain stem, ganglion cells of pontine nuclei, and the Purkinje cells of the cerebellum.[92–95] Early selective infection of the limbic system in the brain may cause a disease characterized by extreme excitability and agitation (furious rabies). The more common syndrome of encephalitis is associated with early, very widespread infection of the brain. Brain infection leads rapidly to death by mechanisms that are poorly understood.[92–95]

The pathologic findings of human rabies are viral encephalitis and neuronal degeneration. Gross changes of the brain include vascular congestion and edema. Evidence of meningitis is not common, but when it does happen, it is almost always in children.

Microscopically, there are lymphocyte and plasma-cell exudates with perivascular cuffing involving most of the brain, but primarily the limbic system. Polymorphonuclear cells may be present in the early stages of the disease. A study of 49 fatal cases of rabies [99] showed that the most common pathologic findings were perivascular cuffing (94%), neuronophagia (57%), and Babès' nodules (focal collections of "embryonal cells" that surround infected neurons) (42%). The same study showed that the most commonly affected areas of the brain were the medulla (38%), pons (38%), and spinal cord (36%). The thalamus, cerebral cortex, and basal ganglia were involved in slightly more than 25% of cases.[99]

Negri bodies are cytoplasmic inclusions seen within human and animal neurons infected with rabies virus (Figure 9.6). They are most commonly seen in the cerebellum and the hippocampus, but can be seen in the medulla, pontine nuclei, spinal cord, cerebral cortex, basal ganglia, thalamus, and peripheral ganglia.[91] They are generally round and surrounded by a halo and exhibit a visible internal structure. Electron microscopy reveals that they are composed of clusters of assembling viral nucleocapsid. Although they are considered pathognomonic of rabies infection, 10–30% of cases of culture-proved rabies do not have evidence of Negri bodies.[92–99]

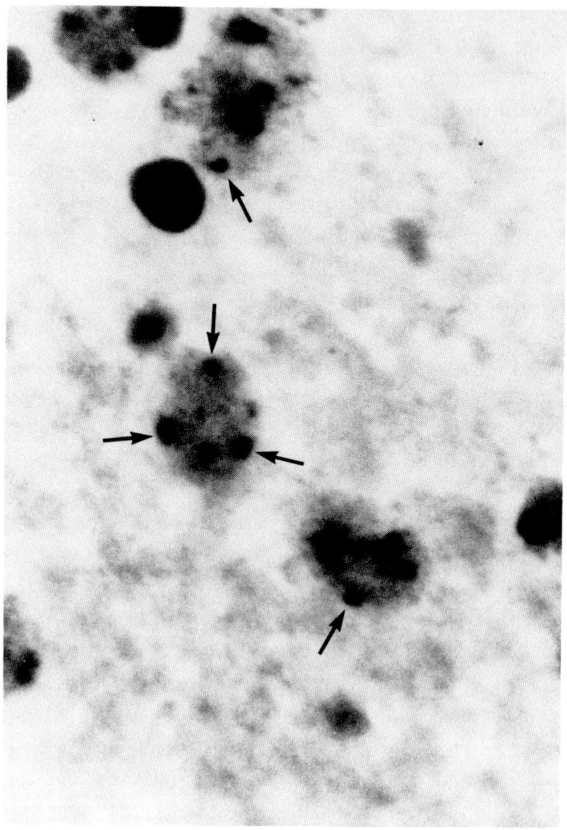

Figure 9.6. Negri bodies in cytoplasm of Purkinje cell in cerebellum. Micrograph courtesy of Dr. Makonnen Fekadu, DVM, PhD. Centers for Disease Control.

Clinical Manifestations

Following infection, rabies can produce five recognized clinical stages in humans: (1) incubation period, (2) prodrome, (3) acute neurologic phase, (4) coma, and (5) death.

As mentioned previously, the severity of the wounds and the site of inoculation will influence the length of the incubation period. Children tend to have shorter incubation periods. Curiously, there is also a trend toward a shorter incubation period in vaccine recipients with vaccine failure. It has been suggested that the presence of acute stress and the use of steroids can also shorten the length of the incubation period.[92–95]

The prodromal period lasts from 2 to 10 days and is characterized by such nonspecific symptoms as malaise, headache, fever, fatigue, anorexia, nausea, vomiting, diarrhea, cough, and sore throat. Anxiety, and occasionally visual or olfactory hallucinations, can occur. The most consistent and specific symptom of this stage, found in up to 50% of the patients, is local pain and paresthesias at the site of inoculation, which may have already healed completely.[1,92–95]

The symptomatology of the neurologic phase can be one of two different types—a "furious" presentation or a "paralytic" or "dumb" presentation.[92–95] The furious type is characterized by agitation, hyperactivity, bizarre behavior, aggressiveness with attempts to bite other persons, disorientation, and hallucinations. Hydrophobia, the most characteristic finding of rabies, occurs in 17–50% of reported cases. It is the result of painful spasms of the pharyngeal and laryngeal muscles when the patient swallows fluids, and may cause pulmonary aspiration. A conditioned response is created, and patients develop "fear" just from looking at water. Other stimuli that may cause similar spasms and bouts of terror are the blowing of air over the patient's face (aerophobia), loud sounds, touching the patient's skin and exposure to bright lights. Among symptoms during this stage are fever, hypersalivation, and paralysis.[1, 92–95] Focal or generalized seizures are frequent and were the cause of death in 28% of the cases in one reported series.[99]

The paralytic or dumb rabies may be the primary presentation or follow the furious stage. It presents in approximately 10–15% of patients, either as a progressive, flaccid, ascending, symmetric paralysis closely mimicking the Guillain-Barré syndrome, or as an asymmetric paralysis involving the exposed extremity. Respiratory and cranial nerves also may be involved, leading to respiratory insufficiency.[1,92–95] Neurologic findings may wax and wane during the acute neurologic phase. Death during the acute phase results from cardiac or respiratory problems. The acute neurologic phase lasts two to ten days, with eventual deterioration of the patient's mental status into coma.

During the coma stage, a variety of phenomena that can arise are focal or generalized seizures, hyperventilation, brain edema, pneumonia, aspiration, atelectasis, and hypersalivation. Hypothalamic involvement may result in diabetes insipidus, inappropriate secretion of antidiuretic hormone, or hypothermia or hyperthermia. Autonomic-nervous-system abnormalities may result in cardiac dysrhythmias, hypotension and hypertension, paralytic ileus, and urinary retention.[92–95] The duration of this stage is variable, and survival depends on the aggressiveness of supportive therapy. Rabies is almost universally fatal and there are only a few isolated reports of recovery from it.[100]

Diagnosis

The importance of the diagnosis of rabies lies in its potential for transmission to close contacts, health-care workers, or transplant recipients exposed to tissues from infected patients.[1] The diagnosis can be made by histopathology, virus cultivation, serology, or detection of viral antigen.[1,81,83,92–95] Unfortunately, there are no known methods to identify rabies infection prior to the onset of clinical signs. The available history of an animal bite in the recent past will help suggest the diagnosis, but the disease should be suspected in any case of rapidly progressive encephalitis, even if there is no history of animal exposure. Other clinical entities to rule out are encephalitides attributable to other viruses, tetanus, botulism, Guillain-Barré syndrome, and poliomyelitis.[92–95,97]

The virus is easily grown from postmortem material, but isolation from saliva, CSF, and urine is possible antemortem, especially during the early phase of the illness. Serologic diagnosis is possible if the patient survives beyond the acute period. Neutralizing antibodies in serum and CSF can be detected by day 6 to 10 in vitro by a rapid fluorescent focus-inhibition test (RFFIT) or in vivo by the mouse-infection neutralization test (MNT). The presence of antibody in either serum or CSF indicates infection in the absence of past immunization. Recently, detection of rabies virus antigens by immunofluorescence from the skin of the neck and/or corneal epithelium has been used, with rapid and reliable results.[1,81,83,92–95] However, in a retrospective review of 28 cases of rabies by Anderson and colleagues,[97] viral isolation was the only test that gave positive results during the first four days of illness, while immunofluorescence testing of skin or corneal specimens was helpful only in 50% of the tested patients within the first 10 days of illness.

Prevention

As mentioned before, the treatment of rabies, once the disease has developed, is mainly supportive. Prevention of potential exposure and adequate treatment of animal bites are the main measures that can be offered. Passive immunization can be accomplished with the human rabies immune globulin (HRIG), which is preferable to antiserum from animals.[92–96]

The only vaccine available in the United States since the duck-embryo vaccine was discontinued in 1981[92–96] is HDCV. It is a killed-virus vaccine that is safe and has been proved to provide excellent immunogenicity.

Persons likely to be exposed to rabies should receive preexposure prophylaxis. Laboratory workers, veterinarians, animal-control officers, and people who travel to areas where rabies is highly endemic should receive initial immunization followed by maintenance boosters with killed-rabies vaccine. A preexposure vaccination schedule would include administration of 1 ml of HDCV on days 0, 7, and 21, with boosters every 2 years while exposure continues.[92–96]

Postexposure treatment is intended to prevent rabies in persons who have been exposed to the virus. Careful assessment of each individual case is important and should include information as to (1) the species of the biting animal, (2) the circumstances of the bite, and (3) the type of exposure. Public-health officers can provide valuable assistance in making decisions. Treatment includes 20 IU/kg of HRIG, with half the dose given intramuscularly and the other half at the wound site. HDCV at 1 ml on days 0, 3, 7, 14, and 28 should be started at the same time that the HRIG is given.[92–96,101]

Enteroviral Encephalitis

The enteroviruses are a group of at least 68 recognized viruses classified as picornaviruses (pico = small + rna, for ribonucleic acid). The enteroviruses include the polioviruses (3 types), the coxsackie A viruses (23 types), the coxsackie B viruses (6 types), the echoviruses (31 types), and 5 recently identified enteroviruses.[102–10] Humans are the only natural hosts of human polioviruses, coxsackieviruses, and echoviruses. Spread is from person to person by fecal–oral and possibly oral–oral and respiratory routes. Attack rates are greatest among those persons with poor personal hygiene.[102–105] During the summer, swimming pools may serve as a means to spread enteroviruses. Children make up the main susceptible cohort, as they lack protective antibody and their unhygienic habits facilitate its spread.[102–103] Approximately 60-70% of enteroviral infections occur in males. These agents are by far the most common pathogens that require hospitalization for suspected sepsis in young infants during the summer and fall in the United States.[102]

The enteroviruses are the etiologic agents for a wide variety of clinical syndromes.[102–105] All the members of this group of viruses can cause a syndrome of encephalitis, and they are the most common identifiable cause of the "aseptic meningitis" syndrome.[2,10,14,102–105] Only a small fraction of the acute encephalitides of known etiology is caused by enteroviruses. The most frequent serotypes causing encephalitis are echovirus 6 and 9 and coxsackievirus A9, B2, and B5.[2,10,14,102–105]

Pathogenesis and Pathology

The upper respiratory tract, particularly the oropharynx, is the portal of entry for most enteroviruses. After the initial acquisition of the virus, it is implanted in the pharynx and the lower alimentary tract and extends to the regional lymph nodes. From here, virus enters the bloodstream and gains access to cells of the reticuloendothelial system and of specific target organs, such as the meninges, brain, spinal cord, myocardium, and skin.[102–104] After entering the bloodstream, polioviruses gain access to the CNS at the level of the medulla oblongata or from passage at the capillary level to lower motor neuron fibers, from where they travel along nerve fibers into the CNS to infect motor neurons.[102–104] Coxsackie B viruses are associated with more severe illness than the type A group or the echovirus group.[102–104]

In the CNS, the enteroviruses can produce meningeal edema, congestion, and occasionally mild infiltration with inflammatory cells. Lesions in the brain and spinal cord are focal rather than diffuse, but frequently involve many different areas. They consist of areas of eosinophilic degeneration of cortical cells, clusters of mononuclear and glial cells, and perivascular cuffing.[102–104]

Clinical Manifestations

Frank encephalitis is a well-described, though unusual, manifestation of CNS infection with coxsackieviruses and echoviruses. Encephalitis is regarded as part of the spectrum of aseptic meningitis and rarely occurs without meningeal involvement.[102–104] Clinical manifestations are indistinguishable from those of other viral encephalitides. Occasionally, some patients present with focal manifestations, such as partial motor seizures, hemichorea, and acute cerebellar ataxia. The course is relatively benign in the vast majority of adult cases, but instances of residual neurologic damage and death have been reported, particularly in children and neonates.[102–105] The main consideration in the differential diagnosis, as with other encephalitides, is herpes simplex encephalitis, because of the availability of specific and effective treatment for the latter.

A syndrome of chronic meningoencephalitis caused by echoviruses has been described in patients with agammaglobulinemia and is associated with a dermatomyositis-like picture.[106]

The development of encephalitis during poliomyelitis is uncommon, and when it does occur, it is most commonly seen in infants. Seizures are a common feature. The paralysis in these patients is spastic, in contrast to the flaccid type seen in spinal poliomyelitis. Clinically, it is indistinguishable from other types of infectious encephalitis. The prognosis for polioencephalitis is poor, with death being the rule.[102–103]

Diagnosis

The CSF findings in enteroviral encephalitis are similar to those seen in enteroviral aseptic meningitis. Pleocytosis in the range of 10–500 cells/mm^3 are usual; mononuclear predominance is seen. Glucose is usually normal, and protein may be normal or slightly elevated.[102-104]

Viral isolation in cell culture is currently the most sensitive and reliable method for detecting enteroviruses in clinical specimens, except for most serotypes of group A coxsackieviruses. These viruses do not grow in cell culture and must be inoculated into newborn mice or guinea-pig embryos. In general, the cytopathic effect produced by enteroviruses in standard cell culture is quite distinctive and can be recognized fairly early and with accuracy by experienced technicians.[81] The isolation rate of enteroviruses from the CSF of patients with presumptive enteroviral meningitis varies from 43 to 77% in different geographic areas and with different predominant enterovirus serotypes.[81] The combined use of three or four different cell-culture types can significantly increase the yield and speed of virus recovery from clinical specimens.[81]

Serologic diagnosis of enteroviral infections depends on a fourfold rise in the titer of NT antibody in acute- and convalescent-phase sera. The main problem is the multiplicity of serotypes that need to be tested. An ELISA test to detect the presence of IgM during acute infection has been used with relatively good sensitivity.[81,102-104] Methodologies for the rapid diagnosis of enteroviral menigoencephalitis other than cell culture are still under development. Immunofluorescent staining of CSF leukocytes for viral antigen has been attempted.[107] The main problem is the low concentration of the virus in the CSF during infection. The use of complementary-deoxyribonucleic-acid probes for the detection of enteroviruses may improve the early detection of these infections, but at the present time the test is not sensitive enough to be used routinely.[50,81]

Mumps Encephalitis

Mumps is generally a self-limited febrile disease of childhood. Its most prominent manifestation is nonsuppurative swelling and tenderness of one or both parotid glands. It is caused by a virus of the paramyxovirus group, which is an RNA virus.[108,109]

Approximately 20–40% of the cases of mumps are subclinical.[108,109] Infections with the mumps virus are seasonal and peak between April and July, but mumps encephalitis occurs all year. It predominates in males.[108]

In the mid-1960s, mumps was the leading cause of viral encephalitis and was responsible for 20–30% of the cases. The widespread use of mumps vaccine in the United States has resulted in a decrease of more than 95% in reported cases of mumps meningoencephalitis. In 1983, the last year for which the CDC collected statistics on mumps encephalomyelitis, seven cases were reported in the United States.[108,109]

The CNS is involved as a complication of mumps in approximately 15% of the patients. Meningitis is far more common than is encephalitis.[105,109-113]

Encephalitis is reported to occur in 1 in 400 to 1 in 6,000 cases of mumps.[113] It has most often been of the postinfectious type, with demyelination the predominant pathologic finding.[108-110,113] A smaller group of patients develop encephalitis during the parotitis episode, and in this case the pathologic findings are those of a primary encephalitis with widespread neuronolysis and no evidence of demyelination.[108-110,113] Encephalitis may occur before the development of parotitis in up to 18% of the patients.[108]

The clinical manifestations of mumps encephalitis are those of a nonfocal encephalitic process not different from other encephalitides.[108-113] Neurologic symptoms and fever gradually resolve over 1 to 2 weeks. Death occurs in less than 2% of reported cases, and neurologic sequelae in only a small percentage.[111-113]

The diagnosis is easily suspected in patients with evident parotitis or in those with a recent history of mumps. In cases where the development of encephalitis precedes the parotitis, the diagnosis is more difficult but can be made readily once parotitis develops. No treatment is available.

CSF findings in mumps meningoencephalitis are the same as for mumps meningitis, with a mononuclear pleocytosis in the range of 10–1,000 cells/mm^3. Abnormally low glucose levels have been reported in 15–30% of the patients.[108-112] Elevation of CSF protein is usually mild.

Isolation of the virus from CSF can be done in primary monkey-kidney-cell lines, human diploid fibroblasts, or HeLa cells.[81] Serologic diagnosis can be made by testing for CF, HI, or NT antibodies.[81,112] Mumps-specific serum IgM has been found by ELISA and by an indirect immunofluorescence test. It develops during the first week of illness and may be found in 80–85% of the patients.[83]

Measles Encephalitis

Measles is a highly contagious disease that is transmitted with high efficiency via the respiratory route. Within family settings, introduction of measles into the household results in infection of nearly 100% of susceptibles.[114]

The measles virus is a member of the family *Paramyxoviridae* and the genus *Morbillivirus;* it is an RNA virus.[114]

In 1962, the year preceding the licensure of the measles vaccine, 481,530 measles cases were reported in the United States.[115] By 1979, reported cases of both measles and measles encephalitis reached all-time record lows of 13,597 and three cases, respectively. The three cases of measles encephalitis represented a greater than 99% reduction from levels in the prevaccine era.[115] During a period of 6 years from 1973 to 1979, 160 cases of measles encephalitis were reported to the CDC.[115] By 1981, only 3,032 cases of measles were reported.[114] More recently, there has been a resurgence of measles, with 2,933 cases reported to the CDC in 1988.[116] Outbreaks occurred mainly in California, Pennsylvania, New Jersey, and Virginia.[116] A decrease in the rate of immunization of children is the likely cause of the recent increase in cases.

Encephalitis occurs in about 0.5 to 1 of every 1,000 measles cases.[79,114,115,117] Symptoms of encephalitis usually are seen during the period of the measles exanthem and within 8 days of the onset of illness.[114,117] The risk of encephalitis rises with the age of the measles patient; the highest incidence is in school-age children.[114,115]

The clinical picture is characterized by a recurrence of the fever and the appearance of headache, lethargy, irritability, confusion, and seizures. Indeed, up to 56% of patients may experience seizures.[114,117] The great majority of patients improve and return to normal after 2 to 3 days, but about 30% of patients progress to a comatose state, which may persist for weeks.[114] Approximately 15% of people who have measles encephalitis die as a result of the illness.[115] In addition, 25% of the patients may develop brain damage, with such sequelae as mental retardation, seizures, severe behavior disorders, deafness, hemiplegia, and paraplegia.[114,115,117]

CSF findings are not different from those of other viral encephalitides. On the other hand, CSF abnormalities may be found in the absence of symptoms of meningoencephalitis. A prospective study of 59 patients with measles showed that CSF pleocytosis occurred in 30% of the patients, and abnormal EEG tracings were found in 11 of 22 patients. None of these patients had clinical evidence of encephalitis.[118]

Although the pathophysiologic mechanism of measles encephalitis was initially thought to be immunologic with predominance of demyelination, as is usual in postinfectious encephalomyelitis,[119] the detection of virus in brain tissue and CSF and the histologic changes of an acute viral encephalitis suggest that the encephalitis of measles can also be the result of direct viral invasion of the CNS.[114,117]

Rapid diagnosis of measles infection during the exanthematous period is achieved by detection of measles antigen by ELISA or immunofluorescence in nasopharyngeal secretions prior to and at the onset of rash and in skin biopsy up to a few days after onset of the rash. The virus is not easily recoverable from CSF or brain biopsy. Specific IgM to measles appears during the first days of the illness, peaks at 10 days, and is detectable for 4 weeks or more.[81,83,114,117]

Rubella Encephalitis

Rubella (German measles) is a mild viral infection characterized by low-grade fever, lymphadenopathy, and exanthematous rash, most commonly observed among school-aged children and susceptible adults. Its major morbidity is related to the severe congenital malformations it can induce when the infection occurs during pregnancy.

The rubella virus is a member of the *Rubivirus* genus of the family *Togaviridae*, and it is physiochemically related to the other members of its family (*Alphavirus*, *Flavivirus*, and *Pestivirus*).

The last large epidemic of rubella in the United

States took place in 1964, when more than 500,000 cases were reported from all over the country.[120] Rubella became a reportable disease in the United States in 1966. Prior to that year, information on the incidence of rubella came from several states that had maintained mandatory surveillance for many years.[121,122] The characteristic epidemic cycle of rubella in the United States was interrupted by the introduction of a live, attenuated rubella vaccine in 1969.[121,122] In 1988, 221 cases of rubella were reported to the CDC, while the median number of cases from 1983 to 1987 was 618.[116]

Encephalitis is a rare complication of rubella.[123,124] Sherman and colleagues[123] reported six cases of encephalitis in an epidemic of rubella during the spring of 1964 that involved approximately 30,000 children. The rate of encephalitis was 1 per 5,000 cases. However, since rubella does not always exhibit the characteristic rash, some cases of acute viral encephalitis of unknown etiology may be due to rubella.

The encephalitis caused by the rubella virus is similar to but less severe than that associated with measles.[123,124] Symptoms arise from 2 to 6 days after the onset of the rash, but occasionally the encephalitis may occur as long as one week after the illness begins, or even precede the exanthem.[123,124] Characteristically, the abrupt onset of headache, lethargy, irritability, and stiff neck is followed by fever, convulsions, and changes in the level of consciousness.[123,124] The duration of the illness is usually brief.

The mortality from rubella encephalitis is variable, with one report showing a mortality of 50% among six children studied in Pittsburgh in 1964,[123] whereas during the same period in Atlanta, another six children recovered uneventfully.[124] Kenny and associates[125] studied seven survivors of rubella encephalitis 1 year after their illness and found no significant intellectual dysfunction or social maladjustment. Five of the seven had abnormal EEG tracings, and two patients had minor neurologic abnormalities.

The CSF examination shows the presence of a mild lymphocytic pleocytosis in the range of 10–300 cells/mm^3, the protein is slightly elevated, and the glucose is normal.[123,124] EEG examination shows generalized dysrhythmia and slowing.[124] Rapid diagnosis of rubella during the exanthematous period is made by detection of rubella antigen by ELISA or IF in the nasopharyngeal secretions. Specific IgM to rubella appears early in the illness, peaks at 10 days and is detectable for 4 weeks or more.[81]

Varicella-Zoster Encephalitis

Varicella-zoster virus (VZV) is a herpesvirus, morphologically indistinguishable from other members of this group. As with other herpesviruses, it contains double-stranded DNA in a protein shell surrounded by a lipid envelope.[16,126-128]

In the United States, contact with VZV is almost universal, and the percentage of seroreactive native-born persons in urban areas approaches 100% by age 60.[126-128] Epidemics of chicken pox take place every winter and spring, but cases are recognized throughout the year.

For most children, varicella is a relatively benign disease; however, it may be associated with serious morbidity or mortality in neonates, immunocompromised patients, or adults.[16,126-129] As is true of other herpesviruses, VZV may produce a latent infection. After the initial infection of varicella, the virus remains in ganglion cells in a latent form without producing clinical manifestations. Reactivation of the virus produces zoster or "shingles."[16,126-129]

For unknown reasons, the major complications of varicella (i.e., pneumonia and encephalitis), are disproportionately common in very young children and in adults over 20 years of age.[126,130] Neurologic complications at the time of primary varicella infection in nonimmunocompromised children are uncommon, although an abnormal EEG was reported in 22% of uncomplicated cases of varicella.[16]

The most common neurologic manifestation of varicella is cerebellitis, found in 0.1– 0.75% of the cases.[81,127,128,131] It usually presents toward the end of the first or at the beginning of the second week after the onset of varicella. This illness is characterized by ataxia, nausea, vomiting, and headaches. Symptoms last from a few days to a few weeks. The prognosis is good. The cerebellar involvement in VZV seems to be more frequently the result of an immunologic reaction, and it is classified as a postinfectious encephalitis.[16]

Varicella encephalitis attributable to direct cerebral infection by the virus is seen in approximately 0.05% of patients.[16,131] Evidence of meningeal inflammation and perivascular cuffing by inflammatory cells in varicella encephalitis has been found at autopsy, although the virus has not been isolated from brain tissue, and the presence of inclusion bodies is uncommon.[16,132] Signs and symptoms typically appear 5 to 6 days after the onset of rash, and include fever, headache, meningeal signs, seizures, and alterations in consciousness.[16,131]

The characteristic lesions of chicken pox or herpes zoster are frequently sufficient for diagnosis of VZV infection. However, HSV will occasionally cause vesicles in apparent dermatomal distribution, with lesions that are indistinguishable from those of VZV infection.[16,81,126-128,131] Detection of VZV antigen in skin eruptions by the IF technique can make an immediate diagnosis of the acute disease.[81,83]

Serology can be performed with numerous assays. Immunofluorescence, immunoperoxidase, and radioimmunoassay are all more sensitive than CF assays.[127] IgM to VZV can be detected by the fluorescent antibody to membrane antigen test (FAMA) as early as the second day of the rash.[127]

VZV can be isolated from the vesicles in cultures of human fetal fibroblasts. The virus grows relatively slowly (4 to 7 days) and may be difficult to isolate because of the presence of antibody or interferon in the vesicle, especially in the case of herpes zoster.[81] Serologic recognition of the presence of specific IgM may be useful for diagnosing primary varicella but is not useful for herpes zoster.[81] DNA probes have shown good sensitivity in initial studies.[50]

Mortality ranges from 15 to 35%.[16,126,131] During the period 1972–1978, 403 cases of varicella-associated encephalitis were reported. There were 64 deaths, for a mortality rate of 15%.[130] Significant sequelae occur in 10–15% of the cases.[16]

Herpes zoster affects approximately 1% of the general population, mainly older persons. Up to 25% of those with underlying neoplasms, particularly lymphomas,[16,126-128] may develop herpes zoster.

Zoster encephalitis is much less common than localized radiculomyelitic disease but is more common than isolated zoster myelitis.[16,132,133] Cerebral symptoms may be due to direct brain infection by the virus. Rarely, a VZV-induced vasculitis with subsequent stroke may occur.[16] Encephalitis predominately is found in patients with underlying immunosuppression and appears to be more frequent after trigeminal zoster than after infection of other sites.[16] The mortality from herpes-zoster encephalitis is difficult to determine, but it seems to be in the range of 20–30%.[16,134]

Abnormal EEGs have been obtained in patients with zoster encephalitis. CSF pleocytosis has been reported in approximately 40% of patients with uncomplicated zoster. In patients with encephalitis, mononuclear pleocytosis up to 500 cells/mm^3 and elevated CSF protein have been commonly reported.[16,134]

Pathology shows mononuclear cell infiltrates in the CNS with perivascular location; demyelination has also been described. CNS inflammation has been reported to be diffuse as well as focal. Granulomatous giant-cell arteritis, intranuclear inclusions, and virus-like particles in endothelial cells in the meninges have been observed, particularly in patients with VZV-induced vasculitis.[16,134]

For the most part, treatment of VZV infections has focused on the prevention and treatment of disseminated disease in immunocompromised patients.[16,126,128,129] Antiviral therapy is available in the form of acyclovir and is indicated for patients with varicella or zoster who have severe immunosuppression. It is also recommended that therapy be given to patients with normal immune systems who develop serious complications of VZV, such as pneumonia or encephalitis. Acyclovir should be given intravenously at a dosage of 30 mg/kg/day in three divided doses for 10 days.[126,128,129]

The use of immunoglobulin prophylaxis with varicella-zoster immune globulin prepared from normal donor plasma selected for high antiviral titers is currently recommended for prevention of varicella in high-risk susceptibles.[126,128]

A live, attenuated varicella vaccine that has been under development for at least 15 years is currently being considered for licensure in the United States.[128] The vaccine is effective but can produce a rash, as well as a mild varicella infection. Therefore, immunocompromised vaccine recipients must be chosen carefully.[138] The vaccines are infectious to other patients, and the vaccine strain can establish latent infection and can reactivate to produce typical zoster. Therefore, one of the main goals of vaccination—the prevention of zoster—is not met.[128]

Epstein-Barr Virus Encephalitis

EBV belongs to the herpesvirus group. It is the etiologic agent for all cases of heterophile-positive infectious mononucleosis (IM) and for some cases of heterophile-negative mononucleosis. In addition, the virus has been associated with African Burkitt's lymphoma, nasopharyngeal carcinoma, and lymphoproliferative diseases associated with immunodeficiency disorders or with immunosupression after organ transplantation.[129,135] EBV has a worldwide distribution, but prevalence of infection varies markedly in different cultural and socioeconomic settings. In some countries, such as China and

Japan, over 90% of children have antibodies to EBV by age 3 to 6 years,[135] whereas infections in developed countries are often delayed into late childhood or early adolescence.[135]

Usually a benign disease, IM is characterized mainly by fever, lymphadenopathy, and tonsillopharyngitis. Hepatomegaly and splenomegaly may also be present.[129,135] Serious nervous-system disorders have been estimated to affect approximately 1–5% of hospitalized patients with IM, and are seen mostly during its clinical course.[135,136] The pathophysiology of the CNS manifestations of EBV is unknown. Lymphocytic infiltration may produce a vasculitis and ischemia or an immunologic mechanism may be responsible.[135] Direct viral invasion of neurons seems probable, and a postinfectious immunologic mechanism is possible.[135-138]

The encephalitis of EBV usually presents at the time of the other manifestations of IM, but can also present before or after typical IM.[135-138] The symptoms are not different from other viral encephalitides, although a syndrome called "Alice in Wonderland" with visual distortion of images may occur. The outcome is usually good, however, some fatalities have been reported.[135-138] The figures for mortality and residual morbidity after neurologic involvement are less than 8 and 12% respectively.[138]

The findings in the CSF vary from normal to a mild mononuclear pleocytosis with or without an increased protein concentration. Almost all survivors recover completely.[135-138]

EBV infection is diagnosed by determination of heterophile antibodies and by EBV specific serology. Antibodies to viral capsid antigen, early antigens, and EBV-associated nuclear antigen are useful diagnostically.[133] Isolation of the virus from the CSF has also been reported.[139]

Approach to the Patient with Suspected Encephalitis

The possibility of encephalitis should be raised whenever a patient presents with a febrile illness associated with an altered mental status, focal neurologic symptoms, or an abnormal behavior.

A careful clinical history will give information regarding possible epidemiologic clues—such as travel to an area with a known active outbreak of arboviral encephalitis, possible exposure to or presence of an illness where encephalitis may be a complicating feature (i.e., mumps, chicken pox), or presence of nonneurologic symptoms—that may direct the clinician to a possible etiologic diagnosis. The time of the year may be helpful in ruling out infections with known seasonal presentation. The time course of the illness may help differentiate a chronic infection from an acute one.

A detailed physical and neurologic examination should help to define the extent of neurologic involvement, if there are focalizing findings, or if there is a diffuse involvement of higher cerebral functions.

Because there is effective treatment for most bacterial "meningoencephalitides," and also for HSVE, these should be the most important diagnoses to be considered and excluded. A lumbar puncture to examine the CSF is the procedure that will be helpful in differentiating a "viral" from a "bacterial" process. It may need to be repeated after 24–48 hours because many viral infections may initially present with a predominately neutrophilic pleocytosis suggestive of a bacterial process. When there is doubt, the patient may be treated for a possible bacterial meningoencephalitis until the appropriate cultures are finalized. The CSF should be sent for Gram stain and AFB stain, as well as for bacterial antigen and cryptococcal antigen detection, bacterial and viral cultures, and glucose and protein determination. The use of serum or CSF to determine the presence of specific viral antibodies or antigens is at best only helpful to make a retrospective diagnosis.

If a viral infection seems to be the cause of the encephalitic syndrome, the main diagnosis to consider is HSVE, and it should be pursued. The presence of focal neurologic findings is in favor of HSVE but other viral encephalitides (mainly La Crosse encephalitis) and bacterial infections (brain abscess or empyema) may also present in this way. HSVE may also present with diffuse involvement of the CNS. Diagnostic tests that may show evidence of localized CNS involvement should be performed as soon as possible. MRI, if available, and an EEG should be the initial tests performed since they are the most sensitive noninvasive tests, followed by CT and technetium scans.

If HSVE is a possibility, a brain biopsy should be scheduled immediately, if the appropriate facilities to obtain the speciment and perform the pathologic and microbiologic studies required are available. Because the morbidity and mortality of HSVE are influenced by the use of acyclovir, particularly when administered early in the course of the disease, treatment with intravenous acyclovir should be started as soon as the diagnosis of HSVE is considered, and may be continued until the biopsy results are finalized. If there is enough evidence of HSVE, therapy should be continued for 10 to 14 days. If the viral cultures are negative at 5 days, acyclovir may be discontinued. If there is evidence of another condition for which treatment is available, specific therapy should be instituted.

In summary, a high index of suspicion and an aggressive diagnostic and therapeutic approach may influence the outcome of the "treatable" causes of encephalitis. Unfortunately, for the vast majority of the cases, no specific treatment is available and supportive therapy is the cornerstone of treatment.

References

1. Benson CA, Harris AA: Acute neurologic infections. *Med Clin North Am* 1986;70:987–1011.
2. Ho DD, Hirsch MS: Acute viral encephalitis. *Med Clin North Am* 1985;69:415–429.
3. Koskiniemi M, Manninen V, Vaheri A: Acute encephalitis: a survey of epidemiological, clinical and microbiological features covering a twelve year period. *Acta Med Scand* 1981;209:6115–120.
4. Meyer HM, Johnson RT, Crawford IP, et al: Central nervous system syndromes of "viral" etiology. A study of 713 cases. *Am J Med* 1960;29:334–347.
5. Cherry JD, Shields WD: Encephalitis and meningoencephalitis, in Feigin RD, Cherry JD (eds): *Textbook of Pediatric Infectious Diseases,* 2nd ed. Philadelphia, WB Saunders, 1987, pp 494–496.
6. Koskiniemi M, Vaheri A: Acute encephalitis of viral origin. *Scan J Infect Dis* 1982;14:181–187.
7. Centers for Disease Control: Encephalitis surveillance, 1978. *CDC Annual Summary,* May 1981.
8. Kennard C, Swash M: Acute viral encephalitis: its diagnosis and outcome. *Brain* 1981;104:129–148.
9. Ho M: Acute viral encephalitis, in Vinken PJ, Bruyn GW (eds): *Handbook of Clinical Neurology: Infections of the Central Nervous System II.* New York, North-Holland Publishing Co, 1978, pp 63–82.
10. Powell KE, Kappus KD: Epidemiology of St. Louis encephalitis and other acute encephalitides. *Adv Neurol* 1978;19:197–215.
11. Monath TP: Arthropod-borne encephalitides in the Americas. *Bull WHO* 1979;57:513–531.
12. Rennels MB: Arthropod-borne virus infections of the central nervous system. *Neurol Clin* 1984; 2:241–254.
13. Centers for Disease Control: Summary of notifiable diseases, United States, 1987. *MMWR* 1988;36:3–11, 18–19, 53–59.
14. Beghi E, Nicolosi A, Kurland LT, et al: Encephalitis and aseptic meningitis, Olmstead County, Minnesota, 1950–1981. I. Epidemiology. *Ann Neurol* 1984;16:283–294.
15. Whitley RJ: *Herpes simplex* infections of the central nervous system. A review. *Am J Med* 1988; 85(supp2A):61–67.
16. Tenser RB: *Herpes simplex* and *herpes zoster*. Nervous system involvement. *Neurol Clin* 1984;2:215–240.
17. Griffith JF, CH'ien LT: *Herpes simplex* virus encephalitis. Diagnostic and treatment considerations. *Med Clin North Am* 1983;67:991–1008.
18. Whitley RJ, Soong SJ, Dolin R, et al: Adenine arabinoside therapy of biopsy-proved *herpes simplex* encephalitis. National Institute of Allergy and Infectious Diseases Collaborative Antiviral Study. *N Engl J Med* 1977;297:289–294.
19. Smith MG, Lennette EH, Reames HR: Isolation of the virus of *herpes simplex* and the demonstration of intranuclear inclusions in a case of acute encephalitis. *Am J Pathol* 1941;17:55–68.
20. Whitley RJ, Alford CA, Hirsch MS, et al: Vidarabine versus acyclovir therapy in *herpes simplex* encephalitis. *N Engl J Med* 1986;314:144–149.
21. Skoldenberg B, Forsgren M, Alestig K, et al: Acyclovir versus vidarabine in *herpes simplex* encephalitis. Randomized multicentre study in consecutive Swedish patients. *Lancet* 1984;2:707–711.
22. Whitley RJ, Soong SJ, Hirsch MS, et al: *Herpes simplex* encephalitis: vidarabine therapy and diagnostic problems. *N Engl J Med* 1981;304:313–318.
23. Whitley RJ, Nahmias AS, Visintine AM, et al: The natural history of *herpes simplex* virus infection of mother and newborn. *Pediatrics* 1980;66:489–494.
24. Whitley RJ, Nahmias AJ, Soong SJ: Vidarabine therapy of neonatal *herpes simplex* virus infection. *Pediatrics* 1980;66:495–501.
25. Kohl S: *Herpes simplex* virus encephalitis in children. *Pediatri Clin North Am* 1988;35:465–483.
26. Whitley R, Lakeman AD, Nahmias A, et al: DNA restriction-enzyme analysis of *herpes simplex* virus isolates obtained from patients with encephalitis. *N Engl J Med* 1982;307:1060–1062.
27. Ellison PH, Hanson PA: *Herpes simplex:* a possible cause of brain-stem encephalitis. *Pediatrics* 1977; 59:240–243.
28. Latronico N, Candiani A: Brainstem herpes virus encephalitis (letter). *Lancet* 1987;19–2(8560):690–691.
29. Sage JI, Weinstein MP, Miller DC: Chronic encephalitis possibly due to *herpes simplex* virus: two cases. *Neurology* 1985;35:1470–1472.
30. Klapper PE, Cleator GM, Longson M: Mild forms

of herpes encephalitis. *J Neurol Neurosurg Psychiatry* 1984;47:1247–1250.

31. Oommen KJ, Johnson PC, Ray CG: *Herpes simplex* type 2 virus encephalitis presenting as psychosis. *Am J Med* 1982;73:445–448.
32. Olson LC, Buescher EL, Artensein MS, et al: Herpesvirus infections of the human central nervous system. *N Engl J Med.* 1967;277:1271–1277.
33. Leider W, Magoffin RL, Lennette EH, et al: *Herpes simplex* virus encephalitis and its possible association with reactivated latent infection. *N Engl J Med* 1965;273:341–347.
34. Davis LE, Johnson RT: An explanation for the localization of *Herpes simplex* encepahlitis. *Ann Neurol* 1979;5:2–5.
35. Drachman DA, Adams RD: *Herpes simplex* and acute inclusion body encephalitis. *Arch Neurol* 1962;7:61–79.
36. Esiri M: *Herpes simplex* encephalitis, an immunohistological study of the distribution of viral antigen within the brain. *J Neurol Sci* 1982;54:209–226.
37. Nahmias AJ, Whitley RJ, Visintine AL, et al: *Herpes simplex* virus encephalitis: Laboratory evaluations and their diagnostic significance. *J Infect Dis* 1982;145:829–836.
38. Johnson RT: Pathogenesis of herpes virus encephalitis. I—Virus pathways to the nervous system of suckling mice demonstrated by fluorescent antibody staining. *J Exp Med* 1964;119:343–356.
39. Johnson RT, Mims CA: Pathogenesis of viral infections of the nervous system. *N Engl J Med* 1968;278;23–30.
40. Barringer JR, Swoveland P: Recovery of *Herpes simplex* virus from human trigeminal ganglions. *N Engl J Med* 1973;288:648–650.
41. Morawetz RB, Whitley RJ, Murphy DM: Experience with brain bipsy for suspected herpes encephalitis. A review of forty consecutive cases. *Neurosurgery* 1983;12:654–657.
42. Whitley RJ, Soong SJ, Linneman C Jr, et al: *Herpes simplex* encephalitis: clinical assessment. *JAMA* 1982;247:317–320.
43. Schlageter, J: *Herpes simplex* encephalitis without CSF lekocytosis. *Arch Neurol* 1984;41:1007–1008.
44. Vaheri A, Keski-Oja J, Salonen EM, et al: Cerebrospinal fluid IgG bands and virus specific IgG, IgM and IgA antibodies in *herpes simplex* virus encephalitis. *J. Neuroimmunol* 1982;3:247–261.
45. Skoldenberg B, Kalimo K, Carlstrom A, et al: *Herpes* simplex encephalitis: a serological follow-up study. Synthesis of *herpes simplex* virus immunoglobulin M, A and G antibodies and development of oligoclonal immunoglobulin G in the central nervous system. *Acta Neurol Scand* 191;63:273–285.
46. Levine DP, Lauter CB, Lerner AM: Simultaneous serum and CSF antibodies in *herpes simplex* encephalitis. *JAMA* 1978;240:356–360.
47. Lakeman FD, Koga J, Whitley RJ: Detection of antigen to *herpes simplex* virus in cerebrospinal fluid from patients with *herpes simplex* encephalitis. *J Infect Dis* 1987;1455:1172–1178.
48. Boerman RH, Raap AK, VD Ploeg M: Rapid diagnosis of *herpes simplex* virus type 1 encephalitis by radioactive genome detection in cerebrospinal fluid (letter). *Lancet* 1987;1:94.
49. Redfield DC, Richman D, Albanil, et al: Detection of *herpes simplex* virus in clinical specimens by DNA hybridization. *Diag Microbiol Infect Dis* 1983;1:117–128.
50. Tenover FC: Diagnostic deoxyribonucleic acid probes for infectious diseases. *Clin Microbiol Rev* 1988;1:82–101.
51. Koskiniemi M, Vaheri A, Manninem V, et al: *Herpes simplex* virus encephalitis: new diagnostic and clinical features and results of therapy. *Arch Neurol* 1980;37:763–767.
52. Cappel R, Thiry L, Clinet G: Viral antibodies in the CSF after acute CNS infections. *Arch Neurol* 1975;32:629–631.
53. Kahlon J, Chatterjee S, Lakeman FD, et al: Detection of antibodies to *herpes simplex* virus in the cerebrospinal fluid of patients with *herpes simplex* encephalitis. *J Infect Dis* 1987;155:38–44.
54. Schoechetman G, Ou C, Jones WK: Polymerase chain reaction. *J Infect Dis* 1988;158:1154–1157.
55. Brodkorb E, Lindqvist M, Jonsson M, et al: Diagnosis of *Herpes simplex* encephalitis. A comparison between electroencephalography and computed tomography findings. *Acta Neurol Scand* 1982; 66:462–471.
56. Smith JB, Westmoreland BF, Reagan TJ, et al: A distinctive clinical EEG profile in *herpes simplex* encephalitis. *Mayo Clin Proc* 1975;50:469–474.
57. Wolman B, Longson M: Herpes encephalitis. *Acta Pediatr Scand* 1977;66:243–246.
58. Davis JM, Davis KR, Kleinman GM, et al: Computed tomography of *herpes simplex* encephalitis, with clinicopathological correlation. *Radiology* 1978;129:409–417.
59. Greenberg SB, Taber L, Septimus E, et al: Computarized tomography in brain biopsy proven *herpes simplex* encephalitis. *Arch Neurol* 1981;38:58–59.
60. Schroth G, Gawehn J, Thron A, et al: Early diagnosis of *herpes simplex* encephalitis in MRI. *Neurology* 1987;37:179–183.
61. Kohl S, James AR: *Herpes simplex* virus encephalitis during childhood. Importance of brain biopsy diagnosis. *J Pediatr* 1985;107:212–215.
62. Whitley RJ: The frustrations of treating *herpes simplex* virus infections of the central nervous system (editorial). *JAMA* 1988;259:1067.
63. Craven RB: Togaviruses, in Belshe RB (ed): *Text-*

book of Human Virology. Littleton, NH, PSG Publishing Co, 1984, pp 599–648.
64. Tsai TF, Monath TP: Viral diseases in North America transmitted by arthropods or from vertebrate reservoirs, in Feigin RD, Cherry JD (eds): *Textbook of Pediatric Infectious Diseases,* 2nd ed. Philadelphia, WB Saunders, 1987, pp 1417–1456.
65. Watts DM, Thompson WH, Yvill TM, et al: Overwintering of *La Crosse* virus in *Aedes triseriatus*. *Am J Trop Med Hyg* 1974;23:694–700.
66. Thompson WH, Beaty BJ: Venereal transmission of *La Crosse* viruse from male to female *Aedes triseriatus*. *Am J Trop Med Hyg* 1978;27:187–196.
67. Potter ME, Currier II RW, Pearson JE, et al: Western equine encephalomyelitis in horses in the northern Red River Valley, 1975. *JAVMA* 1977;170: 1396–1399.
68. Centers for Disease Control: Arboviral infections of the central nervous system, United States, 1987. *MMWR* 1988;37:506–515.
69. Meyer KF, Haring CM, Howitt BF: The etiology of encephalomyelitis in horses in the San Joaquin Valley, 1930. *Science* 1931;74:227–228.
70. Howitt BF: Recovery of the virus of equine encephalomyelitis from the brain of a child. *Science* 1938;88:455–456.
71. Monath TP: Epidemiology, in Monath TP (ed): *St. Louis Encephalitis*. Washington, DC, American Public Health Association, 1980, pp 239–312.
72. Longshore WA, Stevens IM, Hollister AC, et al: Epidemiologic observations on acute infectious encephalitis is California, with special reference to the 1952 outbreak. *Am J Hyg* 1956;63:69–86.
73. Schultz DR, Barthal JS, Garret C: Western equine encephalitis with rapid onset of parkinsonism. *Neurology* 1977;27:1095–1096.
74. Calisher CH, Berardi VP, Muth DJ, et al: Specificity of immunoglobulin M and G antibody responses in humans infected with eastern and western equine encephalitis viruses: application to rapid serodiagnosis. *J Clin Microbiol* 1986;23:369–372.
75. Goldfield M, Sussman O: The 1959 outbreak of eastern encephalitis in New Jersey. *Am J Epidemiol* 1968;87:1–57.
76. Fothergill LD, Dingle JH, Farber S, et al: Human encephalitis caused by the virus of the eastern variety of equine encephalomyelitis. *N Engl J Med* 1938;219:415.
77. McGowan JE, Bryan JA, Gregg MB: Surveillance of arboviral encephalitis in the United States, 1955–1971. *Am J Epidemiol* 1973;97:199–207.
78. Powell KE, Blakey DL: St. Louis encephalitis. The 1975 epidemic in Mississippi. *JAMA* 1977; 237:2294–2298.
79. Southern PM Jr, Smith JW, Luby JP, et al: Clinical and laboratory features of epidemic St. Louis encephalitis. *Ann Intern Med* 1969;71:681–689.
80. White MG, Carter NW, Rector FC, et al: Pathophysiology of epidemic St. Louis encephalitis. I—Inappropriate secretion of antidiuretic hormone. *Ann Intern Med* 1969;71:691–702.
81. Chonmaitree T, Baldwin CD, Lucia HL: Role of the virology laboratory in diagnosis and management of patients with central nervous system disease. *Clin Microbiol Rev* 1989;2:1–14.
82. Monath TP, Nystrom RR, Bailey RE, et al: Immunoglobulin M antibody capture enzyme-linked immunosorbent assay for diagnosis of St. Louis encephalitis. *J Clin Microbiol* 1984;20:784–790.
83. Grandien M, Olding-Stenkvist E: Rapid diagnosis of viral infections. *Scan J Infect Dis* 1984;16:1–8.
84. Hammon WMcD, Reeves WC, Galindo P: Epidemiologic studies of encephalitis in the San Joaquin Valley of California, 1943, with the isolation of viruses from mosquitoes. *Am J Hyg* 1945;42:299–306.
85. Hammon WMcD, Reeves WC: California encephalitis virus: a newly described agent. *Calif Med* 1952;77:303–309.
86. Thompson WH, Kalfayan B, Anslow RO: Isolation of California encephalitis group virus from a fatal human illness. *Am J Epidemiol* 1965;81:245–253.
87. Peters CJ, LeDuc JW: Bunyaviruses, phleboviruses and related viruses, in Belshe RB (ed): *Text of Human Virology*. Littleton, NH, PSG Publishing Co, 1984, pp 547–598.
88. Thompson WH, Evans AS: California encephalitis virus studies in Wisconsin. *Am J Epidemiol* 1965;81:230–244.
89. Balfour HH Jr, Siem RA, Bauer H, et al: California arbovirus *(La Crosse)* infections. I—Clinical and laboratory findings in 66 children with meningoencephalitis. *Pediatrics* 1973;52:680–691.
90. Monath TP: Arboviruses of Central and South America, in Feigin RD, Cherry JD (eds): *Textbook of Pediatric Infectious Diseases,* 2nd ed. Philadelphia, WB Saunders, 1987, pp 1456–1468.
91. Steele JH: Rabies in the Americas and remarks on global aspects. *Rev Infect Dis* 1988;10(S4):S585–S597.
92. Robinson PA: Rabies virus, in Belshe RB (ed): *Textbook of Human Virology*. Littleton, NH, PSG Publishing Co, 1984, pp 485–511.
93. Bernard KW, Hattwick MAW: Rabies virus, in Mandel GL, Douglas RG Jr, Benett JE (eds): *Principles and Practices of Infectious Diseases,* 2nd ed. New York, Wiley Med Publication, 1985, pp 897–907.
94. Atanasiu P, Gamet A: Rabies, in Vinken PJ, Bruyn GW (eds): *Handbook of Clinical Neurology. Infections of the Nervous System II*. New York, North-Holland Publishing Co, 1978, pp 235–274.
95. Plotkin SA, Clark HF: Rabies, in Feigin RD, Cherry JD (eds): *Textbook of Pediatric Infectious Diseases,*

2nd ed. Philadelphia, WB Saunders, 1987, pp 1676–1684.
96. Centers for Disease Control: Surveillance Summaries. Rabies Surveillance, United States, 1987. *MMWR* 1988;37(no.SS-4):1–17.
97. Anderson LJ, Nicholson KG, Tauxe RV, et al: Human rabies in the United States, 1960 to 1979: epidemiology, diagnosis, and presentation. *Ann Intern Med* 1984;100:728–735.
98. Centers for Disease Control: Human rabies—California, 1987. *MMWR* 1988;37:305–308.
99. Dupont JR, Earle KM: Human rabies encephalitis—a study of forty-nine fatal cases with a review of the literature. *Neurology* 1965;15:1023–1034.
100. Hattwick MAW, Weis TT, Stechschulte CJ, et al: Recovery from rabies—a case report. *Ann Intern Med* 1972;76:931,942.
101. Baer GM, Bridbord K, Hui FW: Research towards rabies prevention. *Rev Infect Dis* 1988;10:(S4)S573–S815.
102. Moore M, Morens DM: Enteroviruses, including polioviruses, in Belshe RB (ed): *Textbook of Human Virology*. Littleton, NH, PSG Publishing Co, 1984, pp 407–483.
103. Cherry JD: Enteroviruses: polioviruses (poliomyelitis), Coxsackieviruses, echoviruses, and enteroviruses, in Feigin RD, Cherry JD (eds): *Textbook of Pediatric Infectious Diseases,* 2nd ed. Philadelphia, WB Saunders, 1987, pp 1729–1790.
104. Modlin JE: Coxsackievirus and echovirus, in Mandel GL, Douglas RG Jr, Benett JE (eds): *Principles and Practices of Infectious Diseases,* 2nd ed. New York, Wiley Med Publication, 1985, pp 814–825.
105. Ratzan KR: Viral meningitis. *Med Clin North Am* 1985;69:399–413.
106. McKinney RE, Katz SL, Wilfert CM: Chronic enteroviral meningoencephalitis in agammaglobulinemic patients. *Rev Infect Dis* 1987;9:334–356.
107. Taber LH, Mirkovic RR, Adam V, et al: Rapid diagnosis of enterovirus meningitis by immunofluorescent staining of SCF leukocytes. *Intervirology* 1973;1:127–134.
108. Tolpin MD, Schauf V: Mumps virus, in Belshe RB (ed): *Textbook of Human Virology*. Littleton, NH, PSG Publishing Co, 1984, pp 311–331.
109. Brunell PA: Mumps, in Feigin RD, Cherry JD (eds): *Textbook of Pediatric Infectious Diseases,* 2nd ed. Philadelphia, WB Saunders, 1987, pp 1628–1632.
110. Taylor FB, Toreson WE: Primary mumps meningoencephalitis. *Arch Int Med* 1963;112:216–221.
111. McLean DM, Bach RD, Larke RPB, et al: Mumps meningoencephalitis, Toronto, 1963. *Can Med Assoc J* 1964;90:458–462.
112. Levitt LP, Rich TA, Kinde SW, et al: Central nervous system mumps. *Neurology* 1970;20:829–834.
113. Baum SG, Litman N: Mumps virus, in Mandel GL, Douglas RG Jr, Benett JE (eds): *Principles and Practices of Infectious Diseases,* 2nd ed. New York, Wiley Med Publication, 1985, pp 871–877.
114. Modlin JF: Measles virus, in Belshe RB (ed): *Textbook of Human Virology*. Littleton, NH, PSG Publishing Co, 1984, pp 333–360.
115. Centers for Disease Control: Measles encephalitis—United States, 1962–1979. *MMWR* 1981;30:362–364.
116. Centers for Disease Control: Summary of notifiable diseases, United States, 1988. *MMWR* 1989;37: 802–803.
117. Cherry JD: Measles, in Feigin RD, Cherry JD (eds): *Textbook of Pediatric Infectious Diseases,* 2nd ed. Philadelphia, WB Saunders, 1987, pp 1607–1628.
118. Hanninen P, Arstila P, Lang H, et al: Involvement of the central nervous system in acute, uncomplicated measles virus infection. *J Clin Microbiol* 1980;11:610–613.
119. Johnson RT, Griffin DE, Hirsch RL, et al: Measles encephalomyelitis—clinical and immunologic studies. *N Engl J Med* 1984;310:137–141.
120. Centers for Disease Control: Rubella surveillance. Report No. 1, 1969.
121. Centers for Disease Control: Rubella and congenital rubella, United States, 1984–1986. *MMWR* 1987; 36:664–675.
122. Preblud SR, Serdula MK, Frank JA, et al. Current status of rubella in the United States, 1969–1979. *J Infect Dis* 1980;142:776–779.
123. Sherman FE, Michaels RH, Kenny FM: Acute encephalopathy (encephalitis) complicating rubella. *JAMA* 1965;192:675–681.
124. Walker JM, Nahmias AJ: Neurologic sequelae of rubella infection. *Clin Pediatr* 1966;5:699–702.
125. Kenny FM, Michaels RH, Davis KS: Rubella encephalopathy. Later psychometric, neurologic, and encephalographic evaluation of seven survivors. *Am J Dis Child* 1965;110:374–380.
126. Weller TH: Varicella and *Herpes-zoster*. Changing concepts of the natural history, control, and importance of a not-so-benign virus. *N Eng J Med* 1983;309:1362–1368 and 1434–1440.
127. Brunell PA: *Varicella-zoster* infections, in Feigin RD, Cherry JD (eds): *Textbook of Pediatric Infectious Diseases,* 2nd ed. Philadelphia, WB Saunders, 1987, pp 1602–1607.
128. Straus SE: The management of varicella and zoster infections. *Inf Dis Clin North Am* 1987;1:367–382.
129. Hirsch MS, Schooley RT: Treatment of herpesvirus infections. *N Engl J Med* 1983;309:963–970.
130. Preblud SR: Age-specific risks of varicella complications. *Pediatrics* 1981;68:14–17.
131. Johnson RT, Milbourn PE: Central nervous system manifestations of chicken pox. *Can Med Assoc J* 1970;102:831–834.
132. McCormick WF, Rodnitzky RL, Schochet SS Jr, et

al: *Varicella-zoster* encephalomyelitis. *Arch Neurol* 1969;21:559–570.

133. Appelbaum E, Kreps SI, Sunshine A: *Herpes-zoster* encephalitis. *Am J Med* 1962;32:25–31.

134. Jemsek H, Greenberg SB, Taber L, et al: *Herpes-zoster* associated encephalitis: clinicopathologic report of 12 cases and review of the literature. *Medicine* 1983;62:81–97.

135. Fleisher GR: Epstein-Barr virus, in Belshe RB (ed): *Textbook of Human Virology*. Littleton, NH, PSG Publishing Co, 1984, pp 853–886.

136. Lange BJ, Berman PH, Bender J, et al: Encephalitis in infectious mononucleosis: diagnostic considerations. *Pediatrics* 1976;58:877–880.

137. Silverstein A, Steinberg G, Nathanson M: Nervous system involvement in infectious mononucleosis. *Arch Neurol* 1972;26:356–358.

138. Demey HE, Martin JJ, Leus RM, et al: Coma as a presenting sign of Epstein-Barr encephalitis. *Arch Int Med* 1988;148:1459–1461.

139. Halstead CC, Chang RS: Infectious mononucleosis and encephalitis. Recovery of Epstein-Barr virus from spinal fluid. *Pediatrics* 1979;64:257–258.

10
Postinfection Complications of the Central Nervous System

SHUBHA KERKAR AND ABDOLGHADER MOLAVI

Postinfection Encephalitis

Postinfection encephalitis/encephalomyelitis is an acute disease of the central nervous system (CNS) that occurs while a patient is recovering from an infectious disease, most commonly a viral infection. A clinically and histopathologically similar illness, called postvaccinal encephalomyelitis, may arise following administration of certain vaccines. Both of these syndromes are thought to be caused by some, as yet poorly defined host-immune attack on the brain and/or spinal cord, triggered by the temporally related infected or vaccination. Involvement of the CNS is usually widespread and the term "acute disseminated encephalomyelitis" has been used to describe the entity. Other terms, such as acute perivascular myelinoclasis, perivenous encephalitis, and acute demyelinating encephalomyelitis, have been introduced to describe its pathologic features. Correspondingly, the term "immune-mediated encephalomyelitis" has been used, to indicate its pathogenesis.

Etiology

Postinfection encephalomyelitis occurs most commonly after measles,[1,2] varicella,[1,3] herpes zoster,[4] mumps,[5,6] rubella,[1] influenza,[7,8] infectious mononucleosis,[9,10] and nonspecific acute febrile illnesses (most commonly, upper respiratory infections).[11] In rare cases where there is no history of a preceding illness, it is postulated that a subclinical viral infection may have been present.[12] With the exception of *Mycoplasma* infections,[13] postinfection encephalomyelitis is not a recognized complication of bacterial infections.

Postvaccinal encephalomyelitis has been seen as a complication of vaccinations employing vaccinia virus (smallpox)[14,15] or fixed rabies virus grown in neural tissue.[16] The occurrence of this complication after vaccination with attenuated measles virus is uncertain.[17] The discontinuation of smallpox vaccination and the use of duck-embryo-based (or human-diploid-cell) rabies vaccines, which contain no neural tissue and are not associated with neurologic complications, have left postvaccinal encephalomyelitis a matter of historical interest today.

Pathology

The essential histopathologic lesion is demyelination. This occurs in foci that are typically perivenular and may be distributed throughout the brain and spinal cord. Microglial proliferation is a prominent feature of the foci and is always found with demyelination.

The analysis of the literature on autopsy findings in postmeasles encephalomyelitis is suggestive of the following sequence of events.[18,19] The initial change appears to be infiltration of the walls of small veins in the white matter with mononuclear cells. This is followed by a perivenular inflammatory response, which is predominantly mononuclear. Later in the course, foci of demyelination develop, extending radially from the involved venules in the white matter. When the clinical condition is hyperacute and fulminant, multiple small hemorrhages are seen in the white matter. For such cases, the terms acute hemorrhagic leukoencephalitis and hemorrhagic immune-mediated encephalomyelitis have been used.[20,21]

Pathogenesis

The autoimmune mechanism of postinfection encephalomyelitis is supported by three lines of evidence. First, there is a lag between the infection (or vaccination) and the onset of the neurologic illness. Second, viruses have not been recovered from the brain and viral antigens have not been detected in brain tissue. Third, the neuropathologic findings are identical to those found in experimental allergic encephalomyelitis, a prototype autoimmune disease.

Most of the early research on postvaccinal neurologic complications was done in the 1920s and early 1930s when it became evident that the encephalomyelitis complicating smallpox vaccination had a histopathology similar to that seen after inoculation with rabies vaccine. Since the rabies vaccine used at that time (Semple type) was produced in animal-brain tissue, it was postulated that neurologic complications of the vaccine were due to an immune reaction to the brain tissue. Rivers and colleagues[22] tested this hypothesis by repeated intradermal injections of homogenized brain tissue into animals and produced the first experimental model of allergic encephalomyelitis.[22,23] However, only a minority of animals became ill after months of continued inoculation. Experimental allergic encephalomyelitis became a practical and reproducible experimental disease when Kabat and associates[24] discovered that it could be consistently induced by a single injection of brain homogenate emulsified in complete Freund's adjuvant. This experimental model made it possible to determine various antigens required to induce the disease.[25,26] The use of multiple adjuvants such as complete Freund's adjuvant and pertussis vaccine produced a hyperacute hemorrhagic white-matter disease resembling the human hemorrhagic immune-mediated encephalomyelitis.

The immune response in experimental allergic encephalomyelitis is cell mediated and results from T-cell sensitization to the myelin basic protein. The disease can be passively transferred with cloned T cells reactive with this protein.[27] An antibody to myelin basic protein is also present in experimental allergic encephalomyelitis, but its role is less clear and it will not transfer the disease. The myelin basic protein, which has a molecular weight of 18,500 daltons, constitutes 30% of the CNS myelin protein.[28]

Until the 1950s most rabies vaccines consisted of fixed rabies virus propagated in brain tissue and then inactivated. The vaccination schedule required daily inoculations over a two-week period. From the current understanding of the pathogenesis of experimental allergic encephalomyelitis, it is not surprising that this vaccination was attended by a high incidence of encephalomyelitis. High serum levels of antibody to myelin basic protein and intrathecal synthesis of the antibody have been seen in patients with encephalomyelitis following rabies vaccination, suggesting that myelin basic protein is an encephalitogenic antigen.[29]

Studies of fatal cases of measles encephalomyelitis have demonstrated a pattern of myelin protein loss resembling that seen in experimental allergic encephalomyelitis and an absence of viral antigen by immunoperoxidase staining and of viral RNA by in situ hybridization.[30,31] Lymphocytes from patients with measles encephalomyelitis, varicella encephalomyelitis, and encephalomyelitis following respiratory infections have been shown to proliferate when cultured in the presence of myelin basic protein, indicating affinity between the autoreactive lymphocytes and their antigenic target.[32] Peripheral lymphocytes responsive to myelin basic protein may act as effector cells in the process of demyelination[32] and are found to be considerably higher in patients with postmeasles encephalitis as compared with those with uncomplicated measles.[33] The absence of intrathecally generated antibodies against measles virus further suggests that the virus does not replicate in the brain.[32]

The mechanism by which a viral infection induces a cell-mediated immune response against myelin basic protein is not known. Antigens cross-reacting between virus and myelin protein have not been found, and considering the wide diversity of viruses associated with postinfection encephalomyelitis, this would seem an unlikely mechanism of pathogensis.

Epidemiology

Postinfection encephalitis/encephalomyelitis in the past accounted for nearly one third of the cases of acute encephalitis in the United States. The majority were associated with exanthematous viral infections, particularly measles, and, to a lesser extent, varicella and rubella. The successful immunization against measles, mumps, and rubella in the United States has decreased the incidences of these infections and the associated neurologic complications, Currently, nonspecific febrile illnesses, usually upper respiratory infections, are the most common antecedent infections, particularly in adults.

The incidence of encephalitis following measles is approximately one per 1,000 cases; while that for varicella is one per 2,500 cases.[34] CNS complications occur in one per 6,000 cases of rubella; most represent acute encephalopathy rather than postinfection demyelinating encephalitis.[12] Although some cases of mumps meningoencephalitis are due to direct viral invasion of brain parenchyma, the majority of carefully studied cases have shown perivenular demyelination typical of postinfection encephalitis.

Mycoplasma pneumoniae may cause encephalitis by either direct invasion of the brain parenchyma or an autoimmune mechanism. The observed delay of about two weeks between the respiratory episode and the appearance of neurologic symptoms and the presence of autoantibodies in the brain suggests an autoimmune etiology in some of the cases.

Encephalomyelitis following smallpox vaccination is only of historical interest, with a reported incidence in the United States of one per 300,000 primary vaccinations.[15] The incidence of this complication after vaccination with brain-derived Semple rabies vaccine is approximately 1 per 400.[16] This vaccine is no longer used in the United States.

Postinfection encephalomyelitis is seen more frequently in children and young adults because associated infections, such as measles, mumps, and varicella, are primarily childhood diseases. That which occurs after nonspecific febrile illnesses, however, is seen in all age groups.

Clinical Features

Postvaccinal encephalomyelitis usually develops about 8 to 15 days after inoculation. In the classic postinfection encephalomyelitis, the signs and symptoms of a specific infection appear and run a typical course that need not be unusually severe. Within a period of 3 to 13 days after the onset (i.e., rash in exanthematous illnesses, parotid swelling in mumps, etc.), the symptoms of CNS dysfunction became manifest. The latent period is short in rubella (1–5 days) but longer in varicella, mumps, and influenza, with measles occupying an intermediate position.

The onset is usually abrupt with fever and obtundation, frequently associated with seizures and multifocal neurologic signs. The illness may also begin subacutely with fever, headache, and vomiting. These are followed by symptoms and signs referable to the cerebrum, the cerebellum, the pontobulbar area, or the spinal cord, which may occur in any combination. Generalized convulsions occur in a significant proportion of patients (47–56% of those with postmeasles encephalitis).

The neurologic manifestations are polymorphic and may include hemiplegia, quadriplegia, cranial-nerve palsies, and optic neuritis. The last may occur as an anatomically isolated version of postinfection encephalitis.[36] Acute transverse myelitis has been observed either as part of encephalomyelitis or, occasionally, as the only manifestation of postinfection CNS complication.[1,37] Isolated involvement of the basal ganglia and development of movement disorders such as chorea and myoclonus have been reported, but are rare.

A cerebellar syndrome with ataxia, either unilateral or bilateral, occurs most commonly in varicella encephalitis,[3] but may appear following measles and rubella.[1] It begins abruptly, usually 5 to 6 days after the appearance of the rash. There may be associated vomiting, dysarthria, and nystagmus. Impairment of consciousness is rare, and pyramidal signs are absent. Most of the affected children make a complete recovery.

Acute hemorrhagic leukoencephalitis is a fulminant form of postinfection encephalitis. Most cases follow mild upper respiratory infections or influenza, with occasional cases being seen in association with viral exanthema of childhood. Typically, an ill-defined viral syndrome is followed by sudden headache, high fever, nuchal rigidity, mental confusion, stupor rapidly progressing to coma, generalized convulsions, and frequent focal neurologic abnormalities. Mortality is high, and death usually follows within a few days after the onset of neurologic symptoms.

Diagnosis

No reliable laboratory feature has been found that specifies the nature of the underlying neuropathologic process. The cerebrospinal-fluid (CSF) profile is consistent with aseptic meningitis. There is moderate pleocytosis, usually under 1,000/mm^3, with lymphocyte predominance. In acute hemorrhagic leukoencephalitis, the initial cells are mostly granulocytes, and erythrocytes are also often present. The CSF protein is slightly elevated and the glucose is within normal limits. Rarely, the CSF remains completely normal throughout the course of the illness. The electroencephalogram (EEG) is abnormal in at least 50% of cases, but the findings are nonspecific.

Computed Tomography

Computed tomography (CT) is not sensitive and the findings are nonspecific in postinfection encephalomyelitis. In a series of 11 patients reported by Lukes and Norman,[38] four had normal CT scans despite repeated examinations. Abnormalities were found in seven patients; these included hypodense nonenhancing lesions in the subcortical white matter and patchy or confluent contrast-enhancing cortical lesions. Delay between the onset of clinical signs and the appearance of lesions on CT scan was common, and there was limited correlation between clinical findings and the distribution and type of abnormality seen on the scan. Pasternak and associates[39] reported CT findings in two children with postvaricella encephalomyelitis. The scan was normal in one but showed a low-density cerebellar lesion on the other that correlated with clinical findings.

Magnetic-Resonance Imaging

Magnetic-resonance imaging (MRI) is highly sensitive in detecting white-matter abnormalities; hence it is well suited to demonstrate lesions in postinfection encephalomyelitis.[40,41] In three patients with this disease, MRI revealed multiple foci of demyelination in the brain stem, cerebrum, and cerebellum.[40] The anatomic location of the lesions correlated with the patients' focal neurologic deficits. In patients with acute hemorrhagic leukoencephalitis, MRI shows the presence of various stages of hemorrhage superimposed on areas of demyelination.

Although MRI is the most sensitive and specific modality to show lesions of postinfection encephalomyelitis, the findings are not specific. Progressive multifocal leukoencephalopathy and CNS lymphoma may produce similar white-matter abnormalities.

Differential Diagnosis

Acute Viral Encephalitis

Acute viral encephalitis in the United States is usually caused by arboviruses, herpesviruses (especially herpes simplex type I), and enteroviruses.[42] It is predominantly a disease of gray matter with perivascular and parenchymal infiltration of inflammatory cells. In contrast, postinfection encephalomyelitis is predominantly a disease of white matter with perivenular inflammation and demyelination. In acute viral encephalitis, there is direct invasion of brain parenchyma by the virus, and intrathecal synthesis of antibodies can be demonstrated.[43] The T cells predominate in the brain (helper/suppressor ratio of 4–5 : 1) and are probably involved in the clearance of virus-infected cells.[44] In postinfection encephalomyelitis, there is no evidence that the virus invades the CNS and intrathecal synthesis of antibody does not occur. The cellular response is inappropriately directed against host antigens and the inflammatory cells in the brain may be the effector cells in the process of demyelination.

Other Types of Encephalitis

Although viruses account for the majority of cases of encephalitis, it is important to recognize that encephalitis may be caused by other organisms, such as *M pneumoniae, Borrelia burgdorferi, Toxoplasma gondii,* and *Naegleria* spp. Since the clinical features are not distinctive, a systematic approach is necessary to narrow the list of possibilities and to rule out treatable entities.

In patients with tuberculous or fungal meningitis, the presence of vasculitis or brain edema may produce clinical features suggestive of encephalitis.[45,46] The onset, however, in contrast to postinfection encephalitis, is usually gradual, and the associated clinical and laboratory findings are also distinctive.

Encephalitis/meningoencephalitis, characterized by confusion, stiff neck, headache, and a sterile spinal fluid, is a recognized complication of infective endocarditis and may be the initial presenting manifestation.[47–49] It is caused by cerebral microemboli originating from valvular vegetations—a different pathogenesis than that of postinfection encephalitis.

Multiple Sclerosis

Acute attacks of multiple sclerosis clinically resemble postinfection encephalomyelitis. However, coma and meningismus are common in postinfection encephalomyelitis but are rare in multiple sclerosis, whereas visual loss and diplopia are common in multiple sclerosis and rare in encephalomyelitis. The lesions are demyelinating in both, but in encephalomyelitis they are diffuse and in multiple sclerosis they are focal. Multiple sclerosis recurs whereas postinfection encephalomyelitis is a monophasic disease with only rare episodes of relapse. Finally, autoreactive lymphocytes to myelin basic protein can be demonstrated in postinfection encephalitis but not in multiple sclerosis.

Prognosis

The course of post infection encephalomyelitis is variable and the outcome is unpredictable. Patients with mild illness recover promptly. Those who are severely ill may recover, sometimes dramatically, whereas in others the course may be inexorably downhill. The highest mortality is seen during the first week of the illness, and, in fact, patients who survive the first week usually recover.

The only clinical features of definite prognostic significance are coma and convulsions. The overall mortality of measles encephalitis is around 15%, but in patients with severe disease who have convulsions or become comatose, the mortality rises to 30–40%. Mortality rates for rubella encephalitis are similar, but in varicella encephalitis, the mortality is less than 10%.

With regard to sequelae, children with mild disease usually make a complete recovery. With severe illness, neuropsychiatric sequelae may occur, ranging from disorders of behavior or mild residual weakness to severe emotional disturbance, gross mental retardation, or epilepsy. The severity of the sequelae is related to the duration of coma and the presence of convulsions. Age is also important; children tend to suffer more mental impairment than adults.

Treatment

Treatment consists of supportive care, including the use of anticonvulsants and, when necessary, intensive-care monitoring. Corticosteroids have frequently been used in the management of postinfection encephalomyelitis—the rationale being that the disease has an autoimmune mechanism and, therefore, immunosuppressive therapy must be effective. Several randomized and nonrandomized studies have shown that these agents do not have any beneficial effect.[50–52] A retrospective study of 91 cases of postinfection encephalomyelitis showed higher mortality and sequelae rates among those who had received steroids.[53] On the assumption that the more severe cases may have been treated, the data were reanalyzed to include only those patients admitted in coma. Even in this reanalysis, death rates were still higher in patients treated with corticosteroids.

Reye Syndrome

In 1963, Reye, Morgan, and Baral[54] described the clinicopathologic features of the disease that is now recognized as Reye syndrome. It occurs most commonly following a viral illness and is characterized by an acute noninflammatory encephalopathy associated with fatty infiltration and dysfunction of the liver.

Etiology

The etiology of Reye syndrome remains obscure. An antecedent viral illness appears to be essential for the development of the disease. Upper respiratory infections, predominantly influenza A and B, are the prodromal illness in 60–70% of cases, with varicella present in 20–30% and diarrheal illnesses in 5–15%.[55] Reye syndrome occurs more frequently after influenza B than after influenza A.

Pathogenesis and Pathology

The available evidence indicates that Reye syndrome is the consequence of a primary injury to the mitochondria of multiple organs, especially the liver, with its metabolic consequences.[56] Morphologic studies have confirmed the presence of a characteristic mitochondrial injury in the hepatocytes.[57] Concurrent reductions in mitochondrial enzymes involved in ureagenesis, gluconeogenesis, and the citric-acid cycle have been documented.[58] Further evidence of mitochondrial injury is suggested by the finding of dicarboxylic acids in urine and serum, suggesting that mitochondrial beta-oxidation of fatty acids is compromised. The resulting metabolic abnormalities, particularly hyperammonemia, may have synergistic effects with the CNS mitochondrial injury to produce cerebral edema and encephalopathy through, as yet, incompletely understood mechanisms.[56]

The role of salicylates in the pathogenesis remains unclear. A relationship between Reye syndrome and aspirin exposure during the prodromal viral illness has been documented.[59,60] It is important, however, to realize that the absence of salicylate exposure does not exclude the diagnosis of Reye syndrome. The decline in the incidence of the syndrome in recent years may have been secondary to reduced aspirin usage in children during periods of influenza activity and in the presence of varicella.

The histopathology of Reye syndrome has been studied in considerable detail. Changes in the liver include microvesicular sleatosis, glycogen depletion, and distorted mitochondrea; an inflammatory infiltrate is absent. Mitochondrial abnormalities similar to those seen in the hepatocytes have been noted in neurons and in muscle fibers.

Epidemiology

Reye syndrome occurs most commonly in children, but has been reported in early infancy and, rarely, in adults.[61] The incidence ranges from 0.3 to 6.0 cases per 100,000 children. These statistics are influenced by the periodic coincidence of influenzal epidemics. A temporal relation between the seasonal occurrence of influenza B and epidemics of Reye syndrome has been demonstrated. Regional differences in disease incidence have also been recognized, with higher rates in the western north central and eastern north central states.[56] During the past decade, even with aggressive surveillance efforts, there has been a steady decline in the number of reported cases.[62]

Clinical Features

Characterisitically, 3–5 days after the antecedent viral illness, there is an abrupt onset of intractable vomiting together with lethargy. The mechanism underlying the vomiting remains unexplained. Some patients experience no changes in the level of consciousness but remain lethargic to various degrees. Others may develop agitated delirium (occasionally associated with sympathetic nervous-system overactivity), increasing obtundation, and coma. The intracranial pressure, which is normal in patients without altered consciousness, increases with worsening encephalopathy and may cause brain damage and transtentorial herniation. Hepatic enlargement is present in about one half of the cases.

Encephalopathy typically persists for 1 to 4 days, with a gradual improvement in survivors. Recovery of consciousness in patients with permanent neurologic impairment may require weeks.

Diagnosis

The most significant laboratory findings are elevated transaminases (exceeding three times normal levels), hypoprothrombinemia, and hyperammonemia associated with normal bilirubin. Noncomatose patients may have normal or mildly to moderately elevated serum ammonia concentration. With worsening encephalopathy, the serum ammonia concentratrion increases to up to 20 times normal. The serum levels of free fatty acids are also elevated. Hypoglycemia may occur, especially in children under one year of age.

The CSF is under increased pressure but is ascellular with otherwise normal constituents. A lumbar puncture is recommended as part of the initial evaluation, particularly if the diagnosis is uncertain.[63] The presence in the CSF of white cells or elevation of the protein concentration should cast doubt on the diagnosis and other possibilities should be considered. A lumbar puncture performed later in the course may be hazardous, with an increased likelihood of central herniation.

Percutaneous liver biopsy will confirm the diagnosis, but it is usually not necessary. Hepatic lesion is evanescent and the characteristic alterations are found only during the first 3 to 4 days of the illness. The diagnostic criteria include the following clinical and laboratory elements.[63]

1. The presence of an antecedent viral illness.
2. A latent interval of several days before the onset of pernicious vomiting.
3. The development of diffuse encephalopathy.
4. A threefold or greater elevation of the serum alanine. aminotransferase (ALT, SGPT) and aspartate aminotransferase (AST, SGOT) levels.
5. Prolongation of the prothrombin time.
6. Hyperammonemia.
7. Normal CSF examination.
8. No other explanation for the hepatic and cerebral abnormalities.

A childhood syndrome, distinguishable from Reye syndrome only by the absence of hepatic involvement and a high incidence of acute convulsions, can follow a number of viral illnesses and vaccinations.

Treatment

The therapeutic goal in the management of patients with Reye syndrome is to attenuate the various compounding metabolic insults and achieve a metabolic steady state as soon as possible. Generally accepted as standard treatment is the use of hypertonic glucose and hypertonic mannitol, placement of the patient in an intensive-care unit when significant alterations in the level of consciousness are present, parenteral administration of vitamin K, and monitoring of the intracranial pressure.[63] There is no indication for the use of corticosteroids. Current evidence suggests that corticosteroid therapy may be associated with higher mortality and may contribute to pancreatic involvement.

With proper management, most patients make a full and complete recovery without any neurologic or psychologic sequelae. The mortality rate is around 10%.

References

1. Miller HG, Stanton JB, Gibbons JL: Para-infectious encephalomyelitis and related syndromes. *Q J Med* 1965;25:427–505.
2. La Bocetta AC, Tornay AS: Measles encephalitis: report of 61 cases. *Am J Dis Child* 1964;107:247–255.
3. Appelbaum E, Rachelson MH, Dolgopol VB: Varicella encephalitis *Am J Med* 1953;15:223–230.
4. McAlpine D, Kurcowa Y, Toyokura Y, et al: Acute demyelinating disease complicating herpes zoster. *J Neurol Neurosurg Psychiatry* 1959;22:120–123.
5. Donohue WL, Playfair FD, Whitaker L: Mumps encephalitis: pathology and pathogenesis. *J Pediatr* 1955;47:395–412.
6. Schwartz GA, Yang DC, Noone EL: Meningoencephalitis with epidemic parotitis. *Arch Neurol* 1964;11:453–462.
7. Flewett TH, Hoyt JG, et al: Influenzal encephalopathy and postinfluenzal encephalitis. *Lancet* 1958; 2:11–15.
8. Sulkava R, Rissamen A, Phyhala K: Postinfluenza encephalitis during the influenza A outbreak in 1979–1980. *J Neurol Neurosurg Psychiatry* 1981;44: 161–163.
9. Bergin JD: Fatal encephalopathy in glandular fever. *J Neurol Neurosurg Psychiatry* 1960;23:69–73.
10. Ambler M, Stoll J, Tzamalowkas A, et al: Focal encephalomyelitis in infectious mononucleois. *Ann Intern Med* 1971;75:579–583.
11. Johnson RT, Griffin DE, Gendelman HE: Postinfectious encephalomyelitis. *Semin Neurol* 1985;5:180–190.
12. Christie AB: *Infectious Diseases: Epidemiology and Clinical Practice*, vol 2, 4th ed. Edinburgh, Churchill Livingstone, 1987, pp 782–806.
13. Fischer RS, Clark AW, Wolinsky JS, et al: Postinfectious encephalitis complicating mycoplasma pneumoniae infection. *Arch Neurol* 1983;40:109–113.
14. Spillane JD, Wells CEC: The neurology of Jennerian vaccination. *Brain* 1964;87:1–43.
15. Neff JM, Levine RH, Lane JM, et al: Complications of smallpox vaccination in the United States 1963. II. Results obtained by four statewide surveys. *Pediatrics* 1967;39:916–923.
16. Hemachudha T, Phanuphak P, Johnson RT, et al: Neurologic complications of semple-type rabies vaccine: clinical and immunologic studies. *Neurology* 1987;37:550–556.
17. Fenichel GM: Neurological complication of immunization. *Ann Neurol* 1982;12:119–124.
18. Adams JM: Clinical pathology of measles encephalitis and sequelae. *Neurology* 1968;18:(suppl)52–56.
19. Hart MN, Earle KM: Hemorrhagic and perivenous encephalitis: a clinical-pathological review of 38 cases. *J Neurol Neurosurg Psychiatry* 1975;38:585–591.
20. Johnson KP, Wolinsky JS, Ginsberg AH: Immune-mediated syndromes of the nervous system related to virus infections, in Vinken PJ, Bruyn GW (eds.): *Handbook of Clinical Neurology*. vol 34. Amsterdam, North-Holland Publishing Co, 1978, 391–434.
21. Gosztonyi G: Acute haemorrhagic leucoencephalitis (Hurst's disease), in Vinken PG, Bruyn GW (eds): *Handbook of Clinical Neurology*. vol 34. Amsterdam, North-Holland Publishing Co 1978, pp 587–606.
22. Rivers TM, Sprent DH, Berry GP: Observations on attempts to produce acute disseminated encephalomyelitis in monkeys. *J Exp Med* 1933;58:39–54.
23. Rivers TM, Schwentker FF: Encephalomyelitis accompanied by myelin destruction experimentally produced in monkeys. *J Exp Med* 1935;61:689–702.
24. Kabat EA, Wolf A, Bezer AE: The rapid production of acute disseminated encephalomyelitis in rhesus monkey by injection of heterologous and homologous brain tissue with adjuvants. *J Exp Med* 1947;85:117–130.
25. Whitaker JN, Gupta M, Smith OF: Epitopes of immunoreactive myelin basic protein in human CSF. *Ann Neurol* 1986;20:329–336.
26. Paterson PY: Experimental allergic encephalomyeli-

tis and autoimmune disease. *Adv Immunol* 1964; 5:131–207.
27. Ben-Nun A, Wekerle H, Cohen IR: The rapid isolation of clonable antigen-specific T lymphocyte lines capable of mediating autoimmune encephalomyelitis. *Eur J Immunol* 1981;11:195–199.
28. Itoyama Y, Webster HF: Immunocytochemical study of myelin-associated glycoprotein (MAG) and basic protein (BP) in experimental allergic encephalomyelitis (EAE). *J Neuroimmunol* 1982;3:351–364.
29, Hamachudha T, Griffin DE, Giffels JJ, et al: Myelin basic protein as an encephalitogen in encephalomyelitis and polyneuritis following rabies vaccination. *N Engl J Med* 1987;316:369–374.
30. Moench TR, Griffin DE, Obriecht CR, et al: Acute measles in patients with or without neurologic involvement: distribution of measles virus antigen and RNA. *J Infect Dis* 1988;158:433–442.
31. Gendelman HE, Wolinsky JS, Johnson RT, et al: Measles encephalomyelitis: lack of evidence of viral invasion of the central nervous system and quantitative study of demyelination. *Ann Neurol* 1984; 15:353–360.
32. Johnson RT, Griffin DE, Hirsch RL, et al: Measles encephalomyelitis—clinical and immunological studies, *N Engl J Med* 1984:310:137–141.
33. Johnson RT, Hirsch RL, Griffin DE, et al: Clinical and immunological studies of measles encephalitis. *Trans Am Neurol Assoc* 1981;106:42–45.
34. Preblud SR, D'Angelo LJ: Chickenpox in the United States, 1972–1977. *J Infect Dis* 1979;140:257–260.
35. Sriram S, Steinman L: Postinfectious and postvaccinial encephalomyelitis. *Neurol Clin* 1984;2:341–353.
36. Sebst RG, Selhorst JB, Myer EC: Parainfectious optic neuritis. *Arch Neurol* 1983;40:347–351.
37. Croft JB: Para-infectious and postvaccinal encephalitis. *Postgrad Med* 1969;45:329–400.
38. Lukes SA, Norman I: Computed tomography in acute disseminated encephalomyelitis. *Ann Neurol* 1983; 13:567–572.
39. Pasternak JF, DeVivo DC, Prensky AC: Steroid responsive encephalomyelitis in childhood. *Neurology* 1980;30:481–486.
40. Atlas SW, Grossman RI, Goldberg HI, et al: MR diagnosis of acute disseminated encephalomyelitis. *J Comput Assist Tomogr* 1988;10:798–801.
41. Epperson LW, Whitaker JN, Ashwani K: Cranial MRI in acute disseminated encephalomyelitis. *Neurology* 1988;38:332–333.
42. Ho DD, Hirsch MS: Acute viral encephalitis. *Med Clin North Am* 1985;69:415–442.
43. Kahlon J, et al: Detection of antibodies to herpes simplex virus in the cerebrospinal fluid of patients with herpes simplex encephalitis. *J Infect Dis* 1987;155:38–44.
44. Johnson RT: The pathogenesis of acute viral encephalitis and postinfectious encephalomyelitis. *J Infect Dis* 1987;155:359–364.
45. Molavi A, LeFrock JL: Tuberculous meningitis. *Med Clin North Am* 1985;69:315–331.
46. Sabetta JR, Andriole VT: Cryptococcal infections of the central nervous system. *Med Clin North Am* 1985;69:333–344.
47. Ziment I: Nervous system complications in bacterial endocarditis. *Am J Med* 1968;122:349–352.
48. Pruitt AA, Rubin RH, Karchmer AW, Duncan GW: Neurologic complications of bacterial endocarditis. *Medicine* 1978;57:329–343.
49. Lerner PI: Neurologic complications of infective endocarditis. *Med Clin North Am* 1985;69:385–398.
50. Allen JE: Treatment of measles encephalitis with adrenal steroids. *Pediatrics* 1957;20:87–91.
51. Karelitz S, Eisenberg M: Measles encephalitis. Evaluation of treatment with adrenocorticotropin and adrenal corticoids. *Pediatrics* 1961;27:811–818.
52. Zeigra SR: Corticosteroid treatment of measles encephalitis. *J Pediatr* 1961;59:322–323.
53. Boe J, Solberg CO, Saeter T: Cortcosteroid treatment for acute meningoencephalitis: a retrospective study of 346 cases. *Br Med J* 1965;1:1094–1095.
54. Reye RDK, Morgan G, Baral J: Encephalopathy and fatty degeneration of the viscera: a disease entity in childhood. *Lancet* 1963;2:749–752.
55. Hurwitz ES, Nelson DB, Davis C, et al: National surveillance for Reye syndrome: a five-year review. *Pediatrics* 1982;70:895–900.
56. Heubi JE, Partin JC, Partin JS, Schubert WK: Reye's syndrome: current concepts. *Hepatology* 1987;7:155–164.
57. Partin JC, Schubert WK, Partin JS: Mitochondrial ultrastructure in Reye's syndrome (encephalopathy and fatty degeneration of the viscera). *N Engl J Med* 1971;285:1339–1343.
58. Brown RE, Forman DT: The biochemistry of Reye's syndrome. *Crit Rev Clin Lab Sci* 1982;17:247–297.
59. Halpin TJ, Holzhauer FJ, Campbell RJ, et al: Reye's syndrome and medication use. *JAMA* 1982;248:687–691.
60. Hurwitz ES, Barrett MJ, Bregman D, et al: Public Health Service study on Reye's syndrome and medications. *N Engl J Med* 1985;313:849–857.
61. Nesbitt JAA, Minuk GY, Alberta C: Adult Reye's syndrome. *Ann Emerg Med* 1988;17:155–158.
62. Sullivan-Boylai JZ, Corey L: Epidemiology of Reye syndrome. *Epidemiol Rev* 1981;31:1–26.
63. DeVivo DC: Reye syndrome. *Neurol Clin North Am* 1985;3:95–115.

11
The Cerebellum and CNS Infection

Bruce A. Cohen and Howard L. Lipton

Clinical–Physiologic Correlations

The cerebellum is one of the three basic subdivisions of the brain. It is located in the posterior fossa beneath the tentorial membrane and overlies the pons and medulla. It connects to the brain stem by way of three cerebellar peduncles: the superior (brachium conjunctivum), middle (brachium pontis), and inferior (restiform body). Through complex interconnections and feedback circuits, the cerebellum participates in the initiation of movement, the coordination of complex and sequential muscular activity, and the regulation of motor tone. It also integrates somatic and motor input and coordinates motor output to maintain posture and equilibrium. Cerebellar influences, which are predominately inhibitory, affect the smoothness and precision with which these functions are carried out. Thorough review of the complexity of these interactions is beyond the scope of this chapter and the interested reader is referred to the monograph of Gilman, Bloedel, and Lechtenberg.[1]

Cerebellar disease produces imprecision of speed, range, and force of movement, more prominently in the patient with acute illness. Hypotonia, or decreased resistance to passive movement, is due in part to decreased muscle-spindle activity and tends to improve over time. In unilateral disease, postural asymmetry may be present, with tilting toward the affected side. Muscle stretch reflexes are usually normal or decreased, and may be pendular as a result of the loss of speed of reciprocal muscle activation.

Cerebellar ataxia is most prominently manifested by tremor, which occurs with purposeful movement. When the upper extremities are affected, coarse jerky oscillations accompany the initiation of motion, which may stop short of or move beyond its intended target. As the traget is approached, the amplitude and range of the oscillations may increase. Abnormalities of gait include a widened base and a characteristic reeling or staggering quality with an irregular stride. Truncal ataxia and titubation (anterior-posterior, side-to-side, or rotational oscillations of the head) may be present. The patient may be unable to stand with feet together, even with the eyes open. Milder degrees of ataxia may be demonstrated by an inability to walk with tandem steps or by wavering on heel-knee-shin manuevers.

Loss of coordination and synchronization, or dyssynergy, results in decomposition of movement. Complex movements are broken down into individual components performed in a mechanical sequence. Disturbance in the synchronization of reciprocal firing between agonist and antagonist muscle groups produces impairment of alternating movements, or dysdiadochokinesia, and loss of the "check reflex," or rebound. Although acute cerebellar lesions may be associated with fatigue and a perception of weakness, substantial loss of strength is not a feature of cerebellar pathology. Its presence suggests involvement of other regions of the nervous system.

Ocular movements may be impaired. Loss of smoothness and precision produces a ratchetlike quality with a tendency to overshoot the visual target. Gaze-paretic nystagmus may be seen in which the eyes are deviated away from an acute cerebellar lesion and oscillate with a shift in gaze, most intensely when directed toward the affected side. Rebound nystagmus, a transient reversal of the direction of the fast component, is considered specific for cerebellar localization. Other abnormalities of ocular movement—such as downbeat or sustained horizontal nystagmus, skew deviation, gaze apraxia, ocular myoclonus, ocular flutter, and opsoclonus—may be seen. Speech disturbances are caused by dyssynergy of the muscles of phonation. Speech output may be slow and slurred. In classic cerebellar scanning speech, words have an explosive staccato quality, and are uttered with irregularly variable intonation and meter.

Localization of cerebellar lesions is possible to a limited degree. Medial cerebellar involvement produces a syndrome manifested by truncal ataxia, postural unsteadiness, staggering ataxic gait, titubation, and ocular motor abnormalities, including dysmetria and gaze-evoked and rebound nystagmus. Involvement of the hemispheres produces ipsilateral appendicular symptoms, predominatly involving the upper extremities, with loss of fine motor coordination, (more prominent distally than proximally), ataxia, dysmetria, dysdiadochokinesis, hypotonia, intention tremors, and pendular or decreased reflexes. Gait disorders, dysarthria, ocular motility abnormalities as described for midline lesions, and nystagmus may also be seen.

Infections may present either as localized abscesses or granulomas producing focal cerebellar signs or as a diffuse pancerebellar syndrome. The following discussion focuses on infections that can present with prominent cerebellar symptoms (Table 11.1). Many of these patients have signs of more diffuse neurologic involvement when examined. The specific diseases mentioned here are discussed elsewhere in this book where the full spectrum of their neurologic involvement is reviewed, and where diagnostic and therapeutic information is presented in detail.

Table 11.1. CNS infections presenting with cerebellar syndromes.

Viral	
Varicella-zoster virus	Poliovirus
Measles	Epstein-Barr virus
Mumps	Herpes simplex
Rubella	Influenza
Coxsackie virus	Adenovirus
Echo virus	JC virus
Enterovirus 71	
Agent Unknown	
Creutzfeldt-Jakob disease	Kuru
Bacterial	
Hemophilus	Cat-scratch bacillus
Mycoplasma	Mycobacteria
Legionella	Streptococci
Rickettsia	(aerobic, anaerobic)
Salmonella	Staphylococci
Borrelia	*Proteus*
Brucella	Bacteroides
Bordetella	*Escherichia coli*
Fungal and Parasitic	
Cryptococcus	*Toxoplasma*
Blastomyces	*Taenia*
Histoplasma	*Falciparum*
Coccidioides	*Echinococcus*
Streptomyces	*Schistosoma*
Nocardia	*Trypanosoma*
Aspergillus	

Viral Infections

Acute Viral Infections

Acute cerebellar ataxia can be seen in association with a wide variety of viral infections in both children and adults. The syndrome is characterized by a rapid onset of gait ataxia and varying degrees of upper-limb incoordination, truncal ataxia, dysarthria, and ocular motility disorders. Some patients have marked intermittent tremors of axial or extraocular muscles.[7] Patients are often afebrile and subtle signs of more widespread neurologic involvement may be apparent on examination. Symptoms typically follow a respiratory or gastrointestinal illness or the skin rash of an exanthematous infection by days to weeks. On occasion, they may precede or be the only prominent symptom of the underlying infection. The prognosis for this condition is good, particularly in children, with complete resolution of signs over a period of months. Persistent residua may occur,[7] but because mortality is rare, few pathologic studies are available. The syndrome may represent a limited immune-mediated postinfectious encephalitis or a direct central-nervous-system (CNS) viral infection.

Diagnosis of acute cerebellar ataxia is based on the characteristic clinical presentation in conjunction with the absence of abnormalities on imaging studies. To our knowledge, no reports of the use of magnetic-resonance imaging (MRI) in this condition are available. Cerebrospinal-fluid (CSF) determinations may be normal but usually show a mild, predominately lymphocytic pleocytosis, with normal or mildly elevated protein and normal glucose levels.

Virus can sometimes be isolated from the throat, feces, or CSF, or serum serology may show a rise in titer, reflecting acute infection.

The most common exanthematous eruption associated with acute cerebellar ataxia is varicella,[7–14] however, cases have also been described with measles,[14,16] mumps,[14,26] and rubella.[14] Neurologic symptoms usually follow the appearance of the skin rash but also have been reported to precede it.[12] In a series of 59 cases of varicella encephalitis,[11] cerebellar ataxia occurred in 18, making it one of the most common neurologic complications. Because of the generally benign prognosis, few pathologic studies are available; however, evidence exists to support both immune-mediated demyelination and direct viral invasive mechanisms of disease. Appelbaum and colleagues.[11] reported perivascular inflammation and demyelination in six cases reviewed from the literature, suggesting an immune-mediated postinfectious encephalitis as describved by Johnson and co-workers.[17] Gershon and associates[9] demonstrated CSF antibody to varicella-zoster virus (VZV) in 15 of 16 patients with various neurologic manifestations, but found none in seven patients with clinical VZV infections and no neurologic involvement. Peters and associates[10] demonstrated antigens to VZV virus in CSF cells from two patients with acute cerebellar ataxia by indirect immunofluorescent staining, and suggested that direct viral invasion of the CNS might occur in some cases. In mumps, cerebellar ataxia may be the predominent neurologic manifestation[14] or precede development of a more diffuse encephalitis.[26] Neurologic symptoms may occur with or without the presence of parotitis.[4] Cerebellar symptoms in measles infections are more commonly part of a diffuse encephalitis, but have been described as the only neurologic manifestation.[16]

A number of enteroviruses have been associated with acute cerebellar ataxia, including coxsackieviruses A[19] and B[18] and echoviruses 6[20] and 9.[21] Patients may present with cerebellar symptoms in the absence of a preceding or concurrent respiratory or gastrointestinal illness. Virus is sometimes recovered from throat or fecal swabs and, on occasion, from CSF.[21] Serologic studies may show acute elevations of antibody titer on serial samples. The prognosis in these cases is generally good for complete resolution of symptoms. Enterovirus 71—a cause of hand, foot, and mouth disease—has been associated with an acute cerebellar syndrome in Japan.[27] The neurologic symptoms typically appeared 2–4 days after the onset of illness and resolved within 3 weeks.

Poliovirus has also been associated with cerebellar ataxia.[23,24] Neurologic symptoms follow respiratory, gastrointestinal, or nonspecific constitutional symptoms by several days. The prognosis is similar to that for the other infections described above, with improvement over a period of weeks to months. One fatal case was reviewed by Howe,[25] who noted perivascular inflammation and congestion in the cerebellar white matter. Diagnosis in most of these cases was made by virus recovery from stool samples or on the basis of acute elevations in antibody titers.

Infectious mononucleosis, caused by the Epstein-Barr virus, is associated with varied neurologic manifestations in approximately 1% of cases.[32] An acute cerebellar syndrome developing over hours to days has been described as the predominant neurologic manifestation and may be the presenting feature of the illness[32] or occur in the absence of systemic symptoms.[31] The cerebellar syndrome is similar to those previously described and typically improves over weeks to months. The CSF may show a mild or moderate lymphocytic pleocytosis and increased protein, while glucose and opening pressure are usually normal. Serum antibody titers often are elevated reflecting acute infection. Dolgopol and Husson[28] described a case of meninogoencephalitis in which autopsy examination disclosed selective degeneration of cerebellar Purkinje cells. Herpes simplex virus type 1 usually produces a progressive encephalitis marked by diffuse cerebral involvement with frontotemporal predominance, while type 2 produces an aseptic meningitis in immunocompetent adults. Dano[35] reported a case in which acute cerebellar ataxia in an eight-year-old child was seen three days following an upper respiratory infection and was associated with an increase, and later a decrease, of serial antibody titers to herpes simplex virus. Influenza A and B[36] and adenovirus infections[15] have also been reported to cause cerebellar ataxia.

Persistent Viral Infections

Patients with a number of persistent latent viral infections may initially present to the physician with a subacute cerebellar syndrome. Progressive multifocal leukoencephalopathy (PML) was initially described in immunocompromised patients with hematologic malignancies or collagen-vascular diseases.

Today, it often occurs in the setting of infection with the human immunodeficiency virus (HIV-1). The full spectrum of disease involves demyelinating lesions of the subcortical white matter, brain stem, and cerebellum caused by a papovavirus, called JC virus. Virions can be demonstrated pathologically in oligodendrocytes by electron microscopy. A subacute cerebellar syndrome may be the presenting feature in either the HIV-infected[38] or the non-HIV-infected patient.[37] Computed-tomography (CT) scans may show white-matter attenuation, but MRI is more sensitive and shows high signal lesions on T_2-weighted spin-echo images.[42] The CSF is normal or may show nonspecific inflammatory changes of mild pleocytosis, increased protein, and increased IgG in HIV-1–seropositive patients. Diagnosis is made by tissue examination. Though rare case reports of response to cytarabine have been published,[39–41] no therapy has been shown to be consistently effective and the usual course is one of progressive deterioration and death.

Subacute sclerosing panencephalitis (SSPE) is a late catastrophic infection attributable to a defective measles virus and characterized by progressive dementia, ataxia, myoclonus, and other focal neurologic signs. The disease may start insidiously with mild cognitive changes and irritability, with ataxia and incoordination appearing within weeks or months. Over time, a more diffuse encephalitis evolves with relentless progression. Elevated levels of antibodies to measles virus can be found in both serum and CSF. The CSF pressure is normal, and cell counts are also normal or are mildly increased. Protein is typically normal but IgG content is increased and oligoclonal bands can usually be demonstrated. Measles virus has been isolated from cultures of brain tissue of patients with SSPE.[15]

A late rubella panencephalitis with progressive dementia and pyramidal and cerebellar degeneration has been described[18] that can occur years after the initial infection. Pancerebellar dysfunction is a prominent feature and may represent the initial manifestation of this condition.

Creutzfeldt-Jacob disease is a progressive CNS spongiform degeneration marked by dementia, as well as by pyramidal, extrapyramidal and cerebellar signs, and myoclonus. Though the specific infectious agent has not yet been identified, the disease has been transmitted by contact with infected neurologic tissue or by corneal transplant. Approximately 10% of cases may present with a progressive cerebellar syndrome,[43] followed weeks to months later by more diffuse encephalopathic features. Kuru, a disease found in New Guinea and spread through cannibalism, appears to be similar in character to the ataxic form of Creutzfeldt-Jakob disease. Cerebellar pathology includes spongiform changes, patchy loss of Purkinje cells, kuru plaques, and focal necrosis in the granular layer.[43] The CSF is unremarkable. The electroencephalogram is usually normal or nonspecifically slow in early stages but may evolve to a characteristic pattern of periodic sharp waves. There is no therapy and the disease progresses relentlessly to death in virtually all cases.

Bacterial Infections

Bacterial infections may affect the cerebellum either in the form of a diffuse cerebellitis or by focal granulomatous or abscess formation. Schwartz[45] described six cases of young children with cerebellar ataxia in the setting of acute meningitis, all of whom recovered after treatment with antibiotics. In four of these cases, the ataxia was present at the onset of illness. The infecting organism was *Hemophilus influenzae* in five of the six cases.

Acute cerebellar ataxia has been reported in conjunction with *Mycoplasma pneumoniae*.[46–48] Symptoms typically followed a respiratory illness by a few weeks, and improved over weeks to months. Abramovitz and colleagues[47] report isolation of *Mycoplasma* from the CSF and throat of a patient with cerebellar ataxia and confusion. Sera but not CSF showed elevated IgM titers to *Mycoplasma* antigens by complement fixation and enzyme-linked immunosorbent assay (ELISA). All symptoms resolved after two weeks of antibiotic therapy. The authors suggested that these findings support a theory of pathogenesis by direct *Mycoplasma* invasion of the CNS.

Legionella pneumophila has been associated with neurologic symptoms in a number of reports.[49–55] Cerebellar involvement may occur in conjunction with a more diffuse encephalitis or as an isolated neurologic symptom. Prognosis for resolution of the neurologic signs varies. Schetty and collegues.[49] reported a patient with pancerebellar dysfunction in the setting of Legionnaires' disease. Treatment produced resolution of the pneumonia and constitutional symptoms, but residual dysarthria and mild gait ataxia remained at follow-up seven months later.

Residual ataxia of all limbs after six months was also found in a case of Baker and co-workers.[52] which had both brain-stem and cerebellar features during the acute stage of illness. Lees and Tyrrell's[53] case, had a more diffuse cerebral and cerebellar involvement including aphasia, pyramidal tract signs, and confusion, in addition to severe ataxia. When this patient was followed up three years later, the only neurologic residue noted was some mild word-finding difficulty, suggesting that the neurologic prognosis can be reasonably good in the long term. Other patients recover quickly, as in Friedman's[54] second case, in which the patient showed resolution of cerebellar symptoms within three weeks.

The pathophysiology of neurologic manifestations in *Legionella* infections is uncertain. CT examinations in those cases where available have been unrevealing, and CSF studies have been normal in all of these patients with the exception of Lees and Tyrrell's[53] case, in which a lymphocytic pleocytosis was found. Pendelbury and associates[50] reviewed an autopsy series of 40 patients with Legionnaires' disease, of whom 40% had neurologic signs or symptoms not attributable to any preexisting disease. Most of these patients had changes in mentation. Neuropathologic examination failed to disclose any lesions attributable to *Legionella* and the authors suggested that some mechanism other than direct bacterial invasion, such as a toxic factor, accounted for the neurologic symptoms. Weir and colleagues[55] reviewed clinical and electrophysiologic features of 16 patients with Legionnaires's disease that involved both the peripheral and central nervous systems. They suggested that the multisystem features and absence of evidence for direct bacterial invasion made an endotoxin-like agent the most attractive pathologic mechanism.

Rickettsial infections can also present with cerebellar features. Miller and Price[56] reviewed a series of patients with Rocky Mountain spotted fever and neurologic symptomatology. Typically, this illness manifests as a diffuse encephalitis with headache and fever, alteration of consciousness, and brainstem involvement. Neurologic symptoms occur within a week after onset of the fever, and usually, though not always, after the appearance of the petecchial or macular skin rash. The CSF in these patients may be normal or show a mild to moderate pleocytosis. Pathologically, there are perivascular inflammatory infiltrates. In one of these cases, focal cerebellar ataxia was described that persisted for several months following treatment of the infection.[56]

Acute cerebellar ataxia may be the presenting neurologic symptom in *Salmonella* infections. Sawhney and co-workers[57] reported three cases in which the cerebellar symptoms appeared within 2–3 days after the onset of fever, progressing over the next 24 to 48 hours, and then improving gradually after a 1–2-week period. Salmonellae were cultured from blood in one case and demonstrated by an acute rise in antibody titers in the other two. Chambers and associates[58] reported a case of a man with *Salmonella* paratyphi B who developed an encephalitis characterized by convulsions and pancerebellitis two weeks after the onset of fever and other constitutional symptoms. The CSF was normal and the diagnosis was based on a culture of blood and feces and an increased serum antiboby titer to the *Salmonella* H antigen. His cerebellar signs resolved over a three-week period following therapy with chloramphenicol.

Lyme disease is a spirochete infection caused by *Borrelia burgdorferi,* and is associated with a wide spectrum of neurologic symptoms, including an encephalitis that may have prominent cerebellar ataxia as a feature.[60] Neurologic symptoms may appear within weeks to months of the initial inoculation.[59] The CSF may be normal or show lymphocytic pleocytosis and elevated protein with increased IgG and oligoclonal bands. Antibody to *B burgdorferi* can be found in both the serum and the CSF.[62] Central- and peripheral-nervous-system demyelination has been reported[61] and may reflect an immune-mediated pathophysiology. Alternatively, direct invasion of the brain may occur[59] as in other *Spirochete* infections.

Acute cerebellar ataxia or encephalitis with predominently cerebellar features has also been reported in cat-scratch disease,[64,65] brucellosis,[66] pertussis, and scarlet fever.[63]

Mycobacterium tuberculosis may produce a cerebellar syndrome in association with a posterior fossa meningitis[4,69] or as a result of a tuberculoma or tuberculous abscess.[68–70] In the latter instance, symptoms may be localized in the midline or one of the cerebellar hemispheres with headache, focal cerebellar symptoms, and subacute progression of increased intracranial pressure suggesting a mass lesion that can be demonstrated by CT or MRI.

Bacterial abscesses of the cerebellum are related predominantly to otogenic infections when present as single lesions.[71–75] Typical pathogens include streptococci, staphylococci, and *Proteus* organisms. The most common presenting symptom is headache, and fever may or may not be present. Cerebellar symptoms typically develop subacutely following the onset of the headache, and signs of increased intracranial pressure follow. The diagnosis is readily made by CT scan with contrast infusion. When encapsulization is present, the prognosis is better.[71,74] Treatment generally consists of surgical drainage and excision, as discussed in more detail elsewhere in this book.

Fungal and Parasitic Infections

A number of relatively unusual infections can present with cerebellar symptoms caused by localized abscess or granuloma formation. Ataxia may also be an early feature of chronic meningitis, though it is usually accompanied by other manifestations of the syndrome.

One of the more common CNS fungal infections encountered is *Cryptococcus neoformans*, which is found in both normal people and in patients who are immune suppressed owing to either disease or steroid therapy. It is the most common opportunistic meningitis in HIV-1–infected individuals, and may also present as localized cryptococcomas, seen as enhancing lesions on CT scans.[76,79] These masses can occur anywhere in the brain, including the cerebellum,[76,77] and may or may not be associated with cryptococcal meningitis. In HIV-1–infected patients, CSF cryptococcal antigen and cultures can be negative in the absence of meningitis[79] and diagnosis may require biopsy. Recently, Fujita and associates[76] reviewed their experience and other reported cases, and they recommended surgical resection of accessible lesions greater than 3 cm in diameter.

Blastomycosis can produce cerebellar granulomas or abscesses as isolated masses[80,82] or in association with meningitis.[81] Infection may occur in normal or immunocompromised individuals, with or without systemic infection.[83] The clinical course may be subacute over weeks[80] or months,[82] or chronic.[81] The CSF may reveal elevated protein and a mononuclear pleocytosis. Glucose is sometimes decreased and opening pressures may be normal or elevated.

Histoplasmosis most commonly produces a self-limited pulmonary infection, but it may produce a chronic meningitis or localized CNS mass lesions.[85,91,92] Cerebellar lesions present subacutely with a progressive neurologic deficit over weeks to months. The CSF commonly shows lymphocytic pleocytosis, elevated protein, and occasionally decreased glucose. CNS lesions may be seen in the absence of disseminated disease, and diagnosis usually requires biopsy.

Cerebellar abscesses or granulomas have also been reported as resulting from coccidiodomycosis,[90] *Streptomyces* infection,[93] and nocardiosis.[84] The last infection is notable because of its response to penicillin and emphasizes the importance of reaching a specific diagnosis.

Aspergillosis differs from other fungal infections in its tendency to invade intracerebral blood vessels, often presenting acutely as a hemorrhagic infarction in cerebrum or cerebellum.[83,87,88]. Abscess or granuloma formation may also occur and present as a subacute progressive cerebellar syndrome.[86] Neurologic pathology is seen in both normal and immunocompromised hosts[83] and may occur with or without systemic involvement.[86,87] CT scans readily demonstrate hemorrhages or mass lesions. The CSF may be normal or show a mononuclear pleocytosis with elevated protein and normal or decreased glucose.[87,88] Fungal cultures are often negative, and diagnosis may be difficult in life without a biopsy.[87]

Toxoplasmosis, now seen most commonly in the United States in the setting of HIV infection, may present as cerebellar ataxia.[87,88] Lesions usually enhance on CT scans with contrast infusion. MRI may demonstrate additional areas of involvement not seen on CT. Typically, the presentation is subacute over days to weeks. The CSF may be normal or show mononuclear pleocytosis, elevated protein, and normal or mildly decreased glucose. A specific diagnosis generally requires biopsy and immunoperoxidase staining of tissue specimens for *Toxoplasma* antigens. The rapid improvement commonly seen following therapy with pyrimethamine and sulfadiazine may be diagnostic in patients with multiple lesions; however, mixed opportunistic processes are common in HIV-1–infected patients and any lesions not improving after 2–3 weeks of antibiotic therapy should be biopsied.

Cysticercosis commonly affects the nervous system and is endemic in Mexico and a number of other developing countries.[97,98] Infections are being recognized increasingly in the United States and may present as seizures, meningitis, hydrocephalus, or localized abcess formation with focal symptoms and signs.[97–99] Catapano and Marx[96] have reported a patient presenting with acute headache, ataxia, vertigo, and emesis resulting from a cerebellar cyst. They noted cysts in the cerebellum in up to 18% of cases in an autopsy series. Hydrocephalus attributable to obstruction by intraventricular cysticerci may also produce vertigo and ataxia, with accompanying headaches often provoked by positional changes. McCormick and associates[99] note that the fourth ventricle is the most common site for intraventricular cysts. CT scans show active parenchymal lesions as either low-density nonenhancing lucencies representing viable cysticerci, ring or nodular enhancing lesions representing acute inflammatory reactions to the parasite, or a diffuse encephalitis with multiple areas of nodular or ring enhancement and small ventricles resulting from diffuse cerebral swelling.[98] Therapy includes shunting for hydrocephalus and treatment with praziquantal, using steroids or osmotic diuretics if needed. When a large cyst is life-threatening, decompressive surgery may be required.

Cerebellar ataxia has also been reported in conjunction with falciparum malaria, both during the initial stages of the attack[103] and as a delayed syndrome following treatment by three to four weeks and resolving within several months.[100,101] In the later instance, the question of an ataxic syndrome resulting from chloroquine therapy has been raised as a potential explanation.[102]

Echinococcal cysts may occur in the CNS in up to 2.4% of autopsy cases.[105] They are found more frequently in children and rarely in the cerebellum.[104] The progression is typically subacute or chronic over months, as described by Schijman,[104] mimicking a cerebellar tumor. Subacutely progressive cerebellar syndromes have also been described in schistosomiasis[106,107] and in trypanosomiasis.[108,109]

Differential Diagnosis

Cerebellar syndromes may be seen with many noninfectious pathologic processes. In a young adult, cerebellar disease is often an early feature of multiple sclerosis. Diffuse cerebellar involvement may be paraneoplastic and represent the presenting symptom of an underlying carcinoma—most commonly originating in the lung, breast, or ovary—or a lymphoma. Neoplastic processes may invade the cerebellum directly with metastases, or originate there, particularly in children who may have cerebellar astrocytomas or neuroblastomas.

Vascular disease may present with cerebellar symptoms attributable to infarction or hemorrhage on the basis of atherosclerotic, embolic, or vasculitic mechanisms. Examination will usually reveal signs of focal cerebellar involvement. Noninfectious inflammations such as sarcoidosis also can produce localized cerebellar lesions. A number of drugs and toxins may cause cerebellar symptoms, including alcohol, lead, thallium, solvents, organic mercurials, anticonvulsants, chemotheraputic agents, psychotropics, and isoniazid. Metabolic conditions causing ataxia include hypothyroidism, hyponatremia, hypoglycemia, and, in young patients, a number of metabolic deficiency disorders, including Hartnup's disease, maple-syrup-urine disease, hyperpyruvic acidemias, urea-cycle abnormalities, and Leigh's disease (see Weiss and Guberman[4] and Stumpf[5]).

The interested reader is referred to the general references following this text, particularly to the monograph by Gilman, Bloedel, and Lechtenberg,[1] for a full discussion of the spectrum of noninfectious cerebellar disorders.

References

1. Gilman S, Bloedel JR, Lechtenberg R: *Disorders of the Cerebellum*. Philadelphia, F.A. Davis, 1981.
2. DeJong RN: *The Neurologic Examination*, 4th ed. Hagerstown, Md., Harper & Row, 1979, pp. 318–328.
3. Adams RD, Victor M: *Principles of Neurology*, 4th ed. New York, McGraw-Hill, 1989, pp. 68–75.
4. Weiss S, Guberman A: Acute cerebellar ataxia in infectious disease, in Vinken PJ, Bruyn GW, Klawans HL (eds): *Handbook of Clinical Neurology, Vol 33, Infections of the Nervous System, Part 1*. New York, Elsevier-North Holland, 1978, pp. 619–639.
5. Stumpf DA. Diseases of the brainstem and cerebellum, in Swaiman KF (ed): *Pediatric Neurology, Principles and Practice*. St. Louis, C.V. Mosby Co, 1989, pp. 219–224.
6. Menkes JH: *Textbook of Child Neurology*, 3rd ed. Philadelphia, Lea & Febiger, 1985, pp. 462–463.
7. Weiss S, Carter S: Course and prognosis of acute cerebellar ataxia in children. *Neurology* 1959;9: 711–721.
8. King G, Schwarz GA, Slade HW: Acute cerebellar

ataxia of childhood: report of nine cases. *Pediatrics* 1958;21:731–745.

9. Gershon A, Steinberg S, Greenberg S, Taber L: Varicella-zoster associated encephalitis and detection of specific antibody in cerebrospinal fluid. *J Clin Microbiol* 1980;12:764–767.
10. Peters ACB, Versteeg J, Lindeman J, Bots, GTAM: Varicella and acute cerebellar ataxia. *Arch Neurol* 1978;35:769–771
11. Applebaum E, Rachelson MH, Dolgopol VB: Varicella encephalitis. *Am J Med* 1953;15:223–230.
12. Goldstone AS, Millchap JG, Miller RH: Cerebellar ataxia with pre-eruptive varicella. *Am J Dis Child* 1963;106:111–114 (197–200).
13. McKendall RR, Klawans HL: Varicella-zoster virus complications, in Vinken PG, Bruyn GW, Klawans HL (eds): *Handbook of Clinical Neurology, Vol 34, Infections of the Nervous System, Part II*. New York, Elsevier-North Holland, 1978, pp. 163–164.
14. Miller HG, Stanton JB, Gibbons JL: Para-infectious encephalomyelitis and related syndromes. *Q J Med* 1956;25:427–505.
15. Jubelt B, Harter DH: Viral infections, in Rowland LP (ed): *Merritt's Textbook of Neurology*, 7th ed. Philadelphia, Lea & Febiger, 1984, pp. 79–116.
16. Tyler HR: Neurological complications of rubeola (measles). *Medicine* 1957;36:147–167.
17. Johnson RT, Griffin DE, Hirsch RL, et al: Measles encephalomyelitis: clinical and immunologic studies. *New Engl J Med*. 1984;310:137–141.
18. Wolinsky JS, Berg BO, Maitland CJ: Progressive rubella panencephalitis. *Arch Neurol* 1976;33:722–723.
19. Berg R, Jelke H: Acute cerebellar ataxia in children associated with Coxsackie viruses group B. *Acta Pediatr Scand* 1965;54:497–502.
20. Meyer HM, Johnson RT, Crawford IP, et al: Central nervous system syndromes of "viral" etiology. *Am J Med* 1960;29:334–347.
21. Marzetti G, Midulla M: Acute cerebellar ataxia associated with echo type 6 infection in two children. *Acta Pediatr Scand* 1967;56:547–551.
22. McAllister RM, Hummeler K, Coriell LL: Acute cerebellar ataxia: report of a case with isolation of type 9 echo virus from the cerebrospinal fluid. *N Engl J Med* 1959;261:1159–1162
23. Mendez-Cashion D, Sanchez-Longo LP, Valcarcel M, Rosen L: Acute cerebellar ataxia in children associated with infection by poliovirus I. *Pediatrics* 1962;29:808–815.
24. Curnen EC, Chamberlin HR: Acute cerebellar ataxia associated with poliovirus infection. *Yale J Biol Med* 1961:34:219–233.
25. Howe HS: The pathological changes in the cerebellum in acute anterior poliomyelitis. *Neurol Bull* 1919;2:261–266.
26. Azimi PH, Shaban S, Hilty MD, Haynes RE: Mumps meningoencephalitis. *JAMA* 1975;234: 1161–1162.
27. Ishimaru Y, Nakamo S, Yamaoka K, Takami S: Outbreaks of hand, foot, and mouth disease by enterovirus 71. *Arch Dis Child* 1980;55:583–588.
28. Dolgopol VB, Husson GS: Infectious mononucleosis with neurologic complications: report of a fatal case. *Arch Int Med* 1949;83:179–183.
29. Schnell RG, Dyck PJ, Bowie EJW, et al: Infectious mononucleosis: neurologic and EEG findings. *Medicine* 1966;45:51–63.
30. Dowling MD Jr, Van Slyck EJ: Cerebellar disease in infectious mononucleosis. *Arch Neurol* 1966;15: 270–274.
31. Bajada S: Cerebellitis in glandular fever. *Med J Aust* 1976;1:153–156.
32. Lascelles RG, Longson M, Johnson PJ, Chiang A: Infectious mononucleosis presenting as acute cerebellar syndrome. *Lancet* 1973;2:707–709.
33. Bennett DR, Peters HA: Acute cerebellar syndrome secondary to infectious mononucleosis in a fifty-two year old man. *Ann Int Med* 1961;55:147–149.
34. Gilbert JW, Culebras A: Cerebellitis in infectious mononucleosis. *JAMA* 1972;220:727.
35. Dano G: Acute cerebellar ataxia associated with herpes simplex virus infection. *Acta Pediatr Scand* 1968;57:151–152.
36. Berglund G, Mossberg HO, Rydenstam B: Acute cerebellar ataxia in children. *Acta Pediatr Scand* 1955;44:254–262.
37. Jones HR Jr, Hedley-Whyte ET, Kelleher JE Jr, et al: Primary cerebellopontine progressive mutlifocal leucoencephalopathy diagnosed premortem by cerebellar biopsy. *Trans Am Neurol Assoc* 1980;300–302.
38. Miller, JR, Barrett RE, Britton CB, et al: Progressive multifocal leukoencephalopathy in a male homosexual with T-cell immune deficiency. *N Engl J Med* 1982;307:1436–1438.
39. Peters ACB, Versteeg J, Bots GTAM, et al: Progressive multifocal leukoencephalopathy immunofluorescent demonstration of simian virus 40 antigen in CSF cells and response to cytarabine therapy. *Arch Neurol* 1980;37:497–501.
40. Bauer WR, Turel AP Jr, Johnson KP: Progressive multifocal leukoencephalopathy and cytarabine: remission with treatment. *JAMA* 1973;226:174–176.
41. Marriott PJ, O'Brien MD, Mackenzie ILK, Janota I: Progressive multifocal leukoencephalopathy: remission with cytarabine. *J Neurol Neurosurg Psychiatry* 1975;38:205–209.
42. Berger JR, Kaszovitz B, Post JD, Dickinson, G: Progressive multifocal leukoencephalopathy associated with human immunodeficiency virus infection. *Ann Int Med* 1987;107:78–87.
43. Gomori AJ, Partnow MJ, Horoupian DS, Hirano A:

The ataxic form of Creutzfeldt-Jakob disease. *Arch Neurol* 1973;29:318–323.
44. Roos R, Gajdusek CD, Gibbs CJ Jr: The clinical characteristics of transmissible Cruetzfeldt-Jakob disease. *Brain* 1973;96:1–20.
45. Schwartz JF: Ataxia in bacterial meningitis. *Neurology* 1972;22:1071–1074.
46. Steele JC, Gladstone RM, Thanasophon S, Fleming PC: Acute cerebellar ataxia and concomitant infection with *Mycoplasma pneumoniae*. *J Pediatr* 1972;80:467–469.
47. Abramovitz P, Schwartzman P, Harel D, et al: Direct invasion of the central nervous system by *Mycoplasma pneumoniae:* a report of two cases. *J Infect Dis* 1987;155:482–487.
48. Wyler AR, Harris AB: Cerebellar ataxia with *Mycoplasma pneumonia*. *Ann Int Med* 1974;80:556–557.
49. Shetty KR, Cilyo CL, Starr BD, Harter DH: Legionnaires' disease with profound cerebellar involvement. *Arch Neurol* 1980;37:379–380.
50. Pendlebury WW, Perl DP, Winn WC Jr, McQuillen JB: Neuropathologic evaluation of 40 confirmed cases of *Legionella pneumonia*. *Neurology* 1983; 33:1340–1344.
51. Maskill, MR, Jordan EC: Pronounced cerebellar features in Legionnaires' disease. *Br Med J*. 1981;283:276.
52. Baker PCH, Price TRP, Allen CD: Brain stem and cerebellar dysfunction with Leigonnires' disease. *J Neurol Neurosurg Psychiatry* 1981;44:1054–1056.
53. Lees AW, Tyrrell WF: Severe cerebral disturbance in Legionnaries' disease. *Lancet* 1978;2:1336–1337.
54. Friedman HM: Legionnaires' disease in non-Legionnaires: a report of five cases. *Ann Int Med* 1978;88:294–302.
55. Weir AI, Bone I, Kennedy DH: Neurological involvement in legionellosis. *J Neurol Neurosurg Psychiatry* 1982;45:603–608.
56. Miller JQ, Price TR: The nervous system in Rocky Mountain spotted fever. *Neurology* 1972;22:561–566.
57. Sawhney IMS, Prabhakar S, Dhand VK, Chopra JS: Acute cerebellar ataxia in enteric fever. *Trans Roy Soc Trop Med Hyg* 1986;80:85–86.
58. Chambers ST, Wilson AP, Seal DV, Rogers KB: Paratyphoid fever presenting with grand mal fits and cerebellar signs. *J Infect Dis* 1985;10:48–50.
59. Finkel MF: Lyme disease and its neurological complications. *Arch Neurol* 1988;45:99–104.
60. Reik L, Steere AC, Bartenhagen NH, et al: Neurologic abnormalities of Lyme disease. *Medicine* 1979;58:281–294.
61. Reik L, Smith L, Khan A, Nelson W: Demyelinating encephalopathy in Lyme disease. Neurology 1985;35:267–269.
62. Sindic CJM, Depre A, Bigaignon G, et al: Lymphocytic meningoradiculitis and encephalomyelitis due to *Borrelia Burgdorferi:* a clinical and serological study of 18 cases. *J Neurol Neurosurg Psychiatry* 1987;50:1565–1571.
63. Batten FE: Ataxia in childhood. *Brain* 1905;28:484–505.
64. Hindle J, Pearce JMS: Cerebellar encephalopathy in cat scratch disease. *J Neurol Neurosurg Psychiatry* 1987;50:936.
65. Bruyn GW: Cat scratch disease, in Vinken PJ, Bruyn GW, Klawans HL (eds): *Handbook of Clinical Neurology, Vol 34, Infections of the Nervous System, Part II*. New York, Elsevier-North Holland, 1978, p 471.
66. Sahs AL: Brucellosis, in Vinken PJ, Bruyn GW, Klawans HL (Eds): *Handbook of Clinical Neurology, Vol 34, Infections of the Nervous System, Part I*. New York, Elsevier-North Holland, 1978, p 314.
67. Bouza E, De La Torre MG, Parras F, et al: Brucellar meningitis. *Rev Infect Dis* 1987;9:810–822.
68. Wakisaka S, Soejima T, Matsuoka S: Cerebellar tuberculoma: a case report and review of the literature. *Neurol Med Chir* 1987;27:31–36.
69. Udani PM, Parekh VC, Dastur DK: Neurological and related syndromes in CNS tuberculosis: clinical features and pathogenesis. *J Neurol Sci* 1971; 14:341–357.
70. Yang PJ, Reger KM, Seeger JF, et al: Brain abscess: an atypical CT appearance of CNS tuberculosis. *Am J Neurorad* 1987;8:919–920.
71. Van Dellen RJ, Bullock R, Postma MH: Cerebellar abscess: the impact of computed tomographic scanning. *Neurosurgery* 1987;21:547–549.
72. Chun CH, Johnson JD, Hofstetter M, Raff MJ: Brain abscess: a study of 45 consecutive cases. *Medicine* 1986;65:415–431.
73. Morgan H, Wood MW: Cerebellar abscesses: a review of seventeen cases. *Surg Neurol* 1975;3:93–96.
74. Shaw MDM, Russel JA: Cerebellar abscess: a review of 47 cases. *J Neurol Neurosurg Psychiatry* 1975;38:429–435.
75. Garfield J: Brain abscesses and focal suppurative infections, in Vinken PK, Bruyn GW, Klawans HL (eds): *Handbook of Clinical Neurology, Vol 33, Infections of the Nervous System, Part I*. New York, Elsevier-North Holland, 1978, pp. 138–139.
76. Fujita NK, Reynard M, Sapico FL, et al: Cryptococcal intracerebral mass lesions, the role of computer tomography and nonsurgical management. *Ann Int Med* 1981;94:382–388.
77. Selby RC, Lopez NM: Torulomas (cryptococcal granulomata) of the central nervous system. *J Neurosurg* 1973;38:40–46.
78. Lewis JL, Rabinovich S: The wide spectrum of cryptococcal infections. *Am J Med* 1972,53:315–322.

79. Zuger A, Lovie E, Holzman RS, et al: Cryptococcal disease in patients with the acquired immunodeficiency syndrome: diagnostic features and outcome of treatment. *Ann Int Med* 1986;104:234–240.
80. Leers WD, Russell NA, Laroye G: Cerebellar abscess due to *Blastomyces dermatidis*. *Can Med Assoc J* 1972;107:657–660.
81. Gonyea EF: The spectrum of primary blastomycotic meningitis: a review of central nervous system blastomycosis. *Ann Neurol* 1978;3:26–39.
82. Waisbren BA, Ullrich D: An isolated blastomycetoma of the posterior cranial fossa treated successfully with surgery and amphotericin B. *Am J Med* 1962;32:621–624.
83. Salaki JS, Louria DB, Chmel H: Fungal and yeast infections of the central nervous system: a clinical review. *Medicine* 1984;63:108–132
84. List CF, Williams JR, Beeman LB, Payne CA: Nocardiosis with multilocular cerebellar abscess: report of a cured case. *J Neurosurg* 1954;11:394–398.
85. Le Bourgeois PA: Isolated central nervous system histoplasmosis. *South Med J* 1979;72:1624–1625.
86. Salmon MA: Aspergilloma of the cerebellum. *J Roy Soc Med* 1978;76:611–613.
87. Walsh TJ, Hier DB, Caplan LR: Aspergillosis of the central nervous system: clinicopathologic analysis of 17 patients. *Ann Neurol* 1985;18:574–582.
88. Young RC, Bennett JE, Vogel CL, et al: Aspergillosis: the spectrum of the disease in 98 patients. *Medicine* 1970;49:147–173.
89. Young RF, Gage G, Grinnell V: Surgical treatment for fungal infections in the central nervous system. *J Neurosurg* 1985;63:371–381.
90. Nakazawa G, Lulu RE, Koo AH: Intracerebellar coccidioidal granuloma. *AM J Neurorad* 1983; 4:1243–1244.
91. Bridges WR, Echols DH: Cerebellar histoplasmoma: case report. *J Neurosurg* 1967;26:261–263.
92. Cooper RA Jr, Goldstein E: Histoplasmosis of the central nervous system. *Am J Med* 1963;35:45–57.
93. Clarke PRR, Warnock GBR, Blowers R, Wilkinson M: Brain abscess due to *Streptomyces griseus*. *J Neurol Neurosurg Psychiatry* 1964;27:553–555.
94. Greenlee JE, Johnson WD, Campa JF, et al: Adult toxoplasmosis presenting as polymyositis and cerebellar ataxia. *Ann Int Med* 1975;82:367–371.
95. Navia BA, Petito CK, Gold JWM, et al: Cerebral toxoplasmosis complicating the acquired immune deficiency syndrome: clinical and neuropathological findings in 27 patients. *Ann Neurol* 1986;19:224–238.
96. Catapano MS, Marx JA. Central nervous system cysticercosis simulating an acute cerebellar hemorrhage. *Ann Emerg Med* 1986;15:847–849.
97. Del Brutto OH, Sotelo J: Neurocysticercosis: an update. *Rev Infect Dis* 1988;10:1075–1087.
98. Sotelo J, Guerrero V, Rubio F: Neurocysticercosis: a new classification based on active and inactive forms: a study of 753 cases. *Arch Int Med* 1985;145:442–445.
99. McCormick GF, Zee CS, Heiden J: Cysticercosis cerebri. *Arch Neurol* 1982;39:534–539.
100. Senanayake N: Delayed cerebellar ataxia: a new complication of *Falciparum* malaria? *Br Med J* 1987;294:1253–1254.
101. De Silva HJ: Delayed cerebellar Ataxia: A new complication of *Falciparum* malaria? *Br Med J* 1987;294:1612.
102. James RF. Cerebellar ataxia in patients with malaria treated with chloroquine. *Postgrad Med J* 1988; 64:167.
103. Vietz G: Malaria, in Vinken PJ, Bruyn GW, Klawans HL (eds): *Handbook of Clinical Neurology, Vol 35, Infections of the Nervous System, Part III*. New York, Elsevier-North Holland, 1978, p 146.
104. Schijman E: Hydatid cysts of the posterior fossa. *Neurosurgery* 1985;17:1014–1015.
105. Thomson AF: Other helminthous infections, in Vinken PJ, Bruyn GW, Klawans HL (eds): *Handbook of Clinical Neurology, Vol 35, Infections of the Nervous System, Part III*. New York, Elsevier North-Holland, 1978, pp 347–348.
106. Scrimgeour EM, Gajdusek DC: Involvement of the central nervous system in *Schistosoma mansoni* and *S. haematobium infection Brain* 1985;108:1023–1238.
107. Bambirra E, Alves A, De Sovza J, et al: The tumoral form of schistosomiasis: report of a Case with cerebellar involvement. *Am J Trop Med Hyg* 1984;33:76–79.
108. Dumas M, Girard PL: Human African trypanosomiasis, in Vinken PJ, Bruyn GW, Klawans HL (eds): *Handbook of Clinical Neurology, Vol 35, Infections of the Nervous System, Part III*. New York, Elsevier-North Holland, 1978, pp. 71–72.
109. Spina-Franca A, Mattosinho-Franca LC: American trypanosomiasis (Chagas' disease), in Vinken PJ, Bruyn GW, Klawans HL (eds): *Handbook of Clinical Neurology, Vol 35, Infections of the Nervous System Part III*. New York, Elsevier-North Holland, 1978, p 105.

12
Prions Causing Transmissible Neurodegenerative Diseases

STANLEY B. PRUSINER AND KAREN K. HSIAO

Seven diseases, four of animals and three of humans, are probably caused by prions (Table 12.1). The unusual properties of the infectious pathogens causing scrapie prompted introduction of the term "prion" to distinguish this class of particles from viruses and viroids.[1] The slow infectious agents that cause transmissible mink encephalopathy (TME), chronic wasting disease (CWD), and kuru are not well characterized; thus, further knowledge about the properties of these infectious agents must be obtained before they can be firmly classified as prions. Much more is known about the prion particles that cause Creutzfeldt-Jakob disease (CJD), Gerstmann-Sträussler-Scheinker syndrome (GSS), and bovine spongiform encephalopathy (BSE).[2–4] For ease of discussion, all the diseases listed in Table 12.1 are referred to as prion diseases even though a prion etiology must be considered tentative until the molecular properties of each slow infectious agent are well defined.[5]

All of the prion diseases recognized to date share many features; these are listed in Table 12.2. All known prion diseases are confined to the central nervous system (CNS). Prolonged incubation periods ranging from two months to two decades have been observed. The clinical course in these diseases is usually rather stereotyped and progresses to death. The clinical phase of prion illnesses may last for a few weeks to a few years. A reactive astrocytosis is usually found throughout the CNS in all of these diseases.[6,7] Neuronal vacuolation is also found, but it is not a constant or obligatory feature. The infectious agents, or prions, causing these diseases possess unusual molecular properties that appear to distinguish them from both viruses and viroids.[1,8]

Progress in the purification of the hamster scrapie prion[9,10] led to the detection of a unique protein, PrP 27–30, which was shown to be a major component of the infectious particle.[11–15] PrP 27–30 is a sialoglycoprotein[16] and was found to polymerize into rods possessing the ultrastructural and histochemical characteristics of amyloid.[17] The development of a large-scale purification protocol provided sufficient immunogen for the production of an antiserum to PrP 27–30,[18] which, in turn, has afforded a means for the molecular comparison of the infectious particles causing scrapie in rodents with those causing CJD.[19] We have also used this antiserum to show that amyloid plaques in the brains of scrapie-infected hamsters are composed of paracrystalline arrays of prion proteins.[18,20]

Direct evidence for the presence of protease-resistant prion proteins isolated from the brains of patients dying of CJD and GSS was obtained.[2,3] Purified fractions from the brains of two patients with CJD were found to contain protease-resistant proteins ranging in apparent molecular weight from 10,000 to 50,000. These proteins reacted with antibodies raised against the scrapie prion protein PrP 27–30. Rod-shaped particles were found in sucrose gradient fractions prepared from the brains of these patients that were similar to those isolated from rodents with either scrapie or experimental CJD.[17,19] After being stained with Congo red dye, the protein polymers from patients with CJD exhibited green birefringence when examined under polarized light. The findings suggested that the amyloid plaques found in the brains of CJD patients may be composed of paracrystalline arrays of prions similar to those in prion diseases in laboratory animals. Indeed, that is the case—amyloid plaques in CJD, GSS, and kuru stain with PrP antibodies.[21–23]

Table 12.1. Prion diseases.*

Disease	Natural host
Scrapie†	Sheep and goats
Transmissible mink encephalopathy (TME)	Mink
Chronic wasting disease (CWD)	Mule deer and elk
Bovine spongiform encephalopathy (BSE)	Cattle
Kuru	Humans—Fore
Creutzfeldt-Jakob disease (CJD)†	Humans
Gerstmann-Sträussler syndrome (GSS)	Humans

*Alternative terminologies include subacute transmissible spongiform encephalopathies and unconventional slow virus diseases.[68]
†Prions have been shown to cause scrapie and CJD; they are presumed to cause the other diseases listed.

Table 12.2. Some characteristics of prion diseases.

- Diseases are confined to the nervous system.
- Prolonged incubation period of months to decades precedes the onset of clinical illness.
- Progressive clinical course of weeks to years invariably leads to death.
- All diseases exhibit a reactive astrocytosis and many show vacuolation of neurons.
- The infectious agents (prions) causing these diseases exhibit properties that distinguish them from both viruses and viroids.

Creutzfeldt-Jakob Disease

In 1920, Creutzfeldt[24] described a progressive dementing illness in a 22-year-old woman. The following year, Jakob[25] described four older patients with a clinically similar presentation and course. During the ensuing four decades, numerous cases of CJD were described clinically and pathologically. In 1959, Klatzo, Gajdusek, and Zigas[26] noted the neurologic similarities between CJD and kuru, a degenerative cerebellar disorder of New Guinea natives. That same year, Hadlow[27] described the neuropathologic similarities between kuru and scrapie and suggested that kuru might be transmissible to laboratory animals after a prolonged incubation period. During the next decade, both kuru and CJD were transmitted to apes and monkeys.[28–30]

Clinical Features

The majority of CJD patients present with deficits in higher cortical function.[31–38] These deficits virtually always progress to a state of profound dementia characterized by memory loss, impaired judgment, and a decline in virtually all aspects of intellectual function.[39] A minority of patients present with either cerebellar deficits or visual impairment. Those with cerebellar problems generally exhibit difficulty in walking as well as incoordination. Frequently, the cerebellar deficits are rapidly followed by the onset of a progressive dementia.[40,41] Visual problems often begin with blurred vision and diminished acuity. Like the cerebellar syndromes, the dementia rapidly follows the appearance of visual symptoms.

Generally, patients with CJD are between 50 and 65 years of age; however, patients as young as 17 and as old as 83 have been recorded.[35,37,38,42]

A recent study indicates that lower motor neuron disease in association with a progressive dementing syndrome is not transmissible to apes and monkeys.[43] Based on these findings, the authors argue that the term "amyotrophic Creutzfeldt-Jakob disease" is not a useful label.

Most patients (~90%) with CJD exhibit myoclonus. These jerky, nonrhythmic, irregular involuntary movements can be seen at various times throughout the illness.[34,37,38] Unlike other involuntary movements, myoclonus persists during sleep. Startle myoclonus, which is elicited by abrupt changes in the environment such as loud sounds or bright lights, is frequently seen.

It is important to stress that myoclonus is not confined to CJD. Dementia with myoclonus can also be due to Alzheimer's disease.[44]

The electroencephalogram (EEG) can be useful in the diagnosis of CJD. During the early phase of CJD, the EEG is usually normal or shows only scattered theta activity. In most, but not all, advanced cases, repetitive, high-voltage, triphasic and polyphasic sharp discharges are seen. The presence of these stereotyped periodic bursts of ~200-ms duration occurring every 1 to 2 seconds make the diagnosis of CJD very likely.[39,45–50] These discharges are frequently, but not always, symmetric; there may be a one-sided predominance in terms of amplitude. As CJD progresses, normal background rhythms become fragmentary and slower. The appearance of these periodic electrical complexes during the clinical course of CJD is variable, and in many cases their presence is temporary.

In documented cases of accidental transmission of CJD to humans, an incubation period of 1.5–2.0 years preceded the development of clinical disease.[51,52] In other cases, incubation periods of up to 30 years have been suggested. Most patients with CJD live 6–12 months after the onset of clinical signs and symptoms[37,38,42]; however, some live only a few months from the time of diagnosis, whereas others live for up to 5 years.[53] It is rare to see a patient with CJD who dies in less than 1 month from the onset of symptoms.

Diagnosis

The constellation of dementia, myoclonus, and periodic electrical bursts in an afebrile 60-year-old patient is generally CJD. Clinical abnormalities in CJD are confined to the CNS. Fever, elevated sedimentation rate, leukocytosis in blood, or a pleocytosis in cerebrospinal fluid (CSF) should alert the physician to another etiology to explain the patient's CNS dysfunction.

CJD is one of many CNS disorders to be considered in the differential diagnosis of dementia. In its early stages, CJD generally has no specific clinical characteristics that distinguish it from degenerative dementias such as Alzheimer's disease. As it progresses, its frequently rapid course, coupled with myoclonus and periodic bursts on the EEG, serves to clarify the diagnosis. With the exception of a brain biopsy, there are no specific laboratory tests for CJD; however, negative studies on CSF and blood, as well as normal computed tomography scans except for cortical atrophy, in some cases[54] are important aspects of the dementia workup. Widespread patchy hypometabolism of [^{18}F]-2-deoxyglucose as measured by positron-emission-tomography scanning has been reported in CJD, but the changes are indistinguishable from those in Alzheimer's disease.[55]

If the constellation of pathologic changes frequently found in CJD are seen in a brain biopsy, then the diagnosis is reasonably secure. However, the enthusiasm for brain biopsies in patients with suspected CJD is quite low for two reasons: first, there is no specific effective treatment for CJD, and second, decontamination of surgical instruments requires special protocols as described later.

Epidemiology

Found throughout the world, CJD is a rare disorder with an incidence of approximately one case per million population.[42] Many geographic clusters of CJD have been reported,[42,56–58] suggesting that common exposure to some etiologic agent may play a role, but attempts to identify the offending agent have been unsuccessful to date.

While most cases of CJD are sporadic, 5–10% are familial.[59–61] CJD appears to be inherited as an autosomal dominant trait with variable penetrance. Some families in which there are multiple cases of CJD also have several cases of Alzheimer's disease.[61] The relationship, if any, between CJD and Alzheimer's disease remains to be established.[62] Our recent demonstration of a related human gene that hybridizes with a PrP cDNA[63] makes the future study of familial CJD most important.

Care of CJD Patients

For many years, investigators have tried to implicate the ingestion of scrapie-infected sheep or goat meat in the pathogenesis of CJD in humans. Numerous epidemiologic studies have failed to establish a convincing relationship, but speculation about this potential route of inoculation continues.[42,64–67] It is unknown whether scrapie-infected sheep and goats provide a nonhuman reservoir for CJD prions. On the other hand, there is ample documentation of the transmission of kuru among New Guinea natives after they consumed kuru-infected brain during ritualistic cannibalism.[68] Recent studies provided convincing data that the oral route of inoculation, although extremely inefficient can be a source of prion infection.[69]

Accidental transmission of CJD to humans appears to have occurred with corneal transplantation,[51] contaminated EEG electrode implantation,[52] and surgical operations using contaminated instruments or apparatus.[42,70–72] When corneas unknowingly removed from donors with CJD were transplanted in apparently healthy recipients, the disease, after prolonged incubation periods, also appeared in the transplant recipients. Animals with experimental CJD and scrapie have significant levels of prions in their corneas, making this scenario seem quite probable. The implantation of improperly decontaminated EEG electrodes led to CJD in two young patients with intractable epilepsy. These same electrodes stored in ethanol-formalin for several years were found to cause CJD in a chimpanzee 18 months after their experimental implantation.

Several investigators have suggested that patients undergoing surgical procedures may have been accidently inoculated with prions during their operations.[68,71] Presumably, some instrument or piece of apparatus in the operating theater became contaminated when a CJD patient underwent surgery; subsequent cases were then exposed to CJD prions. Although the epidemiology of these studies is highly suggestive, no proof for such episodes exists.

Human pituitary growth hormone (hGH) has been implicated in seven cases of CJD in young adults who received hGH therapy.[73–79] Presumably, hGH preparations purified from some batches of 10,000 human pituitaries were contaminated with prions. Since CJD occurs at a rate of $\sim 1/10^6$ in the general population and $\sim 10\%$ of the population dies each year, it is probable that 1 in 10,000 deaths are due to CJD. Regulatory agencies have removed hGH purified from human sources and replaced it with recombinant hGH synthesized in bacteria. How many more cases of CJD resulting from pituitary hGH will be found is uncertain. It is noteworthy that the incubation periods may have ranged from 3 to 21 years, and that most cases presented with incoordination and ataxia, followed by dementia in later stages of the disease. PrP^{CJD} was found in brain tissue from one case of CJD in a young man who had received pituitary hGH.[75]

It is important to stress that CJD is neither a contagious nor a communicable disease, but it is transmissible.

While the risk of accidental inoculation by aerosols is very small, procedures involving the production of aerosols should be carried out in certified biosafety cabinets. The Centers for Disease Control/National Institutes of Health manual in "Biosafety in Microbiological and Biomedical Laboratories" recommends biosafety level-2 practices, containment equipment and facilities.[80] Compliance requires standard microbiologic practices in a facility with limited access where all personnel wear laboratory coats. The manual also recommends that gloves be worn for all activities during which the skin might come into contact with infectious tissues or fluids. With a few exceptions, those guidelines developed for care of patients with hepatitis are applicable to CJD patients.

The primary problem in caring for patients with CJD is the inadvertent infection of health-care workers by needle and stab wounds; the possible transmission of contagion through the air has never been documented. Accidental parenteral inoculation, especially with neural tissues and including formalin-fixed specimens, is potentially very hazardous. Extreme care should be taken to avoid autoinoculation or other traumatic inoculations with infectious tissues or body fluids. It is recommended that needles or other sharp instruments not be used except where substitutes cannot be devised. Proper disposal of contaminated needles is mandatory to prevent accidental exposure by supporting hospital personnel. EEG and electromyographic needles should not be reused after their use in studies on CJD patients.

There are no data to indicate that CJD actually has been transmitted from a patient to a health-care worker, however. Thus, patients with CJD should not be ignored or disregarded, but should be accorded the best medical care possible.

While the handling of CJD-infected tissues is potentially dangerous, adequate containment and decontamination procedures are available, as have been outlined here and described in detail elsewhere. Of note, the development of CJD in two histopathology technicians has been anecdotally reported.[81,82] Both technicians had processed brain specimens from patients with CJD. Whether these technicians developed CJD as a result of occupational exposure to prions is unknown. There is no rational, scientific reason for surgeons or nurses to resist performing biopsies on demented patients when this operation is warranted medically. Likewise, there is no reason for pathologists or morgue assistants to resist performing autopsies on patients whose clinical diagnosis was CJD. Progress in the diagnosis, care, and treatment of CJD patients requires the dedicated efforts of physicians, nurses, and other health-care workers. The standard microbiologic practices outlined here, along with specific recommendations for decontamination, would seem to be adequate precautions for the care of CJD patients and the handling of infected specimens.

The extreme resistance of the scrapie prion to inactivation by procedures that are commonly used to destroy viruses has been appreciated for almost four decades.[1,68,83–85] Similar structural features for CJD prions in human brain have recently been described.[2] Earlier studies had shown that many of the unusual properties of the scrapie prion were shared with the pathogen causing CJD.[68,86]

In recent years, many investigators have devoted considerable effort to defining procedures for decontamination of CJD-infected materials.[68,85,87–91] While there is general agreement about the extreme resistance of prions to inactivation, there is some disagreement about the optimal conditions for sterilization. Little is known about the resistance of the human CJD prion to inactivation; most of our knowledge comes from animal models of experimental CJD and scrapie. The most widely studied murine CJD model uses an isolate from a Japanese case of CJD.[92] Whether or not this murine CJD prion accurately reflects the properties of human CJD prions from other racial backgrounds remains to be established. It is noteworthy that human CJD prions from British and American patients can rarely be transmitted to mice,[93] whereas most Japanese cases readily transmit.[94]

Although some investigators recommend treating CJD-contaminated materials once with 1 N NaOH at room temperature,[95] we believe that this procedure may be inadequate for sterilization. We routinely use three 30-minute treatments with 2 N NaOH to yield a final concentration of 1 N for cold sterilization[91]; alternatively, we use 4.5 hours of autoclaving. In some cases, we combine treatment with 1 N NaOH with autoclaving for one and a half hours.[91] One communication reports that 1 N NaOH completely inactivated hamster-adapted scrapie prion preparations, but no data were given in the report.[95] In our experience, a one-time exposure to 1 N NaOH appears to be inadequate for sterilization of scrapie prions.[91,96]

Our recommendations for sterilization of prions are summarized in Table 12.3. A significant number of protocols, such as ethylene oxide, ultraviolet irradiation, ethanol, formalin, and autoclaving for 90 minutes, do not appear to be adequate to accomplish their goal. The term "sterilization" implies *complete* destruction of prions; any residual infectivity can be extremely hazardous.

Since an operating room where a CJD patient undergoing a neurosurgic procedure is the most likely place for hospital equipment to become contaminated,[71] sterilization of surgical instruments by the recommended procedures described in Table 12.3 seems mandatory, especially if the patient's cranium has been opened. Presumably, the human CJD brain has higher titers of prions than any other organ. This seems to be the case in experimental scrapie.[97] It is equally important to consider the efficacy with which prions infect experimental animals. Recent studies with hamster scrapie prions have shown that the intracerebral route of inoculation is approximately 10^9 times more efficient than oral ingestion.[69] These data emphasize the extreme danger of introducing small numbers of prions into nervous-system tissue during neurosurgical procedures. Transmission of CJD to humans from contaminated instruments is well documented.[52,71]

It has been argued that subclinical cases of CJD will harbor high titers of the infectious prions, but that these will not become manifest until the patient develops a neurologic disorder some time after the surgery is completed. Though this observation is particularly disconcerting, the rarity of CJD clearly indicates that very few, if any, patients develop CJD as a result of neurosurgical procedures.

Table 12.3. Sterilization procedures for prions.

A. Recommended procedures
   1. Autoclaving for 4.5 hr (121°C, 15 psi).
   2. 1 N NaOH* followed by autoclaving for 1.5 hr.
   3. 1 n NaOH* for 30 min at 25°C repeated three times.

B. Ineffective procedures
   Ethylene oxide, ultraviolet irradiation, ethanol, formalin, beta-propiolactone, bleach, boiling, detergents, chaotropic salts, acids, ionizing radiation, alcoholic iodine, acetone.

*A 2 N NaOH stock is convenient as it can be diluted to a final concentration of 1 N.

Therapeutic Intervention

There is no known effective therapy for treating or preventing CJD. There are no well-documented cases of patients with CJD recovering either spontaneously or after therapy, with one possible exception.[98] The disease appears to be uniformly fatal.

Amantadine, an antiviral drug, continues to be tried as a therapeutic pharmaceutical[99–101] although, as yet, without documented success. HPA-23, an antiviral drug that inhibits viral glycoprotein synthesis, is also being used to treat CJD patients; however, this experience has been so limited that it is unclear whether or not the drug has any effect in such patients.[38] HPA-23 given to scrapie-infected animals around the time of inoculation profoundly extends the length of the incubation period,[102] but seems to have no effect on the course of scrapie infection when given later. Other chemicals, such as DEAE dextran and cortisone, have also been shown to extend the length of the incubation period in experimental scrapie.[103,104]

Although antibodies have been raised against the scrapie prion protein and these cross-react with prion proteins in CJD human brains,[2] passive immunization, or even vaccination, would seem to be of little value. CJD and scrapie both progress in the absence of any immune response to the offending prions.

Neuropathology

Frequently, the brains of patients with CJD show no recognizable abnormalities upon gross examination. In patients surviving several years, variable degrees of cerebral atrophy are likely to result in brain weights as low as 850 g. In some cases, the sulci may be enlarged, as well as the ventricles, which may show hydrocephalus ex vacuo.

The pathologic hallmarks of CJD at the light-microscopic level are spongiform degeneration and astrogliosis. Generally, the spongiform changes occur in the cerebral cortex, putamen, candate nucleus, thalamus, and molecular layer of the cerebellum.[105–107] The characteristic feature of spongiform degeneration is many small, rounded vacuoles, ranging in size from 1 to 5 mm, in the neuropil between nerve-cell bodies.[108] On electron microscopy, the vacuoles appear to be swollen neuronal processes and to be surrounded by a membrane.[106,109] Frequently, many membrane fragments can be seen within them. In some patients with CJD, we have seen brain sections without any recognizable spongiform degeneration. It is noteworthy that vacuolation in natural scrapie of sheep is very limited,[6] whereas experimental scrapie in rodents is accompanied by widespread vacuolar changes. The brains of mink with TME generally show widespread vaculation, but infected Aleutian mink fail to show any detectable vacuolar change.[110] Thus, vacuolation, while a common feature of prion diseases, does not seem to be an obligatory change.

Astrogliosis seems to be a constant feature, though nonspecific, of prion diseases. Widespread proliferation of fibrous astrocytes is found throughout the gray matter of brains infected with CJD prions. Astrocytic processes filled with glial filaments form extensive networks. Whether or not prions possess some glial growth or maturation activity remains to be established. Alternatively, changes in neuronal function may provoke this attendant gliosis. Generally the white matter is devoid of lesions, but several cases of CJD in Japan have exhibited well-documented vacuolar changes.[111] The lack of an inflammatory response in CJD and other prion diseases is an important pathologic feature of these degenerative disorders.

Amyloid plaques have been found in 5–10% of CJD. Recent studies have shown that purified CJD prions from humans and animals exhibit the ultrastructural and histochemical characteristics of amyloid.[2,17] Amyloid plaques have been found in brains of mice infected with some human Japanese CJD cases.[112] These plaques stain with antisera raised against scrapie hamster PrP 27–30 protein.[22,23,113] Although not yet demonstrated directly at the ultrastructural level, it seems likely that amyloid plaques in human CJD are like those in experimental CJD and scrapie, and thus are composed of filamentous arrays of prions.[20]

The majority of cases of kuru show plaques with cores that are presumably composed of amyloid.[26,107] The kuru plaques differ from senile plaques in that senile plaques have a collection of amorphous material, presumably degenerating dendrites, around their amyloid core. The kuru plaques do not possess such a large halo. Both kuru and senile plaques have been reported in CJD, but they are not a constant feature of the disease.[114,115] Kuru plaques do seem to be a constant feature of GSS.[61,116]

Transmission to Animals

CJD has been transmitted to a variety of laboratory animals (Table 12.2). Until recently, the laboratory diagnosis of CJD required transmission to animals—the most reliable hosts being nonhuman primates—and over 200 cases have been transmitted to apes and monkeys (Gajdusek DC, Gibbs CJ Jr, personal communication). Many fewer cases of CJD have been transmitted to goats, marmosets, cats, and laboratory rodents; most cases cannot be transmitted to nonprimates.[93] The chemical basis for these differences among isolates is unknown. It is of interest that nearly 80% of all Japanese CJD cases are readily transmitted to rats and mice.[94]

Prolonged incubation times ranging from 4 months to more than 4 years have been recorded for CJD in experimental animals. Like CJD patients, the infected animals develop a progressive CNS disorder that leads to death in a comparatively short time. With a few exceptions, the neuropathologic changes in animals with experimental CJD are similar to those described here for humans.

Immunologic and Electron-Microscopic Studies

Recent studies suggest that the rapid and reliable diagnosis of CJD postmortem should be possible using antisera to prions.[2] Partial purification from 1 to 2 g of infected brain tissue using detergent extraction, differential centrifugation, and enzyme digestion has permitted us to detect prion proteins in all cases of CJD analyzed by immunoblots.[2] Antibodies raised against the scrapie hamster prion protein, PrP 27–30, were found to react with protease-resistant proteins in the partially purified fractions prepared from human CJD brain. Brains from control patients with anoxic encephalopathy of Alzheimer's disease did not contain these protease-resistant, immunoreactive prion proteins. It seems likely that this protocol should rapidly replace transmission studies using apes and monkeys.

In fractions containing human CJD prion proteins, rod-shaped particles were also found by electron microscopy after negative staining.[2] Most of the particles were of uniform diameter of ~11 nm; their mean length were ~165 nm, but they varied from 25 to 550 nm. Infrequently, the rods appeared twisted. These rod-shaped particles are of dimensions similar to filamentous structures previously described in thin sections of human CJD brain.[117] More recently, some investigators have reported the presence of highly twisted, helically wound fibrils in detergent extracts prepared from CJD patients and have suggested that these particles are diagnostic.[118–119] We have failed to find such fibrils, which are composed of subfilaments wound with a regular periodicity, in our purified preparations or in tissue sections from CJD patients or scrapie-infected animals.[2,17,20]

Gerstmann-Sträussler-Scheinker Syndrome

GSS is a rare, usually familial, neurodegenerative disease that afflicts patients in the third to seventh decades of life. The exact incidence of GSS is unknown, but it is estimated to be between 1 and 10 per 100 million. Patients present initially with ataxia or dementia and deteriorate inexorably to death over one to ten years. Protease-resistant PrP and PrP-immunoreactive amyloid plaques with characteristic morphology accumulate in the brains of patients with GSS.[2,3,120] PrP is a consituent of cerebral amyloid specific for the transmissible encephalopathies; it is absent in other neurodegenerative diseases.[22,23,113] GSS can be transmitted to experimental animals through intracerebral inoculation of patient-brain homogenates, but positive transmission is variable even between members of a single pedigree[61,93]; current diagnostic criteria for GSS incorporate clinical and neuropathologic features, but exclude animal-transmission studies.

Pedigree studies suggested that GSS and familial CJD may be inherited as autosomal dominent disorders.[61,121] The significance of this observation was uncertain until recently when GSS was demonstrated to be a genetic disease and its development was linked to a missense variant of the prion protein.[122,123] Molecular cloning studies demonstrated a C to T substitution in the second position of codon 102, which may have resulted from deamination of a methylated C situated 5' to G.[124,125] This mutation creates a Dde 1 restriction site, which was used to demonstrate genetic linkage between the PrP codon 102 amino-acid substitution (Pro→Leu) and the development of GSS in two pedigrees. Whether this substitution is the cause of GSS remains to be established.

About 10–15% of cases of CJD are familial whereas most cases of GSS are inherited.[61,121,126] Based on clinical and pathologic criteria, GSS can be classified into three forms: an ataxic form, for which the PrP codon 102 leucine substitution appears to be characteristic; a dementing form; and a dementing form accompanied by pathologic quantities of neurofibrillary tangles. When familial CJD is included, at least four forms of human inherited prion diseases can be deciphered. GSS and familial CJD are the only known human diseases that are both genetic and infectious.

The linkage between the PrP gene and GSS established, for the first time, that GSS is a genetic disorder. These observations parallel earlier studies in which the murine PrP gene was found to be linked to susceptibility (i.e., length of the incubation time) for experimental scrapie.[127] Moreover, the finding of a unique PrP gene amino-acid substitution on the same chromosome as that carrying the GSS locus in two pedigrees also resembles earlier studies in which substitutions of two amino-acid residues at PrP codons 108 and 189 correlate with short and long incubation times in experimental scrapie of mice.[128] If the leucine substitution at codon 102 arose independently in the two pedigrees, then it could represent more than a linked genetic marker and might itself provoke the development of GSS. While the composition of the GSS prion has not been determined directly, by analogy with results from experimental scrapie studies in rodents, it is likely that it is composed largely, if not entirely, of an abnormal isoform of human PrP. The striking and specific correlation between the leucine substitution and the ataxic form of GSS leads us to speculate that other specific mutations in PrP may correlate with the other forms of inherited prion diseases.

Kuru

For many decades, kuru devastated the lives of the Fore highlanders of Papua New Guinea.[68] The high incidence of the disease among women left a society of motherless children raised by their fathers. At present, it is unusual in the Fore region to see an older woman. With the cessation of traditional warfare, older men are now found, many of whom have had a succession of wives, each dying of kuru after bearing several children. Because contamination during ritualistic cannibalism appears to have been the mode of spread of kuru among the Fore people and since cannibalism had ceased by 1960 in the Fore region, the patients now developing kuru presumably were exposed in the kuru agent more than two decades ago.[68,129] In several cases, we obtained direct histories from patients and their families of the episode in which they cannabilized the remains of a near relative who had died of kuru, presumably providing the source of infection. That the kuru agent could remain apparently quiescent in these patients for two decades and then manifest itself in the form of a fatal neurologic disease is suggested by incubation periods of over 7.5 years in some monkeys inoculated with kuru agent.[130]

Clinical Characteristics

In a study of 15 patients with kuru, 13 received detailed neurologic examinations.[131] Ten of the 15 patients were women, and all were adults. The patients ranged in age from 29 to 60, with a mean age of 40.2 years. The mean age of the 10 women was 43.2 years and of the 5 men, 34.2. Five men and 4 women were under 40; all those over 40 were female. The youngest patient, a male, was 29 years old. Twelve of the patients lived in the South Fore, and the other three in the North Fore. The duration of clinical disease ranged from 5 to 22 months, with difficulty in walking considered as marking its onset.

All 15 patients related a history of joint pain preceding difficulty in walking by several months. Eleven of the 15 also reported diffuse headache as a prodomal symptom. The diagnosis of kuru was first made by the patients themselves upon recognizing that they were finding it difficult to walk. The rugged, mountainous terrain, which is frequently muddy from tropical rains, provided an ample test for assessing their balance on a daily basis.

Eleven of the 15 patients showed no signs of dementia at the time of examination, while four were disoriented and confused and had loss of memory. The latter individuals exhibited speech and frontal-lobe release signs consisting of suck, snout, bite, and both hand and foot grasps. Three of the demented patients required a stick to maintain their balance while standing, and one was unable to stand. With advanced kuru, truncal ataxia and tremor were so severe that the stick had to be implanted into the earth, and patients with advanced disease were unable to walk without the assistance of another person. In all patients still able to walk with the help of a stick or an observer, marked truncal ataxia was evident.

All the patients exhibited an apprehensive facial expression, which would remain unchanged for as long as 30 minutes. It could be interrupted, however, by laughter. All patients were able to smile when requested to do so. Examination of the cranial nerves revealed no abnormalities except for ataxic movements of the eyes during tests of conjugate gaze. Optokinetic nystagmus was diminished or absent bilaterally in most kuru patients, even at an early stage of the disease.

There was no evidence of muscle wasting or diminished strength, though one patient had coarse fasciculations intermittently in the triceps, quadriceps, and gastrocnemius muscles. No fasciculations of the tongue were observed.

Of the 13 patients who underwent neurologic examination, four showed increased resistance to passive movements and an additional seven exhibited mild rigidity with demonstrable cogwheeling. The initial clinical descriptions of kuru emphasized this aspect of the disease, as well as the cerebellar dysfunction.[132,133] No patient was hypotonic. Nine of the 15 patients exhibited choreiform movements. All 15 had normal strength. In 8 of 13 patients, hyperactive deep tendon reflexes were demonstrable but were confined to the lower extremities. Seven patients had ankle clonus. Two showed unilateral extensor plantar responses, and two others exhibited bilateral responses. In one case, a unilateral extensor plantar response was accompanied by normal deep tendon reflexes. In five patients in whom clonus at the ankles was readily elicited, no extensor plantar response was seen.

On sensory examination, responses to pinprick, temperature, touch, and vibration were normal. Cortical sensory testing failed to reveal deficits.

Marked ataxia of the upper and lower extremities was pronounced in all patients, and all exhibited a prominent intention tremor. Marked difficulties with all tests for coordination were observed. Rapid alternating movement were of uneven amplitude and rhythm.

Clinical Signs

The uniform clinical presentation of kuru is remarkable.[133–138] The prodromal symptoms and onset of the disease were similar in all the patients in a recent study.[131] Even the interval between the prodromal symptoms of headache and joint pain and the onset of difficulty in walking was always 6 to 12 weeks. In most cases, the disease progressed to death within 12 months, and all patients were dead within 2 years of onset. The average duration of illness for the 15 patients in this study was 16 months.[131] Invariably, signs of cerebellar dysfunction dominate the clinical picture. All patients remain ambulatory with the aid of a stick for more than half of the clinical phase of their illness. These clinical characteristics are similar to those reported for adult patients at the peak of the kuru epidemic.[133–138]

There has been debate about dementia in kuru.[133–138] Our findings of memory loss and disorientation accompanied by primitive reflexes, such as snout, bite, suck, rooting, and hand grasps, leave no doubt but that patients become demented at an advanced stage of the disease. These same patients also exhibited considerable muscle paratonia or gegenhalten.

The uniformity of presentation and clinical course in kuru contrasts with that of CJD, in which a wide spectrum of clinical manifestations is found.[33,34] While most CJD patients exhibit dementia, myoclonus, and pyramidal-tract dysfunction at an early stage of the clinical illness, 10–20% present with an ataxic illness.[41,139] However, the dementia appears at an earlier clinical stage in ataxic CJD than in kuru. During the ambulatory phase of disease, no patients with kuru were found to be as severely demented as are most patients with CJD.

Incubation Periods Exceeding Three Decades

The youngest patient with kuru in the series was about 29 years old at the time of examination.[131] His age is in accord with epidemiologic studies showing that no person born in the South Fore after 1959 has developed kuru. These studies indicate that kuru has disappeared progressively, first among children and then among adolescents. Although the number of deaths in adult females has decreased steadily and adult male deaths have remained almost invariant, 70% of all cases in the past 3 years have been in adult females. No one born in a village since cannibalism ceased has ever developed kuru, although the disease continues to afflict people born earlier in the same villages.[129,140] Each year, the youngest new patients are older than those of the previous year. These observations predict that there will be no kuru victims under the age of 30 within 7 years. Of several hundred orphans born since 1957 to mothers dying of kuru, none has yet developed the disease. More than 300 are now over age 15, and many are past 20. Thus, the many children with kuru seen in the 1950s were not infected prenatally, perinatally, or neonatally by their mothers. At the height of the kuru epidemic 20 years ago in the South Fore, where over 90% of the deaths in adult women were from kuru, almost every woman must have been infected. These observations indicate that there was no individual variation in susceptibility to kuru within this population group. The regular disappearance of kuru is inconsistent with the existence of any natural reservoirs for kuru besides humans. Indeed, there is no evidence for animal or insect reservoirs. In addition, there is no evidence of transmission in utero or by human milk. None of these modes of infection would explain the regular pattern that characterizes the disappearance of kuru.

While patients currently afflicted with kuru exhibit greatly prolonged incubation periods, children with kuru who were observed 20 years ago provide some information on the minimum incubation period. The youngest patient with kuru was 4 years old at the onset of the disease and died at age 5. We do not know at what age young children were infected. Accidental transmission of CJD to humans has required only 18 months after intracerebral or intraoptic inoculation.[51,52] An incubation period of 18 months has also been found in chimpanzees inoculated intracerebrally with the kuru agent.

Neuropathology

The neuropathologic changes in kuru are much like those described for CJD and GSS. Spongiform changes, astrogliosis, and amyloid or "kuru" plaques are the pathologic hallmarks of kuru. Most, but not all, cases of kuru exhibit amyloid plaques.[26]

Transmission

Considerable evidence implicates ritualistic cannibalism as the mode of transmission for kuru among the Fore and neighboring tribes.[68] Oral transmission of kuru to monkeys has been documented[130] and the inefficiency of this route of inoculation in scrapie is well established.[69] Whether the proposed scenarios for transmission of kuru through laceration of the skin and rubbing of the eyes is real or not remains to be established.[68] These suggestions for transmission were put forward when early experiments on oral transmission to apes and monkeys failed. The experimental results from oral transmission of scrapie to hamsters suggests that insufficient doses of the kuru prion were used in those protocols.[69]

Apes, monkeys, and cats have been used in kuru-transmission studies. After a prolonged incubation period, experimental kuru in animals is manifest as a neurologic disorder indistinguishable from experimental CJD and scrapie. To date, kuru has not been transmitted to laboratory rodents.[93]

Origin

It has been suggested that kuru began at the turn of the century as a spontaneous case of CJD that was propagated by ritualistic cannibalism.[68] Whether the Fore people and their immediate neighbors provide an especially permissive genetic background for kuru prions to multiply remains to be established. Noteworthy is a case of CJD outside the kuru region in Papua New Guinea.

Infectious, Sporadic, and Genetic Prion Diseases

The human prion diseases illustrate three mechanisms by which CNS degeneration may arise: slow infection, sporadic disease, and genetic disorder.[14,126,140] That the three diseases can be transmitted to laboratory animals by inoculation is well documented.[28,29,61] As pointed out, kuru is thought to have been spread exclusively through a slow infectious mechanism by means of ritualistic cannibalism.[68,129]

Although a few cases of CJD can be traced to inoculation with prions—that is, injections of hGH,[73,75,141] transplantation of corneas, and implantation of cerebral electrodes—the vast majority appear to be sporadic, despite considerable efforts to implicate scrapie-infected sheep as an exogenous source.[68,142] It is possible, although unlikely, that sporadic CJD results from prions that are ubiquitous in humans but have a very low efficiency of infection. In hamsters, scrapie infection by the oral route has been found to be 10^9 times less efficient than intracerebral inoculation.[69]

The genetic linkage of a missense variant of PrP with GSS constrains further the possible structural models for the prion. If prions contain a small, as yet undetected, nucleic acid, then this molecule must be widespread throughout the world to explain sporadic CJD and yet segregate in rare GSS families with the PrP mutation. It is noteworthy that Huntington's disease, another autosomal dominant genetic disorder, does not manifest clinical illness until the fifth decade in most cases. The delayed onset of both Huntington's disease and GSS is not understood. The genetic-linkage results also suggest an interesting mechanism for sporadic CJD if prions contain only PrP^{Sc} (or PrP^{CJD}). A somatic mutation[143] in the PrP gene, or even an RNA editing error[144–147] in a single cell, might lead to the generation of PrP^{CJD} in that cell; prions would then spread to neighboring cells upon exit of the PrP^{CJD} molecules. In contrast, the PrP mutation of GSS is in the germ line, consistent with its genetic transmission.

While scrapie is readily transmitted by inoculation and has been transmitted orally in an experimental setting,[69,148,149] it is unclear how the disease spreads naturally among sheep and goats. Some investigators have favored infection while others have been proponents of a genetic mechanism.[150,151] In retrospect, it seems that both points of view are probably correct. TME probably occurs in domesticated mink after they consume scrapie-infected sheep meat.[152,153] Scrapie prions administered intranasally to mink produce a disease indistinguishable from TME.[154,155] Interestingly, neither scrapie in mink nor TME can be transmitted to mice, suggesting a significant species barrier for mink prions[156] (Hadlow W; unpublished data).

CWD in captive herds of mule deer and elk may have occurred after oral consumption of prion-contaminated sheep by-products.[157] Whether CWD is a naturally occurring disease is uncertain. Over the past 4 years, over 13,000 dairy cattle in Great Britain have developed a spongiform degeneration.[158,159] Recent studies show that BSE is transmissible to mice after a prolonged incubation periods[160] and that a protease-resistant prion protein accumulates in the brains of these cattle.[4] Epidemiologic studies suggest that BSE began when bonemeal fed to dairy cattle as a protein supplement was produced by a new process; around 1981, the rendering temperature was reduced in order to increase the yield of sheep by-products.[159]

Prions—Novel and Unprecedented

The convergence of experimental results implicating a pivotal role for PrP^{Sc} (or PrP^{CJD}) in animal and human prion diseases is both impressive and persuasive. The wide variety of independent disciplines—including protein chemistry, molecular genetics, immunochemistry, neuropathology, and experimental neurology—employed to obtain these experimental data greatly strengthens the assertion that PrP^{Sc} has a central role in prion diseases.

That PrP is encoded by a cellular gene and not by a putative nucleic acid carried within the prion is a major feature that distinguishes prions from viruses. This discovery, coupled with recent genetic studies showing linkage between a PrP missense variant and GSS, demand that scrapie and CJD no longer be considered virologic disorders. Although prion diseases resemble viral illnesses in some respects, the structure, cell biology, and genetics of prions clearly separate them from viruses.

Just as GSS and familial CJD are unprecedented human illnesses since they are both genetic and infectious, the etiologic prion particles seem equally novel. Learning the chemical mechanisms responsible for converting PrP^{C} or a precursor into PrP^{Sc} will be extremely important. Elucidation of PrP^{C} function may open up new avenues of research into mechanisms of cell homeostasis, recognition, and possibly differentiation. However, it remains unknown whether proteins other than PrP are converted from benign, cellular isoforms into malignant, diseased molecules, resulting in degenerative diseases.

The search for other prion diseases should begin in earnest once the chemistry of PrP^{Sc} formation is elucidated. Whether some of the pathogenic mechanisms operative in prion diseases will give new insights into CNS disorders such as Alzheimer's disease, Parkinson's disease, and amyotrophic lateral sclerosis, or some degenerative systemic diseases, is unknown.

Acknowledgments. This chapter was adapted from an article in *Principles and Practice of Clinical Virology,* 2nd ed (Zuckerman AJ, Banatvala JE, Patttison JR, eds), Chichester, England, John Wiley & Sons Ltd., in press, 1990. The authors thank L. Gallagher and V. Nguyen for excellent editorial assistance. This work was supported by research grants from the National Institutes of Health (AG02132 and NS14069) and a Senator Jacob Javits Center of Excellence in Neuroscience (NS22786), as well as by gifts from the Sherman Fairchild Foundation, Inc., RJR-Nabisco, Inc., and National Medical Enterprises.

References

1. Prusiner SB: Novel proteinaceous infectious particles cause scrapie. *Science* 1982;216:136–144.
2. Bockman JM, Kingsbury DT, McKinley MP, et al: Creutzfeldt-Jakob disease proteins in human brains. *N Engl J Med* 1985;312:73–78.
3. Bockman JM, Prusiner SB, Tateishi J, et al: Immunoblotting of Creutzfeldt-Jakob disease prion proteins: host species-specific epitopes. *Ann Neurol* 1987;21:589–595.
4. Hope J, Reekie LJ, Hunter N, et al: Fibrils from brains of cows with new cattle disease contain scrapie-associated protein. *Nature* 1988;336:390–392.
5. Prusiner SB: Prions—novel infectious pathogens. *Adv Virus Res* 1984;29:1–56.
6. Zlotnik I: The pathology of scrapie: a comparative study of lesions in the brain of sheep and goats. *Acta Neuropathol* [suppl] (Berl) 1962;1:61–70.
7. Beck E, Daniel PM, Davey AJ, et al: The pathogenesis of transmissible spongiform encephalopathy—an ultrastructural study. *Brain* 1982; 105:755–786.
8. Diener TO, McKinley MP, Prusiner SB: Viroids and prions. *Proc Natl Acad Sci USA* 1982;79:5220–5224.
9. Bolton DC, McKinley MP, Prusiner SB: Identification of a protein that purifies with the scrapie prion. *Science* 1982;218:1309–1311.
10. Prusiner SB, Bolton DC, Groth DF, et al: Further purification and characterization of scrapie prions. *Biochemistry* 1982;21:6941–6950.
11. McKinley MP, Bolton DC, Prusiner SB: A pro-

tease-resistant protein is a structural component of the scrapie prion. *Cell* 1983;35:57–62.
12. Bolton DC, McKinley MP, Prusiner SB: Molecular characteristics of the major scrapie prion protein. *Biochemistry* 1984;23:5898–5906.
13. Gabizon R, McKinley MP, Groth DF, et al: Immunoaffinity purification and neutralization of scrapie prion infectivity. *Proc Natl Acad Sci USA* 1988;85:6617–6621.
14. Prusiner SB: Prions and neurodegenerative diseases. *N Engl J Med* 1987;317:1571–1581.
15. Prusiner SB: Scrapie prions. *Ann Rev Microbiol* 1989;43:345–374.
16. Bolton DC, Meyer RK, Prusiner SB: Scrapie PrP 27–30 is a sialoglycoprotein. *J Virol* 1985;53:596–606.
17. Prusiner SB, McKinley MP, Bowman KA, et al: Scrapie prions aggregate to form amyloid-like birefringent rods. *Cell* 1983;35:349–358.
18. Bendheim PE, Barry RA, DeArmond SJ, et al: Antibodies to a scrapie prion protein. *Nature* 1984; 310:418–421.
19. Bendheim PE, Bockman JM, McKinley MP, et al: Scrapie and Creutzfeldt-Jakob disease prion proteins share physical properties and antigenic determinants. *Proc Natl Acad Sci USA* 1985;82:997–1001.
20. DeArmond SJ, McKinley MP, Barry RA, et al: Identification of prion amyloid filaments in scrapie-infected brain. *Cell* 1985;41:221–235.
21. Kitamoto T, Ogomori K, Tateishi J, et al: Formic acid pretreatment enhances immunostaining of amyloid deposits in cerebral and systemic amyloids. *Lab Invest* 1987;57:230–236.
22. Roberts GW, Lofthouse R, Brown R, et al: Prion-protein immunoreactivity in human transmissible dementias. *N Engl J Med* 1986;315:1231–1233.
23. Roberts GW, Lofthouse R, Allsop D, et al: CNS amyloid proteins in neurodegenerative diseases. *Neurology* 1988;38:1534–1540.
24. Creutzfeldt HG: Ober eine eingenartige herdförmige erkrankung des zentralnervensystems. *Z Neurol Psych* 1920;57:1–18.
25. Jakob A. Über eigenartige erkrankungen des zentralnervensystems mit bemerkenswertem anatomischen befunde (spastische pseudoscklerose-encephalomyelopathie mit disseminierten degenerationsherden). Preliminary communication. *Dtsch Z Nervenheilk* 1921;70:132–146.
26. Klatzo I, Gajdusek DC, Zigas V: Pathology of kuru. *Lab Invest* 1959;8:799–847.
27. Hadlow WJ: Scrapie and kuru. *Lancet* 1959;2:289–290.
28. Gajdusek DC, Gibbs CJ Jr, Alpers M: Experimental transmission of a kuru-like syndrome to chimpanzees. *Nature* 1966;209:794–796.
29. Gibbs CJ Jr, Gajdusek DC, Asher DM, et al: Creutzfeldt-Jakob disease (spongiform encephalopathy): transmission to the chimpanzee. *Science* 1968;161:388–389.
30. Gibbs CJ Jr, Gajdusek DC: Infection as the etiology of spongiform encephalopathy. *Science* 1969;165: 1023–1025.
31. Siedler H, Malamud N: Creutzfeldt-Jakob's disease. Clinicopathologic report of 15 cases and review of the literature (with special reference to a related disorder designated as subacute spongiform encephalopathy). *J Neuropathol Exp Neurol* 1963; 22:381–402.
32. May WW: Creutzfeldt-Jakob disease. 1. Survey of the literature and clinical diagnosis. *Acta Neurol Scand* 1968;44:1–32.
33. Kirschbaum WR (ed.): *Jakob-Creutzfeldt Disease*. New York, American Elsevier, 1968.
34. Roos R, Gajdusek DC, Gibbs CJ Jr: The clinical characteristics of transmissible Creutsfeldt-Jakob disease. *Brain* 1973;96:1–20.
35. Brown P, Cathala F, Sadowsky D, et al: Creutzfeldt-Jakob disease in France. II. Clinical characteristics of 124 verified cases during the decade 1968–1977. *Ann Neurol* 1979;6:430–437.
36. Lechi A, Tedischi F, Mancia D, et al: Creutzfeldt-Jakob disease: clinical, EEG and neuropathologic findings in a cluster of eleven patients. *Ital J Neurol Sci* 1983;1:47–59.
37. Will RG, Matthews WB: A retrospective study of Creutzfeldt-Jakob disease in England and Wales 1970–79. I. Clinical features. *J. Neurol Neurosurg Psychiatry* 1984;47:134–140.
38. Cathala F, Baron H: Clinical aspects of Creutzfeldt-Jakob disease, in Prusiner SB, McKinley MP (eds.): *Prions—Novel Infectious Pathogens Causing Scrapie and Creutzfeldt-Jakob Disease*. Orlando, Fla., Academic Press, 1987, pp. 467–509.
39. Nevin S, McMenemy WH, Behrman S, et al: Subacute spongiform encephalopathy—a subacute form of encephalopathy attributable to vascular dysfunction (spongiform cerebral atrophy). *Brain* 1960; 83:519–564.
40. Brownell B, Oppenheimer DR: An ataxic form of subacute presenile polioencephalopathy (Creutzfeldt-Jakob disease). *J Neurol Neurosurg Psychiatry* 1965;28:350–361.
41. Gomori AJ, Partnow MJ, Horoupian DS, et al: The ataxic form of Creutzfeldt-Jakob disease. *Arch Neurol* 1973;29:318–323.
42. Masters CL, Harris JO, Gajdusek DC, et al: Creutzfeldt-Jakob disease: patterns of worldwide occurrence and the significance of familial and sporadic clustering. *Ann Neurol* 1978;5:177–188.
43. Salazar AM, Masters CL, Gajdusek DC, et al: Syndromes of amyotrophic lateral sclerosis and dementia: relation to transmissible Creutzfeldt-Jakob disease. *Ann Neurol* 1983;14:17–26.
44. Watson CP: Clinical similarity of Alzheimer and

Creutzfeldt-Jakob disease. *Ann Neurol* 1979;6:368–369.

45. Burger LJ, Rowan AJ, Goldensohn ES: Creutzfeldt-Jakob disease. An electroencephalographic study. *Arch Neurol* 1972;26:428–433.
46. Lee RG, Blair RD: Evolution of EEG and visual evoked response changes in Jakob-Creutzfeldt disease. *Electroencephalogr Clin Neurophysiol* 1973; 35:133–142.
47. Chiaflo N, Fuentes AN, Galvez S: Serial EEG findings in 27 cases of Creutzfeldt-Jakob disease. *Arch Neurol* 1980;37:143–145.
48. Au WJ, Gabor AJ, Vijayan N, et al: Periodic lateralized epileptiform complexes (PLEDs) in Creutzfeldt-Jakob disease. *Neurology* 1980;30:611–617.
49. Kuroiwa Y, Celesia GG: Clinical significance of periodic EEG patterns. *Arch Neurol* 1980;37:15–20.
50. Traub RD, Pedley TA: Virus-induced electrotonic coupling: Hypothesis on the mechanism of periodic EEG discharges in Creutzfeldt-Jakob disease. *Ann Neurol* 1981;10:405–410.
51. Duffy P, Wolf J, Collins G, et al: Possible person to person transmission of Creutzfeldt-Jakob disease. *N Engl J Med* 1974;290:692–693.
52. Bernouilli C, Siegfried J, Baumgartner G, et al: Danger of accidental person to person transmission of Creutzfeldt-Jakob disease by surgery. *Lancet* 1977;1:478–479.
53. Brown P, Rodgers-Johnson P, Cathala F, et al: Creutzfeldt-Jakob disease of long duration: clinicopathological characteristics, transmissibility and differential diagnosis. *Ann Neurol* 1984;16:295–304.
54. Kovanen J, Erkinjuntti T, Livanainen M, et al: Cerebral MR and CT imaging in Creutzfeldt-Jakob disease. *J Comp Asst Tomogr* 1985;9:125–128.
55. Friedland RP, Prusiner SB, Jagust WJ, Budinger TF, Davis RL: Bitemporal hypometabolism in Creutzfeldt-Jakob disease measured by positron emission tomography with [^{18}F]-2-fluorodeoxyglucose. *J Comput Assist Tomogr* 1984;8:978–981.
56. Goldberg H, Alter M, Kahana E: The Libyan Jewish focus of Creutzfeldt-Jakob disease: A search for the mode of natural transmission, in Prusiner, SB, Hadlow, WJ (eds.). Slow Transmissible Diseases of the Nervous System, vol 1. New York: Academic Press, 1979, pp. 195–211.
57. Mayer V, Mitrova E, Orolin D: Creutzfeldt-Jakob disease in Czechoslovakia and a working concept of its surveillance, in Prusiner, SB, Hadlow, WJ (eds). Slow Transmissible Diseases of the Nervous System, vol 1. New York: Academic Press, 1979, pp. 287–303.
58. Malmgren R, Kurland L, Mokri B, Kurtzke J: The epidemiology of Creutzfeldt-Jakob disease, in: Prusiner, SB, Hadlow, WJ, (eds.). Slow Transmissible Diseases of the Nervous System, vol 1. New York: Academic Press, 1979; pp. 93–112.
59. Rosenthal NP, Keesey J, Crandall B, Brown WJ: Familial neurological disease associated with spongiform encephalopathy. *Arch Neurol* 1976;33:252–259.
60. Neugut RH, Neugut A, Kahana E, Stein Z, Alter M: Creutzfeldt-Jakob disease: Familial clustering among Libyan-born Israelis. *Neurology* 1979; 29:225–231.
61. Master CL, Gajdusek DC, Gibbs CJ Jr, Bernouilli C, Asher DM: Familial Creutzfeldt-Jakob disease and other familial dementias: An inquiry into possible models of virus-induced familial diseases, in: Prusiner, SB, Hadlow, WJ (eds). Slow Transmissible Diseases of the Nervous System, vol 1. New York: Academic Press, 1979; pp. 143–194.
62. Prusiner SB: Some speculations about prions, amyloid, and Alzheimer's disease. *N Engl J Med* 1984;310:661–663
63. Oesch B, Westaway D, Wälchli M, et al: A cellular gene encodes scrapie PrP 27–30 protein. *Cell* 1985;40:735–746.
64. Bobowick AR, Brody JA, Matthews MR, Roos R, Gajdusek DC: Creutzfeldt-Jakob disease: A case-control study. *Am J Epidemiol* 1973;98:381–394.
65. Alter M, Kahana E: Creutzfeldt-Jakob disease among Libyan Jews in Israel. *Science* 1976;192:428
66. Brown P. An epidemiologic critique of Creutzfeldt-Jakob disease. *Epidemiol Rev* 1980;2:113–135
67. LoRusso F, Neri G, Figa-Talamanca L: Creutzfeldt-Jakob disease and sheep brain—A report from central and southern Italy. *Ital J Neurol Sci* 1980; 3:171–174.
68. Gajdusek DC: Unconventional viruses and the origin and disappearance of kuru. *Science* 1977; 197:943–960.
69. Prusiner SB, Cochran SP, Alpers MP: Transmission of scrapie in hamsters. *J Infect Dis* 1985;152:971–978.
70. Kondo K, Kuroina Y. A case control study of Creutzfeldt-Jakob disease: Association with physical injuries. *Ann Neurol* 1981;11:377–381.
71. Will RG, Matthews WB: Evidence for case-to-case transmission of Creutzfeldt-Jakob disease. *J Neurol Neurosurg Psychiatry* 1982;45:235–238.
72. Davanipour Z, Goodmam L, Alter M, Sobel E, Asher D, Gajdusek DC: Possible modes of transmission of Cruetzfeldt-Jakob disease. *N Engl J Med* 1984;311:1582–1583.
73. Brown P: The decline and fall of Creutzfeldt-Jakob disease associated with human growth hormone therapy. *Neurology* 1988;38:1135–1137.
74. Croxson M, Brown P, Synek B, et al: A new case of Creutzfeldt-Jakob disease associated with human growth hormone therapy in New Zealand. *Neurology* 1988;38:1128–1130.

75. Gibbs CJ Jr, Joy A, Heffner R, et al: Clinical and pathological features and laboratory confirmation of Creutzfeldt-Jakob disease in a recipient of pituitary-derived human growth hormone. *N Engl J Med* 1985;313:734–738.
76. Koch TK, Berg BO, DeArmond SJ, Gravina RF: Creutzfeldt-Jakob disease in a young adult with idiopathic hypopituitarism. Possible relation to the administration of cadaveric human growth hormone. *N Engl J Med* 1985;313:731–733.
77. Marzewski. DJ, Towfighi J, Harrington MG, Merril CR, Brown P: Creutzfeldt-Jakob disease following pituitary-derived human growth hormone therapy: A new American case. *Neurology* 1988;38:1131–1133.
78. New MI, Brown P, Temeck JW, Owens C, Hedley-Whyte ET, Richardson EP: Preclinical Creutzfeldt-Jakob disease discovered at autopsy in a human growth hormone recipient. *Neurology* 1988;38: 1133–1134.
79. Weller RO, Steart PV, Powell-Jackson JD: Pathology of Creutzfeldt-Jakob disease associated with pituitary-derived human growth hormone administration. *Neuropathol Appl Neurobiol* 1986;12:117–129.
80. Centers for Disease Control and National Institutes of Health. Biosafety in Microbiological and Biomedical Laboratories, HHS Publication no. (CDC)84-8395, US Department of Health and Human Services, Public Health Service. Richardson JH, Barkeley WE (eds). Washington DC: US Government Printing Office, 1984.
81. Miller DC: Creutzfeldt-Jakob disease in histopathology technicians. *N Eng J Med* 1988;318:853–854.
82. Sitwell L, Lach B, Atack E, Atack D, Izukawa D: Creutzfeldt-Jakob disease in histopathology technicians. *N Eng J Med* 1988;318:854.
83. Gordon WS: Advances in veterinary research. *Vet Res* 1946;58:516–520.
84. Alper T, Cramp WA, Haig DA, Clarke MC: Does the agent of scrapie replicate without nucleic acid? *Nature* 1967;214:764–766.
85. Chatigny MA, Prusiner SB: Biohazards of investigations on the transmissible spongiform encephalopathies. *Rev Infect Dis* 1980;2:713–724.
86. Prusiner SB, Kingsbury DT: Prions—infectious pathogens causing the spongiform encephalopathies. *CRC Crit Rev Clin Neurobiol* 1985;1:181–200.
87. Kimberlin RH, Walker CA, Millson GC, et al: Disinfection studies with two strains of mouse-passaged scrapie agent. *J Neurol Sci* 1983;59:355–369.
88. Walker AS, Inderlied CB, Kingsbury DT: Conditions for the chemical and physical inactivation of the K. Fu. strain of the agent of Creutzfeldt-Jakob disease. *Am J Public Health* 1983;73:661–665.
89. Brown P, Gibbs CJ Jr, Amyx HL, et al: Chemical disinfection of Creutzfeldt-Jakob disease virus. *N Engl J Med* 1982;306:1279–1282.
90. Brown P, Rohwer RG, Green EM, Gajdusek DC: Effect of chemicals, heat, and histopathologic processing on high-infectivity hamster-adapted scrapie virus. *J Infect Dis* 1982;145:683–687.
91. Prusiner SB, McKinley MP, Bolton DC, et al: Methods for assay, purification and characterization, in Maramorosch, K, Koprowski H (eds). Methods in Virology. New York: Academic Press, 1984: pp. 293–345.
92. Tateishi J, Ohta M, Koga M, Sato Y, Kuroiwa Y: Transmission of chronic spongiform encephalopathy with kuru plaques from humans to small rodents. *Ann Neurol* 1979;5:581–584.
93. Gibbs CJ Jr, Gajdusek DC, Amyx H: Strain variation in the viruses of Creutzfeldt-Jakob disease and kuru, in Prusiner, SB, Hadlow, WJ (eds). Slow Transmissible Diseases of the Nervous System, vol. 1. New York: Academic Press, 1979: pp. 87–110.
94. Tateishi J, Sato Y, Ohta M: Creutzfeldt-Jakob disease in humans and laboratory animals, in: Zimmerman, HM (ed). Progress in Neuropathology. New York: Raven Press, 1983: pp. 195–221.
95. Brown P, Rohwer RG, Gajdusek DC: Sodium hydroxide decontamination of Creutzfeldt-Jakob disease virus. *N Engl J Med* 1984;310:727.
96. Prusiner SB, Groth DF, McKinley MP, Cochran SP, Bowman KA, Kasper KC: Thiocyanate and hydroxyl ions inactivate the scrapie agent. *Proc Natl Acad Sci USA* 1981;78:4606–4610.
97. Eklund CM, Kennedy RC, Hadlow WJ: Pathogenesis of scrapie virus infection in the mouse. *J Infect Dis* 1967;117:15–22.
98. Manuelidis EE, Manuelidis L, Pincus IH, Collins WF: Transmission, from man to hamster, of Creutzfeldt-Jacob disease with clinical recovery. *Lancet* 1978;2:40–42.
99. Braham J: Jakob-Creutzfeldt disease: Treatment by amantadine. *Br Med J* 1971;4:212–213.
100. Herishanu Y: Antiviral drugs in Jakob-Creutzfeldt disease. *J Am Geriatr Soc* 1973;21:229–231.
101. Terzano MG, Montanari E, Calzetti S, Mancia D, Lechi A: The effect of amantadine on arousal and EEG patterns in Creutzfeldt-Jakob disease. *Arch Neurol* 1983;40:555–559.
102. Kimberlin RH, Walker CA: The antiviral compound HPA-23 can prevent scrapie when administered at the time of infection. *Arch Virol* 1983;78:9–18.
103. Dickinson AG, Fraser H, Outram GW: Scrapie incubation time can exceed natural lifespan. *Nature* 1975;256:732–733.
104. Ehlers B, Diringer H: Dextran suphate 500 delays and prevents mouse scrapie by impairment of agent replication in spleen. *J Gen Virol* 1984;65:1325–1330.
105. Blackwood, W., McMenemy WH, Meyer A, Nor-

man RM, Russell DS, in Blackwood, W, McMenemy, WH, Meyer, A, Norman, RM, Russell, DS (eds). Greenfield's Neuropathology, 2nd ed. London: Edward Arnold, 1971: pp. 558–567.
106. Lampert PW, Gajdusek DC, Gibbs CJ Jr: Subacute spongiform virus encephalopathies. Scrapie, kuru, and Creutzfeldt-Jakob disease: A review. *Am J Pathol* 1972;68:626–652.
107. Beck E, Daniel PM: Kuru and Creutzfeldt-Jakob disease; Neuropathological lesions and their significance, in Prusiner, SB, Hadlow, WJ (eds). Slow Transmissible Diseases of the Nervous System, vol 1. New York: Academic Press, 1979: pp. 253–270.
108. Masters CL, Richardson EP Jr: Subacute spongiform encephalopathy Creutzfeldt-Jakob disease—The nature and progression of spongiform change. *Brain* 1978;101:333–344.
109. Beck E, Daniel PM, Davey AJ, Gajdusek DC, Gibbs CJ Jr: The pathogenesis of transmissible spongiform encephalopathy—An ultrastructural study. *Brain* 1982;105:755–786.
110. March RF, Sipe JC, Morse SS, Hason RP: Transmissible mink encephalopathy: Reduced spongiform degeneration in aged mink of the Chediak-Higashi genotype. *Lab Invest* 1976;34:381–386.
111. Tateishi J, Doi H, Sato Y, Suetsugu M, Ishii K, Kuroiwa Y: Experimental transmission of human subacute spongiform encephalopathy to small rodents. III. Further transmission from three patients and distribution patterns of lesions in mice. *Acta Neuropathol* (Berl) 1981;53:161–163.
112. Tateishi J, Nagara H, Hikita K, Sato Y: Amyloid plaques in the brains of mice with Cruetzfeldt-Jakob disease. *Ann Neurol* 1984;15:278–280.
113. Kitamoto T, Tateishi J, Tashima I, et al: Amyloid plaques in Creutzfeldt-Jakob disease stain with prion protein antibodies. *Ann Neurol* 1986;20:204–208.
114. Cho HJ: Inactivation of the scrapie agent by pronase. *Can J Comp Med* 1983;47:494–496.
115. Yagishita S. Creutzfeldt-Jakob disease with kuru-like plaques in Japan. *Acta Pathol Jpn* 1981;31:923–942.
116. Seitelberger F: Spinocerebellar ataxia with dementia and plaque-like deposits (Sträussler's disease), in Vinken, PJ, Bruyn, GW (eds). Handbook of Clinical Neurology. Amsterdam: North-Holland, 1981: pp. 182–183.
117. Vernon ML, Horta-Barbosa L, Fuccillo DA, Sever JL, Baringer JR, Birnbaum G: Virus-like particles and nucleoprotein-type filaments in brain tissue from two patients with Creutzfeldt-Jakob disease. *Lancet* 1970;1:964–966.
118. Merz PA, Somerville RA, Wisniewski HM, Manuelidis L, Manuelidis EE: Scrapie-associated fibrils in Creutzfeldt-Jakob disease. *Nature* 1983;306:474–476.
119. Merz PA, Rohwer RG, Kascsak R, et al: Infection-specific particle from the unconventional slow virus diseases. *Science* 1984;225:437–440.
120. Brown P, Coker-Vann M, Pomeroy K, et al: Diagnosis of Creutzfeldt-Jakob disease by Western blot identification of marker protein in human brain tissue. *N Eng J Med* 1986;314:547–551.
121. Baker HF, Ridley RM, Crow TJ: Experimental transmission of an autosomal dominant spongiform encephalopathy: Does the infectious agent originate in the human genome? *Br Med J* 1985;291:299–302.
122. Hsiao KK, Westaway DA, Prusiner SB: An amino acid substitution in the prion protein of ataxic Gerstmann-Stäussler syndrome. *Am J Hum Genet* 1988;43:A87.
123. Hsiao K, Baker HF, Crow TJ, et al: Linkage of a prion protein missense variant to Gerstmann-Stäussler syndrome. *Nature* 1989;338:342–345.
124. Barker D, Schafer M, White R: Restriction sites containing CpG show a higher frequency of polymorphism in human DNA. *Cell* 1984;36:131–138.
125. Bird AP: CpG-rich islands and the function of DNA methylation. *Nature* 1986;321:209–213.
126. Ridley RM, Baker HF, Crow TJ: Transmissible and non-transmissible neurodegenerative disease: similarities in age of onset and genetics in relation to aetiology. *Psychol Med* 1986;16:199–207.
127. Carlson GA, Kingsbury DT, Goodman PA, et al: Linkage of prion protein and scrapie incubation time genes. *Cell* 1986;46:503–511.
128. Westaway D, Goodman PA, Mirenda CA, McKinley MP, Carlson GA, Prusiner SB: Distinct prion proteins in short and long scrapie incubation period mice. *Cell* 1987;51:651–662.
129. Alpers MP. Epidemiology and ecology of kuru, in Prusiner, SB, Hadlow, WJ (eds.). Slow Transmissible Diseases of the Nervous System, vol 1. New York: Academic Press, 1979: pp. 67–90.
130. Gibbs GJ Jr, Amyx HL, Bacote A, Master CL, Gajdusek DC: Oral transmission of kuru, Creutzfeldt-Jakob disease and scrapie to nonhuman primates. *J Infect Dis* 1980;142:205–208.
131. Prusiner SB, Gajdusek DC, Alpers MP: Kuru with incubation periods exceeding two decades. *Ann Neurol* 1982;12:1–9.
132. Zigas V, Gajdusek DC, Kuru: clinical study of a new syndrome resembling paralysis agitans in natives of the Eastern Highlands of Australian New Guinea. *Med J Aust* 1957;2:745–754.
133. Gajdusek DC, Zigas V: Clinical, pathological and epidemiological study of an acute progressive degenerative disease of the central nervous system among natives of the eastern highlands of New Guinea. *Am J Med* 1959;26:442–469.
134. Gajdusek DC, Zigas V: Degenerative disease of the central nervous system in New Guinea—The

endemic occurrence of "kuru" in the native population. *N Engl J Med* 1957;257:974–978.
135. Simpson DA, Lander H, Robson HN: Observations on kuru. II. Clinical features. *Aust Ann Med* 1959; 8:8–15.
136. Alpers M: Kuru: a clinical study, in Mimeographed manuscript, reissued. Bethesda: USDHEW, NIH, NINCDS., 1964:1–38
137. Hornabrook RW: Kuru—a subacute cerebellar degeneration: the natural history and clinical features. *Brain* 1968;91:53–74.
138. Hornabrook RW: Kuru and clinical neurology, in Prusiner, SB, Hadlow, WJ (eds). Slow Transmissible Diseases of the Nervous System, vol 1. New York: Academic Press, 1979: pp. 37–66.
139. Zarranz JJ, Rivera-Pomar JM, Salisachs P: Kuru plaques in the brain of two cases with Creutzfeldt-Jakob disease. *J Neurol Sci* 1979;43:291–300.
140. Alpers M: Epidemiology and clinical aspects of kuru, in Prusiner, SB, McKinley, MP (eds). Prions—Novel Infectious Pathogens Causing Scrapie and Creutzfeldt-Jakob Disease. Orlando, FL,: Academic Press, 1987: pp. 451–465.
141. Goujard J, Entat M, Maillard F, Mugnier E, Rappaport R, Job JC: Human pituitary growth hormone (hGH) and Creutzfeldt-Jakob disease: Results of an epidemiological survey in France, 1986. *Int J Epidemiol* 1988;17:423–427.
142. Kovanen J, Haltia M: Descriptive epidemiology of Creutzfeldt-Jakob disease in Finland. *Acta Neurol Scand* 1988;77:474–480.
143. Hansen MF, Cavenee WK: Genetics of cancer predisposition. *Cancer Res* 1987;47:5518–5527.
144. Chen S-H, Habib G, Yang C-Y, et al: Apolipoprotein B-48 is the product of a messenger RNA with an organ-specific in-frame codon. *Science* 1987; 238:363–366.
145. Feagin JE, Abraham JM, Stuart K: Extensive editing of the cytochrome C oxidase III transcript in trypanosoma brucei. *Cell* 1988;53:413–422.
146. Powell LM, Wallis SC, Pease RJ, Edwards YH, Knott TJ, Scott J: A novel form of tissue-specific RNA processing produces apolipoprotein B-48 intestine. *Cell* 1987;50:831–840.
147. Shaw JM, Feagin JE, Stuart K, Simpson L: Editing of kinetoplastid mitochondrial mRNAs by uridine addition and deletion generates conserved amino acid sequences and AUG initiation codons. *Cell* 1988;53:401–411.
148. Pattison IH, Millson GC: Experimental transmission of scrapie of goats and sheep by the oral route. *J Comp Pathol* 1961;71:171–176.
149. Pattison IH, Hoare MN, Jebbett JN, Watson WA: Spread of scrapie to sheep and goats by oral dosing with foetal membranes from scrapie-affected sheep. *Vet Rec* 1972;90:465–468.
150. Parry HB: Scrapie: a transmissible and hereditary disease of sheep. *Heredity* 1962;17:75–105.
151. Parry HB. Scrapie Disease in Sheep. New York: Academic Press, 1983, 192 pp.
152. Hartsough GR, Burger D: Encephalopathy of mink. I. Epizootiologic and clinical observations. *J Infect Dis* 1965:115:387–392.
153. Hadlow WJ, Karstad L: Transmissible encephalopathy of mink in Ontario. *Can Vet J* 1968;9:193–196.
154. Hadlow WJ, Race RE: Cerebrocortical degeneration in goats inoculated with mink-passaged scrapie virus. *Vet Pathol* 1986;23:543–549.
155. Hadlow WJ, Race RE, Kennedy RC. Temporal distribution of transmissible mink encephalopathy virus in mink inoculated subcutaneously. *J Virol* 1987; 61:3235–3240.
156. Marsh RF, Kimberlin RH: Comparison of scrapie and transmissible mink encephalopathy in hamsters. II. Clinical signs, pathology and pathogenesis. *J Infect Dis* 1975;131:104–110.
157. Williams ES, Young S: Chronic wasting disease of captive mule deer: A spongiform encephalopathy. *J Wildl Dis* 1980;16:89–98.
158. Wells GAH, Scott AC, Johnson CT, et al: A novel progressive spongiform encaphalopathy in cattle. *Vet Rec* 1987;121:419–420.
159. Wilesmith JW, Wells GAH, Cranwell MP, Ryan JBM: Bovine spongiform encephalopathy: Epidemiological studies. *Vet Rec* 1988;123:638–644.
160. Fraser H, McConnell I, Wells GAH, Dawson M: Transmission of bovine spongiform encephalopathy to mice. *Vet Rec* 1988;123:472.

Part III
Spine and Peripheral Nerves

13
Spinal Epidural Abscess

Mark J. DiNubile

Epidural abscesses are uncommon but important causes of back pain.[1–3] Their clinical significance results from their crippling and even life-threatening potential. Fortunately, when these abscesses are suspected, diagnosed, and treated promptly, neurologic sequelae can often be prevented or reversed.[1,2,4–7]

The epidural space can be infected around the brain (cranial epidural abscess) or spinal cord (spinal epidural abscess). Intracranial infections involving the epidural and/or subdural spaces are usually secondary to otorhinologic disease, head trauma, or neurosurgery.[8–10] Spinal epidural abscesses most commonly develop either by direct extension from a contiguous infection, principally vertebral osteomyelitis, or as a metastatic focus seeded hematogenously from a distant, often trivial, infection.[1]

Spinal epidural abscesses may be caused by a variety of pyogenic bacteria, including *Staphylococcus aureus*, as well as *Mycobacterium tuberculosis*, fungi, and occasionally helminths.[2] The nontuberculous bacterial spinal epidural abscess will be the major concern of this chapter.

Functional Anatomy

The epidural space exists between the "visceral" layer of dura covering the spinal cord and the periosteum of the rigid vertebral column (see Figure 13.1). Because it is external to the dural covering of the cord, infection in the epidural space is considered "extradural." Subdural infection (empyema), which is very uncommon in the spinal (as opposed to cranial) subdural space, is often described as an "intradural" but "extra-arachnoid" process. Leptomeningitis implies inflammation in the subarachnoid space. Myelitis and intramedullary abscess involve the parenchyma of the spinal cord itself; intramedullary abscesses are extremely rare.

The dimensions of the spinal cord vary along its vertical axis. The size of the epidural space at any level is inversely related to the cord diameter at that point.[2] The epidural space is largest in the midthoracic region and below the second lumbar disc space where the spinal cord ends. At all levels above the second lumbar space, the epidural space is most prominent posterolateral to the cord. Epidural abscesses usually develop where the epidural space is widest, but typically extend vertically to involve multiple vertebral levels.[1–3] With the exception of cervical epidural infection, most abscesses form posterior to the spinal cord.[2]

Extensive venous anastomoses exist along the length of the spinal cord.[2,11] Vascular connections between the vertebral, epidural, and spinal veins and those draining other organs are potentially important in the pathogenesis of vertebral and epidural infections. In particular, the venous drainage from the pelvis comunicates through Batson's plexus with the lumbosacral vertebral and epidural vessels.[11] Reversal of blood flow toward the spine can follow markedly increased pressure within body cavities.[12]

Pathogenesis

The two most important routes by which microorganisms can reach the epidural space are hematogenous dissemination from a distant infection or direct extension from a contiguous site.[1,2] In many cases, the pathogenesis involves both of these mech-

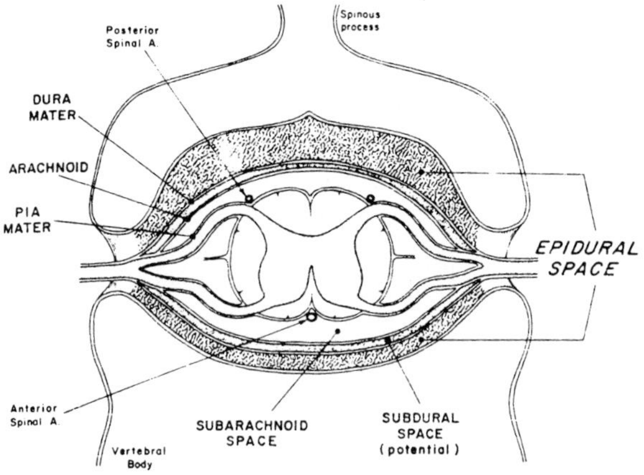

Fig. 13.1. Schematic diagram of the epidural space and surrounding structures. (Reprinted with permission of the *New England Journal of Medicine* from Baker AS, Ojemann RG, Swartz MN, Richardson EP Jr: Spinal epidural abscess. *N Engl J Med* 1975;293:463–468.)

anisms, when hematogenous infection of vertebrae leads to osteomyelitis, which subsequently spreads locally into the surrounding epidural space. With tuberculous infection, vertebral seeding occurs during the primary bacillemia; reactivation of this focus many years later may result in tuberculous osteomyelitis (Pott's disease) and epidural abscess.[13–17] Finally, direct inoculation of organisms into the paraspinal region as a complication of trauma, surgery, lumbar puncture, or epidural anesthesia represents a third but less common mechanism for the development of vertebral osteomyelitis and/or epidural abscess.[18,19]

Any infection or procedure associated with transient or sustained bacteremia may spread to the spine and/or epidural space. The most commonly identified primary foci of infection in patients with epidural abscesses include skin infection, dental abscess, pharyngitis, decubitus ulcer, urinary-tract infection, and endocarditis.[1,2,20–23]. Some of these infections may be trivial, hardly noticed by the patient, and spontaneously resolve before the development of back pain. Intravenous lines, as well as dental, urologic, gastrointestinal, and gynecologic procedures, can result in transient but clinically significant bacteremia.

Prior back trauma predisposes to metastatic seeding of the injured area during bacteremia.[2,24] Patients undergoing chronic hemodialysis and those who use intravenous drugs appear to be at higher risk for vertebral osteomyelitis and its complications than the general population.[25–27] Diabetic, alcoholic, and elderly patients may also be at increased risk.

Vascular anastomoses could allow pathogens causing pelvic and urinary-tract infections to access the lumbosacral spine and epidural space by retrograde flow through Batson's venous plexus.[11,12,23,26]

Direct extension of infection into the epidural space most frequently emanates from vertebral osteomyelitis. As noted earlier, the osteomyelitis itself may be a consequence of hematogenous infection. Other local processes, such as psoas, perinephric, and other retroperitoneal abscesses, occasionally invade the epidural space.[1,2] Wound infections after back surgery or trauma may progress to involve the spine and/or epidural space; alternatively, a superficial wound infection or small sinus tract may actually represent the necessitation of deeper vertebral or epidural infection to the surface.[28]

The mechanisms underlying the neurologic deficits associated with epidural abscesses have not been fully elucidated. Although direct compression of the spinal cord is undoubtedly a major contributing factor, the damage sometimes appears to develop too suddenly or is too extensive to be explained fully by mechanical considerations. Involvement of the vascular supply—with resultant thrombophlebitis, arteritis, or arterial thrombosis causing edema, hemorrhage, and ischemia—may often be the critical pathologic process; however, the relevant experimental data are conflicting and this area remains controversial.[29,30]

Symptoms and Signs

The complete evolution of symptoms in untreated patients with spinal epidural abscess has been classically divided into four stages: (1) spinal ache → (2) root pain → (3) weakness → (4) paralysis.[31] The potentially rapid evolution of this process from apparently innocent backache to neurologic catastrophe compels physicians to consider this entity in the differential diagnosis of all patients with back pain, especially when it is associated with fever and localized spinal tenderness.[1,2,31–35] Other characteristic presenting complaints include root pain (sometimes described as "electric" in character), weakness, and paresthesias.[1,2,31]

Less well recognized presentations of spinal epidural abscesses include meningismus (with cervical involvement), hip pain (with lumbosacral infection), the Brown-Sequard syndrome, and acute abdominal pain.[36–38] Particularly in children, the initial complaints may be misleading, often suggesting an intra-abdominal origin instead of the lower thoracic or lumbar epidural space.[36–41]

The clinical features of spinal epidural abscesses can be somewhat artificially divided into acute and chronic prototypes[1] (Table 13.1). Although these distinctions certainly are not absolute, such a classification provides a useful conceptual schema. The rapidity with which symptoms develop and the clinical course evolves is quite variable, but the actual complaints and physical findings are very similar regardless of the pace of the disease.

Table 13.1. Characteristic clinical presentations of acute and chronic spinal epidural abscesses.

	Acute	Chronic
Duration of symptoms	Less than 2 weeks	More than 2 weeks
Pathogenesis	Hematogenous, frequently from trivial skin infections	Direct extension from vertebral osteomyelitis
Fever	Usually high fever	May be low grade or absent
Systemic toxicity	Sometimes	Infrequently
Back pain ("spinal ache")	Always, typically severe and/or associated with radicular pain	Always, typically severe and/or associated with radicular pain
Localized spinal tenderness	Very common	Almost invariable
Root weakness	Very common	Very common
Peripheral leukocytosis	Usually present	Frequently absent
CSF leukocytes[a] (per mm^3)	Often over 80	Often under 40
CSF protein above 100 mg/dl	Almost invariable	Almost invariable
Etiologic organisms	*S aureus*	*S aureus, M tuberculosis*
Pathology	Frank pus	Granulation tissue, sometimes with pus
Anatomic location	Usually posterior to spinal cord	Occasionally anterior to spinal cord, especially when involving the cervical region
Vertical extent of abscess	Often more than three vertebral spaces	Usually more than three vertebral spaces

[a]Frank pus may be encountered if the abscess is inadvertently entered. Under these circumstances, the spinal needle should not be further advanced, and the aspirated specimen should be promptly submitted for appropriate studies.

Patients with localized back pain, especially when fever has been an associated problem, must be questioned about recent infections, especially of the skin, in the preceding weeks.[1] Minor infections should not be ignored. The presence of genitourinary or other pelvic infections may provide an important historical clue for patients with lumbosacral backache. In addition, epidural involvement should always be suspected when a patient with recent back surgery, epidural anesthesia, lumbar puncture, or vertebral osteomyelitis reports increasingly severe back pain.[19,24]

The physical examination helps to define the location and limits of the spinal tenderness, investigate the possibility of other important etiologies for the back pain (e.g., pancreatitis, aortic aneurysm, pyelonephritis, peptic-ulcer disease), search for residual signs of a possible primary infection, and evaluate neurologic function. Although sensory complaints commonly appear early in the development of epidural processes, objective sensory deficits are almost invariably preceded by significant motor weakness.[1] Obviously, a new or progressive neurologic finding lowers the threshold for investigating the possibility of an epidural collection aggressively.

Any patient with the acute onset or worsening of back pain, fever, and localized spinal tenderness must be evaluated for the possibility of epidural abscess. These patients should be accorded the same concern as patients with known malignancies who develop new back pain.[42] Not all the symptoms and signs classically attributed to an epidural abscess will be present in every patient. Young children and alcoholics are particularly likely to present with atypical syndromes.[35–40] In patients with a subacute or chronic course, the absence of such characteristic findings as fever and systemic complaints is commonplace.[1,2]

Disease processes that may closely resemble spinal epidural abscess include relatively common problems such as disc herniation and vertebral collapse, especially when impingement on the spinal cord or nerve roots ensues.[43] Neoplasms, including lymphoma and metastatic carcinoma, can exactly mimic chronic infection in the epidural space.[42,44] The differential diagnosis of spinal epidural abscess also encompasses intramedullary abscess or tumor, meningitis, hypertrophic spinal pachymeningitis, subdural empyema, epidural hematoma, transverse myelitis, and vertebral osteomyelitis and osteosclerosis.[1,2,26,45–49] This last entity has recently been described as a complication of endemic fluorosis.[48]

Laboratory and Radiologic Findings

Routine laboratory investigation is generally unhelpful in the evaluation of patients with suspected epidural abscesses. Although an elevated erythrocyte sedimentation rate is expected in the large majority of patients with vertebral osteomyelitis and/or epidural abscess, this finding is so nonspecific as to be rarely useful. Since nearly normal sedimentation rates have occasionally been described in many inflammatory conditions, including such infections as osteomyelitis, a normal sedimentation rate should not dissuade a physician from further investigating the possibility of epidural abscess if the clinical circumstances so dictate.[15,26] The sedimentation rate is frequently under 50 mm per hour in tuberculous vertebral osteomyelitis.[15] Leukocytosis is commonly seen in the patient with an acute presentation of epidural abscess associated with systemic complaints and high fever. However, a normal white blood cell count clearly does not exclude the diagnosis of spinal epidural abscess, especially in cases with an indolent course.[1,2] The presence of *S. aureus* bacteremia in a patient with new or increased back pain should always suggest vertebral osteomyelitis and/or epidural infection.

Conventional radiology of the spine may be unrevealing because osseous destruction can be absent or inapparent on routine radiographs. Although patients with chronic epidural abscesses are more likely to have unimpressive fever and systemic symptoms when compared with those with a more acute process, radiographs of the spine are more commonly abnormal in this group of patients. This observation simply reflects the usual pathogenesis of chronic epidural abscess as a consequence of spread from a contiguous focus of vertebral osteomyelitis; in addition, the "chronic" process (by definition) in these patients has usually allowed enough time for osseous changes to become visible on routine radiologic studies.[1] Destruction of the disc space with involvement of adjacent vertebral bodies without osteoporosis is characteristic of pyogenic osteomyelitis; preservation of the disc space with a large paraspinal mass, in a patient with a positive tuberculin skin test, suggests Pott's disease.[13,15,26,45,50] When calcium is present in tuberculous paraspinal abscesses, it is better visualized by computed tomographic (CT) scanning than either conventional radiography or magnetic-resonance imaging (MRI).[15,51–53]

Bone, gallium, and indium scans are frequently positive in areas of vertebral and epidural infection.[26] However, because of their lack of specificity, these scans seldom provide adequate data on which to base therapeutic decisions. Despite unremarkable or equivocal radionuclide studies, the diagnosis of epidural abscess should be further pursued in patients in whom the clinical suspicion of this entity is sufficiently high.

The gold standard for the diagnosis of epidural processes is myelography.[1,2,42] Although a myelogram may rarely be interpreted as normal in the presence of an epidural collection, this study is almost universally abnormal in patients with epidural abscesses at clinical presentation. A complete or partial obstruction is usually evident by myelography, whether done conventionally or with CT scanning. If a virtually complete obstruction is present, the delineation of the upper extent of the abscess will require injection of a contrast medium above the block. At the time of myelography, cerebrospinal fluid (CSF) should be obtained for measurement of protein and glucose concentrations, total and differential cell counts, cytologic examination (if malignancy is suspected), and appropriate stains and cultures. In most cases, a Gram stain and routine culture are adequate as microbiologic investigations. Under certain circumstances, stains and cultures for acid-fact organisms, fungi, and anaerobic bacteria may also be indicated.

The most significant risk of lumbar puncture in the setting of suspected epidural abscess is that the abscess cavity will be inadvertently pierced and bacteria inoculated into the subarachnoid space. If a lumbar epidural abscess is suspected, lumbar puncture must be deferred. A CT scan or MRI should be performed promptly.[53–55] If the possibility of lumbar space involvement is still not excluded and the noninvasive studies have not established the diagnosis, cisternal myelography should be undertaken. Even in the absence of suspicion that the lumbar epidural space is involved, the spinal needle should always be advanced slowly, with frequent aspirations, to detect the possibility that the abscess has extended further than expected.[3,35]

CT scans offer a less invasive, but not infallible, means of detecting epidural collections.[2,53,56] The administration of an intravenous contrast agent may help to define tissue boundaries more clearly, but infrequently yields new or critical information after a nonenhanced study. However, without the intrathecal injection of water-soluble contrast material, the results of CT scanning may frequently be misleading. MRI is the most reliable noninvasive study in patients with suspected epidural abscesses.[54,55,57] Unfortunately, this study may also be inconclusive. Neither CT scanning nor MRI is sufficiently sensitive to exclude the possibility of epidural infection in patients with suggestive clinical syndromes.

A totally normal CSF formula would be very unusual in a patient with epidural abscess.[1] Some authors have suggested lumbar puncture as the initial diagnostic procedure in cases where the clinical suspicion of epidural abscess is relatively low and lumbar involvement is not considered likely.[1] Any abnormalities in the CSF would indicate the need for more definitive evaluation. Occasionally in my experience, cerebrospinal fluid parameters have been only slightly elevated in patients with documented epidural abscesses.

Our recommended approach to most patients with suspected epidural abscesses is the immediate performance of MRI.[57] In the exceptional patient with a nondiagnostic MRI, myelography with high-resolution CT scanning is probably the best sequential study. Conventional myelography is usually an adequate alternative procedure. If the diagnosis is confirmed and surgical exploration undertaken, intraoperative spinal ultrasonography may be useful in locating the epidural abscess and monitoring successful decompression.[57]

Table 13.2. Reported pathogens causing epidural abscesses.

Bacteria
Staphylococcus aureus
Coagulase-negative staphylococci
Enteric gram-negative bacilli
Pseudomonas aeruginosa
Streptococcus pneumoniae
Streptococcus pyogenes
Viridans and other streptococci
Listeria monocytogenes
Salmonella species
Brucella suis
Actinomyces
Anaerobic bacteria
Mycobacteria
Fungi
Aspergillus species
Blastomyces dermatitides
Coccidioides immitis
Cryptococcus neoformans
Mucormycosis
Helminths
Echinococcus granulosus
Dracunculus medinensis (guinea worm)

Microbiology and Treatment

Optimal therapy for epidural abscess includes both appropriate antibiotics and emergent surgical intervention.[1] Antibiotics must initially be chosen empirically, but later adjusted on the basis of stains and eventually cultures. Organisms reported to cause epidural infections are listed in Table 13.2.[27,58]

The clinical circumstances dictate the empiric antibiotic selections. Coverage for *S aureus* is almost always mandatory.[1,2,59,60] A penicillinase-resistant penicillin (e.g., oxacillin or nafcillin) or a first-generation cephalosporin (e.g., cefazolin) will usually be adequate, except in populations at risk for infection with methicillin-resistant staphylococci. These groups may include patients who acquire their infection nosocomially or who inject recreational drugs. When a lumbar epidural abscess follows infection of the urinary tract, knowledge of the urine isolate or microscopic examination of Gram-stained urine can be a valuable aid in selecting antibiotics. Of course, the urinary-tract and epidural-space infections may be unrelated and simply coincidental, but Gram-negative bacilli become a much greater concern in this setting. Gram-negative infections may also complicate intravenous drug use; the exact bacterial species vary regionally across the United States.

Antibiotic therapy should be continued for at least 6–8 weeks in patients whose epidural abscesses complicate pyogenic vertebral osteomyelitis.[26] Shorter courses of therapy are probably adequate when bone infection does not coexist, although the optimal duration of treatment is unknown. As always, care must be tailored for the individual case.

In certain areas of the world, including developing countries, tuberculosis remains a major cause of vertebral osteomyelitis and chronic epidural abscess.[59] *M tuberculosis* has also been increasingly recognized as an important pathogen among patients who use intravenous drugs.[27,58] Short-course treatment regimens may be less effective for tuberculosis involving bones (especially advanced veretebral osteomyelitis) and joints than for infections at other sites.[61] Even when isoniazid and rifampin are used as part of combination chemotherapy, therapy should probably be continued for at least one year.

Most authorities advocate prompt surgery once the diagnosis of epidural abscess is confirmed.[1,2] The standard approach to posterior epidural collections consists of extensive bilateral laminectomy to expose the entire length of the abscess.[62] If pus is found (as opposed to granulation tissue), some surgeons pack the wound completely or partially open and perform delayed closure. More limited procedures have gained wider acceptance recently, especially in children where multilevel laminectomy increases the risk of kyphosis.[40] The adequacy of drainage can be monitored by intraoperative ultrasonography when the entire abscess cavity is not directly visualized.[57]

A small number of successful medical cures of epidural abscesses caused by nontuberculous bacteria have been reported, especially in patients without neurologic signs.[54,62,64] Nevertheless, at present, nonoperative therapy in these patients cannot be recommended.

Vertebral osteomyelitis and epidural abscess resulting from tuberculosis, in contrast to pyogenic infections, are often managed conservatively with chemotherapy and rest.[13,15,16,59,65] Demonstrable neurologic involvement increases the failure rate of purely medical management, as do extensive vertebral destruction and instability. However, even some patients with paraplegia have recovered completely without operative intervention. It is often unclear in these cases whether the neurologic deficits resulted from epidural infection or from other processes. In addition to decompression of epidural abscesses, surgery may be required to confirm the bacteriologic diagnosis, as well as for debridement of infected bone and establishment of spinal stability. In stable patients with minor to moderate neurologic disability, in whom the diagnosis of tuberculosis is certain, nonoperative therapy with careful observation is a reasonable first approach.[15,59] Failure to improve after 4–8 weeks of appropriate medical therapy or progressive neurologic impairment should indicate the need for surgery in patients being managed conservatively. This philosophy of treatment for tuberculous vertebral osteomyelitis has been termed "the middle regime" and clearly underscores individualization of care.[15,66] Radical resection and anterior spinal fusion (instead of a more limited debridement procedure) are often recommended for these patients on the basis of the Medical Research Council trials[15,66–73]

Prognosis

The outcome in patients with nontuberculous bacterial epidural abscess is directly related to the extent of neurologic impairment at the time of operative decompression.[1,2,6,7] The longer weakness is present, the less likely it is that the deficit will be reversible.[1,32,59] Some patients may suffer sudden deterioration, even when the clinical course has previously been indolent. This constant risk underscores the need for prompt surgical intervention in all cases of nontuberculous bacterial epidural abscess, regardless of the neurologic findings and the pace of the disease.

References

1. Baker AS, Ojemann RG, Swartz MN, Richardson EP Jr: Spinal epidural abscess. *N Engl J Med* 1975;293:463–468.
2. Verner EF, Musher DM: Spinal epidural abscess. *Med Clin North Am* 1985;69:375–384.
3. O'Sullivan R, McKenzie A, Hennessy O: Epidural and paraspinal inflammatory conditions. *Aust Radiol* 1988;32:203–206.
4. Russell NA, Vaughan R, Morley TP: Spinal epidural infection. *Can J Neurol Sci* 1979;6:325–28.
5. Danner RL, Hartman BJ: Update of spinal epidural abscess: 35 cases and review of the literature. *Rev Infect Dis* 1987;9:265–274.
6. Peterson JA, Paris P, Williams AC: Acute epidural abscess. *Am J Emerg Med* 1987;5:287–190.
7. Mooney RP, Hockberger RS: Spinal epidural abscess: a rapidly progressive disease. *Ann Emerg Med* 1987;16:1168–1170.
8. Silverberg AL, DiNubile MJ: Subdural empyema. *Med Clin North Am* 1985;69:361–374.
9. DiNubile MJ: Infections of the cranial dura and dural venous sinuses, in Harris AL (ed): *Handbook of Clinical Neurology. Microbial Disease,* vol. 8. Amsterdam, Elsevier, 1988, pp. 167–183.
10. Harris LF, Haws FP, Triplett JN Jr, Maccubbin DA: Subdural empyema and epidural abscess: recent experience in a community hospital. *South Med J* 1987;80:1254–1258.
11. Batson OV: The function of the vertebral veins and their role in the spread of metastases. *Ann Surg* 1940;112:138–146.

12. Wiley AM, Trneta J: The vascular anatomy of the spine and its relationship to pyogenic vertebral osteomyelitis. *J Bone Joint Surg* 1959;44:796–809.
13. Seward DNL: Some problems in diagnosis and management of spinal tuberculosis. *Med J Aus* 1976; 1:822–826.
14. Brashear HR Jr, Rendleman DA: Pott's paraplegia. *South Med J* 1978;71:1379–1382.
15. Gorse GJ, Pais MJ, Kusske JA, Cesario TC: Tuberculous spondylitis. *Medicine* 1983;62:178–193.
16. Shivaram U, Wollschlager C, Khan F, Khan A: Spinal tuberculosis revisited. *South Med J* 1985;76:681–684.
17. Lifeso RM, Weaver P, Harder EH: Tuberculous spondylitis in adults. *J Bone Joint Surg* 1985; 67:1405–1413.
18. Schumtzhard E, Aichner F, Dierck RA, et al: New perspectives in acute spinal epidural abscess. *Neurochirurgica* 1986;80:105–108.
19. Bergman I, Wald ER, Meyer JD, Painter MJ: Epidural abscess and vertebral osteomyelitis following serial lumbar punctures. *Pediatrics* 1983;72:476–80.
20. Elian D, Hassin D, Tomer A, et al: Spinal epidural abscess: an unusual complication of bacterial endocarditis. *Infection* 1984;12:258–259.
21. Clark R, Carlisle JT, Valainis GT: Endocarditis presenting as an epidural abscess. *Rev Infect Dis* 1989;11:338–340.
22. Koopmann CF, Miller RW, Coulthard SW: Retropharyngeal abscess associated with progressive quadriplegia, an epidural abscess, renal failure, and jaundice. *J Otolaryngol—Head Neck Surg* 1948; 92:114–118.
23. Henriques CQ: Osteomyelitis as a complication in urology. *Br J Surg* 1958;46:19–28.
24. Sullivan CR, Bickel WH, Siven HJ: Infections of the vertebral spaces after operations of intervertebral disks. *JAMA* 1958;166:1973–1977.
25. Leonard A, Comty CM, Shapiro FL, Raij L: Osteomyelitis in hemodialysis patients. *Ann Intern Med* 1973;78:651–658.
26. Sapico FL, Montgomerie JZ: Pyogenic vertebral osteomyelitis: report of nine cases and review of the literature. *Rev Infect Dis* 1979;1:754–776.
27. Koppel BS, Tuchman AJ, Mangiardi JR, et al: Epidural spinal infection in intravenous drug abusers. *Arch Neurol* 1988;45:1331–1337.
28. Jamison M, Stanworth P, Maclennan I: An unusual rectal fistula: extradural abscess discharge per rectum. *Br J Surg* 1984;71:651–652.
29. Feldenzer JA, McKeever PE, Schaberg DR, et al: Experimental spinal epidural abscess: a pathophysiological model in the rabbit. *J Neurosurg* 1987; 20:859–867.
30. Feldenzer JA, McKeever PE, Schaberg DR, et al: The pathogenesis of spinal epidural abscess: microangiographic studies in an experimental model. *J Neurosurg* 1988;69:110–114.
31. Heusner AP: Nontuberculous spinal epidural infections. *N Engl J Med* 1948;239:845–854.
32. Phillips GE, Jefferson A: Acute spinal epidural abscess: observations from fourteen cases. *Postgrad Med J* 1979;55:712–715.
33. Bouchez B, Arnott G, Delfosse JM: Acute spinal epidural abscess. *J Neurol* 1985;231:343–344.
34. Chappel R, Verhelst JA, Nagler JM, et al: Epidural abscess causing tetraparesis: a case report. *Paraplegia* 1986;24:364–369.
35. Schlossberg D: Spinal epidural abscess. *South Med J* 1977;70:669–673.
36. Marks WA, Bodensteiner JB: Anterior cervical epidural abscess with pneumococcus in an infant. *J Child Neurol* 1987;2:25–29.
37. Tyson GW, Strachan WE: Spinal epidural abscess presenting as acute abdomen in a child. *Br J Surg* 1979;66:3–7.
38. Sullivan CR, Symmonds RE: Disc infections and abdominal pain. *JAMA* 1964;188:655–658.
39. Baker CJ: Primary spinal epidural abscess. *Am J Dis Child* 1979;17:333–336.
40. Fischer EG, Greene CS Jr, Winston KR: Spinal epidural abscesses in children. *Neurosurgery* 1981; 9:257–260.
41. Smith HP, Hendrick EP: Subdural enpyema and epidural abscess in children. *J Neurosurg* 1983; 58:392–397.
42. Rodichok LD, Harper GR, Ruckdeschel JC, et al: Early diagnosis of spinal epidural metastases. *Am J Med* 1981;70:1181–1188.
43. Keon-Cohen BT: Epidural abscess simulating disc hernia. *J Bone Joint Surg* 1968;50:128–131.
44. Mullins GM: Malignant lymphoma of the spinal epidural space. *Ann Intern Med* 1971;74:416–419.
45. Musher DM, Thorsteinsson SB, Minuth JN, et al: Vertebral osteomyelitis, still a diagnostic pitfall. *Arch Intern Med* 1976;135:105–110.
46. Altrocchi PH: Acute spinal epidural abscess vs. acute transverse myelopathy. *Arch Neurol* 1963;9:17–20.
47. Roberts WA: Pyogenic vertebral osteomyelitis of a lumbar facet joint with associated epidural abscess: a case report with review of the literature. *Spine* 1988;13:948–952.
48. Fisher RL, Medcalf TW, Henderson MC: Endemic fluorosis with spinal cord compression: a case report and review. *Arch Intern Med* 1989;149:697–700.
49. Petty BG, Burrow CR, Robinson RA, Bulkley GB: *Haemophilus aphrophilus* meningitis followed by vertebral osteomyelitis and suppurative psoas abscess. *Am J Med* 1985;78:159–162.
50. Digby JM, Kersley JB: Pyogenic non-tuberculous spinal infection. *J Bone Joint Surg* 1979;61:47–55.
51. LaBerge JM, Brant-Zawadzki M: Evaluation of

Pott's disease with computed tomography. *Neuroradiology* 1984;26:429–434.

52. de Roos A, van Persijn van Meerten EL, Bloem JL, Bluemm RG: MRI of tuberculous spondylitis. *AJR* 1986;146:79–82
53. O'Sullivan R, McKenzie A, Hennessy O: Value of CT scanning in assessing location and extent of epidural and paraspinal inflammatory conditions. *Aust Radiol* 1988;32:203–206.
54. Erntell M, Holtas S, Norlin K, et al: Magnetic resonance imaging in the diagnosis of spinal epidural abscess. *Scand J Infect Dis* 1088;20:323–327.
55. Bertino RE, Porter BA, Stimac GK, Tepper SJ: Imaging spinal osteomyelitis and epidural abscess with short T1 inversion recovery (STIR). *AJNR* 1988; 9:563–564.
56. Kirzner H, Oh YK, Lee SH: Intraspinal air: a CT finding of epidural abscess. *AJR* 1988;151:1217–1218.
57. Post MJD, Quencer RM, Montalvo BM, et al: Spinal infection: evaluation with MR imaging and intraoperative US. *Radiology* 1988;169:765–771.
58. Kaufman DM, Kaplan JG, Littman N: Infectious agents in spinal epidural abscesses. *J Neurosurg* 1980;30:844–850.
59. Editors of the *Lancet:* Tuberculosis of the spine. *Lancet* 1974;ii:137–138.
60. Yang SY: Spinal epidural abscess. *NZ Med J* 1982;95:302–304.
61. Dutt AK, Moers D, Stead WW: Short-course chemotherapy for extrapulmonary tuberculosis: nine years' experience. *Ann Intern Med* 1986;104:7–12.
62. Wright RL: Infections of the spine and spinal cord, in Youmans JR (ed): *Neurological Surgery*. Philadelphia, WB Saunders, 1985; pp. 3449–3458.
63. Messer HD, Lenchner GS, Burst JCM, Resor S: Lumbar epidural abscess managed conservatively. *J Neurosurg* 1977;46:825–829.
64. Leyes D, Lesoin F, Viaud C, et al: Decreased morbidity from acute bacterial spinal epidural abscesses using computed tomography and nonsurgical treatment in selected patients. *Ann Neurol* 1985; 17:350–355.
65. Tuli, SM: Results of spinal tuberculosis by "middle-path" regime. *J Bone Joint Surg* 1975;57:13–23.
66. Medical Research Council Working Party on Tuberculosis of the Spine: First Report—A controlled trial of ambulant out-patient treatment and in-patient rest in bed in the management of tuberculosis of the spine in young Korean patients on standard chemotherapy. *J Bone Joint Surg* 1973;55:678–697.
67. Medical Research Council Working Party on Tuberculosis of the Spine: Second Report—A controlled trial of plaster-of-paris jackets in the management of ambulant out-patient treatment of tuberculosis of the spine in children on standard chemotherapy. *Tuberculosis* 1973;54:261–282.
68. Medical Research Council Working Party on Tuberculosis of the Spine: Third Report—A controlled trial of debridement and ambulatory treatment in the management of tuberculosis of the spine in patients on standard chemotherapy. *J Trop Med Hyg* 1974; 77:72–92.
69. Medical Research Council Working Party on Tuberculosis of the Spine: Fourth Report—A controlled trial of anterior spinal fusion and debridement in the surgical management of tuberculosis of the spine in patients on standard chemotherapy. *Br J Surg* 1974;61:853–866.
70. Medical Research Council Working Party on Tuberculosis of the Spine: Fifth Report—A five-year assessment of controlled trials of in-patient and out-patient treatment and of plaster-of-paris jackets of tuberculosis of the spine in children on standard chemotherapy. *J Bone Joint Surg* 1976;58:399–411.
71. Medical Research Council Working Party on Tuberculosis of the Spine: Sixth Report—Five-year assessments of controlled trials of ambulatory treatment, debridement and anterior spinal fusion in the management of tuberculosis of the spine. *J Bone Joint Surg* 1978;60:163–177.
72. Medical Research Council Working Party on Tuberculosis of the Spine: Seventh Report—A controlled trial of anterior spinal fusion and debridement in the surgical management of tuberculosis of the spine in patients on standard chemotherapy. *Tuberculosis* 1978;59:79–105.
73. Medical Research Council Working Party on Tuberculosis of the Spine: Eighth Report—A 10-year assessment of a controlled trial comparing debridement and anterior spinal fusion in the management of tuberculosis of the spine in patients on standard chemotherapy in Hong Kong. *J Bone Joint Surg* 1982;64:393–398.

14
Myelitis

DOUGLAS R. NORDLI, JACQUELINE A. BELLO, AND DARRYL C. DE VIVO

The term myelitis derives from the Greek roots *myelos* (medulla, marrow), referring to the spinal cord, and *itis*, connoting inflammation. It has been a controversial topic since its initial recognition, with noted authorities debating not only its classification, but also its existence. Leyden[1] classified spinal necrosis under the heading of myelitis and had a bitter dispute with Oppenheim. Oppenheim[2] was more progressive and was responsible for a revision of the classification of diseases of the spinal cord. He considered true myelitis a rare disease, and noted that from 1883 to 1890 he had seen only two cases at postmortem examination. Marie,[3] extending the argument, denied that primary myelitis existed. Subsequently, however, many more cases were described and several large series were assembled. Authors continued to disagree as to the association with acute spinal necrosis and the etiology of myelitis remained obscure. With the advent of modern virology, it became apparent that direct viral invasion of the spinal cord could result in a myelopathy, poliomyelitis being the foremost example. Other viral agents—namely, the echoviruses—were later incriminated, and in more recent times, both herpes simplex virus type 2 (HSV-2) and cytomegalovirus (CMV) have been demonstrated in spinal cord. Still, a large number of cases of myelitis are idiopathic, and now are commonly referred to as acute transverse myelitis.

This chapter will concentrate on acute viral myelitis and transverse myelitis. In the differential diagnosis, other conditions responsible for an acute myelopathy will be mentioned.

Acute Infectious Myelitis

Polio Syndrome

Poliovirus is a member of the picornaviruses, which include both the enteroviruses and rhinoviruses. The enteroviruses include polio-, coxsackie-, and echoviruses, and are so-named for their predilection for the human alimentary tract. Effective immunization has all but eradicated the epidemic disease caused by poliovirus. In the United States, it still occurs in small out breaks in nonimmunized groups and in patients with immunodeficiency who are exposed to attenuated vaccine virus. It is endemic in certain underdeveloped countries.

Polioviruses types 1, 2, and 3 produce acute poliomyelitis, but of the three serotypes, type 1 is responsible for most of the epidemic disease.[4] All of the three serotypes share some common antigens and RNA segments.[5] Surprisingly, only approximately 1–2% of infections have neurologic manifestations.[6] Thus, most patients are unaware of the infection, and even if infected, may dismiss it as a summer cold.

Poliovirus contains a single-stranded RNA genome, and is surrounded by 32 protein subunits with an icosohedral shape. Like most enteroviruses, it is small, about 28 nm in diameter. It is stable at low pH, can withstand temperatures of 60–70°C, and prefers humid environments.

Pathogenesis

Infection is initiated by the ingestion of virus, and it multiplies in the oropharynx and intestinal mucosa.

The virus then drains into deep cervical and mesenteric lymph nodes, and from there into the blood, resulting in a transient viremia.[7] The virus further replicates in various extraneural sites, and is continually reintroduced into the bloodstream, and thus establishes a persistent viremic state.[8] After this stage the virus may gain access to the central nervous system, (CNS), perhaps through direct invasion through capillary walls. Alternatively, it has been suggested that the virus may gain entry to the CNS via the neuromuscular junction, and subsequently ascend along the axon to the neuronal perikaryon.[9]

Clinical Presentation

The disease may have either a mono- or biphasic course. The biphasic course begins with an aseptic meningitis, which may begin to improve when the second phase, the myelitis, begins. This occurs in roughly one third of childhood cases. The myelitis usually presents with painful muscle spasms associated with the development of a flaccid paralysis. The tendon reflexes are lost in involved segments but sensation is unaffected.

The paralysis tends to be multifocal and asymmetric, and has a spotty involvement anywhere from the lower lumbosacral levels of the cord to the brainstem nuclei (bulbar polio). There is a preponderance of dominant limb involvement, with more paralysis occurring in exercising segments at the time of the exposure.[10] This may suggest a role for regional differences in blood flow in influencing the spread of the virus. Furthermore, cervical and lumbar involvement is more common than thoracic involvement.

If the bulbar region is involved, respiratory problems may ensue. Bladder incontinence may occur, as may other types of autonomic dysfunction, including alterations in sweating, gastrointestinal motility, vasomotor control, and temperature stability.[11]

The severity of the disease can vary from fulminating bulbar paralysis requiring intensive respiratory support to mild weakness of a single extremity. Peak involvement occurs within a few days to several weeks, and then recovery slowly takes place. The degree of recovery averages 50% for severely involved muscles and 90% for moderately paralyzed muscle groups. Most recovery occurs within three to six months, but further improvement may be seen within up to two years.[12]

Pathology

The pathology reveals gray, withered ventral-nerve roots in the affected segments of the spinal cord, with a reduction in the size of the anterior horns. This characteristic accounts for the term "polio"—which comes from the Greek *polios,* meaning gray. Microscopically, there is diffuse infiltration of the ventral horns and basilar portions of the dorsal horns with lymphocytes and hypertrophied microglial cells. In acute lesions, there are numerous polymorphonuclear leucocytes. As the process advances, there is a moderate degree of central chromatolysis and dissolution of Nissi substance in the neurons, and neuronophagia is evident. Cases of long duration reveal a striking loss of neurons in the ventral horns.

Most lesions are found in the anterior two thirds of the gray matter, and the distribution may be quite spotty, corresponding to the clinical findings. The lower sacral segments are usually spared. Brainstem involvement is generally most prominent in the medulla. Other CNS sites may be involved, and one may commonly find inflammatory changes in the precentral gyrus with Betz-cell neuronophagia. Furthermore, involvement of deep cerebellar nuclei, the reticular formation, and, rarely, thalamic neurons has been described.[13,14]

Differential Diagnosis

The diagnosis of an acute myelitis is based on the clinical findings described earlier, with examination showing loss of tendon reflexes in the involved muscles without sensory involvement (other than muscle tenderness and pain). The cerebrospinal-fluid (CSF) findings will include pleocytosis and an elevated protein concentration during the acute illness. Virus can be cultured from the CSF in a few instances, and it is present in stool and throat-washing specimens 80–90% of the time.

Acute viral myelitis must be differentiated from acute polyneuritis. Clinically, the spotty and asymmetric flaccid paralysis of a myelitis contrasts with the symmetric ascending paralysis of a neuritis. CSF protein concentrations are elevated in both conditions, but significant pleocytosis occurs more often in myelitis. In infants with poliomyelitis, however, the pleocytosis may be milder than in older children and adults.[15] Other causes of acute flaccid paralysis include spinal-cord compression (tumor, hematoma, spinal arteriovenous malformation, or epidural abscess), botulism, myasthenia, tick-induced paralysis, other causes of neuromuscular blockade, and severe acute myopathies.

Treatment

Immunization against the disease is the only effective medical intervention at the current time. Recently, the development of an enhanced inactivated vaccine (E-IPV) has raised the possibility of an alternative to the live-virus Sabin vaccine.[16] The risk of contracting polio from the latter vaccine is estimated at one case per 2.7 million oral doses. The inactivated vaccine, when properly prepared, should have a lower risk of producing polio, but it will not have the advantage of herd immunity.

Immunization with live virus is contraindicated in those patients with an immunodeficiency. In addition to the typical form of poliomyelitis, an atypical form presenting with a chronically progressive course has been reported in immunodeficient patients. The atypical form may have striking extrapyramidal features, distinguishing it from the more usual presentation of the disease.[17]

There is no specific treatment once the disease has become manifest. In cases of bulbar poliomyelitis, respiratory assistance and intensive care are mandated. Some relief may be given to the painful muscle spasms by massage and warm packs. Rehabilitation therapy may help an individual who is left with permanent muscle weakness.

Other Viruses Responsible for Myelitis

Echovirus (enteric cytopathogenic human orphan viruses) is another enterovirus and approximately 30 types are recognized. Lower-motor-neuron paralysis of the extremities, similar to that noted in cases of poliomyelitis, has been observed in patients infected by various echoviruses, specifically, types 2, 6, and 9.[18]

Additionally, a poliomyelitis-like illness has been associated with coxsackieviruses A7 and A10.[19] Bulbar paralytic disease has been produced by B3 and B5.[20] Transverse myelitis has been observed with coxsackievirus infection, and focal encephalitic and vasculopathic acute hemiplegia has been caused by coxsackievirus A9.

HTLV-1—Tropical Spastic Paraparesis

Tropical spastic paraparesis (TSP) is a disease that usually progresses more slowly than does acute myelitis. The disease begins over a few days in only 13% of cases, and in 4% there is progression to paraplegia and incontinence in less than 1 year.[21] A review of cases worldwide has shown a remarkably homogeneous clinical syndrome dominated by spastic paraparesis with signs of pyramidal tract involvement affecting the legs. Low back pain is a common early symptom. Cutaneous abdominal reflexes and other superficial reflexes are usually absent. There are brisk tendon reflexes, and paresthesias are a common complaint early in the disease. A minimal sensory deficit, mainly involving decreased vibratory sensation in the feet without loss of proprioception, is common. Evidence of peripheral neuropathy has been reported in 14–48% of cases of TSP, depending on the series. The neuropathologic lesion is a chronic inflammatory lesion involving white matter, with perivascular lymphocytic infiltrates, spinal leptomeningitis, small-vessel vasculitis, and astrocytosis. The lesions are mostly in the spinal cord, but also involve the brain stem, cerebrum, and cerebellum.[22]

A recent development has been the association of the human T-lymphotrophic virus type 1 (HTLV-1) and TSP.[23] HTLV-1 is a retrovirus that is considered to be the causative agent of adult T-cell leukemia and non-Hodgkins lymphoma. Osame and colleagues[24] have described more than 250 cases of TSP in associaton with positive HTLV-1 antibodies in serum and in CSF. Gessain and associates[25] in 1985 first noticed the presence of positive HTLV-1 antibodies in the serum and CSF of over 70% of TSP patients in Martinique. These same findings were later verified in other cases of TSP throughout the world. Later, type C viral particles were found, using electron microscopy, in the blood and CSF lymphocyte cultures of patients with TSP. HTLV-1 virus has been isolated from both blood and CSF lymphocytes of TSP patients from Colombia and Jamaica,[26] and intrathecal synthesis of specific IgG monoclonal antibodies to HTLV-1 has been demonstrated.[27]

Myelitis Attributable to Herpesvirus

Herpesvirus—including HSV, varicella-zoster virus (VZV), CMV, and Epstein-Barr virus—has been found in cases of myelitis.[28] There has been at least one autopsy case in the literature documenting direct invasion of the spinal cord by HSV-2 in the setting of the acquired immuno-deficiency syndrome (AIDS). In this report, a 25-year-old man with a history of intravenous-drug use developed an insidiously progressive segmental thoracic myelopathy. Autopsy examination showed an area of dark-gray softening in the ventral portion of the T-7 and T-8 segments. Immune stains demonstrated that most of the cells in this region stained heavily with the monoclonal antiserum to HSV-2 antigen.[29]

In another report, two patients with AIDS developed paraparesis, but these cases revealed CMV polyradiculopathy and a vacuolar myelopathy that occurred in association with brain lesions resembling the Marchiafava-Bignami syndrome.[30] Here, there was no evidence of direct invasion of the spinal cord by virus.

Myelitis Attributable to Lyme Disease

Lyme disease is an infectious disease caused by the spirochete *Borrelia burgdorferi* that may affect the brain, meninges, spinal cord, cranial nerves, and peripheral nerves. Initial attention was drawn to the entity in 1975 when cases appeared in southern Connecticut and the vector, ixodid ticks, was established. The condition usually begins in summer with a typical annular skin rash (erythema chronicum migrans) and is accompanied by systemic symptoms. The neurologic abnormalities occur weeks, or even months, later, followed by the onset of a mono- or oligoarticular arthritis. Neurologic involvement is seen in 11% of patients infected, with the most common manifestation being a lymphocytic meningitis. A characteristic triad of meningitis, cranial neuritis, and radiculoneuritis may occur.

A very similar syndrome is found in Europe, and this has been recognized since 1922 as the meningopolyneuritis of Garin-Bujadoux and Bannwarth.

Acute transverse myelitis (ATM) has been associated with Lyme disease, and probably accounts for approximately 5% of the cases presenting with neurologic findings.[31–33] In an illustrative case report by Rousseau and colleagues,[32] a 19-year-old woman had bilateral motor and sensory involvement of the cord soon after the pathognomonic rash, with positive serologic tests specific for *B burgdorferi*. The patient improved clinically after treatment with intravenous penicillin and the titers concurrently fell. However, this is rarely the prominent or sole neurologic manifestation of the disease, and myelitis more often is associated with meningoencephalitis, which tends to follow a progressive rather than an acute course.

Infection can be documented with appropriate serologic tests. Typically, the CSF shows a lymphocytic pleocytosis with oligoclonal bands and intrathecal antibodies to *B burgdorferi*. The diagnosis of *B burgdorferi* infection should be considered when there are associated cranial polyneuropathies, a painful radiculopathy, or a chronic lymphocytic meningitis.

Myelitis Secondary to Parasitic Infections

A variety of parasitic diseases can affect the spinal cord. Some of these conditions are extremely rare, such as spinal-cord involvement with gnathostoma spinigerum, a parasite common to Thailand, in which a few cases have presented with ascending myelitis. Somewhat more commonly, one may see involvement in cases of toxoplasmosis and cysticercosis.

Spinal cysticercosis constitutes about 5% of all cases of neurocysticercosis and is more frequently extramedullary than intramedullary.[34] The majority of cases are encountered in underdeveloped countries where poor sanitation combined with the ingestion of contaminated pork allows for human exposure. Ingested eggs liberate embryos upon contact with gastric juices that cross the gastric mucosa and migrate to various target organs, including the CNS. There, some limited development of the encysted embryo occurs before the organism dies. In the process, an inflammatory response develops in the surrounding host tissue, which may contribute to the neurologic signs and symptoms. (Figure 14.1) The suspicion is that extramedullary spinal cysticerci are probably the result of the migration of larvae from the brain or cervical region via the subarachnoid space, whereas intramedullary organisms are a result of hematogenous spread.[35] The CSF may show eosinophilia and, currently, antibody detection by Western blot analysis is being performed at the Centers for Disease Control.

Schistosomiasis may also affect the spinal cord and there are two patient groups seen. One group has histiologic proof of granulomas in or around the cord, and the other has unexplained cord or root lesions in the face of florid bilharzial infestation.[36] In the first group, there is usually a progressive asymmetric weakness of the legs with bladder-control and sensory involvement. The examination typically reveals patchy incomplete involvement of the conus and cauda equina. In the second group,

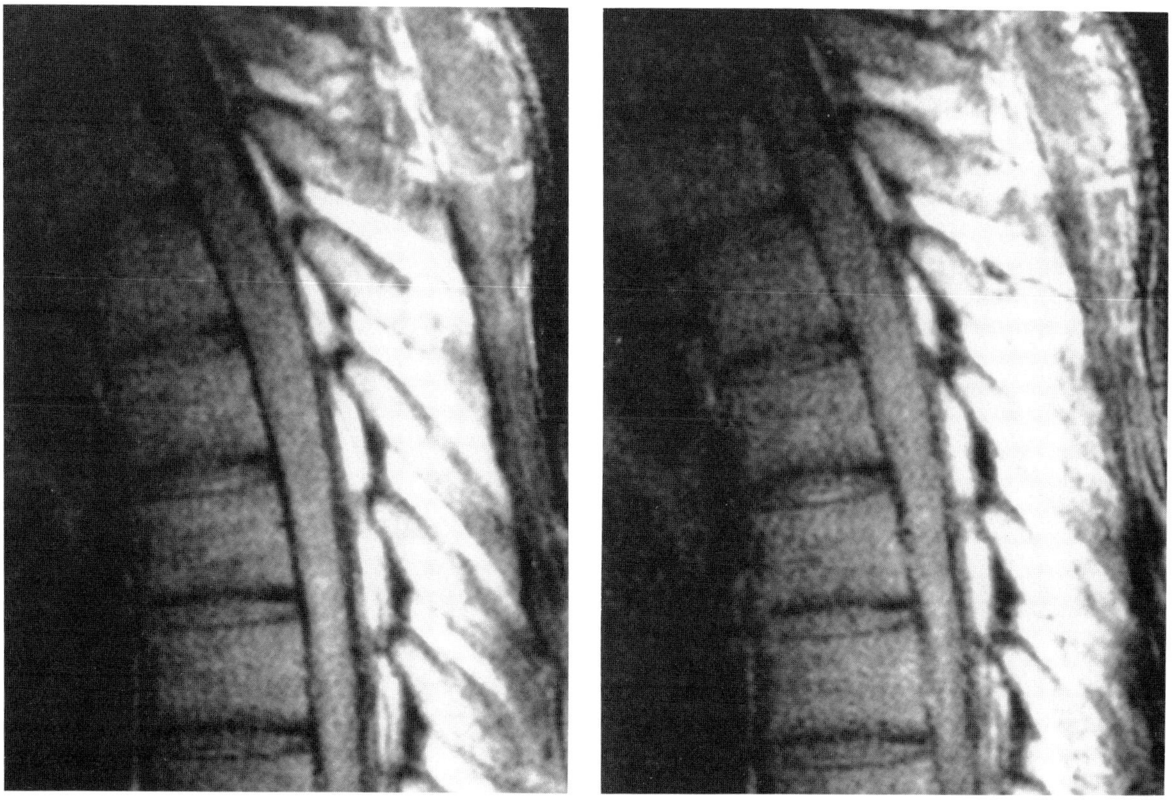

A B

Fig. 14.1. Sagittal T1-weighted MRI scans demonstrate midthoracic cord widening secondary to inflammation—surgically proved cysticercosis. (Courtesy of Drs. J.A. Bello and S.K. Hilal.)

there is a rapid progression of disease quite similar to that seen in transverse myelitis.

Most patients with schistosomiasis show peripheral eosinophilia. Serologic tests may be done, and either *Schistosoma mansoni* or *Schistosoma haematobium* may be found in the stool or in rectal biopsy material. The CSF usually contains a predominantly lymphocytic pleocytosis, generally less than 200 cells/mm^3. The protein is often elevated to 1 g/L or higher. The glucose is normal or minimally reduced. Nearly one half of cases with a subacute or chronic presentation show evidence of conus swelling or a nodular filling defect in the same region.

All reported cases have been exposed in Africa, Central or South America, or the Caribbean countries. The incubation period is anywhere from 2 months to 8 years. It is likely that the ova gain access to the cord via the vertebral venous plexus. The pathology shows granuloma formation, as well as necrosis in some cases. Endarteritis has been reported in association with necrotic features. Circulating immune complexes have been found and implicated in the pathogenesis.

Treatment should consist of a combination of corticosteroids to reduce inflammation and praziquantel, or alternatively oxamniquine, may be used for *S mansoni* infection. With treatment, about one third of patients recover completely, one third improve somewhat, and the final third show no improvement, or even have progression of disease.

HIV Myelopathy

Myelitis has been associated with AIDS and accounts for three of the 366 neurologically symptomatic patients in one series.[37] In cases that have been closely examined, it has been shown to be secondary to infection with other viral agents such as VZV, HSV-2, or CMV.[38] The most common spinal-cord manifestation of human immunodeficiency virus (HIV) infection is a chronic vacuolar myelopathy. This occurs predominantly in adult patients.

In the pediatric population, however, a vacuolar myelopathy is rarely seen, and instead two other patterns of pathology emerge. In some cases, the primary process appears to be a disruption of myelination in the corticospinal tracts. In others, there is apparent axonal degeneration with coincident myelin breakdown, suggesting Wallerian degeneration of the corticospinal-tract fibers. Cord pathology was seen in 14 of the 15 patients studied at autopsy, and it has been suggested that these processes may contribute to the bilateral corticospinal-tract signs that are commonly seen in the pediatric age group.[39] This process results in a chronically progressive course and not the acute presentation of myelitis.

Acute Transverse Myelitis

Transverse myelitis is a clinical syndrome characterized by the acute onset of segmental spinal-cord disease, with both motor and sensory abnormalities at and below the level of the lesion. Synonyms are acute myelomalacia and acute transverse myelopathy. The association with acute necrotic myelopathy is, however, controversial. Transverse myelitis is often associated with respiratory viral infections.

Historical Aspects and Etiology

Although transverse myelitis has been recognized for over a century, and despite several large case series cited in the literature (Paine and Byers,[40] Altrocchi,[41] Ropper and Poskanzer,[42] Berman and associates,[43] and Dunne, Hopkins, and Shield,[44] there is still much ambiguity concerning its etiology. Gowers, in 1884, recognized conditions in which there was "transverse damage to the cord," and knew of cases where the pathology revealed "myelitis" or softening of the cord. In the monograph "The Diagnosis of Disease of the Spinal Cord," the relationship between the onset of illness and its likely etiology is discussed. Diseases that presented with a sudden onset were considered to be of vascular etiology, whereas less acute or subacute presentations were thought to be more likely caused by an inflammatory process, such as myelitis. In a later series by Paine and Byers,[40] it was contended that the vast majority of cases of transverse myelitis were actually of vascular etiology. Miller and co-workers[45] noted the association with viral infection; however, Dunne and associates[44] found no evidence in their cases of direct viral invasion with an antecedant viral infection. Abramsky and Teitelbaum[46] postulated that cell-mediated autoimmune processes may be responsible for the pathology. Lipton and Teasdall[47] concluded that transverse myelitis represented a syndrome of varied etiology. Currently, transverse myelitis is recognized as associated with respiratory viral illnesses, typhoid, and specific viral syndromes, such as mumps, Epstein-Barr virus, and varicella. It has followed immunization with duck rabies vaccine and smallpox vaccine.

Clinical Presentation

Although there are several discrepancies in the series of articles cited above concerning the clinical features of transverse myelitis, some common elements are found. The first neurologic symptom of transverse myelitis is evenly distributed among muscle weakness (25%), sensory loss or paresthesiae (25%), back pain (25%), and root pain (21%). Only 3% of cases present with sphincter disturbance. This distribution roughly holds true for both adult and pediatric cases. Following the initial complaint, there is a rapidly progressive paraparesis, loss of sphincter tone, and loss of pain and temperature sensation below the level of the lesion. Complete anesthesia is, however, rare, and posterior column sensation is usually spared. At the level of the lesion, a zone of painful hyperesthesia often occurs. The motor abnormalities and sensory loss below that level are commensurate with the extent of spinal-cord damage. The exact clinical findings will depend on the location of the lesion, which most commonly is in the thoracic cord. The initial paralysis is of the flaccid type ("spinal shock"), followed over the next days and weeks by progressive spasticity below the level of cord disease. Loss of reflexes may persist at the level of the lesion if the anterior horn cells or root-exit zones are injured.

Pathology and Pathogenesis

On gross examination, cord softening and mild edema may be seen over several segments. Acutely, there will be a predominantly perivascular inflammatory reaction. Later, demyelination with or without necrosis, cavitation, and secondary gliosis will occur. In many cases studied, the differentiation between ischemic cord disease and virus-associated transverse myelitis has been difficult.

Differential Diagnosis

Abscess, hematoma, idiopathic necrosis, radiation myelitis, trauma, herniated intervertebral disks, epidural masses, vascular occlusion attributable to ischemia, syringomyelia, intraspinal cyst, and neoplasm should all be considered in the differential. Transverse myelitis usually does not have multifocal involvement, in contrast to a syrinx. Its onset is acute, which helps distinguish it from tumors and congenital malformations. In the past, contrast myelography was usually indicated to exclude the possibility of a surgically treatable mass lesion. During the acute disease, swelling of the cord may be seen in transverse myelitis in approximately 20% of cases, and, therefore, the differential may be difficult on plain myelography. Currently, however, magnetic-resonance imagery (MRI) may obviate the need for this more invasive procedure.[48] In cases of diffuse fusiform widening of the cord, the area will be isointense on the T2-weighted image in ATM (Figure 14.2), whereas there will often be a higher signal intensity in an intramedullary neoplasm or hematoma. The results of CSF examination may be normal or show mild inflammatory changes, and thus may not be helpful. A lumbar puncture can cause further damage if there is a mass lesion causing spinal-cord compression; therefore, lumbar puncture should be carried out only after neurologic or neurosurgical consultation.

Idiopathic ATM has been attributed to recent viral infection, mutiple sclerosis (MS), and vascular disease. The association with acute viral infections and following vaccinations is well documented. Preceding viral infections occurred in 44% of Paine and Byers'[40] series, and in 21% of Altrocchi's[41] patients. In the study by Lipton and colleagues,[47] a total of 12/34 patients had preceding viral illnesses. Notable also in this study is that in two of the three patients where an autopsy was performed, spinal-cord infarctions were seen, and the authors concluded that vascular disease may be a more frequent cause of ATM than is indicated in the literature. There has been quite a bit of controversy as to the association of acute necrotic myelopathy with ATM. Some believe that this may be an extreme example of inflammation or vascular occlusion; others argue that it is a separate entity.[(49–53)]

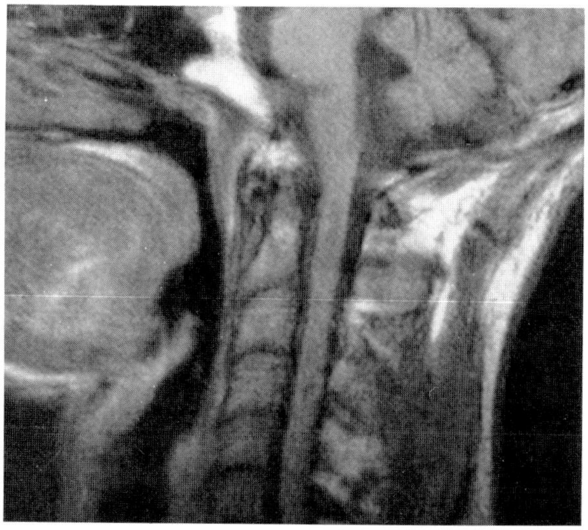

A

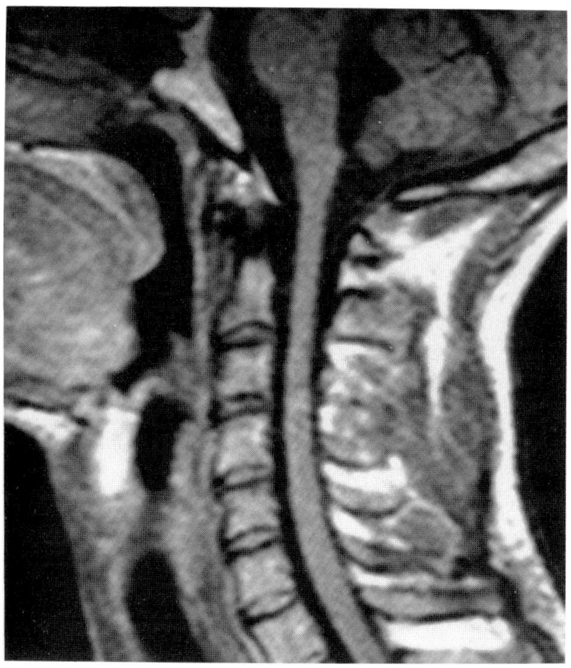

B

Fig. 14.2. (A) Sagittal T1-weighted MRI scan demonstrates diffuse cord swelling without focal lesion—myelitis. (B) Sagittal T1-weighted MRI one week later demonstrates interval decrease in cord size relative to surrounding CSF space (normal widening at C5–C7 persists). (Courtesy of Drs. J.A. Bello and S.K. Hilal.)

Prognosis

Prior to the widespread use of improved respiratory care and antibiotics, nearly all patients with ATM would succumb to its complications. Subsequent studies have shown a more favorable outcome. Lipton and associates[47] reviewed 34 cases (adults) with ATM of unknown cause. Follow-up at 5 to 42 years was done in 29 patients. Only one patient in the series went on to develop MS. Two thirds of the patients recovered and became ambulatory, whereas one third remained paraplegic. Those who retained tendon reflexes and posterior column function had a more favorable outcome. This study agrees with those of Altrocchi[41] and Paine and Byers,[40] both of which demonstrated that patients were almost equally distributed among three groups of recovery: good, fair, and poor. Patients with good recovery had normal gait, normal micturition, and no or minimal neurologic signs. Those with a fair recovery had spastic gait, urgency with occasional incontinence, and minimal neurologic signs. Those with poor outcome were bedridden and incontinent, and had marked neurologic signs.

Treatment

There is no specific treatment for ATM. Supportive measures are most important, and antibiotics, attention to urinary incontinence, and modern respiratory interventions have contributed to the improved survival in modern times. Steroids have been advocated by some authors, but no case-control study exists to prove their efficacy.

Other Causes of Myelitis

Demyelinating Disease

Transverse myelitis and demyelinating diseases are often considered together in discussions of myelopathy syndromes, although it is clear that only a small percentage of cases of transverse myelitis evolve to MS. Nevertheless, MS must always be considered in the differential diagnosis of acute paraparesis.

The precise etiology of the demyelinating process is obscure. There is, however, extensive epidemiologic, pathologic, and experimental data to support the hypothesis that a chronic virus infection acquired during childhood causes clinical symptoms several decades later, secondary to an immune-mediated reaction.[54,55]

The clinical symptoms vary according to the distribution of the lesions. Frequently, there are disturbances in vision, oculomotor function, coordination, and sensation. Transverse myelitis, optic neuritis, or both (Devic's disease) may be the initial presentation.

The diagnosis of MS is based on the presence of neurologic abnormalities that relate to more than one anatomic area of the nervous system and that tend to remit and recur. The spinal fluid may show mild pleocytosis or a slight elevation in total protein during acute exacerbations. CSF immunoglobulins are increased in approximately 75% of proved disease, but neither the presence nor absence of elevated IgG or oligoclonal bands is absolutely diagnostic.

The pathologic examination in the acute stage of MS reveals multiple areas, primarily subcortical in location, in which there are loss of myelin, relative preservation of axons, and perivascular inflammatory cells with edema. Later, a secondary gliosis ensues, resulting in firm, yellowish plaquelike areas—thus the term "sclerosis."

There are some data to support the use of short-term, high-dosage corticosteroid therapy during acute episodes of MS (prednisone at 2 mg/kg/day or adrenocorticotropic hormone at 2–4 units/kg/day). Because chronic problems such as urinary incontinence and spasticity arise, other drugs, such as antispasmodics, may be useful. The prognosis is variable, often with a slowly worsening course over several decades.

Radiation Myelitis

Radiation myelopathy is one of the most severe and devastating of the complications found after radiation therapy. Four general categories have been described.[56] The most acute is the complete paraplegia or quadriplegia that progresses over the course of hours or days. This presents in a fashion similar to that of transverse myelitis and the speculation is that it is related to vascular injury. A second, but rarely seen, complication is of lower-motor-neuron disease presumed to be secondary to anterior-horn-cell damage.

A third complication, believed to be the most common, is the acute transient radiation myelopathy, which becomes manifest usually several months after radiation is finished. Here, in addition to Lhermitte's sign (an electrical sensation elicited by sudden neck flexion), other subjective sensory complaints are found. The neurologic examination is typically normal. This condition is usually observed after cervical irradiation.

The fourth complication is of a chronic progressive myelopathy, which generally begins with a latency of nine to fifteen months after completion of radiation therapy. The first symptoms are paresthesias and diminution of sensations of pain and temperature, which are followed by a steady progression over the ensuing six months to involve all portions of the cord segment included in the field of radiation therapy. The differential diagnosis must include primary-cord lesions or metastases, and radiologic evaluation is imperative. The pathology reveals early spongy demyelination and, later, plasma-cell infiltration and vascular changes. There may be two pathogenetic mechanisms involved—white-matter necrosis at higher doses and vascular damage at lower doses of radiation.

Based on many careful retrospective studies analyzing the radiation data, it has been attempted to arrive at a safe dose for cord radiation. In general, a dose of 5,000 cGy in 25 fractions is considered the upper limit of "safe" exposure. The chance of developing a myelopathy increases with the overall dose, the size of the field, and the fraction size to attain a certain dose. It varies inversely with the total treatment time and the patient's age. That is, children and patients treated over a shorter period are at higher risk for complications. The signs and symptoms are generally irreversible.

There is no specific treatment. Steroids and hyperbaric oxygen treatment have been attempted, and some temporary remissions have been reported with each.

Nutritional and Vitamin-Related Causes of Myelopathy

A syndrome of tropical ataxic neuropathy applies to a myeloneuropathy that affects a large number of people in the tropics, manifested by "burning feet," severe posterior-column dysfunction, and less pronounced pain and temperature perception. Sensory loss is disproportionately greater than the motor defect. This entity has been reviewed in detail,[57] and the multifactorial etiology of most cases has been found to be obscure. Malnutrition, with a deficiency of vitamin B^{12} and folates as a result of postinfectious tropical malabsorption, may contribute. Other neurotoxic, agents such as lathyrus and cyanogenic plants (e.g., cassava), may be responsible for certain outbreaks.

Collagen Vascular Diseases

Transverse myelitis has been reported in various collagen vascular diseases, including mixed connective-tissue disease and systemic lupus erythematosus (SLE).[58,59] At least 36 cases of transverse myelitis have been reported in SLE. The characteristic findings are paraplegia, sensory loss, and bowel/bladder involvement. The CSF characteristically shows an elevation of protein with a concomitant depression of glucose. This pattern is not typically seen in other forms of transverse myelitis. Lupus erythematosus cells were seen in 88% of patients, and a positive Antinuclear antibody (ANA) was almost universal.

The pathogenesis has been ascribed to complement-mediated immune injury. In most of the studied cases at autopsy, ischemic necrosis was found to be the cause of myelopathy, with associated vasculitis, microhemorrhages, myelomalacia, or fresh infarction seen in ten of 11 cases.[60] A notable exception is a case discussed in detail by Johnson and Richardson[61] of a 43-year-old woman afflicted by SLE who presented with a progressive myelopathy. At autopsy, a "remarkable subacute degeneration of the white matter" was seen from the cervical to sacral segments with no occlusion of the blood vessels seen. The authors were uncertain as to the exact pathogenesis of this process.

Sporadic reports of improvement with corticosteroid treatment have been found.

Clinical Approach to the Patient with Acute Myelopathy

In the preceding sections, we have attempted to summarize the major conditions responsible for acute myelopathy. Since there are many conditions that can resemble ATM, the clinical approach to such patients must be comprehensive. (This point is illustrated in the short clinical summary accompanying Figure 14.3). Nevertheless, careful attention to certain clinical clues, the tempo of the illness, and the various associated factors involved may help to eliminate many of the diseases from consideration.

The tempo of the illness may be quite helpful.

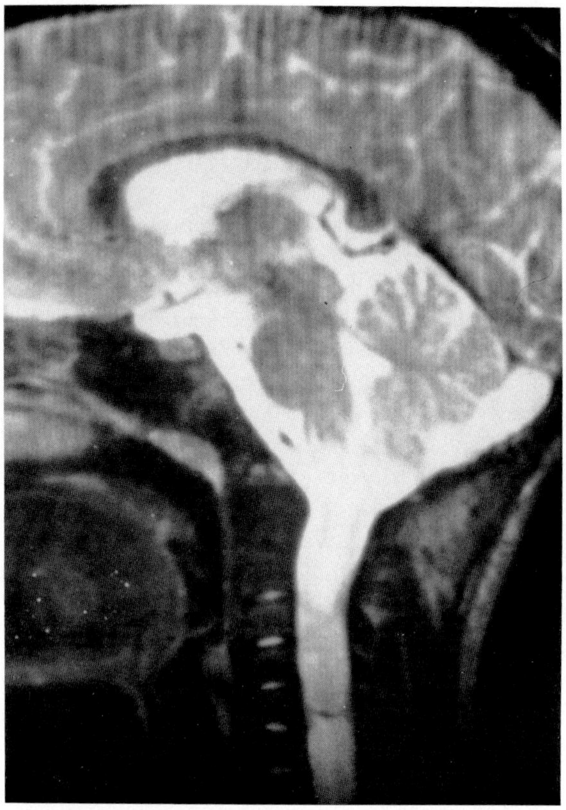

A

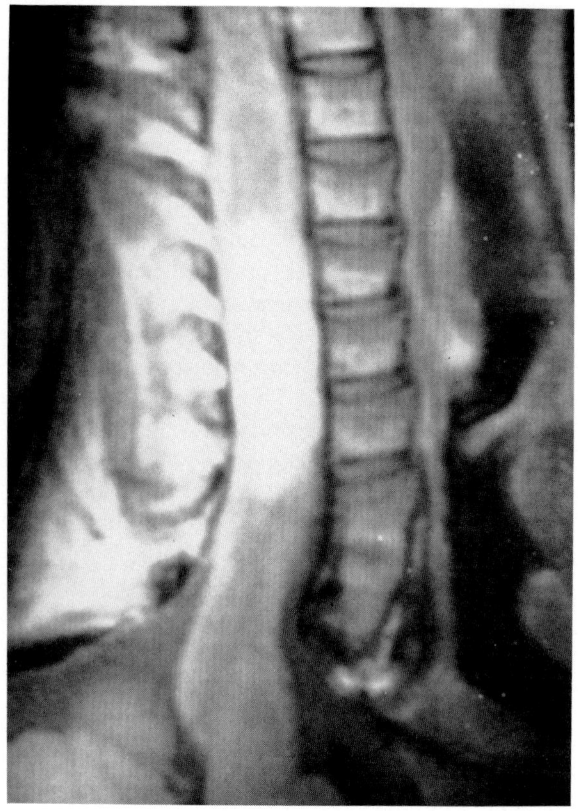

C

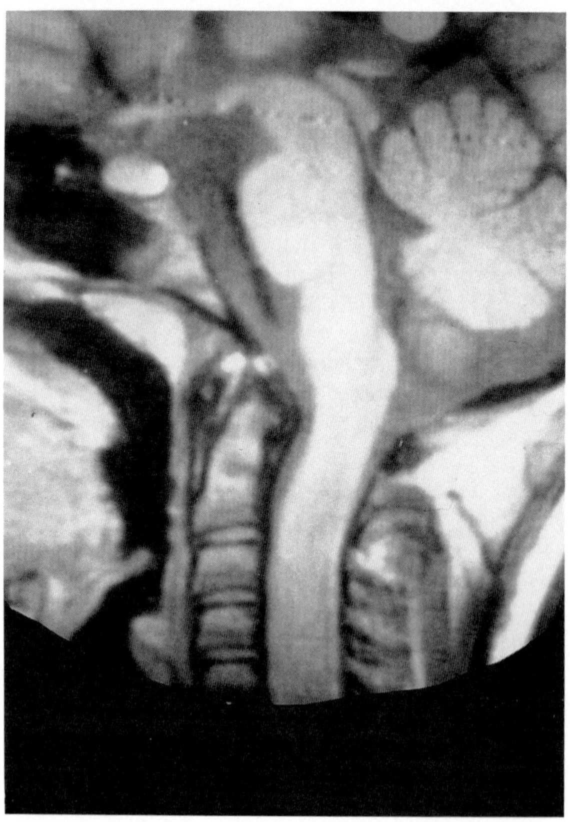

B

Fig. 14.3. MRI films of a 12-year-old girl who presented two weeks after varicella infection with bilateral shoulder pain and arm weakness. Over the following days, she lost the biceps tendon reflexes and had progression of weakness in her arms. The initial sagittal T2-weighted MRI scan (A) demonstrates intramedullary increased signal at the myelomedullary junction extending inferiorly to C2–3. (This represents edema cephalad to the core lesion demonstrated in A and B.) Subsequently, the process evolved, and over the course of the following two weeks, she became progressively weaker in the legs. (This pattern of descending weakness is quite rare in transverse myelitis.) A repeat MRI was obtained and the sagittal T1-weighted image prior to contrast administration (B) demonstrates diffuse cord widening from C1 to C5. The sagittal T1-weighted MRI scan after contrast injection (intravenous gadolinium [diethylenetriamine pentoacidic acid]) (C) separates an enhancing intramedullary lesion extending from C2–3 to C5–6 from the cord edema. Surgery was performed, the lesion was found to be a primitive neuroectodermal tumor, and radiation therapy was begun. Courtesy of Drs. J.A. Bello and S.K. Hilal.)

Table 14.1. CSF values in various forms of myelitis.

	White blood cells	Protein	Glucose	Other
Poliomyelitis	Mild–moderate increase	Normal–mild increase	Normal	Grow virus
Other enteroviruses	Moderate increase	Normal–mild increase	Normal	Viral titer positive
TSP	Normal–mild increase	Mild increase	Normal	+HTLV-1, IgG
Transverse myelitis	Normal–mild increase	Mild–moderate increase	Normal	
Lyme disease	Mild–moderate increase	Moderate increase	—	+Ab *B burgdorferi* +OCB
Parasitic (schisto)	Moderate increase	Moderate increase	Normal or mild decrease	
Demyelinating	Normal–mild increase	Mild increase	Normal	+OCB increased IgG
Collagen vascular disease (SLE)	—	Increase	Decrease	
HIV	Mild increase	Mild–moderate increase	Normal or mild decrease	

Generally, myelitis secondary to viral infection, ATM, demyelinating processes involving the cord, certain forms of radiation myelitis, and trauma to the cord itself will all have either acute or subacute presentations. In contrast, myelopathy secondary to HTLV-1, parasitic disease, and HIV-associated or nutritional and vitamin-related disease will have a more chronic presentation.

Various conditions may be helpful in pointing one in the correct direction. Particular attention should be paid eliciting any history of malignancy, prodromal illness, recent travel, exposure to parasitic diseases, history of tick bites, known risk factors for acquiring HIV, or prior radiation therapy.

The examination is of use to confirm the diagnosis of an acute myelopathy, as well as to suggest its etiology. The function of the posterior columns, in particular, may be informative. These tend to be spared in many cases of transverse myelitis, as well as in cases of vascular occlusion of the anterior spinal arteries. Complete loss of cord function would suggest another process. As mentioned previously, a multifocal, asymmetric, and patchy involvement is more typically seen in viral myelitis.

The localization of the lesion as determined from the history and examination can direct the radiographic studies in a more efficient manner. In most cases, some type of imaging study will be imperative to exclude the possibility of an intrinsic or extrinsic mass. Currently, MRI appears to be supplanting myelography. After the radiographic procedure, CSF analysis is often done. A comparison of the CSF values in various forms of myelitis, however, reveals that routine tests often may not provide a definitive answer (see Table 14.1). Other, more specific tests of the CSF can be more informative, including viral titers, various antibody titers, and oligoclonal bands. Serum tests for HIV, screens for malignancy, specimens for parasite analysis, a collagen-vascular-disease workup, and vitamin levels, including B^{12}, E, and folate may be useful when clinically indicated.

The particular treatment and outcome will vary according to each condition. In general, the outcome for cases of ATM and viral myelitis is favorable, and relates to the severity at the time of presentation. In the case of transverse myelitis, those with good function and preservation of tendon reflexes and posterior-column sensation do well, with fair to good return of function as the rule.

In those cases where treatment is thought to be effective, as in Lyme disease, early treatment is clearly important. For many cases, however, medical treatment may not be clearly efficacious; in these settings, the mainstay of care will be supportive measures and rehabilitation therapy. In most instances, rehabilitation therapy is crucial to prevent contractures, to preserve the mobility of joints, and to enhance recovery.

References

1. Leyden E: Beitrage zur acuten und chronischen myelitis. *Ztschr Klin Med* 1879; 1:1–26. Ueber acute

myelitis. *Deutsche med Wchnschr* 1892;18:621–623,648–653.
2. Oppenheim H. Zum capitel der myelitis. *Berl Klin Wehnschr* 1891;28:761–765.
3. Marie P, quoted by Rhein JHW: A pathological study of acute myelitis. *Univ. Med Bull* 1905;17:373–381.
4. Auld PAM, Kevy SV, Eley RC: Poliomyelitis in children. *N Engl J Med* 1960;263:1093–1100.
5. Young NA: Size of gene sequences shared by polioviruses types 1, 2 and 3. *Virology* 1973;56:400–403.
6. Horstmann DM: The epidemiology of poliomyelitis and allied diseases—1963. *Yale J Biol Med* 1963; 36:5–26.
7. Bodian D: Some physiologic aspects of poliovirus infections, in *The Harvey Lectures*. New York, Academic Press, 1956; pp. 23–56.
8. Nathanson N, Bodian D: Experimental poliomyelitis following intramuscular virus injection. III. The effect of passive antibody on paralysis and viremia. *Bull Johns Hopkins Hosp* 1962; 111:198–220.
9. Price RW, Plum F: Poliomyelitis, in Vinken PJ, Bruyn GW (eds): *Handbook of Clinical Neurology*. Amsterdam, Elsevier North-Holland Biomedical Press, 1978, pp 93–132.
10. Hortsmann DM: Acute poliomyelitis: relation of physical activity at the time of onset to the course of the disease. *JAMA* 1950;142:236–241.
11. Baker AB, Matzke HA, Brown JR: Poliomyelitis. III. Bulbar poliomyelitis: study of medullary function. *Arch Neurol Psychiatry* 1950;63:257.
12. Green WT: The management of poliomyelitis: the convalescent stage, in *Poliomyelitis,* papers and discussions presented at the First International Poliomyelitis Conference. Philadelphia, Lippincott, 1949, pp 165–185.
13. Blackwood W, Corsellis JAN: *Greenfield's Neuropathology*. Edinburgh, Year Book Medical Publishers, 1976, pp 306–308.
14. Bodian D: Poliomyelitis, in Minckler J (ed): *Pathology of the Nervous System,* vol 3. New York, McGraw-Hill, 1972, pp 2323–2394.
15. Abramson H, Greenberg M: Acute poliomyelitis in infants under one year of age: epidemiological and clinical features. *Pediatrics* 1955;16:478–488.
16. Roberts L: Change in polio strategy? *Science* 1988; 240(4856):1145.
17. Davis LE et al: Chronic progressive poliomyelitis secondary to vaccination of an immunodeficient child. *N Engl J Med* 1977;297:241.
18. Foley JF, Chin TDY, Gravelle CR: Paralytic disease due to infection with Echo virus type 9. *N Engl J Med* 1959;260:924–926.
19. Grist NR: Type A7 coxsackie (type 4 poliomyelitis) virus infection in Scotland. *J Hyg* 1962;60:323–332.
20. Jarcho LW, Fred HL, Castle CH: Encephalitis and poliomyelitis in the adult due to coxsackie virus group B, type 5. *N Engl J Med* 1963;268:235–238.
21. Roman GC, Roman LN: Tropical spastic paraparesis: a clinical study of 50 patients from Tumaco (Colombia) and review of the worldwide features of the syndrome. *J Neurol Sci* 1988;87:121–138.
22. Robertson WB, Cruickshank EK: Jamaican (tropical) myeloneuropathy, in Minckler J (ed): *Pathology of the Nervous System,* vol 3. New York, McGraw-Hill, 1972, pp 2466–2476.
23. Roman GC: The neuroepidemiology of tropical spastic paraparesis. *Ann Neurol* 1988;23(S):S113–S130.
24. Osame M, Matsumoto M, Usuku K, et al: Chronic progressive myelopathy associated with elevated antibodies to human T-lymphotropic virus type I and adult T-cell leukemialike cells. *Ann Neurol* 1987; 21:117–122.
25. Gessain A, Barin F, Vernant JC, et al: Antibodies to human T-lymphocytic virus type-I in patients with tropical spastic paraparesis. *Lancet* 1985;2:407–140.
26. Rodgers-Johnson P, St. C Morgan O, Mora C et al: The role of HTLV-1 in tropical spastic paraparesis. *Ann Neurol* 1988;23(S):S121–S126.
27. Vernant J-C, Maurs L, Gout O, et al: HTLV-I associated tropical spastic paraparesis in Martinique: a reappraisal. *Ann Neurol* 1988;23(S):S133–135.
28. Johnson RT: *Viral Infections of the Nervous System*. New York, Raven Press, 1982.
29. Britton CB, Mesa-Tejada R, Fenoglio CM, et al: A new complication of AIDS: thoracic myelitis caused by herpes simplex virus. *Neurology* 1985;35:1071–1074.
30. Singh BM, Levine S, Yarrish RL, et al: Spinal cord syndromes in the acquired immune deficiency syndrome. *Acta Neurol Scan* 1986;73:590–598.
31. Reik L, Burgdorfer W, Donaldson JO: Neurological abnormalities in Lyme disease without erythema chronicum migrans. *Am J Med* 1986;81(1):73–78.
32. Rousseau JJ, Lust C, Zangerle PF, Bigaignow G: Acute transverse myelitis presenting neurological feature of Lyme disease. *Lancet* 1986;2(8517):1222–1223.
33. Bateman LDE, Lawton NF, White JE, et al: The neurological complications of *Borrelia burgdorferi* in the New Forest area of Hampshire. *J Neur Neurosurg Psychiatry* 1988;51:699–703.
34. Trelles JO, Trelles L: Cysticercosis of the nervous system, in Vinkin PJ et al (ed): *Handbook of Clin Neurology* Amsterdam, North-Holland, 1978, pp 291–320.
35. Firemark HM: Spinal cysticercosis. *Arch Neurol* 1978;35:250–251.
36. Cosnett JE, Van Dellen JR: Schistosomiasis (Bilharzia) of the spinal cord: case reports and clinical profile. *Q J Med* 1986;61(236):1131–1139.
37. Levy RM, Bredesen DE, Rosenblum ML: Neurological manifestation of the acquired immunodeficiency syndrome (AIDS): experience at UCSF and review of the literature. *J Neurosurg* 1985;62:475–495.

38. Britton CB, Miller JR: Neurologic complication in acquired immunodeficiency syndrome (AIDS). *Neurol Clin* 1984;2:315–339.
39. Dickson DW, Belman AL, Kim TS, et al: Spinal cord pathology in pediatric acquired immunodeficiency syndrome. *Neurology* 1989;39:227–235.
40. Paine RS, Byers RK: Transverse myelopathy in childhood. *Am J Dis Child* 1953;85:151–163.
41. Altrocchi PH: Acute transverse myelopathy. *Arch Neurol* 1963;9:111–119.
42. Ropper AH, Poskanzer DC: The prognosis of acute and subacute transverse myelopathy based on early signs and symptoms. *Ann Neurol* 1978;4:51–59.
43. Berman M, Feldman S, Alter M, et al: Acute transverse myelitis: incidence and etiologic considerations. *Neurology* 1981;31:966–971.
44. Dunne K, Hopkins IJ, Shield LK: Acute transverse myelopathy in childhood. *Dev Med Child Neurol* 1986;28:198–204.
45. Miller HG, Stanton JB, Gibbon JD: Para-infectious encephalomyelitis and related syndrome. *Q J Med* 1956;25:427–505.
46. Abramsky O, Teitelbaum D: The autoimmune features of acute transverse myelopathy. *Ann Neurol* 1977;2:26–40.
47. Lipton HL, Teasdall RD: Acute transverse myelopathy in adults. *Arch Neurol* 1973;28:252–257.
48. Merine D, Wang H, Kumar AJ, et al: CT myelography and MR imaging of acute transverse myelitis. *J Comput Assist Tomogr* 1987;11(4):606–608.
49. Jaffe D, Freeman W: Spinal necrosis and softening of obscure origin. *Arch Neurol Psychiatry* 1943;49:683–707.
50. Hoffman HL: Acute necrotic myelopathy. *Brain* 1955;78:377–393.
51. Moersch FP, Kernohan JW: Progressive necrosis of the spinal cord. *Arch Neurol Psychiatry* 1934; 31:504–526.
52. Adams RD, Kubik CS: The morbid anatomy of the demyelinative diseases. *Am J Med* 1952;12:510–546.
53. Miller HG, Stanton JB, Gibbons JL: Para-infectious encephalomyelitis and related syndromes. *Q J Med* 1956;25:427–505.
54. Weiner LP, Johnson RT, Herndon RM: Viral infections and demyelinating diseases. *N Engl J Med* 1973;288:1103.
55. Alter M, Cendrowski W: Multiple sclerosis and childhood infections. *Neurology* 1976;26:201–204.
56. Goldwein JW: Radiation myelopathy: a review. *Med Pediatr Oncol* 1987;15(2):89–95.
57. Romsan GC, Spencer PS, Schoenberg BS. Tropical myeloneuropathies: the hidden endemias. *Neurology* 1985;35:1158–1170.
58. Pedersen C, Bonen H, Boesen F: Transverse myelitis in mixed connective tissue disease. *Clin Rheumatol* 1987;6(2):290–292.
59. Warren RW, Kredich DW: Transverse myelitis and acute central nervous system manifestations of systemic lupus erythematosus. *Arthrit Rheum* 1984; 9:1058–1060.
60. Al-Husaini A, Jamal GA: Myelopathy as the main presenting feature of systemic lupus erythematosus. *Eur Neurol* 1985;24:94–106.
61. Johnson RT, Richardson EP: The neurological manifestations of systemic lupus erythematosus. a clinical-pathological study of 24 cases and review of the literature. *Medicine* 1968;47:337–369.

15

Peripheral Nerve Disease Caused by Infection, Toxins, and Postinfectious Syndromes

EDGAR F. SALAZAR-GRUESO AND BARRY G.W. ARNASON

The peripheral nervous system (PNS) is anatomically defined as all neural structures lying outside the pial membrane of the spinal cord and brain stem. The PNS encompasses the spinal roots, the nerve trunks, the dorsal root and autonomic ganglia, peripheral nerves, and the third to 12th cranial nerves. The olfactory and optic nerves are excluded since they are special extensions of the central nervous system (CNS). Consideration of the biology and anatomy of the PNS lies outside the scope of this chapter and interested readers are referred to other reviews.[1,2]

The PNS responds to injury and to disease in a limited number of ways. Traditionally, these are classified in terms of four main processes: (1) Wallerian degeneration, or the response to axonal transection; (2) axonal atrophy and degeneration (axonopathy), or so-called dying-back neuropathy; (3) segmental demyelination (myelinopathy); and (4) primary nerve cell body degeneration (neuronopathy).[2] Sometimes, two or more of these reactions may coexist, making it difficult to decide which is the primary abnormality in a neuropathic process.

Peripheral nerve diseases are also classified in terms of anatomic site or sites of involvement. Focal involvement of a single nerve trunk is defined as a mononeuropathy; focal affliction of cranial nerves is defined as a cranial neuropathy. Mononeuropathy multiplex is a simultaneous or sequential affection of individual noncontiguous nerve trunks. Polyneuropathy connotes a widespread process of the peripheral nerves, usually distal and symmetric. The severity of polyneuropathies varies widely, as does the tempo at which the illness progresses and the mix of motor and sensory involvement. When nerve roots, peripheral nerves, and nerve trunks are all affected, the condition is referred to as a polyradiculoneuropathy. Involvement of nerve roots alone is known as radiculoneuropathy.

Those diseases of the PNS that result from a direct invasion by an infectious organism are usually characterized by an inflammatory reaction—neuritis. Most commonly in infectious neuropathies, the clinical presentation, electrodiagnostic studies, and pathology disclose syndromes of polyneuritis, polyradiculoneuritis, or cranial neuritis. Less often, the presentation may be one of mononeuritis or mononeuritis multiplex. At other times, an infectious organism may produce an exotoxin that damages the peripheral nerves without producing inflammation.

The number of disorders that affect the peripheral nerves is considerable, and their manifestations complex. Several useful strategies have been proposed that permit a logical approach to clinical assessment, correct diagnosis, and management; detailed descriptions of these can be found elsewhere.[2–4] In this chapter, we will consider directly infectious, infection-related but toxin-mediated, and postinfectious syndromes involving the PNS. The pathogenesis and clinical features of these disorders will be reviewed. In addition, selected aspects of diagnosis and treatment of the various conditions will be considered.

Directly Infectious Syndromes

Much of the early literature reporting an association of peripheral nerve disorders with this or that infectious organism suffers from a failure to clearly establish a cause-and-effect relationship. In numerous instances, neuropathies considered to be a direct consequence of invasion by an infectious organism were, in retrospect, postinfectious inflammatory demyelinating polyradiculoneuritis (see later). Criteria that support the proposal that an infectious organism is directly responsible for PNS disease include the following: (1) involvement of peripheral nerves is frequent in seropositive individuals; (2) the organism is observed within and can be cultured from peripheral nerve; and (3) other causes of neuropathy are excluded.[48]

Only a limited number of infectious organisms are currently believed to cause disease of the PNS by direct involvement. These include *Mycobacterium leprae* (leprosy), a limited number of viruses (herpesvirus, retrovirus), and selected parasites.

Leprosy

Leprosy is a chronic disease caused by infection with the acid-fast bacillus M *leprae*. Known since antiquity, leprosy holds an exceptional place in history because of the enduring societal stigma its victims have been forced to bear. The disease reached its peak prevalence in Europe during the Crusades, and for reasons that remain unknown, began to disappear by the 14th century. At present, leprosy is restricted to tropical and subtropical areas,[22] and in the United States, it is encountered in immigrants from those areas. The ease of present-day travel may explain occasional case reports from temperate regions of the world.

Leprosy has a low contagiousness. Transmission occurs as a result of contact with susceptible individuals, usually household members, who carry the bacillus. The portal of entry is most often the skin, but entry can also be via the upper respiratory tract. Infection leads to the invasion of peripheral nerves in all cases. Epidemiologic studies show that leprous neuropathy is the most common treatable neuropathy in the world.[23] Host immunocompetence in response to infection determines the varied and broad clinical and pathologic manifestations of the disease. Probably not more than 10% of infected individuals develop the disease. In this regard, one immunogenetic study reported in abstract form suggests that disease susceptibility is linked to certain HLA genes.[30]

The spectrum of disease is classified into one minor (indeterminate) and three major (lepromatous, dimorphous, and tuberculoid) clinicopathologic entities. At one end of the major-disease spectrum is lepromatous leprosy, which is characterized by a deficient immune response to *M leprae,* as evidenced by a negative lepromin response, and by an extensive invasion of skin and peripheral nerves by blood-borne bacilli. In this form of the infection, peripheral nerve destruction occurs late in the disease, even though the nerves may be teeming with bacilli. At the other end is tuberculoid leprosy, which is characterized by a vigorous T cell-mediated immune response to the lepra bacillus as evidenced by a positive lepromin reaction, the presence of well-localized granulomatous skin and peripheral nerve lesions, and a paucity of bacilli within nerves. The intense immune response in this form of leprosy, while it leads to the destruction of the bacilli, has, as a by-product of this successful defense mechanism, marked peripheral nerve destruction early in the course of the infection. The dimorphous form of leprosy results from an immune response to the bacillus intermediate in its intensity between that of tuberculoid and lepromatous leprosy, with a clinical pattern of disease falling between lepromatous and tuberculoid variants. Indeterminate leprosy is characterized by an indolent solitary macule or papule that is usually hypopigmented. Sensation is often altered within this lesion, and histologically, a mononuclear cell infiltrate surrounding dermal structures and neurovascular bundles is observed. Indeterminate leprosy represents a successful host response to infection with the lepra bacillus. The intensity of the defense response over the course of leprosy may vary. When the response fails, bacilli proliferate and spread; when the response recovers, massive destruction of newly infected nerves may follow.

A number of studies suggest that cell-mediated immunity to *M leprae* plays an important role in the pathogenesis of leprous neuropathy. In lepromatous leprosy, a predominance of cytotoxic/suppressor (CD8) T cells is found in the peripheral blood and in lesions of affected individuals.[24,25] Furthermore, macrophages derived from lepromatous lesions are noted to be engorged with bacilli, which they are unable to kill or degrade. This defect is thought to be a result of either a lack of sensitized T cells capable of releasing gamma interferon (IFN), a product of activated macrophages, or a defect in the mechanism that triggers release of gamma IFN.[25] Other investigators claim that clonally derived CD8 T cells from lepromatous patients appear to exert a suppressive effect on effector functions of *M leprae*–reactive CD4 T cells.[26,27] These findings are to be contrasted with tuberculoid leprosy in which overrepresentation of T cells of the helper/inducer

(CD4) phenotype is found,[24] and in which macrophages activated by the CD4 T cells kill leprae bacilli, but at the price of tissue destruction. The role of the Schwann cell in the presentation of *M leprae* antigens has recently been brought to the forefront by studies that report that *M leprae*–infected Schwann cells express major histocompatibility (MHC) class II antigens after treatment with gamma IFN.[31] If Schwann cells are indeed able to process and present *M leprae* antigens to T cells, such a mechanism may in part explain the cell-mediated immune response in tuberculoid leprosy.

While antibodies to the lepra bacillus are found in leprosy, there is no evidence for a humoral immune response directed against antigens of peripheral nerve myelin.[31] Antineural antibodies directed against intermediate filaments have been detected in serum from infected patients and may be generated from breakdown products of damaged nerves.[32] They are not thought to have a role in disease pathogenesis. Antilepra antibodies appear to have at best a minor role in the control of the bacillary infection or the pathogenes is of leprous neuropathy, except in one circumstance. When patients are first treated, large numbers of bacilli are killed and bacillary degradation products are released to the circulation. At these times, antigen–antibody immune complexes form and may be deposited in vessel walls that develop fibrinoid necrosis. Crops of painful red, indurated cutaneous lesions develop, and the process is known as erythema nodosum leprosum. Vasculitic lesions occur at sites where bacilli are most numerous, which includes nerves. Acute painful focal neuritis with destruction of intraneural elements is frequent.

Segmental demyelination is the pathologic hallmark in all forms of leprosy, and Schwann cells are a prime target. At the microscopic level, copious foamy bacillus-laden macrophages are found invading the endoneurium and perineurium of peripheral nerves of patients with lepromatous leprosy. In contrast, the microscopic picture in tuberculoid leprosy reveals destruction of peripheral nerves by giant-cell granulomas, and bacilli are rare. The lesions in this form of the disease arise as a consequence of a T cell-mediated delayed type hypersensitivity reaction to bacillary antigens. The T cells do not react to peripheral nerve myelin antigens.[28,29] The mechanism that underlies myelin destruction is poorly understood. One possibility is that myelin destruction may be mediated by products of activated macrophages such as tumor necrosis factor (TNF). This protein has been shown in vitro to be toxic to oligodendrocytes causing them to divest themselves of their myelin[53]; it is distinctly possible that TNF is toxic to Schwann cells as well.

In the tuberculoid variant, enlargement of cutaneous nerves and nerve trucks is clinically apparent. On occasion, a mononeuritis or a mononeuritis multiplex is clinically and electrophysiologically evident. The widespread invasion of cutaneous nerves in the lepromatous variant leads to a symmetric loss of pain and temperature sensation. In this form of the disease, the bacilli have a propensity to infiltrate the cooler body parts, such as the pinnae of ears; the dorsal surfaces of hands, forearms, and feet; and the anterolateral aspects of legs. Patchy regions of anesthesia and local areas of dysautonomia develop, indicating destruction of cutaneous nerves. In chronic cases, frank orthostatic hypotension may occur. Skin ulcers at pressure sites (soles and ankles) often develop. In contrast to other polyneuropathies, tendon reflexes are preserved, an indication of the fact that the more deeply situated muscular nerves are usually unaffected. Nonetheless, in chronic and markedly advanced cases, motor dysfunction with weakness, muscular atrophy, and diminished or absent reflexes may be present. Cranial nerve involvement may be present in both tuberculoid and lepromatous leprosy. Extensive destruction of the fifth and seventh cranial nerves leads to the development of the so-called "leonine face." Damage and weakness are most pronounced around the eyes and eyelids. Direct invasion of the eye may lead to keratitis, with subsequent blindness.

The treatment of leprosy is complex and may require the expertise of multiple medical specialists, public health officials, and, at times, rehabilitation and social service professionals. The slow growth of the organism, coupled with the difficulty in obtaining adequate antimicrobial levels in affected tissues, dictates a prolonged course of drug treatment, usually of several years' duration. Diaminodiphenylsulfone (Dapsone) is currently used as a single agent in the treatment of tuberculoid leprosy. Treatment is continued until the patient has been negative for bacilli for a period of 2 years. The treatment of lepromatous leprosy requires administration of Dapsone in combination with other drugs that may include rifampicin, clofazimine, and/or thioamide derivatives (ethionamide and protionamide), followed by several years of monotherapy with Dapsone until the patient tests negative for bacilli.[52,53] The emergence of resistant strains in 10% of lepromatous cases[54] may require a change in drugs and dosage schedules, tailored to local and individual needs.

The leprosy reactions (reversal and downgrading reactions and erythema nodosum leprosum) are severe flareups of the illness that may be life threatening, and at times are associated with drug therapy. In these situations, high-dose corticosteroids (prednisone 60 mg/day) are the drugs of choice and lead to the most effective clearing of symptoms; untoward side effects of prolonged therapy limit their usefulness. At times, discontinuation of antimicrobial drug therapy may be necessary. For erythema nodosum leprosum, thalidomide is recommended, but one must be mindful of the teratogenic side effects of this drug.

Other complications of leprosy include neuralgia or phantom pain. Effective treatment may require use of analgesics, anticonvulsants (in combination or as single agents), and/or transcutaneous electrical nerve stimulation. Acute nerve compression may require surgical decompression. Careful and well-planned cosmetic surgery to correct disfiguring results of the illness is an important adjunct to therapy.

Herpesvirus

Varicella-zoster (VZ) virus is a member of the herpesvirus group. These viruses share common ultrastructural, biochemical, and biophysical characteristics. VZ virus has the ability to infect both the CNS (encephalomyelitis, myelitis, cerebral angiitis) and the PNS (sensory, motor, and cranial neuritis, and neuralgia). VZ virus is currently believed to be transported retrogradely via peripheral axons to the nerve-cell soma, remaining in a latent state in ganglia for prolonged periods of time. Host immune factors are believed to play a leading role in reactivation of the virus. In this section, we will limit our focus to peripheral nerve disorders produced by infection with this virus.

VZ virus is similar to other herpesviruses (herpes simplex virus, cytomegalovirus [CMV] and Epstein-Barr virus [EBV]) in that it contains DNA. VZ virus has a structure that consists of four major components arranged in concentric layers. The innermost layers form the nucleocapsid, which consists of a core surrounded by a capsid composed of 162 capsomeres arranged in two-, three-, and five-fold icosahedral symmetry. The nucleocapsid is, in turn, surrounded by a granular proteinaceous material (tegument). The outermost layer is the envelope, which is composed of a lipid bilayer derived from the host cell membrane into which are inserted radially oriented viral glycoproteins that project to the outer surface.

VZ virus is the etiologic agent of both varicella (chickenpox) and zoster (shingles).[33] Varicella is a generalized exanthem commonly occurring in children, but it also occurs, although less frequently, in adults. In contrast, zoster is a painful exanthem limited to one or more dermatomes and is restricted to adults, except when it occurs against a background of immunosuppression. Varicella is known to arise after exposure to cases of zoster. Much less common is zoster after exposure to cases of varicella or to other cases of zoster. Among the neurologic complications of infection with VZ virus is postinfectious inflammatory demyelinating polyradiculoneuritis, which is more properly considered in the section on Postinfectious syndromes.

Our current view concerning the pathogenesis of VZ virus infection of the nervous system is derived from observations made by Hope-Simpson.[35] He proposed that viremia occurring during primary varicella infection permits virus to migrate up sensory nerves to the ganglion, where it remains in a dormant state, isolated from host immune surveillance, and ready to be reactivated under permissive conditions. This theory is quite consistent with a number of different observations. The hypothesis, however, fails adequately to explain the prolonged latent period that is observed between the initial attack of varicella during childhood and the first attack of zoster, usually in late adult life.

The Hope-Simpson hypothesis derives considerable support from clinical and virologic studies. From clinical observations, the preferential distribution of varicella eruption on the trunk and face would appear to correlate well with the predilection of zoster for thoracic and trigeminal dermatomes. The role of cell-mediate immunity in virus reactivation is demonstrated by the frequency of zoster in immunocompromised patients, particularly those with reticuloendothelial neoplasms and other malignancies and in the acquired immunodeficiency syndrome (AIDS). Immune function declines with age, and the increased incidence of zoster in the elderly also supports this concept. Pathologic studies of dorsal root ganglia in cases of zoster that have come to necropsy show acute ganglionitis,[36] findings consistent with Hope-Simpson's hypothesis. More recently, molecular biologic studies have detected viral DNA[37] and RNA[38] in ganglia from cases of acute zoster, but also in a substantial proportion of asymptomatic individuals.

As previously mentioned, pathologic studies have shown an inflammatory cellular infiltrate in ganglia and the nerve roots of patients suffering from acute illness with VZ virus infection (reviewed by Kennedy[44]). In addition to the involvement of ganglia, others have observed focal poliomyelitis, localized leptomeningitis, and mononeuritis.[45] In patients dying with acute or recent zoster, viral particles resembling VZ virus have been detected in neurons and satellite cells of ganglia by electron microscopy,[46] and in Schwann cells and perineurial and endoneurial cells by immunofluorescence.[47]

Clinically, zoster presents as a vesicular eruption in the distribution of a sensory dermatome. The illness is preceded by paresthesias and pain that may begin up to three weeks before the eruption occurs. Systemic symptoms and signs, such as fever, malaise, headache, and lymphadenopathy, are apt to occur in younger patients. The lesions begin as areas of erythema that develop into vesicles, erupting to form pustules that eventually crust over. The skin lesions evolve over a period of a week to ten days, and healing typically is complete by two to three weeks. The rash may spread to contiguous dermatomes, and is commonly distributed in those head and trunk areas that are usually involved by varicella. Occasional eruptions distant from the affected dermatones (satellite lesions) suggest that viremia may be a concomitant occurrence.

Cranial nerves are affected in 30% of cases, singly or in combination. Involvement of the ophthalmic branch of the trigeminal nerve may lead to blindness. The facial nerve is frequently affected, and the resultant facial paresis usually takes place in association with an otic eruption (Ramsay-Hunt syndrome[52]). Motor neuritis leading to a segmental motor weakness has been found in up to 5% of cases.[51] Motor symptoms typically develop within two weeks, but may be seen as early as one day and as late as four months after infection. The major complication of zoster is postherpetic neuralgia, a condition characterized by intense pain in the distribution of a healed herpetic eruption.

Zoster is a self-limited disease and is not ordinarily treated with antiviral agents. Analgesics or local application of lotions or ointments suffices in most instances. More aggressive antiviral therapy is required to prevent dissemination and complications in immunocompromised patients. The virus is sensitive to the nucleoside analogue acycloguanosine (acyclovir), which selectively inhibits herpes-specific DNA polymerase. This mechanism of action accounts for the lack of toxicity of the drug, which gives it an advantage over other chemotherapeutic agents. However, early treatment with this drug has not been shown to lessen the frequency of postherpetic neuralgia (reviewed by Jolleys[72] and by McKendrick, McGill, and Wood[73]). Treatment of the intractable pain of postherpetic neuralgia is difficult and frequently unsatisfactory. Corticosteroids are of no benefit. Analgesics, anticonvulsants (such as carbamazepine), antidepressants (such as amitriptyline), acupuncture, and/or transcutaneous nerve stimulation may be tried, singly or in combination. In exceptionally difficult cases, surgical intervention (rhizotomy) may be considered; however, this approach may make the pain worse.

Herpes simplex virus type 1 is also a member of the herpesvirus family. It causes the well-known cold sore. As with VZ virus, the virus remains latent in trigeminal ganglia and viral DNA can be demonstrated at autopsy in the ganglia of most normal individuals, even in the absence of a history of herpetic eruptions. Treatment of the cutaneous sores with acyclovir is believed to improve the rate of healing and decrease the period of pain.

Retrovirus

The human immunodeficiency virus (HIV) is a retrovirus and is the etiologic agent of AIDS. The lack of a component immune system in AIDS leads to the development of frequent and unusual opportunistic infections. Infection with HIV frequently affects both the CNS and the PNS. Nervous system abnormalities are detected in 75% of AIDS cases that come to pathologic examination (reviewed by Rosenblum, Levy, and Bredesen[55]) and clinically apparent neuropathy in about 20% of cases. In this section, we will briefly describe the various neuropathies associated with HIV infection.

Four neuropathies have been described in patients with recent HIV seroconversion, with AIDS-related complex (ARC), and in frank AIDS. These include (1) an inflammatory demyelinating polyradiculoneuritis (IDP), (2) a distal symmetric peripheral neuropathy, (3) a mononeuritis multiplex, and (4) a progressive radiculoneuropathy.

Inflammatory Demyelinating Polyradiculoneuritis

IDP occurs most commonly shortly after HIV seroconversion, and less commonly in ARC and

AIDS. Peripheral nerve involvement may present as either a postinfectious inflammatory demyelinating polyradiculoneuritis that is clinically (save for a mild CSF pleocytosis,[58] mean 23 cells/mm^3), electrophysiologically, and pathologically indistinguishable from the Guillain-Barré syndrome (see later), or in a more indolent form, resembling chronic inflammatory demyelinating polyradiculoneuropathy (CIDP).

A number of observations have led to the suggestion that HIV-related IDP is an autoimmune process. The temporal relationship of HIV seroconversion and the development of IDP is similar to the association of a preceding viral infection with the development of the Guillain-Barré syndrome, a putative autoimmune disease that is thought to be T cell-mediated (see postinfectious syndrome). AIDS patients are prone to developing opportunistic infections, including CMV infection; infection with CMV is a known antecedent of the Guillain-Barré syndrome. The IDP of HIV infection generally responds favorably to treatment with plasmapheresis or corticosteroids, an outcome that persuades many investigators that a circulating humoral factor, such as antibody, is involved in its pathogenesis. In this regard, one study reported in abstract form showed high titers of circulating antiperipheral nerve antibodies in affected patients.[57] The additional possibility that direct HIV virus invasion of peripheral nerves or nerve roots is involved in the pathogenesis of IDP cannot be discounted. Reports of HIV isolation from peripheral nerve[56] and detection of HIV particles by electron microscopy[58] argue in support of this latter view.

Distal Symmetric Peripheral Neuropathy

Distal symmetric peripheral neuropathy is common in frank AIDS. In some series, from 30% to as many as 80% of cases of AIDS developed this complication; other series report a lower incidence. Distal symmetric peripheral neuropathy has an insidious onset and is characterized by dysesthesias (occasionally painful), symmetric distal sensory impairment, variable distal muscle weakness and wasting, and depressed or absent tendon reflexes.[59] Electrodiagnostic studies reveal decreased amplitude of sensory nerve action potentials and normal nerve conduction velocities. Nerve biopsy reveals axonal dropout without inflammation. The cause of distal symmetric peripheral neuropathy remains unknown. A preliminary report of improvement of distal symmetric peripheral neuropathy with azothymidine (AZT) treatment remains to be confirmed.[61]

Mononeuritis Multiplex

The pathogenesis of HIV-associated mononeuritis multiplex remains obscure, although some investigators have demonstrated a necrotizing vasculitis.[62] Some patients evolve from mononeuritis multiplex to CIDP, and seem to respond to treatment with plasmapheresis.

Progressive Radiculoneuropathy

Accumulating evidence suggests that the fourth neuropathic syndrome associated with AIDS progressive radiculoneuropathy may be a result of CMV infection. Several studies[62–64] have demonstrated CMV inclusions by electron microscopy and CMV genome by *in situ* hybridization in nerve roots of patients with AIDS with progressive radiculoneuropathy that have come to necropsy. Effective therapy for progressive radiculoneuropathy is not yet available. Success in treating CMV retinitis with ganciclovir (DHPG) suggests that this drug should be considered as a treatment for progressive radiculoneuropathy.

Human T-cell lymphotropic virus type I (HTLV-I) is also a retrovirus. Infection with HTLV-I leads to adult T-cell leukemia and lymphoma. In addition, HTLV-I infection is associated with a chronic myelopathy known both as HTLV-I–associated–myelopathy and as tropical spastic paraparesis (HAM/TSP). Case reports of PNS involvement (radiculoneuropathy) in association with HAM/TSP have begun to appear.[65,66] No effective therapy for peripheral nerve disease is known, although the fact that HAM/TSP can be ameliorated with corticosteroids suggests that corticosteroids may also be of benefit in HTLV-I–associated radiculoneuropathy.

Parasites

Two intracellular protozoan parasites are believed to affect peripheral nerves by direct invasion. Infection with *Trypanosoma cruzi* causes Chagas' disease, an inflammatory disease with cell-mediated destruction of peripheral nerves. In the second instance, infection with *Nosema connori,* a microsporidian intracellular protozoan parasite, is reported to have produced peripheral nerve disease in one immunocompromised patient.

Chagas' disease (American trypanosomiasis) is a

common infectious disease in Central and South America. Parasites are transmitted in feces from insects of the triatomina species. Humans are infected by contamination of insect-induced skin wounds with insect feces. Other modes of infection include ingestion of food contaminated with insect feces, blood transfusions from infected donors, and transplacental spread. Chagas' disease is characterized by acute and chronic phases. In the acute phase, parasites are sequestered in a number of tissues, including the nervous system. Variable systemic symptoms and signs of infection and inflammation are observed, and include fever, sweating, myalgias, tachycardia, lymphadenopathy, hepatosplenomegaly, peripheral blood lymphocytosis, and occasionally emesis and diarrhea. The chronic phase of illness is characterized by a capricious and an indolent destruction of visceral organs, as well as nerve cells in the walls of the viscera. In this phase of the illness, lesions in Auerbach plexus and other peripheral autonomic ganglia develop into acute ganglionitis with subsequent massive degeneration of ganglia. This results in gastrointestinal (megacolon and megaesophagus) and cardiac (chagasic cardiomyopathy) disease. Peripheral nerve disease leads to motor neuropathies, usually affecting the lower extremities. Electrodiagnostic studies demonstrate denervation in the majority of asymptomatic and clinically affected patients.[68]

The pathology in the acute phase of Chagas' disease discloses parasites in Schwann cells, satellite cells, and pericapsular fibroblasts. Perivascular infiltrates are observed in neural sheaths and interfascicular spaces in humans and in an experimental disease in mice.[67] With regard to the experimental model, histologic examination of peripheral nerves of mice chronically infected with *T cruzi* showed granulomatous infiltrates and multifocal demyelinative lesions. When T cells isolated from chronically infected mice and enriched for the helper/inducer phenotype ($L3T4^+$) were adoptively transferred to naive mice, the recipients developed perivascular endoneural inflammatory infiltrates without parasites. In contrast, intraneural injection of serum from chronically infected animals into peripheral nerve of naive animals produced no disease. These results suggest that the pathogenetic mechanism of neuropathy in Chagas disease may be similar to that of experimental allergic neuritis (see "Postinfectious Syndromes[11]).

The treatment of Chagas' disease remains suboptimal. Nitrofuran (nifurtimox) and Imidazole (benznidazole) derivatives are currently recommended.[69] However, cure rates with both agents are low and undesirable side effects are frequent, including a drug-induced peripheral neuropathy. A vaccine for populations-at-risk is still in development.

An association of nosematosis *(N connori),* a parasitic disease of invertebrates and certain vertebrates (felines and rodents), and peripheral nerve disease in humans remains to be established. To date, one case report detailing necropsy findings of an infant with thymic atrophy and hypogammaglobulinemia who died from complications of infection with *N connori* has been reported.[71] This five-month-old infant had evidence at autopsy of extensive dissemination of the parasite in all organs of the body, including autonomic ganglia and peripheral nerves.

Infectious Toxin-Mediated Syndromes

In the previous section, we discussed direct invasion of peripheral nerves by infectious organisms. In this section, we will consider infection-related peripheral nerve disease caused by toxins elaborated by microorganisms.

Diphtheric Neuropathy

Diphtheria, an acute bacterial illness caused by *Corynebacterium diphtheriae,* is now rare in the West. However, the disease remains common in underdeveloped countries, where neurologic complications of infection are still observed. The acute illness, in its most common presentation (faucial infection), leads to the formation of an inflammatory exudate in the throat and trachea. At this site, the bacteria elaborate and secrete an exotoxin that is toxic to the cardiac and nervous systems.

The toxin is made by bacteria lysogenic for corynephages whose genome carries the toxin *(tox)* structural gene (reviewed by Pappenheimer[70]). The toxin is secreted in a proenzyme form as a single polypeptide chain (molecular weight [MW] 57 kDa). Proteolytic cleavage ("nicking") yields a two-chain (dichain) polypeptide held together by a disulfide bridge. The dichain polypeptide is composed of A and B fragments and is both toxic to sensitive cells and enzymatically active. Fragment A (light chain; MW 21 kDa) possesses adenosine-5'-diphosphate–(ADP) ribosyl transferase enzyme activity, while fragment B (heavy chain; MW 37 kDa) binds to cell-membrane receptors.[5] The noxious effect of the toxin resides in fragment A, which enzymatically catalyzes the transfer of an ADP-ribose moiety from oxidized NAD (NAD^+) to elongation factor 2 (EF-2). This reaction inactivates EF-2, leading to termination of peptide elongation in the cell, inhibition of protein synthesis, and eventually cell death.[6] Fragment B, while not toxic, is essential since binding of it to the cell membrane permits internalization of fragment A.

The neurologic attack in diphtheria falls on cranial and peripheral nerves. Tissues of the CNS are not usually affected because the blood–brain barrier prevents toxin entry.[7] The PNS is most susceptible in those areas where the blood–nerve barrier is absent, such as the nodose ganglion of the vagus nerve, dorsal root ganglia, and nerve roots; peripheral nerves are also affected. In the latter site, histologic studies of human disease and of experimental animal models show segmental and paranodal demyelination, a consequence of the death of Schwann cells.[7,8,10] Slowing of conduction and conduction block are the physiologic correlates of segmental demyelination as detected by electrodiagnostic studies.[9]

The frequency of neurologic complications in diphtheria varies widely. The incidence of neuropathy has been reported to range from 8 to 66%, with an overall average of 20%. The wide range perhaps reflects the variable severity of illness. Palatal paralysis occurs early because of the high local concentration of toxin. Within days, the trigeminal, facial, vagal, and hypoglossal nerves are affected. Ciliary paralysis with attendant loss of accommodation and blurring of vision appears by the third week. On occasion, paralysis of extraocular muscles occurs.

Peripheral neuropathy usually appears within two to three months of infection and is of a mixed motor and sensory type with weakness; paresthesias; loss of superficial, joint, and position sense; and impaired or lost tendon reflexes. The neuropathy varies in severity from a mild deficit with maximal distal involvement to a rapidly ascending paralysis. The cerebrospinal fluid (CSF) usually contains an increased protein; CSF lymphocytosis has also been reported but is not usual. The long latency between the acute illness and subsequent development of neuropathy has no clear explanation.

It is generally accepted that antitoxin administered within 48 hours of the onset of infection lessens the incidence and severity of diphtheritic complications, especially neuropathy.[11] This treatment is, however, of no value once neuropathic complications appear and therapy in these situations is chiefly supportive.

Botulism

Botulism is caused by the ingestion of a food-borne exotoxin produced by *Clostridium botulinum*. The disease preferentially affects axon terminals, leaving myelin and axons intact. Food-borne illness is usually the result of consumption of home-canned products (most often acidic vegetables), which are easily infected with *C botulinum*. Other forms of botulism result from endogenous production of exotoxin by bacteria growing either in the intestine (infant botulism) or in a wound (wound botulism).

C botulinum is composed of a heterogeneous group of bacterial strains that produce eight antigenically distinct but related toxins identified as types A, B, C_1, C_2, D, E, F, and G.[12] Although most strains of bacteria produce one toxin type, others are capable of producing more than one type. Epidemiologic studies have shown that toxin type A is responsible for 60% of cases of botulism, type B for 30%, and type E for 10%.[19]

All of the botulinum toxins, with the exception of C_2, are known to be neurotoxins.[13,14] The seven neurotoxins are synthesized as single polypeptide chains with molecular weights ranging from 140 to 167 kDa. There is evidence that specific bacteriophages and plasmids contain the genetic information for the production of toxin in disease-producing strains of *C botulinum*.[15] Further processing of botulinum neurotoxin by nicking near the N-terminus, either by host or bacterial proteases, produces a dichain molecule composed of a light chain and a heavy chain. The heavy chain is three times the size of the light chain; the two are linked by a disulfide bridge.[16] It is believed that entry to the cell is gained by receptor-mediated binding of the heavy chain, and that toxicity is mediated via the light chain.[17] The toxin interferes with release of acetylcholine quanta at the presynaptic nerve endings of the neuromuscular junction,[17,18] as well as at other cholinergic synapses, by a mechanism that is not fully understood. The defect in neuromuscular transmission produced by the toxin is similar in nature to that observed in the myasthenic syndrome of Lambert-

Eaton, but quite different from that observed in myasthenia gravis. As a consequence of toxin action, the terminal axon is permanently damaged and unable to release transmitter. Sprouts grow from the axon at sites proximal to the site of the blockade. These sprouts make new connections with the muscles, new neuromuscular junctions form, and this is followed by recovery.

The effects of the toxin are usually experienced within 12–36 hours of ingesting contaminated food. Autonomic dysfunction is the first abnormality, with the appearance of dry mouth, blurred vision, urinary difficulties, and diarrhea or constipation. Ptosis, strabismus, and extraocular muscle palsies occur next and may suggest a diagnosis of myasthenia gravis; the presence of poorly reactive or unreactive pupils secures a diagnosis of botulism. Bulbar dysfunction rapidly ensues and is followed by weakness of the muscles of the neck, trunk, and limbs. In severe cases, the tendon reflexes are lost. The entire clinical picture may take 2–4 days to evolve and may lead to an erroneous diagnosis of postinfectious demyelinating polyradiculoneuritis. In contrast to this syndrome, sensation remains intact and the CSF shows no abnormalities. Diagnosis is aided by electrodiagnostic studies, which characteristically show reduced compound-muscle-action potentials (CMAP) during low-frequency repetitive stimulation (2 Hz), with an increase in CMAP during high-frequency repetitive stimulation (10 Hz). The diagnosis is confirmed by showing that serum, stool, and suspect food are toxic to mice.

The aims of treatment are to remove nonabsorbed toxin, neutralize the effects of absorbed but not yet internalized toxin, and provide supportive care. Enemas or induction of emesis may serve to remove any remaining toxin from the gastrointestinal tract. Antimicrobial drugs may be administered to eliminate bacteria from the gut (food-borne or infant botulism) or in a wound (wound botulism). Aminoglycoside and tetracycline antimicrobials should be avoided, if possible, since these tend to potentiate neuromuscular blockade. If botulism is suspected, prompt administration of trivalent equine antitoxin (Connaught Laboratories) is recommended, even before laboratory confirmation of the diagnosis is made; however, antitoxin is expensive ($500/day), its efficacy remains unproved, and it causes a hypersensitivity reaction in about 9% of cases. The recommended dose is one vial given intravenously and one vial given intramuscularly, once the result of intradermal testing for sensitivity to horse serum is known. The same dose is repeated in two to four hours if symptoms and signs progress.[20] In patients who have a history of atopy or demonstrate a hypersensitivity reaction to antitoxin, desensitization to antitoxin should be carried out. Guanidine hydrochloride (14–50 mg/kg) or aminopyridines (4-aminopyridine or 3,4-diaminopyridine) are reported to help by promoting release of acetylcholine at the neuromuscular junction; however, questionable efficacy of the former[21] and adverse side effects of both (bone-marrow suppression and renal and neurologic dysfunction with guanidine and seizures with aminopyridines) limit the usefulness of these agents.

Postinfectious Syndromes

In the previous sections, we discussed peripheral nerve diseases that either result from direct infection of nerves or are caused by toxins released by infectious organisms. These entities should be contrasted with peripheral nerve disease that occurs during recovery from a recent infectious illness. Here we will discuss the acute ascending paralysis, usually referred to as postinfectious demyelinating polyradiculoneuritis or as the Guillain-Barré syndrome.

Postinfectious demyelinating polyradiculoneuritis is an acutely evolving paralytic disease of unknown cause. It occurs throughout the world and at all ages. The characteristic pathologic feature is one of scattered inflammatory cellular infiltrates within nerves and roots composed primarily of T cells and macrophages. At sites of inflammation, there is destruction of peripheral nerve myelin.

Approximately two thirds of patients recall an antecedent acute infectious illness that had usually abated by the time neuropathic symptoms began. The interval between the prodromal infectious episode and the onset of neuropathic symptoms is most often from 1 to 3 weeks, occasionally longer. In most cases, the agent responsible for the prodromal illness, which is usually either an acute influenza-like respiratory illness or an acute dysenteric episode, remains unidentified. Perhaps 10% of cases follow the glandular fever-like syndrome caused by CMV. At times, IgM antibody to CMV, the presence of which argues strongly for infection in the immediate past, may be detected even when no recent illness can be recalled. It follows that the severity of the infection in no way correlates with the occurrence of a complicating polyneuritis. About 5% of cases begin following a surgical procedure. Usually, blood transfusions have been given in such cases, and it is distinctly possible that CMV was introduced in the transfused blood. An additional 5% of cases have been convincingly associated with infectious mononucleosis, a disease caused by EBV. Some 1–2% of cases follow varicella (chickenpox) or zoster (shingles). Note that CMV, EBV, and VZ virus are all herpesviruses. Numerous reports of postinfectious demyelinating polyradiculoneuritis following measles, rubella, mumps, hepatitis and influenza A and B, as well as echovirus and coxsackievirus infections, have been recorded over the years. The difficulty in evaluating these reports relates to the frequency with which infections with these agents occur and the rarity of postinfectious demyelinating polyradiculoneuritis. The associations remain highly problematic in our opinion.[40]

More firmly established is a tie to antecedent mycoplasma pneumonia infection. Approximately 5% of postinfectious demyelinating polyradiculoneuritis cases have serologic evidence of active or recent mycoplasmal infection. In recent years, a link with *Campylobacter jejeuni* enteritis has been noted by several observers (reviewed by Ropper[39]). In some series, 15–20% of cases of postinfectious demyelinating polyradiculoneuritis have had evidence of recent infection with this organism. Polyneuritis in association with HIV infection has been discussed in a previous section. It follows from what has preceded that a substantial proportion of cases of postinfectious demyelinating polyradiculoneuritis can be accounted for by infection with a limited number of organisms. The question then becomes: How do these infections cause the disease or predispose to it? There is reason to believe that postinfectious demyelinating polyradiculoneuritis is an autoimmune process, although the antigen or antigens of myelin against which the immune attack is directed remain totally unknown.

A model for postinfectious demyelinating polyradiculoneuritis known as experimental allergic neuritis (EAN) has been developed. Animals immunized with a protein of peripheral myelin known as P_2 develop an acute demyelinating disease that faithfully mimics the human one clinically, pathologically, and electrophysiologically. EAN is a T-cell–mediated disease and P_2 is the antigen. Polyneuritis patients, however, do not demonstrate T-cell or antibody responses to P_2, so the model is imperfect.

There has been considerable interest in the concept of molecular mimicry.[34] It is hypothesized that there are close sequence similarities between small regions of proteins of infectious agents and small regions of host proteins. The infection triggers an immune response to the sequence on the infectious organism, which then cross-reacts with the analogous region of the host protein. In this way, tolerance to self is broken and a tissue-destructive autoimmune response ensues. As molecular mimicry has been demonstrated in several autoimmune diseases, the concept is an attractive one in postinfectious demyelinating polyradiculoneuritis; unfortunately, firm evidence in support of it is lacking at the present time.

As previously mentioned, EAN is a purely T cell-mediated process. The situation in postinfectious demyelinating polyradiculoneuritis may be more complex. It has been established that plasmapheresis exerts a beneficial effect on the course of the human illness.[41,42] Since plasmapheresis removes circulating immunoglobulin, among other plasma components, the possibility that circulating antibody may have a role in the pathogenesis of postinfectious demyelinating polyradiculoneuritis has been suggested. Forssman-type IgM antibodies that bind to myelin have been detected in the serum of patients with the disease, particularly early in the course of the illness—a finding that lends credence to this suggestion.[43] At the same time, the process is unlikely to be purely and simply antibody mediated since this will not account for the inflammatory cellular infiltrates that are the pathologic hallmark of the disease. A synergism between an antibody-mediated process and a T cell–mediated one is distinctly possible.

The clinical diagnosis usually presents little difficulty. The onset of symptoms is subacute; evolution is complete after 2 weeks in 50% of cases, after 3 weeks in over 80%, and after 4 weeks in over 90%. A stable period, which is usually brief, is followed by a recovery period that proceeds to completion within a period of weeks to a few months. Perhaps 5% of cases are left with a permanent handicap.

The major complaint is of weakness, which covers a wide spectrum from mild ataxia to total paralysis of every motor and cranial nerve. In most instances, weakness begins in the legs, more commonly distally at first and then proximally, but the arms may be involved before the legs. The process is characterized by relative but seldom absolute symmetry. Facial weakness, usually bilateral, is noted in half the cases. In 20% of cases, weakness becomes so profound that respiratory assistance is required. Tendon reflexes are generally abolished. Ataxia may be prominent early in the disease and can cause confusion as to the diagnosis. Sensory symptoms are in general less prominent than motor ones, although almost all patients complain of subjective tingling or numbness, usually of a distal symmetric glove- and stocking-like type. Objectively demonstrable sensory loss is less extensive than the subjective complaints would lead one to anticipate and may even be absent. Significant muscular or neuropathic pain is felt in 30% of cases. Autonomic function is frequently abnormal and may cause wide fluctuations in blood pressure, pulse, abnormalities of sweating, and gastric atony.

The CSF protein is normal during the first few days of the illness, but then rises, sometimes reaching very high values after 3 to 4 weeks. Cells in the CSF are not prominent, but a few cases may show 20–30 cell/mm^3. Conduction of nerve impulses through areas of segmental demyelination is severely compromised. Conduction velocity is characteristically slowed, though not invariably so, and prolonged distal latencies are frequent. Nerve-conduction studies, if carefully performed, reveal abnormalities in 90% of cases.

In severe cases, the major effort in terms of clinical management must be devoted to the prevention of complications. Seriously ill patients are best cared for in intensive-care or respirator units. A course of vigorous plasmapheresis treatment has been shown to lessen the time of hospital confinement, and in severe cases, the time spent on a respirator. Immunosuppressive and glucocorticoid treatments are not recommended.

Acknowledgments. The excellent secretarial assistance of Edwina Wharfe in the preparation of this chapter is greatly appreciated.

References

1. Dyck PJ, Thomas PK, Lambert EH, et al (eds): *Peripheral Neuropathy,* 2nd ed. Philadelphia, W.B. Saunders, 1984.
2. Asbury AK, Gilliatt RW: The clinical approach to neuropathy, in Asbury AK, Gilliatt RW (eds): *Peripheral Nerve Disorders: A Practical Approach,* London, Butterworths, 1984, pp 1–20.
3. Dyck PJ: Diseases of peripheral nerves, in Engel AG, Banker BQ (eds): *Myology: Basic and Clinical.* New York, McGraw-Hill, 1986, pp 2069–2108.
4. Spencer PS, Schaumberg HH (eds): *Experimental and Clinical Neurotoxicology.* Baltimore, Williams & Wilkins, 1980.
5. Middlebrook JL, Dorland RB: Bacterial toxins: cellular mechanism of action. *Microbiol Rev* 1984;48: 199–221.
6. Morris RE, Saelinger CB: Entry of bacterial toxins into mammalian cells, in Simpson LL (ed): *Botulinum Neurotoxin and Tetanus Toxin.* San Diego, Calif, Academic Press, 1989, pp 121–152.
7. Waksman BH: Experimental study of diphtheritic polyneuritis in the rabbit and guinea pig. Part III. The blood-nerve barrier in the rabbit. *J. Neuropathol Exp Neurol* 1961;20:35–77.
8. Fisher CM, Adams RD: Diphtheritic polyneuritis: a pathological study. *J. Neuropathol Exp Neurol* 1956;15:243–268.
9. Bostock H, Sears TA, Sherratt RM: The spatial distribution of excitability and membrane current in normal and demyelinated mammalian nerve fibers. *J. Physiol* 1983;341:41–58.
10. Webster H, Spiro D, Waksman B, et al: Phase and electron microscopic studies of experimental demyelination. *J Neuropathol Exp Neurol* 1961;20:5–13.
11. Paley RG, Truelove SC: Diphtheria in the army in the United Kingdom. A study of its complications. *J R Army Med Corps* 1948;90:109–116.
12. Smith LDS: *Botulism: The Organism, Its Toxin, The Disease.* Springfield, Ill, Charles C Thomas, 1977.
13. Simpson LL: A comparison of pharmacological properties of *Clostridium botulinum* type C_1 and C_2 toxins. *J. Pharmacol Exp Ther* 1982;223:695–701.
14. Simpson LL: The pathophysiological actions of the binary toxin produced by *Clostridium botulinum,* in Eklund MW, Dowell VR Jr (eds): *Avian Botulism: An International Perspective.* Springfield, Ill, Charles C Thomas, 1987, pp 249–264.
15. Eklund MW, Poysky FT, Habig WH: Bacteriophages and plasmid in *Clostridium botulinum* and *Clostridium tetani* and their relationships to production of toxins, in Simpson LL (ed): *Botulinum Neurotoxin and Tetanus Toxin.* San Diego, Calif, Academic Press, 1989, pp 25–51.
16. DasGupta BR: Structure and structure function relation of botulinum neurotoxins, in Lewis GE (ed): *Biomedical Aspects of Botulism.* New York, Academic Press, 1981, pp 1–19.
17. Wright GP: The neurotoxins of *Clostridium botulinum* and *Clostridium tetani. Pharmacol Rev* 1955; 7:413–465.
18. Baroff DA, Del Castillo J, Evoy WH, et al: Observations of the action of type A botulinum toxin on frog neuromuscular junctions. *J Physiol* 1974;240:227–253.

19. MacDonald KL, Cohen ML, Blake PA: The changing epidemiology of adult botulism in the United States. *Am J Epidemiol* 1986;124:794–799.
20. Centers for Disease Control: *MMWR* 1986;35:490–491.
21. Kaplan JE, Davis LE, Narayan V, et al: Botulism, type A, and treatment with guanidine. *Ann Neurol* 1979;6:69–71.
22. Bechelli LM, Martinez-Dominguez V: Further information on the leprosy problem in the world. *Bull WHO* 1972;46:523–536.
23. Sabin TD, Swift TR: Leprosy, in Dyck PJ, Thomas PK, Lambert EH, et al (eds): *Peripheral Neuropathy*, 2nd ed., Philadelphia, WB Saunders, 1984, pp 1955–1987.
24. Van Voorhis WC, Kaplan G, Sarno EN, et al: The cutaneous infiltrates of leprosy. *N Engl J Med* 1982;307:1593–1597.
25. Noguera N, Kaplan G, Levy E, et al: Defective gamma-interferon production in leprosy. Reversal with antigen and interleukin 2. *J Exp Med* 1983;158:2165–2170.
26. Ottenhoff THM, Elferink DG, Klatser PR, et al: Cloned suppressor T cells from a lepromatous leprosy patient suppress *Mycobacterium leprae* reactive helper T cells. *Nature* 1986;322:462–464.
27. Modlin RL, Kato H, Mehira V, et al: Genetically restricted suppressor T cell clones derived from lepromatous leprosy lesions. *Nature* 1986;322:459–461.
28. Mshana RN, Humber DP, Harboe M, et al: Immune responses to bovine neural antigens in leprosy patients. *Lepr Rev* 1983;54:217–227.
29. Mshana RN, Humber DP, Harboe M, et al: Nerve damage following intraneural injection of *Mycobacterium leprae* into rabbits pre-sensitized to mycobacteria. *Clin Exp Immunol* 1983;52:441–448.
30 Kikuchi I, Ozawa T, Sanada K, et al: Immunogenetic analysis of leprosy in the Japanese; second report (abstract). *Int J Lepr* 1984;52:617.
31. Mshana RN, Harboe M, Stoner GL, et al.: Immune responses to bovine neural antigens in leprosy patients. I. Absence of antibodies to an isolated myelin protein. *Int J Lepr* 1983;51:33–40.
32. Estis-Turf EP, Benjamins JA, Lefford MJ: Characterization of the antineural antibodies in the sera of leprosy patients. *J Neuroimmunol* 1986; 10:313–330.
33. Weller TH, Witton HM: The etiologic agents of varicella and herpes zoster: serologic studies with the viruses propagated *in vitro*. *J Exp Med* 1958; 108:869–890.
34. Oldstone MBA: Molecular mimicry and autoimmune disease (minireview). *Cell* 1987;50:819–820.
35. Hope-Simpson RE: The nature of herpes zoster: a long-term study and a new hypothesis. *Proc R Soc Med* 1965;59:9–20.
36. Ruppenthal M: Changes of the central nervous system in herpes zoster. *Acta Neuropath* 1980;52:59–68.
37. Gilden DH, Vafai A, Shtram Y, et al: Varicella-zoster virus DNA in human sensory ganglia. *Nature* 1983;306:478–480.
38. Hyman RW, Ecker JR, Tenser RB: Varicella-zoster virus RNA in human trigeminal ganglia. *Lancet* 1983;2:814–816.
39. Ropper AH: Campylobacter diarrhea and Guillain-Barré syndrome. *Arch Neurol* 1988;45:655–656.
40. Arnason BGW: Acute inflammatory demyelinating polyradiculoneuropathies, in Dyck PJ, Thomas PK, Lambert EH, et al (eds): *Peripheral Neuropathy*, 2nd ed, Philadelphia, WB Saunders, 1984, pp 2050–2100.
41. McKhann GM, Griin JW, Cornblath DR, et al: Plasmapheresis and Guillain-Barré syndrome: analysis of prognostic factors and the effect of plasmapheresis. *Ann Neurol* 1988;23:347–353.
42. McKhann GM, Griffin JW, Cornblath DR, et al: Role of therapeutic plasmapheresis in the acute Guillain-Barré syndrome. *J Neuroimmunol* 1988;20:297–300.
43. Koski CL, Chou DK, Jungalwala FB: Anti-peripheral nerve myelin antibodies in Guillain-Barré syndrome bind a neutral glycolipid of peripheral nerve myelin and cross-react with Forssman antigen. *J. Clin Invest* 1989;41:280–287.
44. Kennedy PGE: Neurological complications of varicella-zoster virus, in Kennedy PGE, Johnson RT (eds): *Infections of the Nervous System*. London, Butterworths, 1987, pp 177–208.
45. Denny-Brown D, Adams RD, Fitzgerald P: Pathologic features of herpes zoster: a note on "Geniculate" herpes. *Arch Neurol Psychiatry* 1944;51:216–231.
46. Ghatak NR, Zimmerman HM: Spinal ganglion in herpes zoster. A light and electron microscopic study. *Arch Pathol* 1973;95:411–415.
47. Esiri MM, Tomlinson AH: Herpes zoster demonstration of virus in trigeminal nerve and ganglion by immunofluoresce, and electron microscopy. *J Neurol Sci* 1972;15:35–48.
48. Swift TR, Rivner MH. Infectious diseases of nerve, in Vinken PJ, Bruyn GW, Klawans HL (eds): *Handbook of Clinical Neurology, Vol 51, Revised Series 7: Neuropathies* (Mathews WB, co-ed). Amsterdam, Elsevier Science Publishing, 1987; pp 179–194.
49. Thomas JE, Howard FM Jr: Segemental zoster paresis—a disease profile. *Neurology* 1972; 22:459–466.
50. Hunt JR: On herpetic inflammations of the geniculate ganglion. A new syndrome and its complications. *J. Nerv Ment Dis* 1907;34:73–96.
51. Seljma KW, Raine CS: Tumor necrosis factor mediates myelin and oligodendrocyte damage *in vitro*. *Ann Neurol* 1988;23:339–346.
52. WHO Study Group: Chemotherapy of leprosy for control programmes. WHO Technical Report Series No. 675, 1982.

53. WHO Geneva: Treatment and patient care, in *A Guide to Leprosy Control,* Ch 6. WHO, Geneva, 1988, pp. 30–46.
54. Jacobson RR, Trautman JR: The treatment of leprosy with the sulfones. I. Faget's original 22 patients; a thirty year follow-up on sulfone therapy for leprosy. *Int J Lepr* 1971:39:726.
55. Rosenblum ML, Levy RM, Bredesen DE (eds): *AIDS and the Nervous System.* New York, Raven, 1988.
56. Cornblath DR, McArthur JC, Kennedy GE, at al: Inflammatory demyelinating peripheral neuropathies associated with human T-lymphotropic virus type III infection. *Ann Neurol* 1987;21:32–40.
57. Miller RG, Parry G, Lang W, et al: AIDS-related inflammatory polyradiculoneuropathy: prediction of response to plasma exchange with electrophysiologic testing. *Muscle Nerve* 1985;8:626.
58. Bailey RO, Singh JK, Bishop MB: AIDS neuropathy: the role of axoplasmic transport. *Neurology* 1987; 37(suppl 1):356.
59. So YT, Holtzman DM, Abrams DI, et al: Peripheral neuropathy associated with acquired immunodeficiency syndrome: prevalence and clinical features from a population-based survey. *Arch Neurol* 1988;45:945–948.
60. Yarchoan R, Brouwers P, Spitzer AR, et al: Response of human-immunodeficiency-virus-associated neurological disease to 3'-azido-3' deothymidine. *Lancet* 1987;1:132–135.
61. Said G, Lacroix-Ciaudo C, Fujimara H, et al: The peripheral neuropathy of necrotizing arteritis: a clinicopathological study. *Ann Neurol* 1988;23:46–465.
62. Eidelberg D, Sotrel A, Vogel H, et al: Progressive polyradiculopathy in acquired immune deficiency syndrome. *Neurology* 1986;36:912–916.
63. Behar R, Wiley C, McCutchan JA: Cytomegalovirus polyradiculoneuropathy in acquired immune deficiency syndrome. *Neurology* 1987;37:557–561.
64. Grafe MR, Wiley CA: Spinal cord and peripheral nerve pathology in AIDS: the roles of cytomegalovirus and human immunodeficiency virus. *Ann Neurol* 1989;25:561–566.
65. Salazar-Grueso EF, Dawson G, Wollman R, et al: HTLV-I infection associated with a familial spastic paraparesis (FSP) syndrome (abstract). *Ann Neurol* 26(1):152, 1989.
66. Vernant J-C, Buisson G, Bellance R, et al: Pseudo-amyotrophic lateral sclerosis, peripheral neuropathy and chronic polyradiculoneuritis in HTLV-I-associated paraplegias, in Román GC, Vernant J-C, Osame M (eds): *HTLV-I and the Nervous System.* New York, Alan R Liss, 1989; pp 361–365.
67. Said G, Joskowicz M, Barreira Antunes A, et al: Neuropathy associated with experimental Chagas disease. *Ann Neurol* 1985;18:676–683.
68. Pagano MA, Basso S, Aristimuño GG, et al: Electromyographical findings in human chronic Chagas disease. *Arq Neuro-Psiquiatr* 1978;42:316–318.
69. Brener Z: Recent advances in the chemotherapy of Chagas disease. *Mem Inst Oswaldo Cruz* 1984; 79(suppl):149–155.
70. Pappenheimer Jr AM: Diphtheria toxin. *Ann Rev Biochem* 1977;46:69–94.
71. Margileth A, Strano A, Chandra R, et al: Disseminated nosematosis in an immunologically compromised infant. *Arch Pathol* 1973;95:145–150.
72. Jolleys JV: Treatment of shingles and post-herpetic neuralgia (editorials). *Br Med J* 1989;298:1537–1538.
73. McKendrick MW, McGill JI, Wood MW. Lack of effect of acyclovir on postherpetic neuralgia. *Br Med J* 1989;289:431.

Part IV
Problematic Pathogens and States

16
Central-Nervous-System Tuberculosis

John E. Kasik

Pathogenesis

Many of the symptoms, signs, and sequelae of tuberculous meningitis (TBM) are the result of an immunologically directed inflammatory reaction to the infection.[1] Although a mycobacterial infection is the inciting cause of the illness, it is the resulting inflammation of the meninges—which is responsible for the damage to blood vessels, scar formation, edema, and exudate in the central nervous system—that produces the clinical manifestations of this disease.

The clinical events in TBM, as with all forms of tuberculosis, usually begin with inhalation of an infected droplet of aerosolized sputum generated by the cough of a person with active pulmonary tuberculosis. In the nonimmune host, the inhaled organisms multiply in the lung and are then dispersed throughout the body, carried by the lymphatics of the lung to the thoracic duct into the general circulation. While phagocytic cells may ingest the organism, in the nonimmune host they often fail to destroy it. As a result, multiple small emboli of mycobacteria escape from their original pulmonary focus and are spread to various organs in the body, including the meninges.[2–4]

These metastatic mycobacteria form small tuberculids; in most instances, as immunity develops, they become dormant, regress, and become quiescent, usually for the life of the patient. In some instances, however, a tuberculid may persist, enlarge, and caseate. Caseation occurs as a part of the immune response, and only after the development of immunity in tuberculosis does the disease produce its classic pathologic picture of caseating granuloma containing epithelioid cells, macrophages, giant cells, and acid-fast bacilli, as are found in a typical tuberculous lesion.[2]

When the caseous contents of a tuberculid in a meninges leaks into the cerebral spinal fluid (CSF), the material dispersed contains a significant amount of mycobacterial antigen, as well as immunologically competent individual produces an intense immune reaction, not unlike the reaction to a large dose of purified protein derivative (PPD) in the skin of a PPD-positive person. As a result, severe inflammatory changes occur with accumulation of cells and the production of hyperemia, edema, capillary damage, and fibrosis. This inflammatory reaction damages nerves, blocks the circulation of CSF, and obstructs small blood vessels, which produces multiple cerebral infarcts. Because of the predilection of these changes for the basilar portion of the brain, the inflammatory reaction tends to interfere with the function of cranial nerves, to produce hydrocephalus and injure blood vessels in that area.[5–7]

Because of the diversity in these pathologic changes and differences in intensity, there can be a wide variation in the clinical presentation of TBM, and there can be a further variation in clinical presentation imposed by the immunologic status of the patient.

It has been known for over a quarter of a century that immunosuppression can modify, and even prevent, some sequelae of TBM.[8] If TBM were to occur in an immunosuppressed patient, a further modification of the clinical picture could arise and cause additional difficulties in establishing the diagnosis. In addition, it should also be mentioned that an intact tuberculoma, if sufficiently large and located in a crucial area, may produce localized symptoms and signs, as would any intracranial space-occupying lesion.[9–11] In this condition, the general inflammatory responses and the associated symptoms and signs noted in TBM can be absent.

The recent changes in the incidence and epidemiology of tuberculosis in the United States further underscore these observations.[12] As documented elsewhere in this book, tuberculosis has emerged as another, important complication of the acquired immunodeficiency syndrome (AIDS). Either typical or atypical mycobacteria can be present and involve the CNS.[13,14]

While the total number of cases of tuberculosis involving patients with AIDS in western nations is still small, the alarming incidence of AIDS in certain regions of Africa, coincident with a high prevalence of latent tuberculosis infection, will be a very serious public-health problem. Even in the United States, where the incidence of skin-test reactivity to tuberculin is rapidly approaching zero, certain localized areas have had remarkable increases in tuberculosis in immunosuppressed individuals.[15,16]

In immunosuppressed patients, the presentation, symptoms, signs, and progression of TBM may be very different from those in a patient with reasonably intact immunity. As a result, at least in a subset of patients who might have TBM, a very large element of uncertainty has been introduced. Even that simple marker for tuberculous infection, a positive reaction to intradermal tuberculin, may be absent, and the only reliable mechanism for identifying an infection in these circumstances is to identify the organism. Biopsy, another mechanism to identify tuberculous infection, is also less useful in immunosuppressed persons than in others, because the pathology is atypical.

Occurrence

In general, it can be said that in the developed countries, there has been a steady decline in the incidence of active tuberculosis for almost a century and that all forms of tuberculosis, including TBM, have reached the status of a rare disorder.[17]

Unfortunately, this is not entirely accurate. As mentioned above, there was a small but very disconcerting increase in reported cases of tuberculosis in the United States in 1987,[12] which appears to be connected to the prevalence of AIDS, especially in certain subsets of the population.[15] These changes were not dramatic and seem to be related to well-recognized social and medical problems, such as intravenous-drug abuse.[16] In other countries where AIDS is a very serious matter, the impact of AIDS on tuberculosis control may pose a very serious public-health question resistant to solution and have long-term implications for other nations. Any increase in the prevalence of tuberculosis will increase the incidence of skin-test conversion and attendant TBM. Considering the presence of isonizid-resistant organisms in some developing countries that also have a serious AIDS problem, there may also be an increase in the difficulty of treating tuberculosis, as compared with the current status of tuberculosis therapy.

As mentioned previously, a serious problem with tuberculous infection in patients with AIDS is the progressive disease produced by certain atypical mycobacteria, such as *Mycobacterium avium intracellularae* complex (MIC).[13,18] Atypical mycobacteria have been the cause of lung disease in patients with apparently normal immunity in the past with some frequency, but extrapulmonary infection in these individuals is rare. In immunosuppressed persons, MIC produced a widespread disseminated disease that is unresponsive to therapy. Despite the spread of the organisms throughout the body, meningeal involvement has been reported to be only a minor feature of this devastating situation.[18]

When CNS tuberculosis has occurred in patients with AIDS, it has been reported as a part of disseminated disease and appears as cerebral abscesses or tuberculomas,[19,20] and the usual manifestation of classical TBM are muted, obscured, or absent.

Bishburg and colleagues[21] have reported that in 4,200 patients with AIDS and the AIDS-related complex, 52 had tuberculosis in some form, ten of whom had CNS involvement. In most of the patients, there was cutaneous anergy to PPD and the presentation of their illnesses was modified by their immunosuppressed state. Most of these patients were intravenous-drug abusers, a group of individuals known to have a high risk of exposure to tuberculosis as well as the AIDS virus. Other studies have yielded similar results.[14,16]

Clinical Presentation

A tuberculoma usually presents with the symptoms of a space-occupying lesion. As a result, the clinical picture depends on the size and location of the tumor and the pressure it produces on adjacent structures. Headache, seizures, paralysis, personality changes, all symptoms compatible with a space-occupying lesion, may be seen.[10,11] Laboratory findings, including abnormalities in the CSF, may be minor and often absent, especially if the lesion is parenchymal. Elevation of CSF protein is common, but pleocytosis and low CSF sugars are rare unless the subarachnoid space is also involved. The PPD skin test should be positive unless immunosuppression is present.

Radiographic studies, including computerized axial tomography (CT scanning), are useful in establishing the presence of this space-occupying lesion, but identification of the lesion as a tuberculoma can be difficult and usually requires a high index of clinical suspicion. Attempts at biopsy or removal create the risk of contaminating the meninges but frequently must be carried out because of the inherent difficulties in establishing a definitive diagnosis. Coverage with antituberculous drugs and steroids may limit the risks incurred with a biopsy and these drugs probably should be used routinely in this situation. Removal of the mass, as opposed to biopsy, depends on the surgical risks involved.

TBM generally has an insidious onset.[6,7,17,22,23] Apathy, lethargy, headache, malaise, mental changes such as an inability to comprehend, personality changes, confusion, sometimes fever, and increasing obtundation are common presenting complaints. Seizures may occur, and symptoms of increased intracranial pressure, such as vomiting, may be present. Occasionally diplopia, photophobia, anorexia, neck stiffness, or speech problems predominate. The course of TBM before the patient seeks help is usually downhill, but occasionally there may be remissions and exacerbations of symptoms during this period.[22–25] These difficulties usually exist for days or weeks, but on occasion can develop more rapidly. There is evidence that an abrupt onset and rapid course of the disease are more common in children than in adults.[24]

Findings on physical examination can range in severity from no objective findings to an obtunded patient with multiple neurologic defects, depending on the stage of the disorder. Common findings are a blunted sensorium, a stiff neck, and cranial-nerve defects, particularly of the fourth (trochlear) nerve. The second (optic), third (oculomotor), sixth (abducens), and eighth (acoustic) cranial nerves may also be involved. Cerebellar and pyramidal tract signs may be present.[17,22]

Examination of the retina in patients with suspected TBM can be difficult because of poor cooperation, but the findings can be sufficiently important to warrant perseverance by the clinician. Papilledema, especially in the adult, may be the only indication of increased intracranial pressure, for example. In addition, patients with TBM occasionally have a retinal tuberculid, a small, grayish-white, choroidal nodule. This is an important finding[22] since it is highly suggestive of tuberculosis. These lesions are said to be more common in miliary disease than in other types of tuberculosis (up to 80% in one report) and as a result are not necessarily diagnostic of TBM.[26–28] Very occasionally, they can also be seen in pulmonary tuberculosis, usually during the hematogenous phase of a primary infection.

The remainder of the examination is usually limited to various neurologic defects related to the diffuse and patchy nature of the damage to the brain that can occur in TBM. Nystagmus or other features of cerebellar involvement may be noted.[17,24] Because the disorder is progressive, in the later stages of TBM, patients may develop decorticate or decerebrate posturing or the signs of cerebral herniation as a result of their increased intracranial pressure. Thus, the important considerations on physical examination are reasonably straightforward but variable. The salient features to look for in suspected TBM are the signs of meningitis, cranial-nerve damage, patchy neurologic defects, and signs of increased intracranial pressure.

Laboratory Diagnosis

The methods used in the laboratory diagnosis of TBM are not complex, but the definitive diagnosis can be difficult to establish. Because of the variety in the clinical presentations and its potential for misdiagnosis, it is one of those disorders that requires a high index of suspicion and clinical vigilance in order to obtain useful data to confirm the diagnosis.[22]

Although the patient's chest x-ray is often negative in TBM, it should be carefully evaluated. Klein and colleagues[7] found abnormalities suggestive of tuberculosis in 11 of 21 patients with TBM, at least retrospectively. In primary tuberculosis, the findings on chest X-ray often appear as a simple pneumonia, usually as a small infiltrate in a lower lobe. Hilar adenopathy may be present, especially in children. Occasionally, TBM may be present in patients with reactivation tuberculosis with the classical findings of a fibronodular infiltrate and cavities most commonly in the apical posterior portion of the upper lobe or in the superior segment of the lower lobe. A pleural effusion or a pleural scar suggestive of old pulmonary disease can be another useful clue to the diagnosis. If an effusion is present, a tap with a biopsy of the pleura should be done.

Miliary tuberculosis is difficult to identify on chest film unless it is specifically looked for by an experienced observer. It presents as a generalized fine nodular pattern.[28,29]. Remote inactive pulmonary disease usually appears as fibrotic scarring, calcification of regional lymph nodes, or as a primary complex (Ghon complex).

The tuberculin skin test is of limited diagnostic value. It is very useful if it is positive,[30] but it does not rule out TBM if it is negative. It must always be done when tuberculosis of any kind is suspected; and in TBM, it must be applied with the recognition that it is often negative despite the presence of active disease. Two studies have reported that approximately 40% of patients with TBM had a negative tuberculin test when using 5 TU of PPD.[31,32] If the 5-TU test is negative, it is useful to repeat the test with 250 TU (second-strength PPD), but frequently this test is also nonreactive[33] in TBM.

It is common practice to apply a tuberculin test with another skin test using an antigen of a type that is usually reactive in the normal general population. These control tests are used in an attempt to assess the state of delayed-type, cell-mediated immunity in these patients, and the results may have some value in the assessment of patients under consideration here.[33] Mumps and monilia antigens appear to be most commonly used for this purpose. Despite its widespread use, the data to support the value this practice are sparse. Even if a patient were found to have a positive mumps or monilia skin test and a negative reaction to second-strength PPD, the clinician could not eliminate TBM from the differential diagnosis.

Evidence has been presented to indicate that an initially negative reaction to tuberculin may become positive after therapy.[34] This sequence of events appears to be logical if one considers the course of the disorder. In the instances where the disease occurs as a part of a primary infection with mycobacteria, later testing may allow time for cell-mediated immunity to tuberculin to develop. In other instances, individuals whose skin test has been suppressed because of the severity of their illness or other medical problems should have sufficient improvement in their general condition to allow their suppressed cell-mediated immunity to be restored. In cases where therapy has been instituted without the confirmation of the diagnosis by biopsy or bacteriologic examination, a positive PPD skin test obtained after a few weeks of treatment would be of very considerable diagnostic importance and a significant inducement to continue therapy in a patient who is also improving on appropriate antituberculous therapy.[35,36]

The PPD skin test can be suppressed as a part of overwhelming tuberculosis, in malnutrition, as a side effect of immunosuppressive drugs, irradiation, or as the result of certain tumors, particularly the lymphomas, or of some of the viral exanthems such as measles.[33–35,37] Suppression may not be complete, but it may be sufficient to diminish the size of the reaction to a point where the clinician considers it negative. It has been generally accepted that the PPD test is positive if the diameter of the induration at the test site is greater than 10 mm, but the clinician should remember that this criterion is not absolute. Any swelling at the test site should be measured and recorded in the chart, and its presence and size should be weighed in the differential diagnosis. While a weakly positive test or a reaction to second-strength PPD can be the result of previous exposure to atypical mycobacteria and of little diagnostic value, one should also remember that the weak reaction may represent the most vigorous response the patient's immune system can develop under the stress of TBM, immunosuppressive drugs, lymphoma, or AIDS.

Cerebrospinal Fluid

An examination of the spinal fluid is usually the most valuable diagnostic procedure in TBM. Although the results may not be definitive, the basic studies are simple, use commonly available equipment, and can be repeated as often as needed to either establish the diagnosis or follow the progress of therapy.[24,38]

As in any instance where an increased intracranial pressure may exist, a spinal puncture carries some risk of herniation, but it meningitis is suspected, the procedure must be done regardless of risk. The physician should be aware of the complications of a spinal puncture, use suitable precautions, and obtain informed consent.

Spinal fluid in TBM is usually a clear or slightly opalescent fluid under increased pressure with an elevated CSF protein, as may be found in a number of other intracranial diseases. In individuals with a tuberculoma of the CNS, as opposed to meningitis, this may be all that is found.[9,10]

When tubercle bacilli and their cellular products are first leaked into the CSF, segmented cells, or polymorpholeukocytes, often appear initially, usually in low to moderate numbers. These are replaced by mononuclear cells within a few days, and this cell type is the one classically found in TBM. The cell count is usually in the low hundreds and seldom above 1,000 cells/mm^3.

The initial appearance of polymorpholeukocytes in the CSF of some patients with TBM may be a significant trap for the unwary and illustrates the degree of caution and perseverance needed to evaluate patients suspected of having TBM, as well as the importance of not relying on a single spinal puncture in suspected cases when the initial evaluation is inconclusive.

CSF glucose is low in TBM, often less than half of normal, in the range of 45–50 mg/dl.[7,17,22–24] CSF glucose should be determined after the CSF and blood glucose levels have had an opportunity to equilibrate, and a blood glucose should always be simultaneously obtained to allow comparison with the CSF value. A useful rule of thumb is to consider the normal CSF glucose values as greater than half the level of the serum. A ratio of CSF to blood glucose below 1:2 is a significant abnormality, particularly if the CSF value is marginally low. In addition, a small percentage of individuals with TBM may have CSF glucose levels that are in the normal range, particularly during the early stages of the disease. In one series, over 10% had levels above 50 mg/dl, and in another study four of 21 patients had CSF sugar above 60 mg/dl.[7,20,24,38] The presence of hyperglycemia, a glucose infusion, or the administration of insulin can obscure the diagnosis by causing rapid changes in serum glucose levels, and these problems must be considered in the evaluation of the CSF findings.

The presence of acid-fast bacilli (AFB) in the CSF should be diagnostic for the disease. Unfortunately, AFB can be found in the CSF on smear only in a small minority of the patients who have subsequently been shown to have TBM.[39] Klein and coworkers[7] have reported that in a major teaching hospital, only four positive smears for AFB was found in 36 examinations of spinal fluid submitted from 21 patients with TBM. This fact is not surprising. The number of bacilli, usually present in the CSF in tuberculous meningitis is never large,[1] the volume of the sample obtained at tap for examination is small, and the fraction of the sample viewed through an oil-immersion lens is minuscule. Centrifugation of the CSF to concentrate the bacilli in a sediment is helpful, and a diligent examination of the stained slides by a skilled microbiologist is essential.[14] The technique of placing a drop of unconcentrated CSF on a slide that is then stained and briefly examined by an inexperienced observer is not satisfactory.

Unfortunately, the reduction in the incidence of tuberculosis has been accompanied by a general decline in clinical microbiologists' in mycobacteriology. This decline has imposed an additional handicap for the physician, who must make a prompt and accurate diagnosis of TBM based on the evaluation of the spinal fluid. The routine submission of all specimens of CSF for AFB to the laboratory, especially as a part of the routine evaluation of immunosuppressed patients, also has created problems. Identification of mycobacteria on smears is difficult and time consuming, and also requires diligence, with a high resistance to boredom. A continuous succession of negative specimens will certainly lead to the boredom and reduce the diligence. The automatic submission of spinal-fluid specimens to a laboratory for acid-fast smear and mycobacterial culturing when there is little or no suspicion of the disease must be discouraged.

Cultures of the CSF for mycobacteria in suspected TBM are of limited value since they are retrospective. Unfortunately, four to eight weeks are needed for cultures to become positive because of the slow in vitro growth of *Mycobacterium tuberculosis*. Reports indicate that 50–80% of cases of TBM have positive CSF cultures.[6,7,17,22]

Allowing the CSF to stand overnight in a sterile test tube may lead to the formation of a small wisplike pellicle in the bottom of the tube that can be seen if the tube is rotated abruptly in a circular manner. This pellicle can be transferred onto a slide, stained, and examined for AFB. It has been said that this procedure can increase the incidence of positive smears. If a larger volume of CSF is submitted to centrifugation, the likelihood of finding AFB on smears, if they are present, is increased.

The measurement of the CSF chloride is no longer considered to be of diagnostic value in TBM, and it is a good example of a formerly used test that is now recognized to be dependent on metabolic factors unrelated to the infection.

The widespread availability of CT has provided another valuable diagnostic instrument for the evaluation of patients with suspected TBM.[40–42] While it cannot establish the diagnosis of TBM, it can be used to rule out other serious CNS diseases in patients who have an obscure illness or evidence of increased intracranial pressure. The tomogram in TBM with contrast enhancement often shows dilated ventricles, an exudate with thickened meninges, particularly in the basilar areas of the brain. The vasculitis and thrombosis associated with TBM are seen on CT scan as multiple areas of radiolucency secondary to ischemia. These changes are usually located in the basil ganglia and adjacent to the sylvian fissure (Figure 16.1).

Another technique useful in TBM that has become increasingly available in the United States and other developed countries is magnetic-resonance imaging (MRI). It has a significant advantage over CT because it allows better visualization of the base of the brain, where TBM is most likely to occur. (See Figure 16.2.)

It has been reported[44] that TBM produces focal infarcts with circumscribed edges, usually in gray matter, together with thickened meninges, often at the base of the brain, with dilated ventricles. White-matter infarcts and infarction of the midbrain and brain stem are also visible. Obstruction of CSF circulation can be identified and followed, and the response to therapy quantified.

While these findings, both CT and MRI, can be produced by a variety of other infectious meningeal diseases such as cryptococcal meningitis,[45] they are sufficiently distinct to add useful information and may allow the clinician enough information to institute chemotherapy, obtain tissue by craniotomy, or install a shunt.

Meningeal biopsy is another approach to establishing the diagnosis of TBM by obtaining tissue and submitting the specimen to the laboratory for histologic and bacterial study. Although this procedure may seem overly aggressive, one should remember that in some instances, particularly where immunosuppressive drugs have been used, the diagnosis of TBM can be difficult and a delay in therapy can be followed by deterioration of the condition of the patient and permanent CNS damage.

There are other tests that have been offered as helpful for diagnosing TBM. One of these, the bromide partition test, once held to be of value in the early diagnosis of TBM, never became widely used and is no longer considered useful.[17] This procedure measures the permeability of the blood–brain barrier by comparing CSF and blood bromide ion and noting their ratio. The test can also be done with radioactive bromide. Since the blood–brain barrier

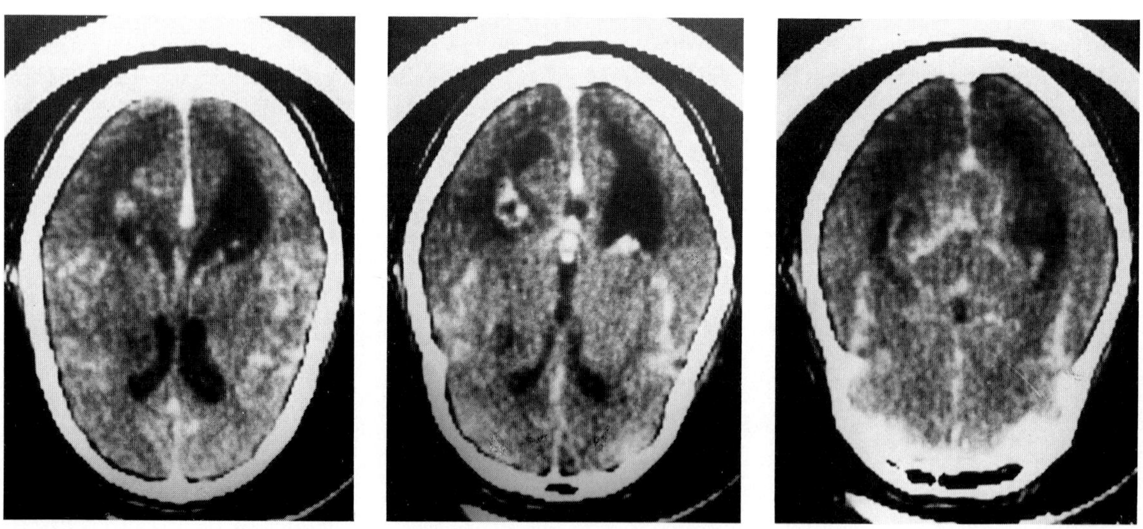

Fig. 16.1. CT scans of an adult with TBM. Note the enlarged ventricles indicating internal hydrocephalis. There is contrast enhancement of the gyral patterns, sylvian fissures, cerebral convolutions, and thickening of the meninges, especially at the base of the brain. [Reprinted with permission from Kasik JE: p. 92 In Schlossberg, D (ed.). *Tuberculosis,* 2nd ed. (In the series *Clinical Topics in Infectious Diseases*. New York, Springer-Verlag, 1987.]

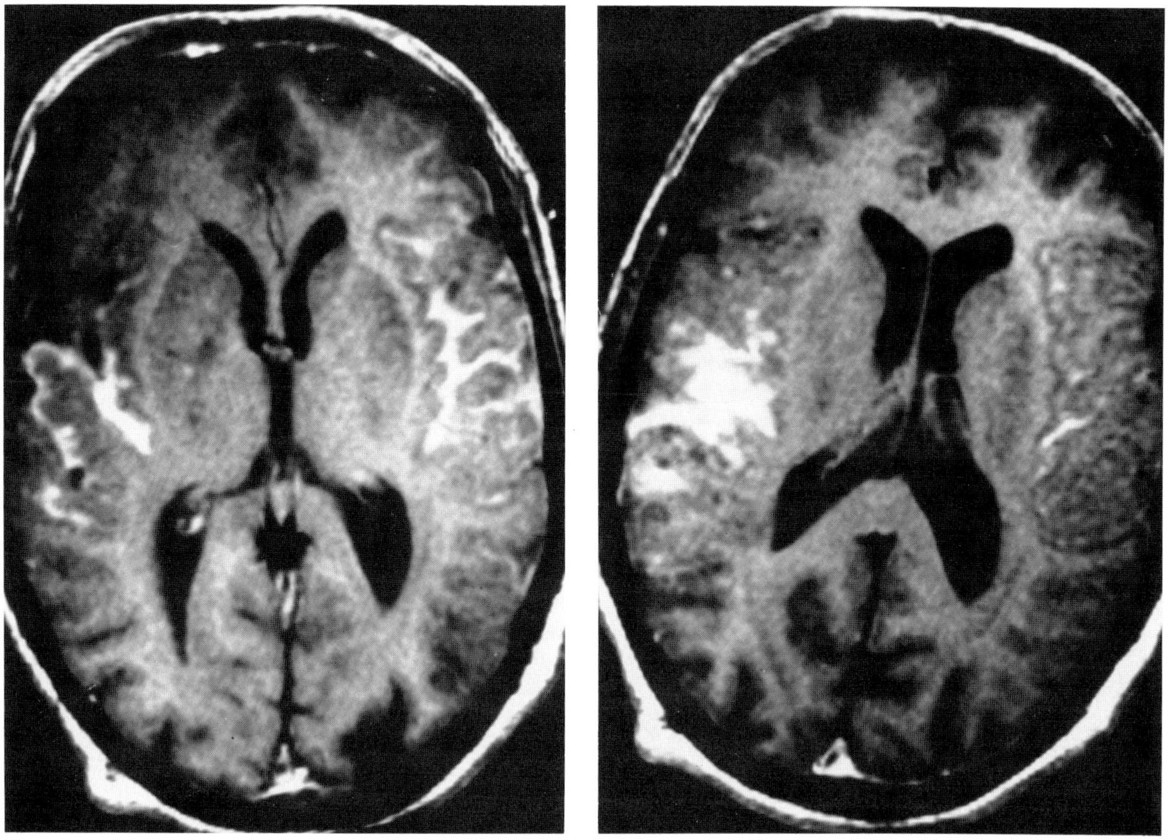

A B

Fig. 16.2. A 33-year-old male institutional patient presented with fever and rapid change of mental status. (A) Axial T1-weighted image obtained immediately after intravenous injection of gadolinium contrast medium (gadolinium/diethylenetriamine pentoacetic acid shows bilateral leptomeningeal enhancement, especially in the region of sylvian fissure. Effacement of the cortical gyrus is also noted. Linear dural/meningeal enhancement is again demonstrated. (B) Axial image 1.5 cm cranial to (A) shows intraparenchymal involvement near the temporoparietal lobe.

should be intact in viral meningitis, this test could discriminate between these infections and others such as TBM. Unfortunately, in practice, the discrimination of this test is less than perfect, and its value is obscured by the fact that other infections of the CNS, such as crypotoccal and bacterial meningitis, also disturb memingeal permeability.

Since cryptococcal meningitis is a clinical problem that can be as difficult to diagnose at TBM and can be confused with that disorder,[44] the successful development of a diagnostic test that identifies cryptococcal antigen in the CNS has proved very useful. It has also increased interest in developing tests to identify mycobacterial antigen in CSF, and this effort appears to have been rewarding.

These newer tests are largely serodiagnostic in nature, either detecting antimycobacterial antibodies in sera or mycobacterial antigen in specimens of body fluid. In the instance of TBM, the detection of mycobacterial antibodies in blood would be helpful.[46]

The same kind of assay, using CSF, has been reported to be of greater value[46–48] than tests using blood. Using an enzyme-linked immunoabsorbent assay (ELISA) to both CSF mycrobial antigen and antibodies, it has been reported that the assay was rapid and specific, with a low false-positive rate.[48] Latex agglutination tests have also been reported to be useful.[49,50]

Another approach that has been claimed to be of help is the determination of adenosine deaminase activity in CSF.[51] The adenosine deaminase is apparently largely derived from thymus-dependent lymphocytes (T cells), which might be a problem if the individual were leukopenic or had AIDS. One very small study in patients with both AIDS and TBM has been reassuring in this regard since this test was positive despite low lymphocyte counts.[51]

All of these new tests appear promising, but their usefulness is limited because of their unavailability, especially in geographic areas with a high incidence of TBM. As stated earlier, general interest in TBM is very low in the developed countries because of its rarity. It is not unusual for hospital laboratories to screen hundreds, or even thousands, of specimens for CSF mycobacteria without yield. Introduction of new tests may be restricted because of a perceived lack of need.

Differential Diagnosis

The list of diseases that should be considered in the differential diagnosis of TBM is long, but in reality the number of those that create major diagnostic problems for the clinician is limited. Certain groups of clinical problems can be discarded using simple, well-defined criteria[22] (see Tables 16.1 and 16.2).

For example, acute bacterial meningitis such as a meningococcal infection can be included in the differential diagnosis of TBM, but bacterial infections usually occur as acute illnesses with large numbers of polymorphic leukocytes and identifiable bacteria in the CSF. In general, this diagnosis can also be almost completely eliminated from consideration by the patient's history and results of culture of the CSF. Partially treated bacterial meningitis can be a diagnostic problem on some occasions, but again the type of cells in the CSF, the history, and an element of caution on the part of the clinician should suffice to identify this problem. Another bacterial illness that can be a more serious problem is subacute bacterial endocarditis (SBE), which often results in multiple mycotic arterial emboli that produce successive infected infarcts of the brain that mimic some of the findings in TBM. The disease is associated with low-grade fever and meningeal signs. In this instance, the symptoms and signs of SBE, such as a heart murmur and evidence of mycotic emboli elsewhere, should be evident. The CSF sugar should be normal unless there is a cerebral abscess that has contaminated the subarachnoid space. Echocardiography of heart valves and blood cultures would identify this abscess in most instances.

Table 16.1. Differential diagnosis for TBM.

Infectious	Fungal (cryptococcal, histoplasmosis, etc.)
	Viral (herpes, mumps, encephalitis, et al)
	Bacterial (partially treated, brain abscess, leptospirosis
	Trypanosomal
Vascular	Multiple emboli, subacute bacterial meningitis, thrombosis of sagital vein
Collagen vascular	Lupis erythematosis, polyarteritis, other collagen vascular diseases
Other meningeal diseases	Sarcoid, metastatic carcinoma, lymphoma, acute hemorrhagic leukoencephalopathy

Table 16.2. Points to stress in evaluating a patient with suspected TBM.

Medical and social history
1. History of significant tuberculosis contact or residence in an area with a high incidence of tuberculosis.
2. A known history of positive PPD skin test, especially a recent conversion.
3. A history of diseases or therapy associated with immunosuppression.
4. Absence of a history of baullus Colmette-Guérin (BCG) immunization.

Physical examination
1. Search for BCG scar.
2. Funded examination for tuberculids and papilledema.
3. Neurologic examination, with special reference to signs of meningeal irritation, state of consciousness, and demonstration of focal signs.

Laboratory
1. Hematocrit, hemoglobin, urinalysis, sedimentation rate, serology for syphilis, 6/60, 12/60, complement fixation test (or equivalent) for fungal infections.
2. Chest x-ray, CT scan of head, MRI.
3. Spinal puncture
   a. Manometrics.
   b. Gross inspection.
   c. Specimens for cell count, differential, and cytology.
   d. CSF glucose with a simultaneous blood sugar. Avoid administration of high concentrations of glucose for two or four hours before the tap.
   e. CSF protein.
   f. Specimen for AFB smear and culture. Gram stain of smear and appropriate bacteriologic culture.
   g. Fluid for India-ink preparation and appropriate assay for cryptococcal and herpes antigen.
   h. Submit specimen for mycobacterial antigen analysis where available.
   i. CSF for syphilis serology.
4. Tuberculin skin test 5 TU;/ if negative, apply 250 TU.

The major clinical problems that must be seriously considered in the differential diagnosis of TBM are the viral and fungal infections of the CNS and infiltration of the meninges by metastatic carcinoma, particularly a lymphoma, or leukemic cells.

Viral infections of the CNS must always be considered in the differential diagnosis of TBM. Viral meningoencephalitis can be caused by herpes simplex, mumps, or eastern equine encephalitis, and has been reported to be sometimes associated with a low CSF sugar. Herpes encephalitis produces focal neurologic deficits, CSF lymphocytosis, and seizures. This disorder can be difficult to eliminate from consideration without a biopsy of the brain. The facts that antiviral therapy for this serious disease has been found to be effective and that both tuberculosis and this viral infection can be opportunistic diseases are factors that must be added to the recommendation that obtaining a biopsy of the brain and meninges may be prudent on some occasions.

While fungal infections of the CNS are rare, they are becoming more common since they are one of the many infectious complications of immunosuppression. They, like TBM, are associated with a low sugar and the appearance of lymphocytes in the CSF. The key points in eliminating this group of infections from consideration in this context would appear to be to consider the history, to search for a potential source of fungal infection, and to identify the organism in the CSF on smear, by culture, or by appropriate serologic tests. Cryptococcal meningitis is an excellent example. It mimics the clinical picture of TBM,[44] including the history of relatively slow progression with occasional partial remissions and the CSF findings. It can be identified by obtaining appropriate cultures or by performing an India-ink preparation of a centrifugal specimen of CSF and obtaining an immunoassay for cryptococcal antigen. The latter test has been shown to be very useful.

Ambic infections, rickettsial diseases, trypanosomiasis, echinococcus, or leptospirosis might be considered in the differential of TBM, but only in unusual circumstances. Again, a history of exposure to the organism and the spinal-fluid findings should be helpful in deciding to do so. Other disorders to remember in the differential diagnosis of TBM are the collagen vascular diseases, sarcoidosis with involvement of the meninges (associated with a low spinal-fluid sugar on occasion), venous thrombosis of superior longitudinal sinus, and neurosyphilis. These possibilities should be dealt with by evaluating the history, doing appropriate laboratory testing, and, in the case of a suspected venous thrombosis, obtaining an angiogram or MRI scan.

In those instances where there is meningeal involvement by a malignant tumor or a lymphoma or leukemic infiltration is suspected, a CSF cytology can be very helpful in establishing a diagnosis. It should be recalled that malignant involvement of the meninges often produces a low CSF glucose and the cells of the tumor can be misidentified as lymphocytes.

Acute hemorrhagic necrotizing leukoencephalitis, a rare and special condition, may be associated with meningeal signs, a low CSF sugar, and pleocytosis. It presents clinically as an acute, rapidly progressive disorder without the more protracted features of TBM. It is also reported to produce a lower CSF protein value in association with internal hydroenphalus than does TBM. Because it has been reported as a complication of leukemia, lymphomas, sarcoidosis, and immunosuppressive therapy, it could be confused with TBM in certain instances.

Clinical Course and Prognosis

The result of untreated TBM is the death of the patient, usually in four to six weeks. While there were sporadic reports of survivors in the era before specific antituberculous therapy, these cases were reported because of their distinct rarity. Patients with CNS tuberculosis can have temporary partial remissions of their symptoms, but their usual course is downhill with worsening of their condition and increasing disability. The partial improvement in the patient's condition can be another trap for the unwary since it may mimic the expected clinical course of other infections producing meningitis where recovery is expected. This may lead to delays in the diagnosis of a disease whose prognosis is adversely affected by delays in therapy.

In the recent past, treated meningeal tuberculosis has been reported to have an overall mortality of between 15 and 30%.[7,52–54] Unfortunately, residual damage is common in the survivors.

The prognosis for the patient with TBM, either death or severe and permanent brain damage, has been clearly related to the patient's status at the time therapy is initiated. Here, the critical factor is the level of consciousness on admission and the number of evident focal neurologic signs noted before effective therapy is begun.[7,24,52] Since it is usual for patients with TBM to have continued worsening of their symptoms, at least for some days after the initiation of adequate chemotherapy, those admitted with severe CNS damage will have much poorer prognosis. The multiple infarctions of the brain, the inflammatory exudate, and the associated nerve damage are often permanent and illustrate the widely held opinion that a patient with serious neurologic deficits on admission will probably be left with serious residual cerebral nervous damage. Patients who are obtunded on admission have a very poor prognosis.

Assessment of the sequelae of patients who have recovered from TBM has indicated that postinfection cranial-nerve palsies, blindness, seizures, impairment of cognitive function, and hydrocephalus are common. These reports[7,27,52,54] indicate that overall about half of patients with TBM who survive will have some residual damage.

Taken together, the incidence of serious sequelae of this infection and the clear correlation between the amount of CNS damage evident at the time appropriate chemotherapy is started emphasize the need for prompt initiation of adequate chemotherapy whenever the diagnosis of TBM is seriously considered. In view of the penalties that result if there is a delay in treatment of TBM, if an error is to be tolerated in treatment, it should be the error of instituting early chemotherapy while continuing efforts to establish a definitive diagnosis.[7,17,55]

Therapy of TBM

The chemotherapy of TBM is, in most circumstances, simple and straightforward. Since the number of tuberculous organisms involved in TBM are small, two-drug therapy is usually sufficient. At present, isoniazid (INH), 300 mg a day (in adults), and 600 mg rifampin, are sufficient. Therapy using more than two drugs can be limited to infections with suspected drug-resistant organisms or atypical mycobacterial infections.

In comatose individuals, injectible INH and, soon to be available, parenteral rifampin can be used. In the absence of injectible drugs, oral drugs by nasogastric tube can be used. Injectible streptomycin and ethambutal, in parenteral form, are available and are suitable companion drugs to INH. Adjunctive therapy is also important in TBM.

Intrathecal PPD tuberculin, commonly used for skin testing of tuberculosis exposure, has been used to limit the destructive inflammatory response in TBM that is the cause of much of the damage to the CNS. This is a relatively old idea[8,56] and has been fairly well documented as being effective.[57] In light of more recent understanding of immunology, the effect of intrathecal PPD would appear to be related to producing an antigen overload in the CSF and suppressing the immune reaction. Limitation of the immune reaction and its inflammatory response and prevention of internal hydrocephalus would be very useful.[58]

Despite these known benefits, the use of intrathecal PPD as adjunct therapy has declined, and there is little enthusiasm for it at present. There is no question that its administration is complicated, and there are concerns about its safety,[59] a factor that may explain its current lack of popularity. In addition, other immunosuppressive drugs have become available. These anti-inflammatory, immunosuppressive drugs should have the same effect as PPD if used appropriately. Steroids have been widely employed in this context, particularly in cerebral edema, as, for example, dexamethasone in patients with head injuries.

Although the use of steroids in TBM has been widely advocated, no definitive, well-controlled study has demonstrated a clear response to such use. Anecdotal evidence suggests that they reduce the inflammatory response and prevent CSF block. Certainly, steroids are known to suppress both immunity and inflammation, an action that would be desirable in patients with TBM if it could be achieved. Against their use are the known complications of steriods in large doses, especially in complex clinical situation such as meningitis where the diagnosis may not have been established. In general, it seems best to use steroids and accept the risk, especially if the situation appears fairly clear and the patient's condition is critical. Prednisone, 60 mg/day, given in two divided doses, is usually employed in adults[60] and then tapered over a period of weeks as the patient improves. Diuretics also may be useful.

In general, other supportive measures in TBM are those normally used in severely ill patients, including careful fluid management, protection of the airway, and support of ventilation. Anticonvulsant therapy may be necessary. It should be recalled that inappropriate antidiuretic hormone (ADH) production often occurs in TBM. Fluid restriction and diuretics may be helpful in this case.

It should be pointed out that TBM is not contagious unless obvious simultaneously active pulmonary disease is present. The care of such patients is greatly simplified if they are not kept in unnecessary isolation.

Other Mycobacteria

TBM produced by species of mycobacteria other than *M tuberculosis* has been reported in people with presumed normal immunity, most commonly *Mycobacterium kansasii*.[61] Unfortunately, these rare mycobacterial infections can be identified only on culture, and probably could not be identified until the patient had either survived on conventional chemotherapy or died. Most species of the so-called atypical mycobacteria are resistant to conventional chemotherapy, but clinical treatment of pulmonary tuberculosis caused by *M. kansasii* with INH and rifampin has had reasonable results despite this species' frequently demonstrating in vitro resistance to these drugs. The problem of MIC infections has not been solved although several new drugs have been introduced, and the prognosis remains very poor when they occur in patients with HIV infection.[14,15]

Drug Resistance

There have been reports of cases of TBM involving organisms resistant to one or more of the commonly used antituberculous drugs. This situation usually arises when a child or a nonimmune adult is exposed to a patient with infectious tuberculosis who is excreting a strain of mycobacterium resistant to one or more antituberculous agents. As a result, the primary infection and subsequent meningeal disease would involve resistant organisms.

Identification of this serious condition is not easy. A careful history of the patient's tuberculous contacts must always be obtained and evaluated. An example of such a contact would be an alcoholic person who had been in and out of tuberculosis therapy for many years and who recently has been living in the same home with the patient.

If there is a suspicion of this problem, initial therapy for TBM should include at least two drugs to which there is reasonable evidence that the organism is sensitive. This sensitivity can be ascertained by carefully evaluating the contact's history, including drug therapy, and obtaining the most recent drug-sensitivity profile from the source case, if available.

Acknowledgment. The author wishes to acknowledge the help of E. A. Franken, Jr., M.D., and Frank M. Behkle, M.D., in providing the CT scans, and of William T. C. Yuh, M.D., for the MRI reproductions. He also wishes to express his gratitude for the help of Patricia K. Foster with the manuscript.

References

1. Rich AR: *The Pathogenesis of Tuberculosis,* 2nd ed. Springfield, Ill, Charles C Thomas, 1951.
2. Myers JA: The natural history of tuberculosis in the human body. *JAMA* 1965;194:1084–1092.
3. Stead WW: Pathogenesis of the sporadic cases of tuberculosis. *N Eng J Med* 1967;227:1008–1012.
4. Stead WW, Kenby GR, Schleuter DP, Jordahl A: The clinical spectrum of primary tuberculosis. *Ann Int Med* 1968;68:731–745
5. Rich AR, McCord HA: The pathogenesis of tuberculous meningitis. *Bull Johns Hopkins Hosp* 1933; 52:5–27.
6. Meyes, BR: 1982; Tuberculous meningitis. *Med Clin North Am* 66:155–162.
7. Klein NC, Damskr B, Hirschman SZ. Mycobacterial meningitis: retrospective analysis 1970 to 1983. *Am J Med* 1985;79:29–34.
8. Smith HV, Vollum RL: Effects of inthrathecal tuberculin and streptomycin in tuberculous meningitis. *Lancet* 1950;2:275–286.
9. Descuns P, Garre H, Pheline C: Tuberculoma of the brain and cerebellum. *J Neurosurg* 1954;11:243–250.
10. Demergis JA, Liftwitch EL, Curtin JA, Witorsch P: Tuberculoma of the brain. *JAMA* 1978;239:413–415.
11. Hildebrant G, Agnoli AL: Differential diagnosis and therapy of intracerebral tuberculomas. *J Neurol* 1982;118:201–208.
12. Rieder HL, Couthen GM,, Kelly GD, et al: Tuberculosis in the United States: Mortality and morbidity. *JAMA* 262:385–389.
13. Kelhn TE, Edward FF, Brannen P, et al: Infections caused by *Mycobacterium avium* complex in immunocompromised patients. *J Clin Microbiol* 1985; 21:168–173.
14. Rieder HJ, Cauthen GM, Block AB, et al: Tuberculosis and acquired immunodeficiency syndrome—Florida *Arch Intern Med* 1989;149:1268–1273.
15. Stoneburner RL, Des Jarlais DC, Deneza D, et al: A larger spectrum of severe HIV_1-related disease in IV drug users. *Science* 1988;242:916–918.
16. Selwyn PA, Hartel D, Lewis VA, et al: A prospective study of the risk of tuberculosis among intravein drug abuses with immunodeficiency virus infection. *N Eng J Med* 1989;320:545–550.
17. Molovi A, LeFock JL: Tuberculous meningitis. *Med Clin North Am* 1985;69:315–331.

18. Hawkin CC, Gold JWM, Whimbey E, et al: Mycobacterium avium complex infection in patients with acquired immunodeficiency syndrome *Ann Int Med* 1986;105:184–188.
19. Sunderam G, McDonald RJ, Manatis T, et al: Tuberculosis as a manifestation of the acquired immunodeficiency syndrome (AIDS). *JAMA* 1986;256: 362–366.
20. Mann J, Sinder D, Francis H, et al: Association between HTLV III/LAV infection and tuberculosis in Zaire (letter to editor). *JAMA* 1986;256:346.
21. Bishburg E, Sunderam G, Reichman L, Kapila R: Central nervous system tuberculosis with acquired immunodeficiency and its related complex. *Ann Int Med* 1986;105:210–213.
22. Parsons M: Diagnosis not to be missed, tuberculosis meningitis. *Br J Hosp Med* 1982;27:682–684.
23. Crocco JA, Bleckel MJ, Rooney JJ, et al: Tuberculous meningitis in adults, *NY State J Med* 1980; 80:1231–1234.
24. Dostur KD, Lalitha VS: The many facets of neurotuberculosis: an epitome of neuropathology. *Prog Neuropathol* 1973;2:351–408.
25. Castleman B (ed.): Weekly clinicopathological exercise. *N Eng J Med* 1974;290:1130–36.
26. Illingsworth RS, Wright T: Tubercles of the choroid. *Br Med J* 1948;2:365–370.
27. Kocen RS, Parsons M: The neurological complications of tuberculosis: some unusual manifestations. *Q J Med* 1970;34:17–31.
28. Munt PW: Miliary tuberculosis in the chemotherapy area. *Medicine* 1971;51:139–155.
29. Gelb AF, Leffler C, Brewin A, et al: Miliary tuberculosis. *Am Rev Respir Dis* 1973;108:1327–1333.
30. Kasik JE, Schuldt S: Why tuberculosis is still a health problem in the aged. *Geriatrics* 1977;3:63–72.
31. Haas EJ, Modhaven T, Quinn EL, et al: Tuberculous meningitis in an urban general hospital. *Arch Int Med* 1977;137:1518–1521.
32. Fitzsimons JM: Tuberculous meningitis: a followup study on 198 cases. *Tubercle* 1963;44:87–102.
33. Barret-Connor, E: Tuberculous meningitis in adults. *South Med J* 1967;60:1061–1067.
34. Rooney JJ, Crocco JA, Kramer S, Lyons HA: Further observations on tuberculin reactions in active tuberculosis. *Am J Med* 1976;60:517–522.
35. Schacter EH: Tuberculin negative tuberculosis. *Am Rev Respir Dis* 1972; 106:587–593.
36. Grieco MH, Chmel H: Acute disseminated tuberculosis as a diagnostic problem. *Am Rev Respir Dis* 1974;109:554–560.
37. Collins FM: The immunology of tuberculosis. *Am Rev Respir Dis* 1982;125:42–49.
38. Seren T, Beus I: Characteristics of cerebral spinal fluid in tuberculous meningitis. *Acta Cytol* 1982; 26:678–680.
39. Kennedy DH, Fallon RJ: Tuberculous meningitis. *JAMA* 1979;241:264.
40. Teah R, Humphries MJ, Hoare RD, O'Mahony G: Clinical correlation of CT changes in 64 Chinese patients with tuberculous meningitis. *J Neuro* 1989; 236:48–51.
41. Nai-Shin C. Tuberculous meningitis. Computerized tomographic manifestations. *Arch Neurol* 1980; 37:458–460.
42. Bullock MR: Diagnostic and prognostic features of tuberculous meningitis on CT scanning. *J Neurol Neurosurg Psychiatry* 1982;45:1098–1101.
43. Price HI, Danziger A: Computerized tomograph in cranial tuberculosis. *Am J Roentgenol* 1978;130:769–771.
44. Schoeman J, Hewlett R, Donald P: MR of childhood tuberculous mengingitis. *Neuroradiol* 1988;30:473–477.
45. Stockstill MT, Kauffman CA. Comparison of cryptococcal and tuberculous meningitis. *Arch Neurol* 1983;40:81–85.
46. Daniels TM: Antibody and antigen detection of immunodiagnosis of tuberculosis. Why not, What more is needed, Where do we stand. *J Infect Dis* 1988; 158:678–680.
47. Soda E, Ruiz-Palacios GM, Lopez-Vidal Y: Detection of mycobacterial antigens in cerebral spinal fluid of patients with tuberculous meningitis by enzyme-linked immunoabsorbant assay. *Lancet* 1983;2:651–652.
48. Duboczy BO, White FC: Latex agglutination test for tuberculosis. *Am Rev Respir Dis* 1986;94:94–98.
49. Watt G, Zaraspe G, Boutista S, Laughlin L: Rapid diagnosis of tuberculous meningitis by using an enzyme-linked immunoabstract assay to detect mycobacterial antigen and antibody in cerebral spinal fluid. *J Infect Dis* 1988;158:681–686.
50. Rebera E, Martinez-Vasquez JM, Ocana I, et al: Activity of adenosine deaminase in cerebral spinal fluid for diagnosis and followup of tuberculous meningitis in adults. *J Infect Dis* 1987;155:603–607.
51. Era J, Crespo MJ, Valls V, De Salamanca RE: Adenosine deaminase activity in cerebral spinal fluid: a useful test for meningeal tuberculosis, even patients with AIDS. *J Infect Dis* 1988;158:896.
52. Shah AK, Gandhi VK: Prognosis of tubercular meningitis. *Indian Pediat* 1984;21:791–795.
53. Kennedy DH: Tuberculous meningitis (letter). *Lancet* 1981;1:261.
54. Fallon RJ, Kennedy DH: Treatment and prognosis in tuberculous meningitis. 1981;3:39–44.
55. Kasik JE: Tuberculosis and other mycobacterial diseases, in Rakel RE (ed): Conn's Current Therapy. Philadelphia, WB Saunders, 1984, p 125.
56. Smith HV, Vollum RL: The treatment of tuberculous meningitis. *Tubercle* 1956;37:301–320.

57. Acheson RM, Smith RV: Radiological technique in the management of tuberculous meningitis. *Q J Med* 1958;27:83–101.
58. Lorber J: Treatment of tuberculous meningitis. *Br Med J* 1960;1:1309–1312.
59. American Trudeau Society: A statement by the Committee on Therapy: tuberculous meningitis. *Am Rev Tubc* 1970;70:756–758.
60. Weg JG: Tuberculosis and other mycobacterial disease, in Conn WE (ed): *Conn's Current Therapy* Philadelphia, WB Saunders Co, 1981, p 137.
61. Wolinsky E: Nontuberculous mycobacterial infections of man. *Med Clin N Am* 1974;58:639–648.

17
Cryptococcal and Other Fungal Infections of the Central Nervous System

PAUL D. HOEPRICH

Any fungus that becomes blood-borne might be expected to lodge in the central nervous system (CNS) and cause disease. Yet, only relatively few fungi cause infections of the CNS with sufficient frequency to merit thorough consideration. For example, in 8,975 complete autopsies carried out from 1964 to 1976 in the southeastern United States,[1] *Candida* spp accounted for 19 of 39 cerebral mycoses. However, candidosis of the CNS is rarely diagnosed premortem despite the fact that candidemia is the most common fungemia.[2] In this chapter, discussion will be limited to the three most frequent mycoses of the CNS in the United States—those caused by *Cryptococcus neoformans,* Zygomycetes, and *Coccidioides immitis*.

Cryptococcal Infections of the CNS

Mycology

Although there are at least seven species in the genus *Cryptococcus,* infections in humans are almost always caused by *C neoformans* (and very rarely, and only in immunocompromised persons, by *Cryptococcus albidus* and *Cryptococcus laurentii*). Cryptococci are primarily saprobes, and infection of humans and other mammals is a dead end.[3,4]

As they cause disease, *C neoformans* are yeastlike, haploid, anamorphic (asexual, imperfect) fungi composed of two varieties: *C neoformans* var *neoformans* and *C neoformans* var *gattii*.[3] There has been laboratory demonstration of a diploid, teleomorphic (sexual, perfect) form shown to arise only from intravariety mating, yielding basidiospores—*Filobasidiella neoformans*[5] (Table 17.1).

In clinical specimens, and as isolated in the clinical laboratory, *C neoformans* measure 3.5–7.0 μm by 3.7–8.0 μm; they reproduce by forming buds that are typically connected to the parent cell by a narrow pore (Figure 17.1).

Encapsulation of *C neoformans* is minimal, if evident, in the saprobic state, minimal to large in cultures, and invariably evident when parasitic. The capsules are acidic, highly viscous polysaccharides consisting primarily of glucuronoxylomannans that vary in structure as reflected in the four serotypes, A–D. The serotypes do not differ in virulence[6]; however, they differ in other properties (Table 17.1), enabling presumptive separation of serotypes A and D (*C neoformans* var *neoformans*) from serotypes B and C (*C neoformans* var *gattii*).

The recognition of *C neoformans* in fixed tissues is facilitated by special stains such as the Mayer mucicarmine stain, where the capsules are colored a deep rose-red and neither *Blastomyces dermatitidis* nor *Histoplasma capsulatum* take up the stain; and the Fontana-Masson stain, which is virtually specific through reaction with melaninlike compounds to reveal dark, brown-black cryptococci against a pink background.[7] The periodic acid-Schiff (PAS) and methenamine silver stains are less specific.

In cultures, the white to tan colonies are mucoid and glistening if composed of encapsulated cryptococci and dry and dull if made up of noncapsulated forms. The cryptococci rarely from pseudophyphae. They do not ferment sugars, but assimilate carbon from several sugars (glucose, galactose, sucrose, maltose, inositol, dulcitol, and inulin, but not lactose). The utilization of certain dicarboxylic acids by serotypes B and C, but not by serotypes A and D (Table 17.1), enables presumptive typing. Nitrogen

Table 17.1. Some characteristics of *C neoformans*.[a]

	Serotypes A and D	Serotypes B and C
Distribution	A—global D—uncommon in the United States, common in Europe	Both rare, except in southern California and southeastern Oklahoma
Reservoir	Bird feces, especially pigeon	Unknown
Dicarboxylic acids	Not assimilated	*l*-malic, fumaric, and succinic utilized
Relative resistance to		
Cycloheximide	Susceptible	Resistant
Canavanine	Susceptible	Resistant

[a]Although *C neoformans* constitutes a valid species, the relationship between serotypes and properties has led to the proposal to designate varieties: *C neoformans* var *neoformans* (serotypes A and D); *C neoformans* var *gattii* (serotypes B and C).
(Reprinted with permission from Hoeprich PD, Jordan MC (eds): *Infectious Diseases*, 4th ed. Philadelphia, Lippincott–Harper & Row, 1989, p 1134.)

is assimilated from several amino acids and from urea and creatinine, but not from nitrates. Cryptococci are urease positive and possess phenol oxidases active on certain phenols to yield melanin or polymers of melaninlike pigments. The detection of *Cryptococcus* spp in contaminated species is aided by use of a culture medium containing inositol (a source of carbon), urea (a source of nitrogen), caffeic acid and ferric citrate (formation of pigment), and gentamicin (suppression of bacteria).

Epidemiology

Serotype A *C neoformans* is global in distribution and accounts for about 95% of isolates in the United States. Type B has been reported from tropical and subtropical (Southeast) Asia and Australia, type C has been isolated from patients in southern California and southeastern Oklahoma, and type D is a frequent clinical and environmental isolate in most of Europe and other temperate regions.

The apparent predilection of types A and D *C neoformans* for avian feces has received the most careful study and the greatest notoriety with regard to pigeon droppings; *C neoformans* may be isolated from the contents of the gut of pigeons and from freshly passed feces. The birds are not ill[8] but the fact that pigeons retain their offal in their nests may contribute to the replication of *C neoformans* to densities as great as 5×10^7/g of feces. Cryptococci may remain viable in avian feces for as long as 2 years (drying and exposure to sunlight are inimical), and it is probable that few other microorganisms find pigeon feces as hospitable; indeed, *C neoformans* of serotypes A and D may be unable to compete as successfully in other environments. It has been suggested that the characteristically high concentrations of creatinine in bird feces favors cryptococcal growth; however, in the laboratory, creatinine does not stimulate growth. While serotypes A and D *C neoformans* appear to occupy an ecologic niche in pigeon feces, and perhaps the feces of other avians, the niche of serotypes B and C *C neoformans* has yet to be discovered.

Human and nonhuman mammals are thought to become infected primarily through inhalation of particles containing live *C neoformans;* that is, the vector appears to be air currents.[9] However, proof is lacking; for example, there are no reports of clusters of cases, and a history of exposure to pigeon feces is rarely obtained. Moreover, *C neoformans* is not an airborne contaminant in clinical laboratories. Human-to-human or animal-to-human transmission has not been documented.

There are but rough estimates of the frequency of cryptococcal meningitis in the United States—some 200–400 cases per year.[10] The disease is rare before puberty, and thereafter there is no relation to age (although most patients are 30–60 years old) or to occupation. Whites appear to be infected more often than blacks and males more often than females (by a ratio of 3:1).

Many patients with cryptococcosis have no detectable underlying disease. Yet noninfectious diseases that in some way compromise cell-mediated host defenses predispose to cryptococcosis. The risk of developing cryptococcosis is increased in patients, whether or not they are under treatment with glucosteroids, if they have malignant neoplasms (particularly of the lymphoreticular system), collagen vascular diseases (particularly disseminated lupus erythematosus), sarcoidosis, or diabetes mellitus (perhaps also in persons who chronically abuse ethanol or are pregnant).[11] There is a markedly increased susceptibility to infection with *C neoformans* in patients who are infected with the human immunodeficiency virus (HIV); in about 13% of patients with the acquired immunodeficiency syndrome (AIDS), *C neoformans* is a major pathogen.[12]

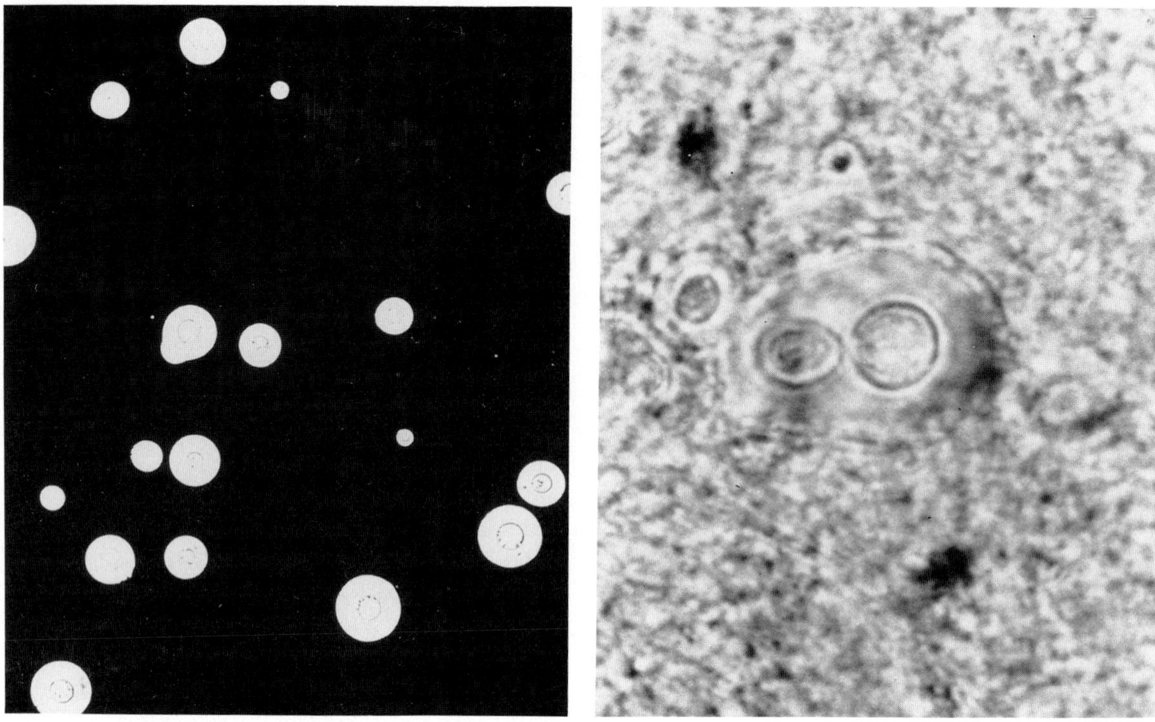

A B

Fig. 17.1. *C neoformans.* (A) India-ink preparation of sediment from CSF of a patient with cryptococcal meningoencephalitis. Note the characteristic thin-pore connecting daughter to mother cell in the left lower field. (Original magnification approximately × 500.) (B) Crush preparation of brain of a mouse inoculated by intracerebral injection 5 days earlier. (Lactophenol cotton blue stain, original magnification approximately × 1,000.) [Reprinted with permission from Hoeprich PD, Jordan MC (eds): *Infectious Diseases,* 4th ed. Philadelphia, Lippincott—Harper & Row, 1989, p 1133.]

Pathogenesis and Pathology

Cryptococci inhaled by normal persons either fail to survive intracellularly or are quickly contained so that either no disease appears or mild, subclinical illness occurs. Factors favoring proliferation leading to disease include infection with a heavily capsulated strain, an inoculum so large that normal cellular defenses are overwhelmed, and the presence of a defense-crippling underlying disease. If access is gained to the circulation, the CNS is a preferred target—for reasons that are quite unclear. In apparently normal persons, the course tends to be chronic, but it may be acute in immunocompromised patients.

Cryptococci do not elaborate toxins or engender hypersensitivity. However, their capsules are primary determinants of virulence, and the titers of capsular polysaccharide in the cerebrospinal fluid (CSF), blood, and other body liquids are directly proportional to the severity of disease.[10,11] Phagocytosis is impaired by capsules; the sloughed capsular polysaccharides may induce immunologic tolerance, diminishing opsonization because little or no humoral antibody is available.[13]

Cell-wall components (but not capsular polysaccharides) may activate complement—with little benefit to the host if the infecting strain is heavily capsulated. The importance of the T-lymphocyte-mediated immune response to killing cryptococci is affirmed by the usual failure of cure of cryptococcosis in patients with AIDS.[12]

While infection of the CNS is at once the most commonly diagnosed and the most often lethal form of cryptococcosis, there is no satisfactory explanation for the apparent predilection of *C neoformans* for the CNS. Infection of the meninges leads to seeding of the CSF and spread throughout the subarachnoid space. A grayish, mucinous exudate accumulates, most often at the base of the brain and over the cerebellum; leptomeningitis is most pronounced in the same areas, and the adjacent convolutions may be flattened. In many patients, there are lesions in both the brain and the meninges—truly a meningoencephalitis.[14] Intracerebral space-occupying lesions may form, tending to occur in the gray matter around the ventricles and the aqueduct, the basal ganglia, the cerebral white matter, and the cerebellar dentate nucleus.

Manifestations

Insidious in onset and slowly progressive, cryptococcal meningitis is a classic chronic meningitis. In most patients, there are manifestations of encephalitis as well as meningitis, but in some there are no symptoms referable to the CNS. Headache is the most common symptom, occurring in more than 75% of patients; while the pain may be referred to frontal, temporal, or retroorbital regions, progression from episodic and mild to constant and severe is more characteristic. Signs of meningeal irritation may not be prominent and are detected in about 50% of patients. Behavioral changes may occur, varying from irritability to psychotic behavior and from lethargy to coma. There may be peripheral motor dysfunctions manifested as altered reflexes or paralyses. Aphasia, visual disturbances, hearing loss, cerebellar signs, and evidences of increased intracranial pressure may be present. About two thirds of the patients are afebrile.

Cryptococcal infection of the substance of the CNS leads to signs and symptoms of a space-occupying lesion. The evolution of disease is typically slow, with or without fever. As many as 25% of the patients are subjected to neurosurgery with the expectation that a neoplasm will be found.[15]

Diagnosis

Cryptococcal lesions in the parenchyma of the CNS may be found by computed tomographic (CT) scanning and magnetic-resonance imaging (MRI). As they are space-occupying lesions, proof of causation requires biopsy, although detection of cryptococcal antigen in the serum and CSF may be suggestive.

In more than 90% of patients with symptomatic cryptococcal meningoencephalitis, the CSF is under increased pressure, the protein is elevated in concentration, and there are 40–400 leukocytes/μl (mostly mononuclear). The concentration of glucose is less than 45% of the simultaneously obtained blood sugar in at least half of the patients. In patients with asymptomatic cryptococcal meningitis, the CSF may be entirely normal (except for the growth of *C neoformans* in cultures).

Detection of *C neoformans* by microscopic examination of the CSF will exceed 50% if sediment obtained by centrifuging at least 5 ml of CSF is prepared with India ink or nigrosin. Confirmation by culture is essential.

The isolation of *C neoformans* is favored by centrifuging 5–10 ml of CSF for culture of the sediment; 3–5 specimens should be collected on different occasions. CSF from the cisternal subarachnoid space is more likely to yield *C neoformans* than CSF from either the lumbar space or the cerebral ventricles. While blood cultures may be positive for *C neoformans* in extensively infected patients, urine, sputum, bone marrow, and expressed prostatic secretions should be cultured in all patients suspected of having cryptococcal meningitis, even if there are no abnormalities of the urinary or respiratory tracts.

Serodiagnosis by assaying for humoral antibody is generally not of great value owing to the possibility of false-positive reactions and to the very low titers, either because of the immunoincompetence of the host or because the copious production of antigen by heavily capsulated *C neoformans* leads to immunologic tolerance. There is no skin-test reagent of proved value.

The capsular polysaccharide antigen of *C neoformans* is detectable in the serum and the CSF in 90% or more of patients with cryptococcal meningoencephalitis, with the height of the titer directly proportional to the severity of the illness. Confirmation of serodiagnosis by culture must be attempted, but therapy should be undertaken without the isolation of *C neoformans* if the titer exceeds 1:8 (latex agglutination test) in CSF obtained from a vulnerable patient.

Scanning, either by CT or MRI, enables assessment of the size of the cerebral ventricles, which is important because low-pressure hydrocephalus may result from impaired absorption of CSF. There will be delayed removal of radioisotope (e.g., colloidal ^{111}In), slow transit over the cerebral convexities, and possibly retrograde entry into the lateral ventricles after injection into the lumbar space.

Cryptococcal mass lesions of the CNS (cryptococcomas) that cause headache, papilledema, abnormal CSF, and no localizing signs may not be differentiable from malignancies without craniotomy. The demonstration of cryptococcal antigen in the serum and CSF is helpful.

The several arboviral meningoencephalitides have epidemiologic characteristics, including time of year and geography, that are helpful in differentiation from cryptococcal disease. The enteroviral meningoencephalitides are usually seasonal and less severe; other viruses may cause characteristic skin rashes. Other fungi, such as *C immitis,* may also cause a chronic meningoencephalitis, whereas protozoa, such as free-living amebae, usually cause more rapidly evolving disease. With all of these possibilities, cultures and serologic tests are definitive aids to specific diagnosis.

Prognosis

Rarely, patients may survive for three or more years with proved cryptococcal infection of the CNS without antifungal chemotherapy.[16] However, untreated disease almost always leads to death: 80–90% within 1 year, 70% within 3 months. Cerebral edema causes brain-stem compression, with or without hydrocephalus; coma, or the complications of coma, may be lethal.

Inability to concentrate, irritability, lethargy, and personality changes, lumped as chronic brain syndrome, may persist for years after an apparent cure. Organic sequelae include optic atrophy and deafness.

Relapse is common in cryptococcosis and antifungal therapy may be curative in no more than 75% of patients; there is, however, no proof of exogenous reinfection. When cryptococcal infection of the CNS complicates AIDS, cure is not possible with currently available therapy; suppression of disease is the most that can be accomplished.

Therapy

Amphotericin B (AmB) given by intravenous (IV) injection is the treatment of choice. The *C neoformans* is typically killed (testing in vitro) by less than 1 μg/ml; native resistance apparently does not occur. The usual total dose is 30–45 mg/kg body weight (2–3 g); if relapse occurs, larger doses may be employed in an effort to control the disease. Particulars of treatment with AmB by IV injection are given in Table 17.2; both cryptococcoma and meningoencephalitis are treated according to this regimen.

The IV injection of AmB causes immediate and transient adverse effects, as well as permanent dam-

Table 17.2. Protocol for the IV administration of amphotericin B (AmB) deoxycholate.

Pharmacy preparation

1. The desired dose is added to sufficient 5% glucose solution for IV injection to provide a final concentration of $\leq$ 10 mg/dl for peripheral-vein injection, 15–20 mg/dl for central-vein injection.
2. Sufficient heparin solution is added to yield a final concentration of 50 U/dl.

Premedication—given 30 min before giving AmB

1. Aspirin (or acetaminophen), 10–15 mg/kg body weight, p.o. (repeat dose every 3 hours for two additional doses).
2. *One* of the following (repeat dose once, 4 hours after initial dose):
    a. Prochlorpromazine, 0.2–0.3 mg/kg body weight, p.o. or IV
    b. Metaclopramide, 2 mg/kg body weight, p.o. or IV
    c. Meperidine, 0.5–1.0 mg/kg body weight, p.o. or IM

Injection

1. The patient should be supine in bed.
2. The temperature, pulse, and blood pressure must be recorded before starting treatment.
3. The infusion assembly should include a Y tube or similar arrangement (to provide access to both 5% glucose solution without additives and the dose of AmB) and an infusion pump.
4. First day—0.25 mg/kg body weight.
    a. Inject 5–10 mg over a period of 15 min, then switch to the 5% glucose solution without additives.
    b. Measure blood pressure at 5 min, 10 min, and 20 min.
        i. If there has been no fall in blood pressure, give the remainder of the dose of AmB within 20 min.
        ii. If there has been a fall in blood pressure:
            (A) Without symptoms: elevate the foot of the bed, inject 0.9% NaCl solution (10 ml/kg body weight) over 30 min, and then give the remainder of the dose of AmB within 45 min.
            (B) With symptoms: elevate the foot of the bed, inject 0.9% NaCl solution (10 ml/kg body weight) over 30 min, and give ephedrine, 0.3–0.6 mg/kg, by intramuscular injection. If there is prompt restoration of the blood pressure and subsidence of symptoms, repeat the 5–10-mg dose.
                (1) If hypotension does not recur, give the remainder of the dose over 45 min.
                (2) If hypotension recurs, put off therapy for 2–3 days before trying again.
5. Second day—0.50 mg/kg body weight.
    a. If there was no hypotension with the first dose, inject the second dose over a period of 30–45 min (measure the blood pressure at 5 min, 15 min, 45 min).
    b. If there was transient hypotension with the first dose, again assess the effect of injection of 5–10 mg, as with the first dose, before giving all of the second dose.
6. Third day—0.75 mg/kg body weight.
   If there was no hypotension with the second dose, inject the third dose over a period of 45–60 min (measure the blood pressure at 5 min, 15 min, 45 min).

Table 17.2. *(continued)*

7. Fourth day—no AmB.
8. Fifth day—0.75 mg/kg body weight.
9. Sixth day—no AmB.
10. Seventh day—0.75 mg/kg body weight:
    a. Pretherapy, obtain blood (low, or trough specimen) for assay of the concentration of AmB.
    b. Inject dose, noting exact duration of administration.
    c. Two hours after infusion is completed, obtain blood (high, or peak specimen) for assay of the concentration of AmB.
11. Continue alternate-day regimen of treatment, adjusting the dose to yield a 2-hour postdose concentration of 2.0–3.0 μg/ml serum (trough of 0.5–1.0 μg/ml).
12. When the appropriate dose is determined, continued therapy on alternate days for inpatients and thrice weekly (Monday, Wednesday, Friday) for outpatients.

Surveillance (in addition to clinical evaluations):

1. Before therapy:
    a. Obtain pictures of lesions—radiographic, MRI, radionuclude, and ultrasound examinations; cultures; and serologic studies within 1 week before treatment.
    b. Determine creatinine clearance, urea nitrogen, creatinine, K^+, and Mg^{++} within 48 hours before treatment.
    c. Carry out urinalysis and complete blood count on the day treatment is started.
2. During therapy:
    a. Weekly—perform studies of 1b and 1c, above. If treatment goes smoothly, shift to biweekly to monthly observations after 4 weeks of therapy.
    b. Monthly—perform studies of 1a, above, plus assays of peak trough concentrations of AmB in blood.
3. After therapy:
   The studies of 1a, b, and c, above, should be repeated monthly for 3 months, then quarterly for 6 mos, and finally semiannually for a period of years appropriate for the mycosis.

Adapted with permission from Hoeprich PD: Candidosis, in Hoeprich PD, Jordan MC (eds): *Infectious Diseases,* 4th ed. Lippincott–Harper & Row, Philadelphia, 1989, pp 476–477.

age. The reversible ill effect of thrombophlebitis may be avoided by infusion through a central venous catheter. Unfortunately, prolonged administration over several hours, long advocated to avoid chills and fever, is not significantly better tolerated than infusion over 1 hour (double-blind comparison).[17] Moreover, infusion within 1 hour offers the advantages of establishing a more favorable gradient, blood to the site of infection,[18] and reducing the cost of outpatient therapy.[19]

Permanent morbidity from the IV administration of AmB most often takes the form of irreversible nephropathy.[20] The extent and severity of nephrotoxicity may be diminished by limiting the total dose[20] and making certain that the patient is eunatremic.[22] Because the nephropathology appears to be related to anoxic damage to the tubules,[23] alternate-day or thrice-weekly administration—a rational schedule in view of the half-life of AmB in the blood (Figure 17.2)—should be beneficial in allowing for at least partial recovery between doses.

Direct damage to the CNS from AmB has also been documented.[23,24] Limitation of the total dose may prevent such adverse effects.

Because AmB is virtually completely excluded from the CSF after IV injection, intrathecal (IT) injection, with or without concurrent IV administration, has been suggested. The value of adding such topical therapy in cryptococcal meningoencephalitis has not been proved, although it may be undertaken in patients with persistent, active meningoencephalitis despite IV therapy; relapse; or severely reduced renal function. Details regarding the administration of AmB by IT injection are given in Table 17.3. Three routes are in use:

1. *Intracisternal* injection is the route that delivers AmB closest to the basilar site of the most intense meningitis; however, immediate adverse effects of severe headache, nausea and vomiting, and tinnitus may foreshadow loss of hearing. As drug-induced arachnoiditis develops, the hazard of iatrogenic subarachnoid bleeding increases.
2. *Intraventricular* injection by means of a subcutaneous reservoir catheter[25] is technically easy

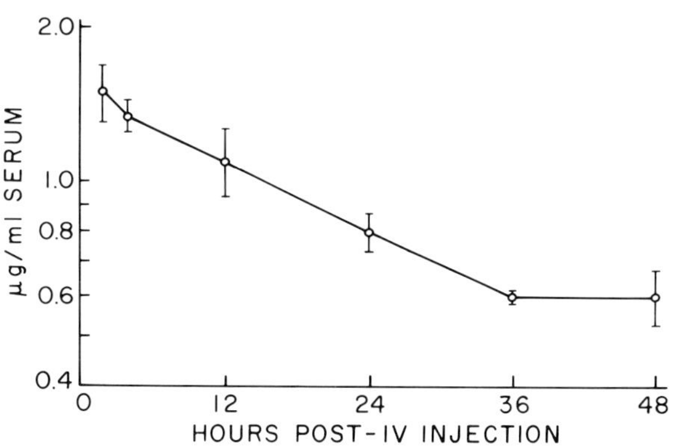

Fig. 17.2. The half-life of amphotericin B in the serum of a patient under long-term treatment for disseminated coccidioidomycosis was 21.5 hours for the beta phase (after mixing). The data points are arithmetic means, ± the standard error, of values obtained following three separate doses of 0.5 mg/kg body weight given over 60 minutes. [Reprinted with permission from Hoeprich PD, Jordan MC (eds): *Infectious Diseases,* 4th ed. Philadelphia, Lippincott—Harper & Row, 1989, p 474.]

Table 17.3. Protocol for the IT administration of amphotericin B (AmB) deoxycholate.

Pharmacy preparation

1. Make AmB-deoxycholate to a concentration of 0.25 mg/ml in 5% glucose solution (in 10% glucose solution for hyperbaric therapy).

Premedication—given 30 minutes before giving AmB.

1. Codeine, 30–45 mg, p.o. (repeat once after 4 hours).
2. *One* of the following (repeat dose once after 4 hours).
   a. Prochlorpromazine, 0.2–0.3 mg/kg body weight, p.o. or IV.
   b. Metaclopramide, 2 mg/kg body weight, p.o. or IV.

Injection

1. The patient should be supine in bed.
2. The temperature, pulse, and blood pressure must be recorded before starting therapy.
3. A volume of CSF equal to the planned dose should be removed before each dose.
4. First day—0.025 mg (0.10 ml).
   a. Inject over 30–60 seconds.
   b. Measure vital signs 15 and 30 minutes postinjection.
5. Second day—same as first day.
6. Third day—0.05 mg (0.20 ml).
   a. Inject over 30–60 seconds.
   b. Measure vital signs 15 and 30 minutes postinjection.
7. Continue to advance dose at 2-day intervals as tolerated by the patient:
   5th day—0.10 mg (0.40 ml)
   7th day—0.20 mg (0.80 ml)
   9th day—0.30 mg (1.20 ml)
   11th day—0.40 mg (1.6 ml)
   13th day—0.50 mg (2.0 ml)
8. When the maximum tolerated dose is attained (usually 0.20–0.50 mg), change to alternate-day or thrice-weekly injections. Continue until evidence of active meningitis has disappeared.
9. Maintenance therapy, one or two injections a week, is continued for periods appropriate to the causative fungus, for example, until a fourfold drop in titer of antigen (in CSF) occurs in cryptococcal meningoencephalitis; for a year or more after CF nonreactivity in coccidioidal meningitis.

Surveillance (in addition to clinical evaluations)

1. Before therapy:
   a. Routine culture and serologic studies of CSF during week before treatment.
   b. Audiogram during week before treatment.
2. During therapy:
   a. Weekly—routine and culture examination of CSF.
   b. Monthly—serologic study of CSF; repeat audiogram.
3. After therapy:
   Repeat examination of CSF and audiogram after 1 month, 3 months, and quarterly for 1 year, then semiannually for a period of years appropriate for the mycosis, for example, 2 years for cryptococcosis, 5 years for coccidioidal meningitis.

and repetitive dosing is facilitated. Unfortunately, the AmB is delivered far from the site of infection and is immediately diluted in CSF; moreover, attaining a therapeutic effect depends on the normal flow of the CSF. Further, there is a definite morbidity from insertion and use; the catheter may become malpositioned, clogged, or infected (usually with *Staphylococcus epidermidis,* and rarely with the causative *Cryptococcus* spp).

3. *Lumbar* injection, while a familiar procedure, delivers AmB far from the basilar site of meningitis, a problem that may be partially overcome by injection of AmB suspended in hyperbaric (10%) glucose solution with immediate postinjection placement of the patient in a 15-degree head-down position. Such hyperbaric therapy[26] may also minimize exposure of the lumbar CNS to high concentrations of AmB and thus minimize arachnoiditis; also, radiculitis may be less because of the lower concentration of AmB in the liquid that leaks extradurally.

Because of the toxicity of AmB, alternatives have been evaluated. Foremost is flucytosine (5-FC), an orally administrable antimicrobic that penetrates all body water, including that of the CNS and CSF. While native resistance occurs in *C neoformans,* most pretreatment isolates are susceptible to less than 25 μg/ml by testing in vitro. Used alone to treat cryptococcal meningitis, 5-FC brought about cure in about two thirds of the patients, without permanent damage from the drug.[27] Failures resulted from (1) inadequate dosage, both in daily dose and duration of treatment; (2) failure of recognition of native resistance (the susceptibility of isolates must be determined before treatment); and (3) the development of resistance during therapy. Adequate dosage of 5-FC yields peak concentrations (one hour after a by mouth dose) of 80–100 μg/ml of serum. With normal renal function, 200 mg/kg body weight per day, given orally in four equal portions, every 6 hours, is usually adequate. With renal dysfunction, the dose must be decreased in direct proportion to the reduction of the creatinine clearance—with verification by measurement of the peak concentration in the serum. Leukopenia and/or thrombocytopenia may occur, typically in patients simultaneously treated with antineoplastic agents, irradiation, and other antimicrobics, including AmB, or in patients with renal dysfunction. Increases in the hepatic transaminases are less frequent and usually resolve completely on withdrawal of the drug.

Combination therapy consisting of AmB (0.3 mg/kg body weight per day, IV) plus 5-FC (150 mg/kg body weight per day, given by mouth in four equal portions every 6 hours), with both drugs given for 6 weeks, was suggested as a means of shortening therapy through an additive or synergistic effect, while reducing toxicity from AmB.[28] By itself, the low dose of AmB in this regimen would provide virtually no clinically significant anticryptococcal activity, whereas the dose of 5-FC recommended for combined therapy has cured patients with cryptococcal meningitis. Such combination therapy is as successful as using AmB alone. Because the success of the two-drug regimen is so highly dependent on the action of the 5-FC, failures will occur in patients infected with strains of *C neoformans* resistant to 5-FC. In addition, if renal function is impaired (preexisting dysfunction plus the adverse effect of the AmB), the excretion of 5-FC will decrease and its body burden will increase, leading to both increased catabolism of 5-FC by intestinal bacteria and retention of the products of catabolism, notably, 5-fluorouracil and derivatives.[29] This may be the explanation for the adverse reactions (e.g., suppression of the bone marrow) seen in 30–40% of patients given combination therapy.

While all of the antifungal azole derivatives for systemic treatment, including the newer triazoles itraconazole and fluconazole, are virtually always inhibitory to *C neoformans* by testing in vitro, they are not cryptococcidal. However, fluconazole is licensed for the treatment of cryptococcal disease, including meningoencephalitis. The utility of fluconazole is best established in the suppression of chronic meningoencephalitis. With an elimination half-life from the blood of about 30 hours in persons with normal renal function, the recommended dose in adults is 200 mg/day. Preparations for peroral and intravenous administration are available; because absorption from the gut is quantitative, without requirement for gastric acid, dosage does not vary with the route of administration. About 80% of the dose of fluconazole is eliminated in antifungally active form in the urine; if the creatinine clearance falls below 50 ml/min/1.73 m^2, the dose should be decreased by 25–50%, in proportion to the excretory deficit. A dose of 200 mg should be given after each hemodialysis. Adverse effects are usually not severe, e.g., gastrointestinal (nausea, vomiting, diarrhea, abdominal pain), headache, skin rash, necessitating cessation of therapy in about 3% of patients. Two deaths from hepatic necrosis, and one with Stevens-Johnson syndrome, have been associated with treatment with fluconazole.

Surveillance is an essential component of therapy. During treatment, the CSF should be examined at least weekly by culture, microscopy (nigrosin or India-ink preparations; cell count with differential), and determination of the concentration of glucose and protein. Although forms consistent in appearance with *Cryptococcus* spp may persist in the CSF on microscopic examination, cultures should become sterile promptly. With effective therapy, there should be a fall in the number of leukocytes, a decrease in the concentration of protein, and a rise in the concentration of glucose, with, most important, a fall in the titer of capsular polysaccharide (also in the serum). The titers need be assayed only at three- to four-week intervals and should fall at least four dilutions during therapy. The CSF will usually become entirely normal within 3 months of termination of treatment; cure should not be declared until surveillance by examination of the patient and the CSF at 2–3-month intervals for at least 2 years following therapy has confirmed that relapse has not occurred.

With currently available treatment, cure of cryptococcosis is not possible in patients with AIDS. After the control of acute disease has been attained, long-term suppression may be attempted using AmB (weekly injections of either 1 mg/kg body weight IV, or 0.25–0.50 mg IT through a subcutaneous reservoir-catheter device. However, adverse reactions limit the acceptance of such treatment and relapse often occurs. Of the newer triazoles, fluconazole is effective for the suppression of cryptococcal meningoencephalitis.

Zygomycotic Infections of the CNS

Mycology

Of the three orders in the class Zygomycetes (fungi that produce zygospores), only two, the Mucorales and the Entomophthorales, contain families of fungi pathogenic for humans[30,31] (Table 17.4). The families Mucorales and Cunninghamellaceae are of particular importance because they contain the genera that cause rhinocerebral zygomycosis[32]: *Rhizopus, Absidia, Mucor,* and *Cunninghamella*.

In tissues, the hyphae of Zygomycetes are broad (6–50 μm in transverse diameter), nonseptate,

Table 17.4. Pathogenic members of the class zygomycetes.

Order Mucorales[a]		
Family	Species†	Synonyms
Mucoraceae	*Rhizopus oryzae*	*Rhizopus arrhizus*
	Rhizopus rhizopodiformis	*Rhizopus cohnii, Rhizopus equinus*
	Rhizopus microsporus	
	Absidia corymbifera	*Absidia ramosa*
	Mucor circinelloides	
	Mucor pusillus	*Rhizomucor pusillus*
	Mucor miehei	*Rhizomucor miehei*
Mortierellaceae	*Mortierella wolfii*	
Cunninghamellaceae	*Cunninghamella elegans*	
	Cunninghamella bertholletiae	
Saksenaeceae	*Saksenaea vasiformis*	
Syncephalastraceae	*Syncephalastrum* spp	
Order Entmophthorales[b]		
Family	Species	
Entomophthoraceae	*Entomophthora cornata*	
	Basidiobolus haptosporus	

(Reprinted with permission from Hoeprich PD, Jordan MC (eds): *Infectious Diseases,* 4th ed. Philadelphia, Lippincott—Harper & Row, 1989, p 1193.)
(Howard DH: Classification of the Mucorales, pp 93–94. In Lehrer RI (moderator): Mucormycosis. *Ann Intern Med* 93:93–108, 1980)
[a]Several other members of the order are capable of growth at 37°C and thus represent potential pathogens of warm-blooded animals. A few examples include *Rhizopus oligosporus, Rhizopus homothallicus, Absidia hyalospora, Mucor rouxii,* and *Syncephalastrum racemosum.* (Scholer HJ, Muller E, Schipper MAA: The Mucorales. In Howard DH (ed): *The Fungi Pathogenic to Humans and Animals: Part A, Biology,* pp 9–59. New York, Marcel Dekker, 1983).
[b]Other species reported as pathogens were misidentifications or have been reduced to synonomy.

and form branches at or near right angles (Figure 17.3). While the Zygomycetes grow readily in the usual laboratory culture media, they are inhibited by cycloheximide, an antifungal agent commonly added to media to prevent overgrowth of nonpathogenic fungi.

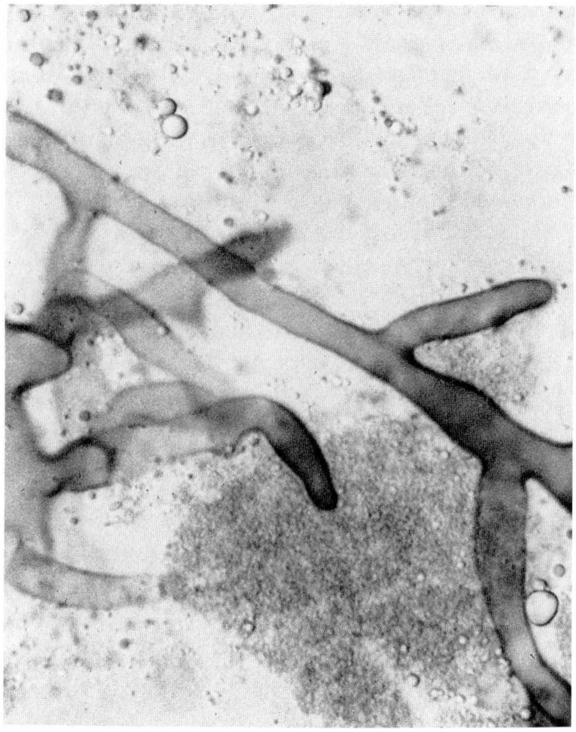

Fig. 17.3. *Rhizopus oryzae.* Crush preparation of a biopsy specimen of palatal lesion from a patient with rhinocerebral zygomycosis complicating diabetic ketoacidosis. (Parker blue-black fountain-pen ink, original magnification approximately × 750.)

Epidemiology

Ubiquitous in nature, the Zygomycetes frequently grow on decaying organic matter. Zygospores readily become airborne and air currents may be the vectors.

Pathogenesis and Pathology

Serum from humans with diabetic ketoacidosis enhances the growth of *Rhizopus* spp and ketoacidotic experimental animals are more susceptible to invasion than normal animals. The Mucorales characteristically invade blood vessels, causing thrombosis and hemorrhagic infarctions. The process is nearly unique among fungi pathogenic for humans (the *Aspergillus* spp may cause a similar picture), and it may be rapidly progressive.

Manifestations

Rhinocerebral disease typically occurs in a patient with diabetic ketoacidosis or with leukemia.[33] The infection often begins as ulcerations in the paranasal sinuses or in the palate (Figure 17.4). Progression may be either slow or rapid to involve the nose, ocular orbits, base of the skull, or intracranial structures.

Patients complain of lethargy, headache, loss of vision, and difficulty in moving the eyes—symptoms that do not improve but may advance although the ketoacidosis appears to be responding to therapy. Black, eschar-like lesions of the palatal mucosa are sometimes seen (Figure 17.4), and there may be proptosis with or without periorbital cellulitis. Roentgenographic examinations, including CT scanning, may reveal only soft-tissue swelling, but may show involvement of the sinuses. The CSF is usually normal, or there may be a modest neutrophilic pleocytosis.

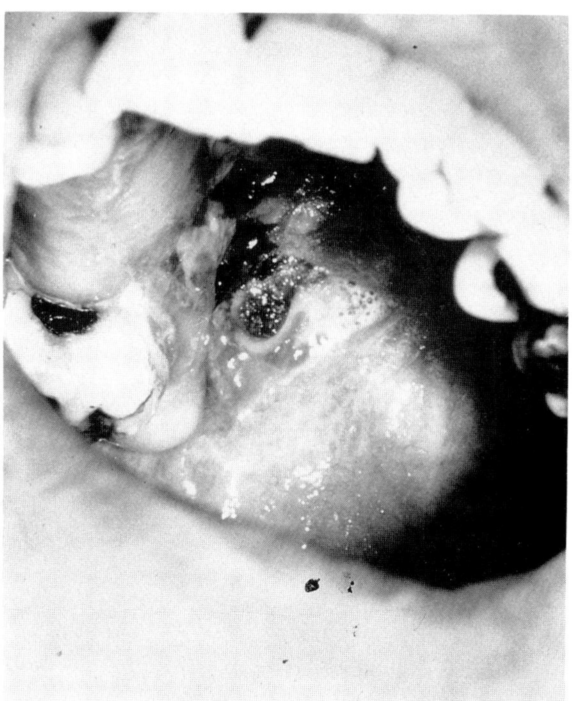

Fig. 17.4. Right palatal lesion in a patient with rhinocerebral zygomycosis caused by *R oryzae* complicating diabetic ketoacidosis. (Courtesy of Michael G. Rinaldi, Ph.D.)

Diagnosis

Because of the ubiquity of the Zygomycetes, isolation in cultures is not diagnostic. There are neither serologic nor skin tests. Demonstration of the characteristic hyphae invading tissues is essential to diagnosis.

Pyogenic bacteria and other fungi must be excluded. Neoplasms, the ophthalmopathy of malignant Graves' disease, and primary neurologic diseases may be confused with rhinocerebral zygomycosis.

Prognosis

Possibly because of a delay in diagnosis, most patients with progressive rhinocerebral zygomycosis die of the disease. Aggressive surgical debridement, rapid correction of the ketoacidosis, and prompt application of AmB are necessary to secure survival.[35]

Therapy

Surgical excision of infected tissues is paramount and cannot be put off while correction of acidosis and initiation of treatment with AmB are carried out. Wide excision is necessary because the extent of invasion is not grossly apparent. Thus, excision of sinuses, drainage of abscesses, ocular enucleations, and palatectomies may be necessary.

Amphotericin B is the antimicrobic of choice and ascent to a therapeutic dose must be pursued rapidly. There are no data confirming the optimal duration of treatment, but total doses of 30 mg/kg body weight are generally advocated.

Coccidioidomycosis of the CNS

C immitis is normally a saprobic inhabitant of the soil in certain semiarid regions of the Americas.[35-37] Infection of humans is virtually always acquired accidentally by inhalation of air contaminated with coccidioidal arthroconidia. Usually, no disease results, but extrapulmonary spread, particularly when the CNS is involved, may be lethal.

Mycology

Coccidioides immitis is the only species in the genus. In its normal habitat in the soil[38] and in cultures in the laboratory, *C immitis* grows as mycelia composed of septate hyphae. Certain hyphae form arthroconidia, thick-walled, barrel-like, generally cylindrical structures that are separated from each other by apparently empty cells (Figure 17.5A). While the arthroconidia are essential to the survival of the fungus, they are also key to the disease, for they are at once the units of dissemination and the infectious elements.

Arthroconidia that gain access to a susceptible host and survive phagocytosis grow in the tissues as globoid structures, 20—100 μm in diameter, called spherules[39] (Figure 17.5B). Spherules go through internal nuclear divisions and cytoplasmic cleavages to yield as many as 10^5 uninucleate endospores that are 2–3 μm in diameter. Some endospores grow inside phagocytes to form new spherules, continuing the parasitic tissue cycle.[40]

Cottony-white colonies form 7–10 days after any morphologic form of *C immitis* is inoculated onto ordinary agar-culture media. While they may become tan to brown as they age, colonial morphology is not characteristic. For this reason, and especially because arthroconidia form as cultures age, it is absolutely essential that clinicians always alert the laboratory when specimens are submitted that may contain *C immitis*.

Demonstration of the spherule form of *C immitis* is essential to laboratory diagnosis. This is done reliably, directly, and quickly by microscopic exumination of tissues obtained by biopsy or by aspiration of closed-space lesions (pus, exudates, and other body liquids, including CSF). Other approaches to diagnosis—such as inoculation of special culture media or experimental animals, or extraction of specific antigens from agar cultures—require weeks for completion.

Antigenic determinants in the cell walls of *C immitis* are present in the coccidioidin and spherulin[41] preparations used for skin testing.

Epidemiology

A disease of the Americas, coccidioidomycosis is endemic from about 40°N, 120°W in California to

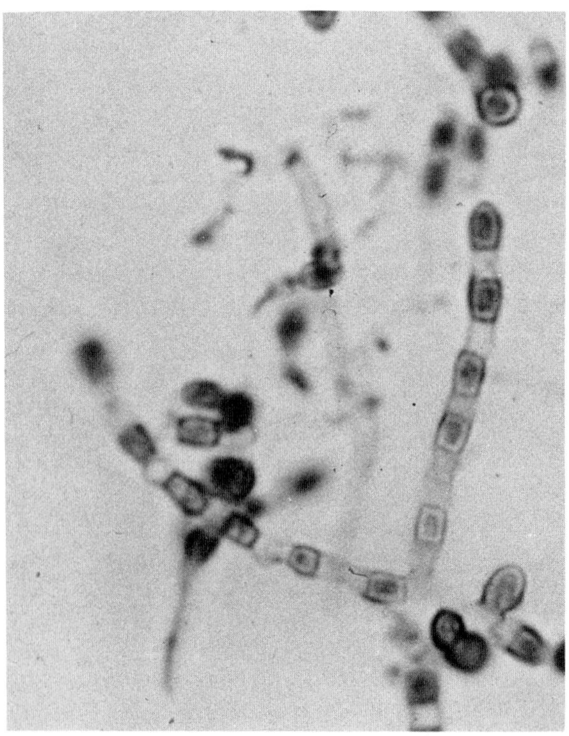

A

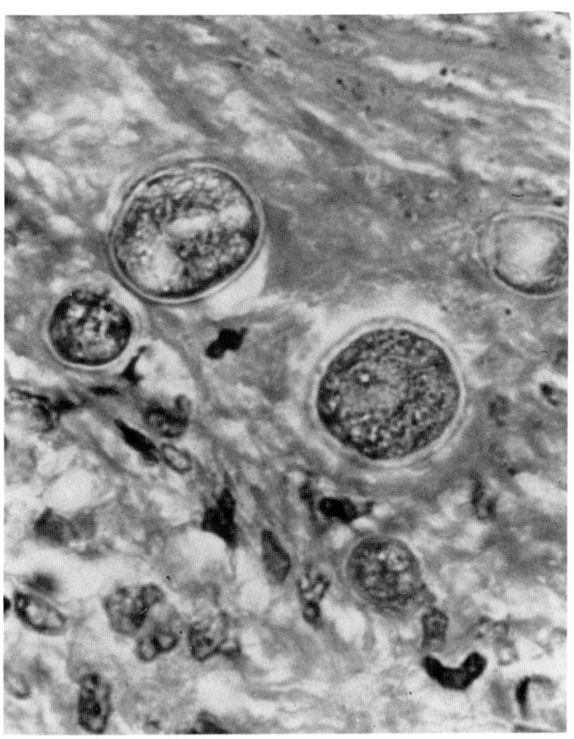

B

Fig. 17.5. *C immitis*. (A) Mould form in culture showing hyphae with heavy-walled arthroconidia. (Lactophenol cotton blue, original magnification approximately × 50; provided by M.G. Rinaldi, Ph.D.) (B) Spherules containing endospores in crush preparation from mouse experimentally infected by intraperitoneal injection of arthroconidia. (Lactophenol cotton blue, original magnification approximately × 450.)

about 40°S, 65°W in Argentina. However, the disease may occur in areas remote from endemic foci when infected persons travel while incubating the infection, and in rare instances when arthroconidia are carried on inanimate objects.

In general, major endemic areas of coccidioidomycosis coincide with the bioclimatic lower Sonoran life zone: arid or semiarid climates of low altitude, alkaline soil, hot summers, moderately wet winters, and infrequent freezes. Perhaps the ecologic niche of *C immitis* is defined primarily by conditions inimical to the growth of competitor saprobes in the soil.

Because the natural route of infection is by inhalation of air contaminated with arthroconidia, air currents are the vectors of *C immitis*.[9,42] That is, the risk of infection is greatest when the soil is dry and arthroconidia become airborne by winds, or when soil containing arthroconidia is disturbed, as by earth-moving machines, archeologic digging, or children at play.

Using case finding by testing for reactivity to coccidioidin, about 80% of infections are clinically inapparent[43] (Figure 17.6). There is no sex preference. While women in general are less likely to develop coccidioidal disease than are men, a woman who is pregnant is at greater risk than a man.

Race is important. Extrapulmonary disease occurs 5–10 times more often in blacks and Filipinos than in whites, whereas Asians and Mexicans may not be at substantially higher risk. The risk of coccidioidal

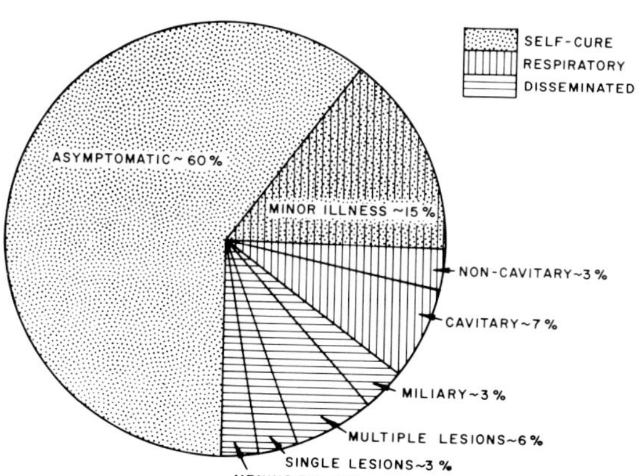

Fig. 17.6. An overview of the outcome of coddidioidomycosis in humans who did not receive specific chemotherapy. [Reprinted with permission from Hoeprich PD, Jordan MC (eds): *Infectious Diseases*, 4th ed. Philadelphia, Lippincott—Harper & Row, 1989, p 499.)

meningitis is about five times greater in blacks and ten times greater in Filipinos than in whites. About five times more blacks than whites die from coccidioidomycosis, whereas Mexicans do not appear to be at higher risk.

Children are neither more susceptible nor more resistant to acquisition of occidioidomycosis or to extrapulmonary spread of the disease.[44] Sex becomes a determinant after puberty.

Pathogenesis and Pathology

If inhaled arthroconidia deposit in alveolar ducts and alveoli and survive phagocytosis, they metamorphose into spherules. Whether intracellular or extracellular, typically a mixed suppurative–granulomatous reaction is elicited. If the host response fails to contain the infection in the lungs, endospores exiting in the lymph become blood-borne.[39] If endospores lodge in the meninges, a proliferative, granulomatous inflammatory reaction is elicited that is patchy in distribution, but is most severe at the base of the brain. Noncommunicating hydrocephalus may result if compression of the aqueduct or obstruction of the foramina prevents outflow of the CSF.

Both humoral and cell-mediated immune responses are elicited. Humoral antibodies are not protective and appear to be of little value in fighting the infection, whereas a vigorous cell-mediated response is essential to recovery. Detection and measurement of humoral antibodies are helpful in diagnosis and assessment of the course of the disease.

Manifestations

Coccidioidal meningitis is insidious in onset and runs a chronic course that typically begins about 3 months after the first manifestation of coccidioidal disease.[45] In about half of the patients with meningitis, no other site of disease can be found. Severe, bilateral headache, often associated with nausea and vomiting, is the prominent complaint of virtually all patients. Also common are altered mental status (changed affect, disorientation, lethargy, confusion, hallucinations); disturbed vision (photophobia, anisocoria, diplopia, nystagmus); and neurologic signs (papilledema, hyperreflexia, cranial-nerve palsies). In about half of the patients, mild to moderate signs of meningeal irritation may be detected. Progression of the disease with increased intracranial pressure results in constant headache, vomiting that is often projectile, and papilledema, with or without seizures, obtundation, stupor, and coma.

Diagnosis

Given the clinical manifestations of meningitis, the epidemiologic history and the course of the disease may be highly suggestive of coccidioidal infection. However, additional evidence is necessary. While isolation of *C immitis* from the CSF is common, it takes time for growth and certain identification of an isolate, and is also hazardous for laboratory personnel. Detection of complement-fixing antibody is diagnostic of coccidioidal infection of the CNS. While low titers (e.g., 1:4, or less) may be engendered by vicinal disease, such as coccidioidal osteomyelitis of vertebrae, titers are generally higher in untreated disease. Antibody titers decrease as a function of the site of collection of CSF: lumbar > cisternal > ventricular (if there is no ventriculitis, and the flow of CSF is normal). While patients with coccidioidal meningitis are usually reactive to coccidioidin, skin testing is of no particular diagnostic value.

Prognosis

Without treatment, patients with coccidioidal meningitis usually die within 2 years of diagnosis.[46] Therapy generally lengthens survival, but cure too often is elusive.

Therapy

Blood-borne AmB is so successfully excluded from the CNS/CSF that therapeutic concentrations cannot be attained by IV administration; IT administration is, in fact, topical therapy. Details regarding IT therapy are given in Table 17.3. The problems of IT therapy with AmB are the same in coccidioidal meningitis as in cryptococcal meningoencephalitis, but are more urgent because of the lack of therapeutic effect of IV therapy and the absence of any other agent with proved utility. Fluconazole is under evaluation for the treatment of coccidioidal meningitis as an investigational agent because it is well absorbed from the gut and enters the CNS/CSF freely.[47]

References

1. Parker JC Jr, McCloskey JJ, Lee RS: The emergence of candidosis. The dominant postmorten cerebral mycosis. *Am J Clin Pathol* 1978;70:31–36.
2. Roberts GD: Detection of fungemia. *Infect Dis Newslet* 1985;4:19–21.
3. Hoeprich PD: Cryptococcosis, in Hoeprich PD, Jordan MC (eds): *Infectious Diseases,* 4th ed. Philadelphia, Harper & Row, 1989, pp 1132–1141.
4. Rippon JW: Cryptococcosis, in Rippon JW: *Medical Mycology. The Pathogenic Fungi and the Pathogenic Actinomycetes,* 3rd ed. Philadelphia, Saunders, 1988, pp 582–609.
5. Kwon-Chung KJ: A new genus *Filobasidiella,* the perfect state of *Cryptococcus neoformans. Mycologia* 1975;67:1197–1200.
6. Bennett JE, Kwon-Chung KF, Howard DH: Epidemiologic differences among serotypes of *Cryptococcus neoformans. Am J Epidemiol* 1977;105:582–586.
7. Yo JY, Lee SS, Ayala AG: Advantage of the Fontana-Masson stain in capsule-deficient cryptococcal infection. *Arch Pathol Lab Med* 1977;111:53–57.
8. Littman ML, Walter JE: Cryptococci: current status. *Am J Med* 1968;45:922–932.
9. Campbell CC: (Philosophical) review of air currents as a continuing vector. *Ann NY Acad Sci* 1980; 353:123–139.
10. Kaufman L, Blumer S: Cryptococcosis: the awakening giant, in *Proceedings of the Fourth International Conference on Mycoses. The Black and White Yeasts-Brasilia.* Washington, DC, Pan American Health Organization, 1977, pp 176–182.
11. Diamond RD: Immunology of invasive fungal infections. *Comp Immunol* 1981;8:585–633.
12. Eng RHK, Bishburg E, Smith SS: Cryptococcal infection in patients with acquired immune deficiency syndrome. *Am J Med* 1986;81:19–23.
13. Kozel TR, Gulley WF, Cazin J Jr: Immune response to *Cryptococcus neoformans* soluble polysaccharide: immunologic responsiveness. *Infect Immunol* 1976; 18:701–707.
14. Littman ML, Zimmerman LE: *Cryptococcosis.* New York, Grune & Stratton, 1956, pp 71–82.
15. Carton CA, Mount LA: Neurosurgical aspects of cryptococcosis. *J Neurosurg* 1951;8:143–156.
16. Campbell GD, Currier RD, Busey JF: Survival in untreated cryptococcal meningitis. *Neurology* 1981; 31:1154–1157.
17. Cleary JD, Weisdorf D, Fletcher CV: Effect of infusion rate on amphotericin B-associated febrile reactions. *Drug Intell Clin Pharm* 1988;22:769–772.
18. Fields BT Jr, Bates JM, Abernathy RS: Effect of rapid intravenous infusion on serum concentrations of amphotericin B. *Appl Microbiol* 1971;22:615–617.
19. Campbell GD: Blastomycosis, in Cherniak R (ed):

Current Therapy of Respiratory Diseases 1984–1985. St. Louis, Mosby, 1984, pp 69–74.
20. Winn WA: Coccidioidomycosis and amphotericin B. *Med Clin North Am* 1963;47:1131–1148.
21. Heidemann HT, Gerkins JF, Spickard WA, et al: Amphotericin B nephrotoxicity in humans decreased by salt repletion. *Am J Med* 1983;75:476–481.
22. Brezis M, Rosen S, Silva P, et al: Polyene toxicity in renal medulla: injury mediated by transport activity. *Science* 1984;224:66–68.
23. Schaffner CP: Polyene macrolides in clinical practice: pharmacology and adverse and other effects, in Omura S (ed): *Macrolide Antibiotics, Chemistry, Biology and Practice*. New York, Academic Press, 1984, pp 457–507.
24. Devinsky O, Lemann W, Evans AC, et al: Akinetic mutism in a bone marrow transplant recipient following total-body irradiation and amphotericin B chemoprophylaxis: a positron emission tomographic and neuropathologic study. *Arch Neurol* 1987;44:414–417.
25. Ratcheson RA, Ommaya AK: Experience with the subcutaneous cerebrospinal-fluid reservoir. *N Engl J Med* 1968;279:1025–1031.
26. Alazraki NP, Fierer J, Halpern S, et al: Use of a hyperbaric solution for administration of intrathecal amphotericin B. *N Engl J Med* 1974;290:641–646.
27. Utz JP, Garriques IL, Sande MA, et al: Therapy of cryptococcosis with a combination of flucytosine and amphotericin B. *J Infect Dis* 1975;132:368–373.
28. Bennett JE, Dismukes WE, Duma RJ, et al: A comparison of amphotericin B alone and combined with flucytosine in the treatment of cryptococcal meningitis. *N Engl J Med* 1979;301:126–131.
29. Polak A, Eschenhoff E, Fernex M, et al: Metabolic studies with 5-fluorocytosine-6-^{14}C in mouse, rabbit, dog and man. *Chemotherapy* 1976;22:137–153.
30. Lehrer RI, Howard DH, Sypherd PS, et al: Mucormycosis. *Ann Intern Med* 1980;93:93–108.
31. Rippon JW: Zygomycosis, in Rippon JW (ed): *Medical Mycology, the Pathogenic Fungi, and the Pathogenic Actinomycetes,* 3rd ed. Philadelphia, WB Saunders, 1988, pp 681–713.
32. Edwards JE Jr: Zygomycosis, in Hoeprich PD, Jordan MC (eds): *Infectious Diseases*. Philadelphia, Harper & Row, 1989, pp 1192–1199.
33. Meyers BR, Wormser G, Hirschman SZ, et al: Rhinocerebral mucormycosis: premortem diagnosis and therapy. *Arch Intern Med* 1979;139:557–560.
34. Parfrey NA: Improved diagnosis and prognosis of mucormycosis. A clinicopathologic study of 33 cases. *Medicine* 1986;65:113–123.
35. Fiese MJ: *Coccidioidomycosis*. Springfield, Ill, Charles C Thomas, 1958, pp 1–253.
36. Rippon JW: Coccidioidomycosis, in Rippon JW (ed): *Medical Mycology: The Pathogenic Fungi and the Pathogenic Actinomycetes,* 3rd ed. Philadelphia, WB Saunders, 1988, pp 433–473.
37. Hoeprich PD: Coccidioidomycosis, in Hoeprich PD, Jordan MC (eds): *Infectious Diseases,* 4th ed. Philadelphia, Harper & Row, 1989, pp 489–502.
38. Swatek FE: Ecology of *Coccidioides immitis*. *Mycopathol Mycol Appl* 1970;40:3–12.
39. Forbus WD: Coccidioidomycosis: a study of 95 cases of the disseminated type with special reference to the pathogenesis of the disease. *Milit Surg* 1946;99:653–719.
40. Baker EE, Mrak EM, Smith CE: The morphology, taxonomy and distribution of *Coccidioides immitis* Rixford and Gilchrist 1896. *Farlowia* 1943;1:199–244.
41. Reiss E: *Molecular Immunology of Mycotic and Actinomycotic Infections*. New York, Elsevier, 1986, pp 53–76.
42. Flynn NM, Hoeprich PD, Kawachi MM, et al: An unusual outbreak of windborne coccidioidomycosis. *N Engl J Med* 1979;301:358–361.
43. Drutz DJ, Cantazaro A: Coccidioidomycosis. *Am Rev Resp Dis* 1978;117:559–585, 727–771.
44. Kafka JA, Cantazaro A: Disseminated coccidioidomycosis in children. *J Pediatr* 1981;98:355–361.
45. Bouza E, Dreyer JS, Hewitt WL, et al: Coccidioidal meningitis: an analysis of thirty-one cases and review of the literature. *Medicine* 1981;60:139–172.
46. Einstein HE, Holeman CW Jr, Sandidge LL, et al: Coccidioidal meningitis. The use of amphotericin B in treatment. *Calif Med* 1961;94:339–343.
47. Saag MS, Dismukes WE: Azole antifungal agents: emphasis on triazoles. *Antimicrob Agents Chemother* 1988;32:1–8.

18
Parasitic Infections of the Central Nervous System

THOMAS F. PATTERSON, JAN E. PATTERSON, MICHELE BARRY, AND FRANK J. BIA

Within the past decade, it has become all too evident that parasitic infections of the central nervous system (CNS) are increasingly relevant to the differential diagnostic process. This trend can only be expected to continue. It depends on several new facts of life for physicians practicing in temperate climates, as well as in the tropics. The current acquired immunodeficiency syndrome (AIDS) epidemic has underscored the ubiquitous distribution of latent and reactivated toxoplasmosis infection, particularly in the CNS. Immunosuppressive regimens for the prevention of transplant rejection are increasingly capable of disseminating an otherwise quiescent and chronic nematode infection, such as intestinal strongyloidiasis. Rapid air travel for business and vacation, migration of refugee populations, and the exposure of long-term health-care workers in developing countries to parasitic infections also emphasize their importance in the differential diagnosis of CNS lesions.

Toxoplasmosis of the CNS

CNS toxoplasmosis has been a relatively uncommon disease confined largely to immunocompromised patients, the fetus with congenital CNS infection and patients with toxoplasma-associated retinitis.[1] However, with the advent of AIDS, the frequency of CNS infection has dramatically increased.[2,3] CNS toxoplasmosis is the most frequent cause of focal intracerebral lesions in patients with AIDS.[3] It has been estimated that by 1991, in the United States alone, there will be 20,000–40,000 cases of CNS toxoplasmosis in AIDS patients.[3] Patients with AIDS, immunocompromised cancer patients, and immunosuppressed transplant recipients represent expanding populations at high risk for CNS toxoplasma infection. It is now essential to understand the pathogenesis of CNS toxoplasmosis and to recognize its clinical features when evaluating patients such as these.

Toxoplasma gondii is an obligate intracellular parasite found throughout the world in many species of warm-blooded animals, both domestic and wild.[4] When humans or other carnivores ingest raw or undercooked meat, toxoplasma tissue cysts in infected skeletal muscles carry the infection to a susceptible host.[4] Tachyzoites are released from each tissue cyst in the host's gastrointestinal tract. Active infection and tissue invasion follow. Members of the cat family serve as definitive hosts for the organism; they can transmit infection directly to humans by shedding infective oocysts. Ingestion of oocysts also causes acute infection in susceptible hosts (Figure 18.1). Congenital toxoplasmosis results from acute toxoplasmosis in a previously seronegative mother. Even if not apparent at birth, congenital infection may later reactivate to cause retinitis or toxoplasmic encephalitis in immunocompromised patients.[1]

The prevalence of toxoplasma infection varies greatly according to geography, ranging from 20 to 70% in the United States to as high as 96% in parts of France.[3,5] Prevalence reflects the density of cats, intermediate hosts, and the consumption of raw or undercooked meats.[1] These epidemiologic differences are important since the prevalence of toxoplasma antibodies indicates the risk of reactivation

This chapter has been updated with permission from a previous article. Parasitic infections of the central nervous system. *Neurol Clin* 1986;4(1):172.

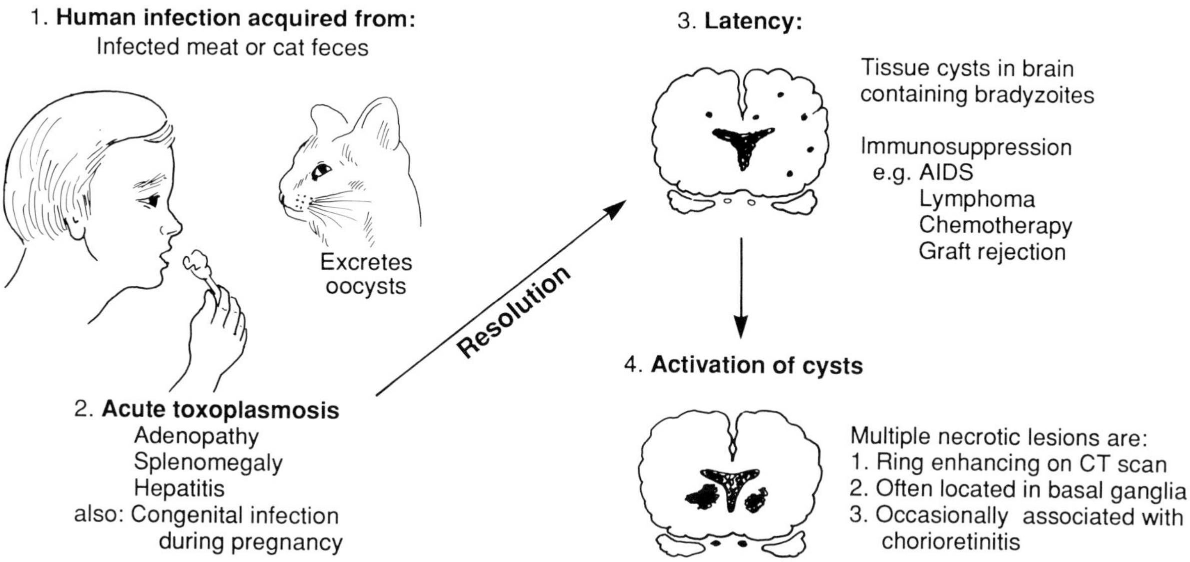

Fig. 18.1. Pathogenesis of cerebral toxoplasmosis by reactivation of latent organisms present in parenchymal brain cysts and retina. Basal ganglia are often involved. [Adapted with permission from Bia FJ, Barry M: Parasitic infections of the central nervous system. *Neurol Clin* 1986;4(1):172.]

in a population of immunosuppressed patients. While toxoplasma infections are common in most parts of the world, such infections are usually asymptomatic or result in an acute self-limited lymphoproliferative syndrome.[4] However, in immunocompromised patients, the acute clinical syndrome is more severe and reactivation of latent tissue cysts is an additional threat. Tissue cysts can rupture and release invasive trophozoites (tachyzoites) within any organ of patients with compromised cell-mediated immunity. These tachyzoites are responsible for destroying cells and producing necrotic foci of infection.[1] When latent tissue cysts are present in the brain, their activiation results in toxoplasmic encephalitis or brain abscess.

CNS involvement during acute infection is seen in 36–60% of patients with compromised immune function.[6,7] These patients have underlying neoplasms (most notably hematologic malignancies) or collagen vascular diseases, or have received corticosteroids, either alone or in combination with other immunosuppressive drugs.[6] Patients undergoing organ transplatation are at significant risk for CNS toxoplasmosis.[8–12] In a review of toxoplasma infections at Memorial Sloan–Kettering Cancer Center from 1972 to 1978 (prior to the AIDS epidemic), 42 cases were identified.[13] In 17 patients without neoplasms, CNS involvement by *T gondii* was not seen. In contrast, 8 of 25 patients with toxoplasmosis and an underlying neoplasm had CNS infections, all of which were fatal.

Townsend and colleagues[14] reviewed the clinical presentation of CNS toxoplasmosis prior to the AIDS epidemic and found three characteristic patterns: (1) a diffuse encephalopathy characterized by confusion, delirium, and obtundation; (2) meningoencephalitis with stiff neck, headache, and focal or generalized seizures; (3) focal signs consistent with a single or multiple space-occupying lesions being the most common presentation.

T gondii is the second most common cause of meningoencephalitis and brain abscess in transplant recipients.[15,16] The growing population of patients undergoing cardiac transplantation is at significant risk for severe toxoplasma infection[8] from cysts present in transplanted cardiac tissues as a result of previous acute infection.[15,17] CNS infection has been documented as a consequence of disseminated acute infection in seronegative recipients of hearts from seropositive donors.[15,18] Immunosuppressive regimens also vary in their ability to reactivate infection.[19] Toxoplasma infection usually becomes evident 1–4 months posttransplantation at a time when active cytomegalovirus (CMV) infection is also seen.[8] An association among toxoplasmosis, CMV, and other DNA virus infections has been described.[8] Immunosuppressed patients with CNS toxoplasmosis may also have other opportunistic infections, which complicates the clinical diagnosis.[20]

Before the AIDS epidemic, 2% of intracerebral infections reported from the Massachusetts General Hospital and 5% from Memorial Sloan-Kettering Cancer Center, were caused by *T gondii*.[6,21] In contrast, toxoplasma infection was documented in 25% of patients with AIDS and CNS infection at Memorial Sloan-Kettering Cancer Center and New York Hospital.[22]

Levy and colleagues,[23,24] at the University of California in San Francisco, reviewed neurologic complications of AIDS, and *T gondii* accounted for nearly one third of all CNS complications. Most CNS toxoplasma lesions in AIDS patients are caused by reactivation of latent infection. In New York City, 2.6% of *all* AIDS patients were reported to have CNS toxoplasmosis. The risk that a patient with AIDS and positive toxoplasma serology will develop CNS toxoplasmosis may be as high as 6–12%.[25] In other AIDS populations, particularly Haitians, the risk of CNS toxoplasmosis is even higher.[26] In the United States, CNS toxoplasmosis has been the initial manifestation of AIDS in 2.1% of patients, if based on biopsy-proved disease.[3] However, in areas of high toxoplasma seroprevalence, such as Germany and France, toxoplasma encephalitis is frequently an initial manifestation of the syndrome, and found in at least 25% of patients with AIDS.[3]

Focal neurologic deficits are present in up to 90% of AIDS patients with toxoplasmosis; most frequently this is a mild hemiparesis.[2] Diffuse encephalopathy, characterized by confusion and lethargy, may be seen initially in approximately 60–70% of patients.[2,3] More than half the patients reviewed by Navia and colleagues[2] presented with both focal signs and diffuse encephalophathy. Headaches and fever are also common, but meningeal signs, even in patients with cerebrospinal fluid (CSF) pleocytosis, are rare. Toxoplasma chorioretinitis may precede or accompany CNS disease.[3]

Laboratory findings in CNS toxoplasmosis are nonspecific and may show a mononuclear pleocytosis, moderate evaluation of protein, and normal or slightly decreased glucose concentration.[20] In patients with AIDS, CSF pleocytosis may be absent during active CNS toxoplasmosis.[27] Trophozoites can be isolated from CSF, blood, and tissue samples by mouse incoulation.[5] However, the diagnosis is definitively established by direct histopathologic examination of brain tissue for free trophozoites and cysts.[5,21] Peroxidase-antiperoxidase stain is more sensitive than conventional hemotoxylin-eosin staining techniques for identifying *T gondii*.[21]

Serologic responses indicative of acute toxoplasma infection will not occur in patients with AIDS, since CNS toxoplasmosis nearly always results from reactivation of latent infection. A rise in specific IgG titer is also uncommon.[3] In areas with a high prevalence of toxoplasmosis, IgM antibody has been demonstrated in the serum of AIDS patients presenting with encephalopathy, indicating an acutely acquired infection. That response has been quite rare in the United States.[3] Local CSF antibody production may indicate active CNS infection.[28] This was demonstrated in 11 of 16 AIDS patients with toxoplasma encephalitis but not in 4 without infection. Serologic testing is more important in establishing previous exposure and risk of reactivation in immunocompromised patients.[3] While a negative serology reduces the likelihood of toxoplasma infection, negative results have occasionally been obtained in patients with AIDS and documented CNS toxoplasmosis.[21]

Computed tomography (CT) scans typically demonstrate multiple, bilateral, hypodense, enhancing lesions that are located in deep subcortical structures, such as the basal ganglia, in over 50% of the cases (Figure 18.2).[3] Double-dose contrast gives maximal enhancement of the lesions and may detect lesions not otherwise seen.[3] CT scans do not provide a specific diagnosis. A typical scan in a high-risk patient with a positive toxoplasma serology is highly suggestive of the disease.[29] Even patients with normal scans, or scans showing only atrophy, have had biopsy-proved disease.[29] Other disease processes, particularly CNS lymphoma, can mimic or coexist with CNS toxoplasmosis.

Magnetic-resonance imaging (MRI) appears to be a sensitive indicator of this disease. In one study, CT showed lesions in 22% of patients, as compared with 42% demonstrated by MRI.[3] There are usually three or more lesions present on MRI in toxoplasmosis; a single lesion suggests other etiologies for disease. MRI has localized a lesion at the C2-4 level secondary to toxoplasmic myelitis,[30] the first reported case of myelitis caused by *T gondii*.

Not only immunosuppressed patients, but also those undergoing organ-transplant evaluation, should have baseline toxoplasma serology performed because there is risk of infection in seronegative patients who receive organs from seropositive donors.[3–12] Pyrimethamine prophylaxis has been

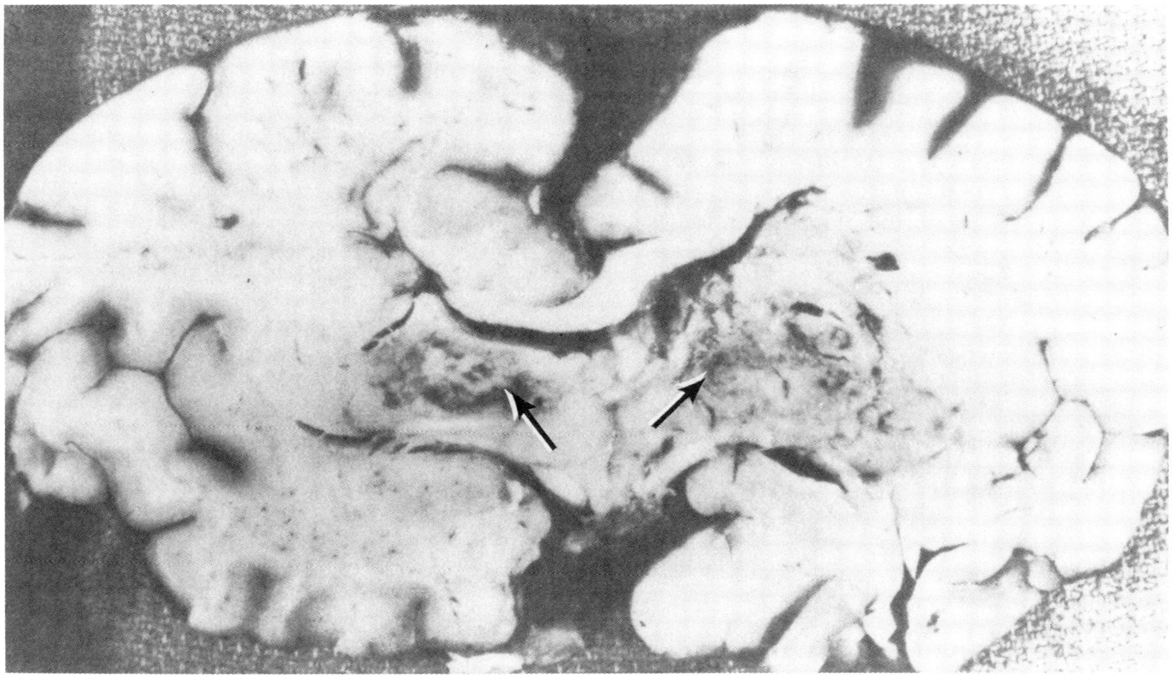

Fig. 18.2. Brain coronal cross section through mamillary bodies. Tissue obtained from a 28-year-old homosexual man who died with extensive CNS lesions from toxoplasmosis. This section demonstrates considerable necrosis (arrows) of midline and periventricular structures (corpus callosum, septum pellucidum, fornix, and basal ganglia), with microhemorrhages in surrounding white matter and cortex. (Reprinted with permission from Horowitz SL, Benston JR, Benson, F, et al: CNS toxoplasmosis in acquired immunodeficiency syndrome. *Arch Neurol* 1983;40:649–652. Copyright 1983, American Medical Association.)

successful in preventing acute infection in seronegative cardiac-transplant recipients who received hearts from seropositive donors.[18] Pyrimethamine and sulfadiazine treatment, at the time seroconversion occurs in these patients, has also been advocated.[9]

In the past, brain biopsy was recommended for diagnosis of all CNS lesions in patients with AIDS. This approach was often hindered by the deep-seated location of the lesions, so empiric therapy was attempted. Considerable data now support an empiric approach to the treatment of CNS toxoplasmosis.[26,31] In a recent study by Cohn and colleagues[31] at Bellevue Hospital in New York, patients with multiple, enhancing, deep-seated lesions on CT scan were so treated. They responded as well as those with biopsy-confirmed disease. These investigators recommend biopsy only if the scan is atypical, or if there is no response to therapy within 10–14 days. Their population did include many patients from the Caribbean, for whom empiric therapy may be more successful owing to the high rates of letent toxoplasma infection.[31] Current therapy for CNS toxoplasmosis includes the combination of pyrimethamine (100 mg loading dose following by 25 mg/day) with sulfadiazine (6–8 g/day).[3,20] Some investigators perfer to give larger doses (75–100 mg/day) of pyrimethamine for the first 6 weeks of therapy because of reported failures with lower doses.[3]

Folinic acid (leukovorin calcium), 10 mg daily, is added to prevent bone-marrow suppression and can be increased to 50 mg daily, if needed. Rash and leukopenia from sulfadiazine are particularly common in AIDS patients,[32] often necessitating discontinuation of the drug. Therapy with pyrimethamine alone has been associated with both failures and relapses.[32] Clindamycin has been substituted for sulfadiazine and has been successful in treatment and prophylaxis.[33] Comparative trials using these drugs are in progress.[3] Initial responses of 80–90% are reported in AIDS patients with CNS toxoplasmosis, but lifelong suppressive therapy for these patients is necessary because of the clear risk of reactivation.[32]

Cerebral Malaria

Malaria is transmitted to humans by Anopheles mosquitoes infected with protozoa of the genus *Plasmodium*. The four species pathogenic for humans are *Plasmodium vivax, Plasmodium ovale, Plasmodium malariae,* and *Plasmodium falciparum,* the cause of cerebral malaria. Falciparum malaria is also associated with drug resistance and high mortality rates.[34]

When the female anopheline mosquito bites, she releases infective sporozoites from salivary glands into the human circulation. They enter hepatocytes, mature, and multiply asexually. Each sporozoite yields thousands of merozoites that are capable of infecting human erythrocytes. During the erythrocytic phase of infection, the clinical manifestations of malaria, such as paroxysmal fever, chills, nausea, and headache, become apparent. Such signs as hepatomegaly, mild icterus, and rapid onset of splenomegaly are also evident. Untreated falciparum malaria can quickly progress to severe anemia, decreased circulating blood volume, and capillary blockage in such organs as the brain. The complications of fulminant, "pernicious" malaria occur during *P falciparum* infections when more than 5–10% of red blood cells are infected. Organ failures such as shock liver or lung, mesenteric ischemia, renal failure, or cerebral malaria are due to capillary blockage by infected erythrocytes.[34] Some parasites differentiate into gametocytes, which can infect another anopheline mosquito, thus completing the cycle.

The pathogenesis of cerebral malaria is not entirely understood.[35] It is thought to involve the sequestration of erythrocytes, caused by surface projections or "knobs" on parasitized erythrocytes, which interact with capillary endothelial cells.[36] An animal model of cerebral malaria has also implicated tumor-necrosis factor as a possible mediator of cerebral malaria.[37] Inflammation does not appear to play a role.[38]

CNS manifestations of malaria are diverse and can be divided into five categories: (1) disturbances of consciousness, (2) acute organic syndromes, (3) movement disorders, (4) focal neurologic signs, and (5) personality changes.[39] Disturbances of consciousness are very common and range from stupor and lethargy to coma. Acute organic syndromes may produce disorientation, confusion, and intellectual deterioration without depression of consciousness. Movement disorders include mild tremors, myoclonus, and severe chorea. Focal signs such as sensory disturbances, hemiplegias, grand mal, and focal seizures have also been described. Acute psychosis or mild neurologic deficits detected by psychometric testing may also occur.[37] In fact, this disease can cause almost any neurologic sign or symptom.[40]

The lumbar puncture is remarkable only for a slight to moderate elevation of opening pressure. Indeed, CSF pleocytosis warrants suspicion of another disease process. A peripheral blood smear showing the characteristic parasitic forms of falciparum malaria confirms the diagnosis of cerebral malaria in the appropriate clinical setting. Therapy is determined by the geographic areas of malaria exposure, since chloroquine-resistant falciparum malaria is becoming the rule in many endemic regions.[41]

Areas where resistant malaria is prevalent now include sub-Saharan Africa, Southeast Asia, South America, Oceania, and the Indian subcontinent.[42] The Centers for Disease Control (CDC) should be contacted for the most up-to-date information (CDC Malaria Hotline: 404/332-4555). Parenteral therapy is usually necessary for adequate treatment of cerebral malaria. For chloroquine-sensitive *P falciparum,* parenteral quinine or chloroquine may be used. Chloroquine-resistant *P falciparum* strains are also becoming resistant to other currently available agents, including quinine, a standard parenteral agent for serious infection with these strains. Intravenous *quinidine* may be used for chloroquine- or quinine-resistant malaria,[43] and has the advantage of being more readily available than parenteral quinine. Therapy should not be delayed because of inavailability of parenteral quinine.[43] Intravenous corticosteroids have been used in the past, but new data suggest they may actually worsen outcome.[44] Neurologic recovery is almost always total if patients are treated promptly with antimalarials.[39,44]

The utilization of malaria chemoprophylaxis when traveling to endemic areas will help to prevent cerebral malaria. Regimens for travel to areas where multiresistant strains exist are becoming more difficult to construct. Medication is started one week before travel and continued for four weeks afterwards.[42] Personal protection measures against mosquito bites are most important and include the use of mosquito netting, appropriate clothing, and insect repellents.

Primary Amebic Meningoencephalitis and Amebic Brain Abscess

Primary amebic meningoecephalitis (PAM) is a rare, usually fatal, infection most connonly caused by *Naegleria fowleri*.[45] Other species of free-living ameba, including *Acanthamoeba* species and *Entamoeba histolytica,* can also cause CNS infection, but with each organism, distinctive clinical and pathologic features of CNS disease are present.[46–49]

Although *N fowleri* is found worldwide, most reported cases have occurred in the United States;[50] most disease occurs in young adults or children who swim in freshwater pools or lakes. Ameba gain access to the CNS by direct penetration through the nasal mucosa, the cribiform plate, and along the olfactory nerves into brain. Inhalation of cysts on dust is the presumed mode of inoculation in arid regions.[51] The clinical course of *Naegleria* infections is rapid, dramatic, and usually fatal within 72 hours of onset.

Symptoms mimic acute bacterial meningitis with severe headache, fever, and anorexia, followed by nausea, vomiting, and meningeal signs. Disturbances in smell or taste may be clues to the diagnosis, before progression to generalized seizures and death.[50] Pathologic features of PAM include cerebral edema with grossly purulent meninges. The olfactory bulbs show areas of hemorrhage and purulent necrosis.[46]

The diagnosis of PAM is made by demonstration of either living amebae on wet mounts of CSF or stained organisms using Wright or Giemsa methods. Organisms are not detected on routine Gram stain; they are destroyed by heat fixation.[50] Amebae could also be grown in culture. CSF examination during PAM reveals a grossly purulent process. Leukocyte cell counts, mostly neutrophils, range from 200 to 20,000 cells/mm^3.[50]

There is no reliable therapy for PAM associated with *N flowleri*. Amphotericin B, given intravenously and intrathecally, has been effective.[46] Another patient was successfully treated with amphotericin B, in combination with micronazole and rifampin.[52] Prevention of infection through adequate chlorination of water (10 ppm) and education of the public remain the most effective means of controlling the disease. A fatal *Naegleria* infection was acquired from a freshwater swimming pool in which traditional chlorination had been replaced by an electronic cleaning device.[53]

In contrast to PAM caused by *N fowleri, Acanthamoeba* spp produce chronic, granulomatous, necrotizing encephalitis with minimal involvement of the meninges. The infection is fatal after weeks to months of CNS infection.[49,54] As with *Naegleria, Acanthamoeba* is found in moist soil and brackish, warm water. The portals of entry for *Acanthamoeba* are the upper respiratory tract and eyes.[54] *Acanthamoeba* keratitis and skin infections occur and healthy persons have been shown to be asymptomatic carriers. Symptomatic CNS infections have been seen in debilitated or immunocompromised patients, including patients with AIDS.[49,55]

Pathologically, *Acanthamoeba* causes a characteristic parenchymal brain lesion, which is a subacute necrotizing or chronic granulomatous encephalitis. Trophozoites and cysts are found together with giant cells, monocytes, and plasma cells. Arteritis may occur in association with aneurysm formation produced by amebic trophozoites located in vascular walls.[54] Clinical symptoms are mainly those of encephalopathy—fever, headache, nausea, vomiting, changes in mental status, and seizures. Other neurologic symptoms include evidence of a space-occupying lesion, ataxia, hemiparesis, visual disturbances, and papilledema, with progression to coma and death. The clinical course and duration of the illness range from one week to about 120 days.[49]

The CSF findings in *Acanthamoeba* infections show a mixed polymorphonuclear and lymphocyte pleocytosis with elevated protein and slightly decreased glucose concentrations.[49] The CSF is not as purulent as in *Naegleria* infections.[49,54] A histologic diagnosis can be confirmed using specific immunofluorescent or peroxidase antibody straining techniques. If keratitis is persent, the organisms can be demonstrated in a corneal scraping. Indirect fluorescent antiboby testing of serum may be helpful in making the diagnosis. The chronic course of *Acanthamoeba* infections differs from the rapidly evolving *Naegleria* infections that fail to induce a serologic response.[54] A chronic progressive *Acanthamoeba* infection must be distinguished from pyogenic brain abscess, tuberculoma, an expanding fungal lesion, or tumor.[55]

Therapy for *Acanthamoeba* meningoencephalitis has not been successful. *Acanthamoeba* species are resistant to amphotericin B.[54] Sulfadiazine has only been shown effective in experimental infections, but ketoconazole and miconazole have been used to treat keratitis.[54,56] The usual course of human infection is progression to coma and death.

Entamoeba histolytica is occasionally responsible for brain-abscess formation. Although *E histolytica* is the etiologic agent of classic amebic dysentery, other syndromes ranging from asymptomatic carriage to hepatic abscess formation and rare hematogenous dissemination do occur. Amebiasis is acquired through ingestion of cysts in contaminated food or water. During intestinal infection, trophozoite penetration of the colonic mucosa may take place.

After trophozoites pass through the portal system they can cause abscesses in the liver, lungs, pleural or pericardial spaces, and, rarely, the brain. The incidence of amebic brain abscess has ranged from 0.6 to 5% of those patients with liver abscesses.[51] In one autopsy series, brain involvement was seen in 8% of patients with liver abscess,[57] but in the absence of liver disease, brain lesions are distinctly uncommon. Although liver lesions are usually single, multiple brain abscess can occur.[58]

Neurologic signs may be minimal despite extensive brain involvement. Hemiplegia and signs of meningeal irritation are present. Pathologically, the lesions are often found in the basal ganglia and the frontal lobes. They range from discrete zones of petechiae formation to large areas of necrosis caused by amebic tissue destruction. A capsule may form around older lesions. Meningeal involvement may produce a purulent, fibrinous exudate.[59]

The diagnosis of amebic brain abscess is best established by determining the etiology of lesions in the liver or lung. Serologic tests are usually positive because extraintestinal disease is usually extensive by the time a brain abscess appears. Examinations of stool for amebic cysts or trophozoites are usually negative. *E histolytica* infection must be distinguished from pyogenic brain abscess, toxoplasmosis, and fungal and mycobacterial disease, as well as disease caused by other amebae.[59]

As opposed to CNS disease caused by *Naegleria* or *Acanthamoeba,* soft-tissue infections due to *E histolytica,* including those in the brain, can be treated successfully with metronidazole and, when necessary, surgery.[51] Because patients with CNS amebiasis frequently have far advanced disease, the mortality rate remains high despite therapy.[59]

Neurocysticercosis

To understand the relationships between human pork-tapeworm infection and neurocysticercosis, one must keep in mind that human ingestion of ova passed by such tapeworms is what poses the threat of neurocysticercosis. This is the most common parasitic infection of the CNS in patients who are not overtly immunosuppressed. Humans acquire pork-tapeworm infection by eating undercooked pork containing larvae of *Taenia solium.*[60–62] Each adult tapeworm has a head (scolex) equipped with suckers and hooklets attaching it to small bowel. Often several meters of ova-containing segments (proglottids) are attached to the scolex. These proglottids continuously break off and are passed in human stool daily. (Figure 18.3). When swine ingest ova, oncospheres are released into their intestine. They enter the venous system and encyst as larvae in other porcine organs. These are cysticerci, and they can also form in humans who ingest *T solium* ova. They have a strong predilection for brain, eyes, and skeletal muscle. The ova that humans ingest could have been passed in their own feces, thereby resulting in an autoinfection. To reiterate the epidemiologic problem, infected pork poses the problem of human tapeworm infection. Infected humans who contaminate food, water, or themselves with the ova of *T solium* pose the treat of cysticercosis, a highly neurotropic infection. (Figure 18.4). Some infected patients have been shown to have over 100 documented brain cysts.

The presence of larva-containing cysticerci in the CNS, is associated with several disease patterns, which depend on their number, size, and location, and the intensity of immunologic reactions to them. Patterns include meningeal infection and inflammation, individual parenchymal cysts causing focal symptoms such as seizures, multiple cysts producing intracranial hypertension, ventricular cysts that obstruct CSF flow, mass lesions of the spinal cord, and asymptomatic infection.[63] However, when cysticerci either die or are destroyed by antiparasitic therapy, cyst expansion and an associated inflammatory response pose a major threat to infected patients. In contrast, living embyos cause very little tissue reaction.

The natural history of parenchymal brain cysts is one of slow expansion, death of larvae, an inflammatory response, and ultimately calcification of the involved area. This process often results in seizure disorders, cysticercosis being one of the most common causes of epilepsy in the tropics. When seizures occur in patients near open fires, they are often associated with burn injuries. Intraventricular cysts may suddently block passage of CSF. When acute obstructive hydrocephalus occurs, it may be catastrophic. Keane[64] reported seven Latin American patients who died from acute obstructive hydrocephalus caused by cysticercosis. Appropriate evaluation occured too late in their course to be helpful. Approximately 20% of neurocysticercosis cases involve the ocular system.[61] Sudden focal

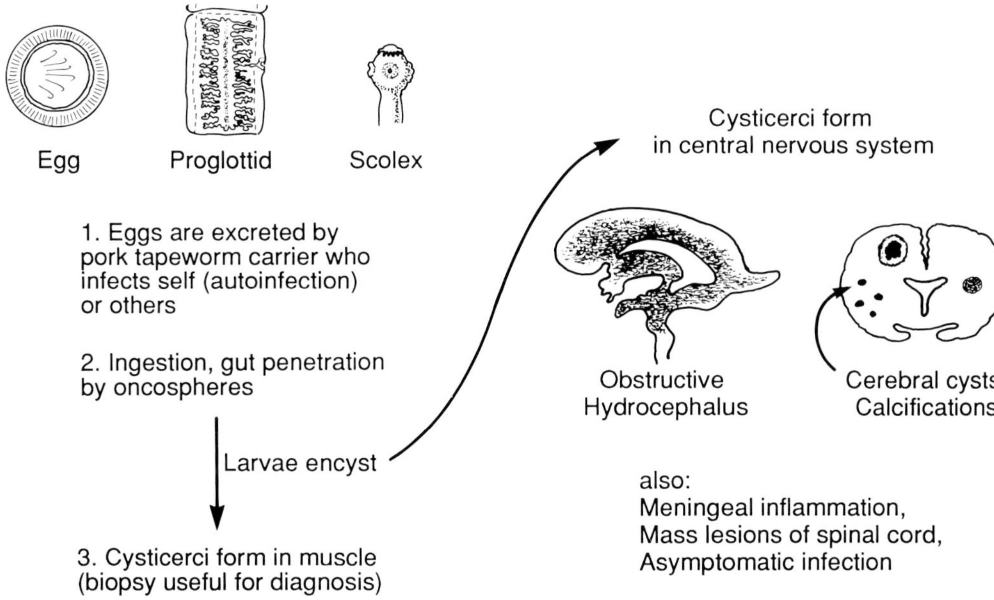

Fig. 18.3. Pathogenesis of neurocysticercosis following ingestion of *T solium* ova. Cysts in ventricles can cause acute obstructive hydrocephalus. Death of larvae is associated with acute exacerbations of CNS disease. [Adapted with permission from Bia FJ Barry M: Parasitic infections of the central nervous system. *Neurol Clin* 1986;4(1):182.]

neurologic deficits, or stroke syndromes, were the major presentations for nearly 12% of patients in one series.[65] In the ventricular system or subarachnoid spaces, multilobulated cysts, free of larval forms, can grow in a racemose form of infection. Such infections can be quite extensive and, in one case, resulted in occlusion of the right internal carotid artery.[66]

The diagnosis of neurocysticercosis does not depend on finding the ova of *T solium* in stool samples since a minority of patients, particularly older patients, harbor adult tapeworms (Table 18.1). Half of infected patients will demonstrate subcutaneous cysts, which are often calcified and visible on soft-tissue radiographs. Serologic tests of serum and CSF for specific antibody are useful, particularly in areas of low prevalence, where cross-reactivity between cysticercosis, echinococcus, schistosomiasis, and other cestode infections may not be a problem.[60] CSF antibodies may not be present in patients with single parenchymal cysts. Otherwise, CSF findings reflect chronic meningitis with lymphocytic pleocytosis (83%), elevated CSF pressures (74%), increased protein concentration (45%), and depressed CSF glucose (82%).[60] In a report of 30 adults and 15 children with suspected neurocysticercosis by Byrd and colleagues[67] in Los Angeles, nearly all presented with seizures. Plain skull films showed calcifications in four adults and one child. Nearly all radionuclide brain scans and most angiograms (80%) were normal.

However, CT scanning (Figure 18.5) has clearly altered the diagnosis and evalution of patients with suspected and treated neurocysticercosis.[68] Adults with neurocysticercosis are more likely to demonstrate older lesions, with little contrast enhancement and considerable calcification, as indicated in Table 18.1. Adults generally will not demonstrate *Taenia* ova in their stools as often as children, whose lesions are more acute and more likely to show contrast enhancement on CT scanning. In the latter group, corticosteroids become an important part of therapy, and response to therapy is inversely related to the duration of CNS infection.

With regard to the treatment of cysticercosis, given the granulomatous, fibrotic, calcific, and hydrocephalic complications of neurocysticercosis and their anatomic distribution, it would be unlikely that one therapeutic agent could control these events. Praziquantel is extremely effective in destroying parenchymal lesions containing larval forms and in destroying adult *T solium* in the bowel.

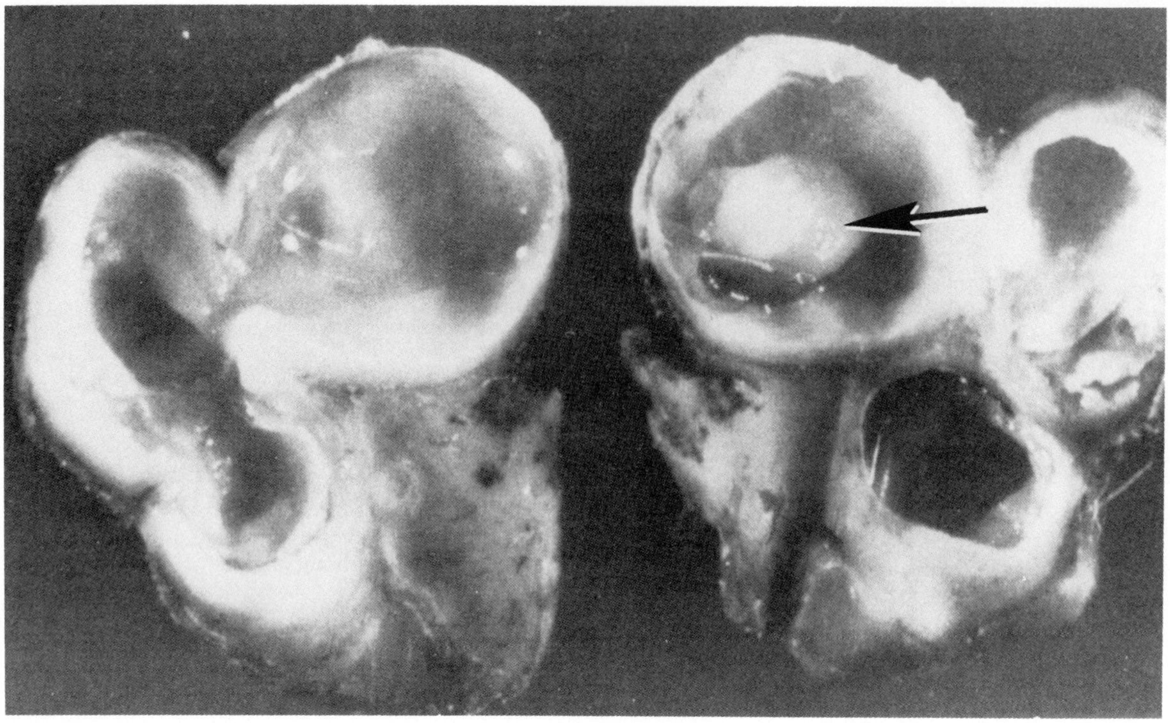

Fig. 18.4. Surgical specimen of cerebral cysticercosis cysts showing clear fluid and a scolex (arrow). (Reprinted with permission from Byrd SE, Locke GE, Biggers S, et al: The computed tomographic appearance of cerebral cysticercosis in adults and children. *Radiology* 1982;144:819–823. Radiological Society of North America.)

During therapy for neurologic disease, most patients (over 90%) will develop apparent clinical exacerbations of their disease as a result of the death of larvae and increased inflammation.

Seizures, headaches, and vomiting are common. CSF pleocytosis and protein concentration may increase, occasionally associated with a conversion of CSF cysticercosis antibody to positive.[69] These changes likely reflect degeneration of the parasite and an inflammatory response; CT scanning at this time will usually show an increase in ring enhancement. Most investigators agree that short-course corticosteroid and anticonvulsant therapy is beneficial in preventing the CNS consequences of effective anticestodal therapy, and this has been our experience in treating parenchymal disease.[70]

Sotelo and co-workers[69] have shown that in untreated control patients with neurocysticercosis followed for a mean interval of nine (plus or minus two) months, there was definite progression of disease—that is, a 12% increase in the total number of brain cysts and a 14% increase in the size of lesions. In contrast, three months after praziquantel therapy (50 mg/kg/day for 15 days), the mean diameter of all cysts had been reduced by 72% and two thirds (101 of 152) of original cysts had disappeared.[69] In their series, headaches and increased neurologic symptoms during treatment were usual in the absence of corticosteroid therapy. One-year follow-up was reported in 35 of these patients.[71] The mean number and diameter of cysts showed reductions of 67% and 73% respectively. In 19 patients (54%), total remission of all cysts occurred. Only three patients were considered treatment failures and 91% of patients with parenchymal disease improved (Figure 18.5).

These results did not apply to all patients. Nine of their 17 patients (53%) with chronic arachnoiditis continued to show CSF findings reflecting meningitis. Five developed hydrocephalus and approximately 25% of cysts were replaced by apparent granuloma formation. Intraventricular cysts may not be amenable to antiparasitic therapy alone.[72] It is not known what effects scarring and residual lesions will have on the development of subsequent seizure disorders. A new imidazole, albendazole, is less expensive than praziquantel and may prove to be

Table 18.1. CT scanning in 171 cases of neurocysticercosis reported from Brazil.

Type of lesion shown on scan	No. of cases	(%)
Nonacute lesions that may show little or no contrast enhancement[a]		
Calcifications alone	82	(48)%
Calcifications and cysts	31	(18)%
Calcifications and hydrocephaly	12	(7)%
Brain cysts	10	(6)%
Posterior fossa cysts	4	(2)%
Acute lesions with edema and postcontrast enhancement[b]		
Diffuse acute lesions	19	(11)%
Single acute lesions	6	(4)%
"Tumoral" lesions	7	(4)%
Total, all cases	171	100%

[a]Stool examination for *Taenia* often negative. Pattern seen in older patients.
[b]31 of 32 patients showed *Taenia* in stool. Pattern often seen in children and more likely to respond to corticosteroids.
(Adapted with premission from Minguetti G, Ferreira MVC: Computed tomography in neurocysticercosis. *J Neurol Neurosurg Psychiatry* 1983;46:936–949.)

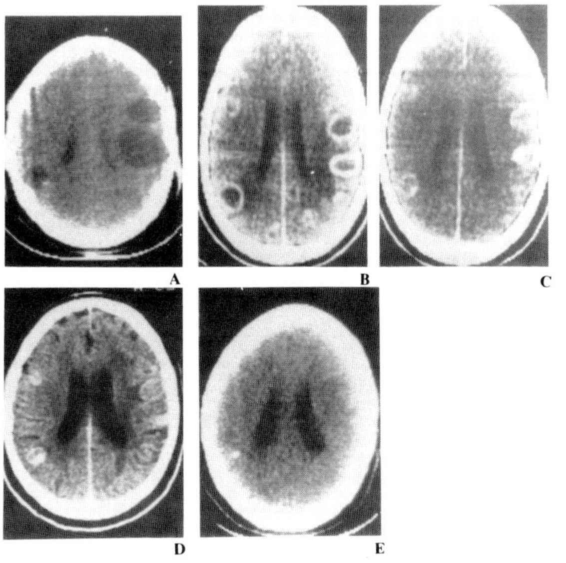

Fig. 18.5. CT images of a patient with neurocysticercosis treated with praziquantel. (A) Before treatment, three large cysts were found. (B) On the last day of treatment, cysts are notably reduced in size, and are surrounded by inflammation, as disclosed by intense concentration of contrast medium around cysts. (C) Three months after treatment, hypodense areas have disappeared, but there is still concentration of contrast medium around lesions. (D) Six months after treatment, inflammation is notably reduced; the same CT slice without contrast did not show evidence of lesion. Note the discrete enlargement of lateral ventricles. (E) After one year of treatment, all lesions have remitted; only one cyst was replaced by granuloma and the ventricles show residual hydrocephalus (authors' interpretations). (Reprinted with permission from Sotelo J, Torres B, Rubio-Donnadieu F, et al: Praziquantel in the treatment of neurocysticercosis: long-term follow-up. *Neurology* 1985;35:752–755.)

slightly more efficacious, but it has been associated with hepatotoxity.[62,73] Corticosteroids may decrease plasma levels of praziquantel.[74] Agapejev and co-workers[75] have combined albendazole therapy with an antihistamine that penetrates the CNS well as an alternative approach to corticosteroids for preventing side effects of therapy.

Stools may not always demonstrate *Taenia* ova in patients with neurocysticercosis (25%). However, Richards and Schantz[76] have shown that only 20–40% of their patients with cysticercosis were adequately examined for ova in stools. They suggest that the yield would reach 50% if appropriate examinations were performed, especially in young patients whose CT findings suggest acute disease.[68] Family members, particularly children, should be included in screening because therapy is most effective in early disease.

Echinococcosis (Hydatid Disease) of the CNS

Hydatid disease, or echinococcosis, is unusual in North America, but it is frequently encountered in travelers to or immigrants from endemic areas, such as Greece, Italy, central Europe, South America, Iraq, Australia, New Zealand, and Africa. Although echinococcal disease of the CNS is rare, patients with expanding mass lesions of the brain or evidence of spinal-cord compression may have important epidemiologic information in their medical histories pointing toward this diagnosis. This includes close contact with dogs or sheep while in an endemic geographic area at any time in the past. Several species of cestodes in the genus *Echinococcus* may infect carnivores, such as dogs. In the canine gastrointestinal tract, parasites grow into adult tapeworms. Dogs become infected with adult tapeworms by eating infected viscera of intermediate hosts, usually sheep. Humans become infected by accidental ingestion of ova excreted by an infected dog.[77]

Three species of parasite cause human infection. *Echinococcus granulosis* results in "typical" or simple cystic hydatid disease. However, in north central United States, Canada, and Alaska, dogs and foxes are potential sources of *Echinococcus multilocularis* infection.[78] *E multilocularis* is a more aggressive and potentially damaging form of hydatid disease causing an invasive "alveolar" or multicystic process. *Echinococcus vogeli,* which has been found in areas of Central and South America, produces "polycystic" hydatid disease.

Infection with *E granulosis* closely resembles human cysticercosis. Oncospheres, released from ova in human gut, travel to other sites, predominately the liver and lungs. Rarely, cerebral or vertebral deposition occurs.[77] Hydatid cysts containing protoscolices slowly develop from the larval form, resulting in organ compression and dysfunction attributable to slow cyst expansion (Figure 18.6).

Rupture of cysts could induce anaphylactoid reactions or spread infective protoscolices, which then develop into secondary cysts in other organs. The larval form of *E multilocularis* does not produce single, large cystic lesions as does *E granulosis,* but maintains an aggressive, proliferative stage in the human host. Masses of small alveolar cysts, associated with dense fibrosis, invade hepatic tissue locally, often mimicking malignancy, with tissue necrosis and occasional metastasis to the lung, pancreas, or spinal cord.[79]

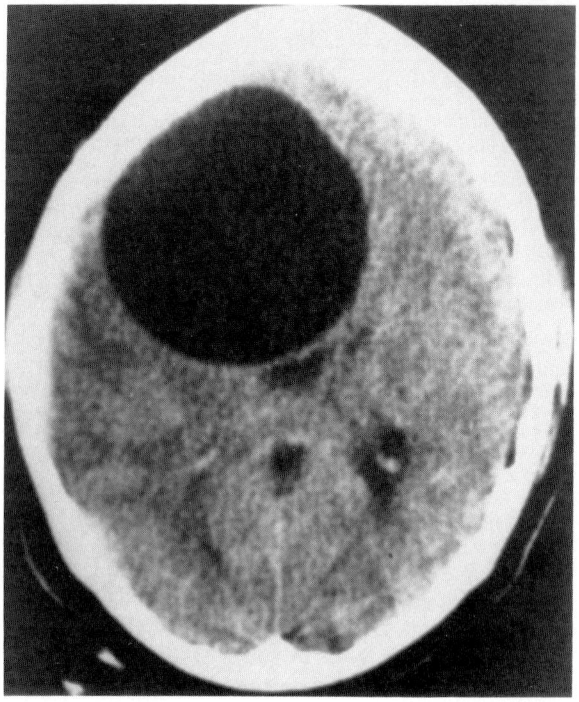

Fig. 18.6. Case of a giant left frontal cerebral echinococcal cysts. CT scan of brain shows a large, well-delimited cyst in the left frontal region displacing the ventricular system. Edema is not present. The cyst was removed intact, with clinical resolution of hemiparesis, papilledema, and galactorrhea with three months. (Reprinted with permission of the publisher from Giant cerebral Echinococcus cysts with galactorrhea and amenorrhea. By Tiberin P, Heilbroon YD, Hirsch, M, et al: *Surg Neurol* 1984;21:505–506. Copyright 1984 by Elsevier Science Publishing Co., Incorporated.)

CNS Lesions

Hydatid involvement of the CNS occurs in 1–2% of documented cases caused by *E granulosis*. Of these 50–75% are found in children.[80,81] Unlike neurocysticercosis, echniococcal cysts rarely localize within cerebral parenchyma. They have a greater tendency to infect and destroy vertebral bone, resulting in spinal-cord compression by continuous expansion.[82,83] When cerebral localization occurs, focal neurologic deficits, obstructive hydrocephalus, and pseudotumoral manifestations are the most common neurologic presentations.[84] Parenchymal brain lesions are not distinguishable from those of neurocysticercosis, based on plain films or CT scan; however, echinococcal cysts tend to be larger and fewer in number (Figure 18.6).

Alveolar echinococcal disease generally does not involve cerebral parenchyma. However, Honma and associates[79] have described a fatal case of alveolar echinococcal disease in a 68-year-old man who was thought to have acquired his infection in the Kurile Islands, 38 years earlier, during World War II. The patient ultimately died with echinococcal invasion of extradural and intradural spaces and subarachnoid extension to the medulla oblongata and cerebellar hemispheres.

Spinal-cord compression is the most common CNS manifestation of hydatid disease, albeit relatively rare. The disease most commonly localizes to the thoracic region. In one series, 82% of lesions were in the thoracic region and only 18% were in the lumbar area.[83] Cysts are usually epidural, causing intradural and extramedullary extension; bony involvement of the spine is frequent.[85] Clinical signs and symptoms are consistent with spinal-cord compression—radicular pain followed by paraparesis and paraplegia, often associated with a sensory level.

Diagnosis of Echinococcal Infections

Radiologic techniques for diagnosis of echinococcal disease may include plain films, CT scanning, myelography, and MRI.[85] Vertebral radiographs often show osseous lesions, such as moth-eaten vertebral bodies, surrounded by sclerosis and soft-tissue calcifications. Extramedullary cord compression can usually be demonstrated by myelography. CT scans and MRI offer noninvasive means to delineate both spinal-cord and vertebral involvement while confirming the cystic nature of lesions. Both can detect cystic lesions in the brain, but defining the etiology of any cystic lesion in the brain is more difficult. Needle biopsy must be avoided since spillage of cyst contents may cause anaphylactoid reactions or spread of infection.

Serologic testing for diagnosis is of limited value. As many as 50% of echinococcal cyst carriers may be seronegative and antibody titers may fluctuate. Only a minority of infected patients demonstrate peripheral blood eosinophilia.[77] Serologic tests for echinococcal antibodies may be positive in patients with cysticercosis.[77] In areas of low endemicity, such as North America, a positive antibody titer coupled with the typical appearance on CT scan and an appropriate epidemiologic history would make a presumptive diagnosis of echinococcal disease. Often surgical extirpation and examination of cyst contents offer only definitive approach to diagnosis.

Treatment of Echinococcal Infections

For patients with cystic hydatid disease causing organ compromise, surgery is often the treatment of choice. Surgical procedures must include techniques that prevent spillage of cyst contents. Surgeons have developed various means to limit spillage, including scolicidal agents, such as 0.5% silver nitrate, in operative packs.[86,87,89] Injecting scolicidal agents such as formalin, ethanol, hypertonic saline, or silver nitrate into liver cysts prior to surgical resection has been associated with a significant risk of ascending cholangitis.[89] Large-diameter suction curettes (such as those used in the termination of pregnancies) can successfully remove the contents of cysts without damage to the pericyst cavity.[88]

The role of antiparasitic chemotherapy in the management of hydatid disease is growing. Encouraging results have been obtained with the benzimidazole carbamate compounds, mebendazole and albendazole, the latter drug achieving the best cyst concentrations.[90] Praziquantel has shown activity against *E granulosis* protoscolices, and either praziquantel or albendazole may have a role in preoperative therapy to destroy viable protoscolices.[91,92] For nonsurgical candidates, the decision to treat patients with albendazole or praziquantel must be made on an individual basis. Neither drug has yet been approved by the Food and Drug Administration (FDA) for the treatment of hydatid disease, and there are no controlled prospective studies or large series upon which to base a decision. Both the CDC and the FDA are helpful in obtaining agents such as albendazole and in planning guidelines for long-term patient monitoring. Prevention programs for echinococcal disease include strict control over livestock slaughtering and disposal of viscera, and limiting access of stray dogs to infected viscera.

Trichinosis Causing CNS Syndromes

CNS infections caused by the nematode *Trichinella spiralis* have been documented at least since 1906.[93] By 1914, Van Cott and Linz[94] had recovered viable larvae from the CSF of a 21-year-old woman who later died of trichinosis. Such events are possible whenever trichina-infected undercooked meat is consumed.

Infective trichina larvae are located in the striated muscles of pigs and other animals, such as boars, horses, and bears. Larvae are consumed by humans eating infected meat. In the small bowel, they develop into adults, which are excreted within weeks. However, newborn larvae leave the intestine and migrate to striated muscle, and occasionally to the CNS. Cardiac muscle is rarely involved.[95]

The symptoms of trichinosis are variable, occurring mainly during larval migration. They include fever (92%) headache (56%), myalgias (86%), and subconjuctival hemorrhages (42%). When larvae reach the CNS and its smaller vessels, they may cause thrombosis, meningoencephalitis, seizures, or focal neurologic findings. In 1935, Most and Abeles[93] reviewed the pathology resulting from CNS trichinosis. Cerebral infarction was evident. Larvae were observed in brain, either surrounded by inflammation or associated with perivascular inflammation. Distinct granulomatous nodules were observed within parenchyma.

In severe cases of CNS trichinosis, the amount of

hemorrhage and edema is considerable. Gay and associates[96] reported a fatal case of CNS trichinosis in which CT scanning documented the following findings. A 50-year-old woman presented with headache, photophobia, myalgias, and fever associated with periorbital edema and eosinophilia. Larvae were present in a quadriceps muscle biopsy. Seizures, left-upper-extremity paresis, and brain-stem compression preceded death. CT scans demonstrated expanding areas of hemorrhage (Figure 18.7). Ellrodt and colleagues[97] have reported three patients from France with CNS trichinosis acquired from infected horse meat. CNS presentations included quadriparesis and cerebellar dysfunction in one, encephalitis and multifocal motor impairment in the second, and confusion with monoplegia in the third. In their second patient with CNS trichinosis, an MRI scan was reported for the first time and demonstrated multifocal brain infarcts.

The diagnosis of trichinosis is based on history and a constellation of laboratory findings that includes eosinophilia (over 90%), a rise in serum muscle enzymes, and a muscle biopsy that demonstrates larvae. Brain biopsy is not indicated, since muscle biopsy is safer and more likely to demonstrate the organisms. Serologic tests for antibodies against *T spiralis* are not useful in the acute situation. Examination of centrifuged CSF for larvae may be helpful. When Van Cott and Lintz[94] first reported their cases in 1914, they described six moving larvae in CSF, which were kept alive for five days in the cold.

The rare case of CNS trichinosis represents a major management problem. Thiabendazole (25 mg/kg twice a day for 1 week) has a greater effect on adult worms than it does on the migrating larvae that cause the problem. It may not be effective for CNS disease.[98] Thiabendazole also has significant gastrointestinal side effects. Ellrodt and associates[97] suggest flubendazole, a mebendazole derivative, 40 mg/kg/day for 10 to 15 days, in addition to high-dose corticosteroids for severe CNS disease. If unavailable they would use mebendazole, 5 mg/kg/day, instead. The use of corticosteroids is probably indicated in patients with severe disease associated with CNS infection.[98] It is not known whether steroids could potentially cause larval dissemination. Agents such as aspirin, that might increase cerebral hemorrhage should be avoided. Prevention of trichinosis is based both on quality control of commercial pork products and adequate cooking to avoid eating trichina-infected pork and infected wild game.

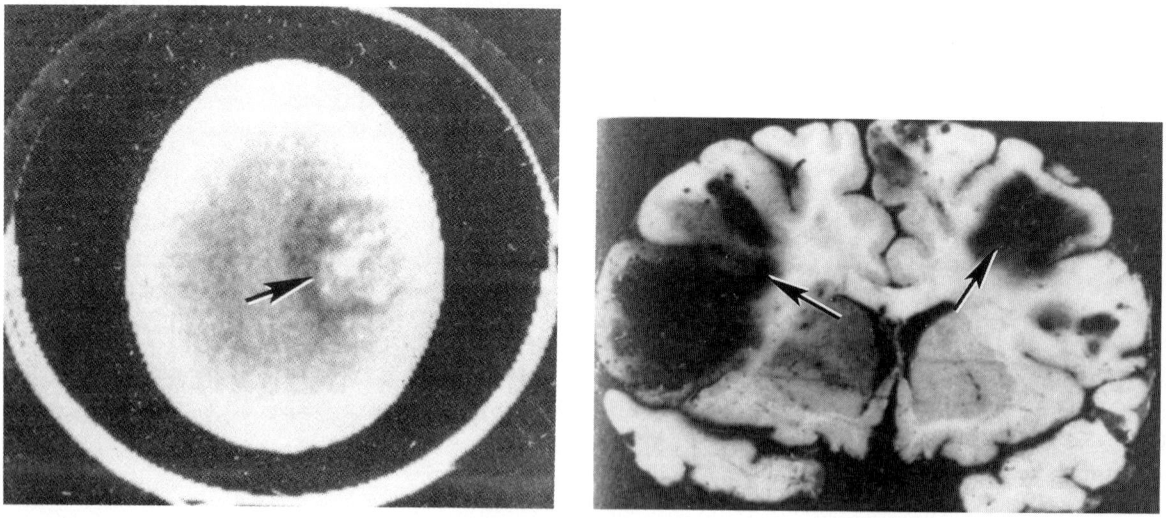

A B

Fig. 18.7. Fatal CNS trichinosis in a 50-year-old woman. Original CT scan showed a small, high-density parietal lobe lesion on right, consistent with hemorrhage and edema. (A) One week later, CT scan shows larger area of right parietal hemorrhage (arrow), surrounding edema, and mass effect. (B) Coronal section of brain shows several hemorrhagic infarcts (arrows) thought to have resulted from venous occlusion. Microscopic examination showed several linear tracts in brain parechyma probably secondary to migrating larvae. (Reprinted with permission from Gay T, Pankey GA, Beckman EN, et al: Fatal CNS trichinosis. *JAMA*, 1982;247:1024–1025. Copyright 1982, American Medical Association.)

Disseminated Strongyloidiasis

Infection associated with the small intestinal nematode of humans, *Strongyloides stercoralis,* should not be considered a tropical disease.[99] This nematode is worldwide in its distribution and the reservoir of infected humans can harbor the organism for at least 30 years.[100] This is possible because of human autoinfection, which also predisposes immunocompromised patients to overwhelming hyperinfection and dissemination.[100,101,102]

The life cycle of *S stercoralis* has either direct or indirect routes for human infection. Usually, humans harbor egg-laying adult nematodes in the upper small intestine. Ova hatch in the gastrointestinal tract and free-living rhabditiform larvae are passed in human feces. They begin their soil phase, and mature into filariform larvae that can penetrate human skin. Alternatively, free-living adults in soil mature and lay eggs that produce infective filariform larvae.

Parasites that have penetrated skin (bare feet) and entered the venous circulation pass through lungs, up the trachea, and down to the duodenum and jejunum, where they mature into egg-laying adults. Under conditions of immunosuppression, the transformation of rhabditiform larvae into filariform larvae within the human host is enhanced. Internal "autoinfection" occurs by direct larval penetration of the gut wall and external autoinfection takes place through skin surfaces.

Azathioprine and cyclophosphamide enhance autoinfection and corticosteroids facilitate bowel penetration. Larve reach the CNS by hematogenous spread. Here they may occlude small vessels, causing microinfarcts, or traverse perivascular spaces, causing granuloma formation in the meninges or CNS.[103] Brain abscesses containing strongyloides larvae have also been described.[104] One patient with systemic lupus erythematosus was reported to have CNS vasculitis that responded to therapy for strongyloidiasis and tapering of corticosteroids.[105]

During early *S stercoralis* infection, cough, epigastric pain, diarrhea, and skin eruptions (larva currens) may occur, often accompanied by eosinophilia. With dissemination, filariform larvae may reach any organ system, including the CNS. This can happen in any debilitated, malnourished, or immunocompromised patient, and eosinophilia may no longer be present. Once within the CNS, clinical manifestations of infection range from mental-status changes to stupor and coma as a result of capillary obstruction and microinfarction. It is not known why disseminated strongyloidiasis is also associated with gram-negative bacteremia, pneumonia, and meningitis. Possibly a hematogenous spread of bacteria occurs during episodes of enteric bacteremia that follow larval penetration of bowel. Also, larvae may carry their own adherent or gut flora with them (piggyback theory) during their invasion of the CNS.[101,103]

For diagnosis, stool, sputum, and duodenal aspirates are examined for characteristic larvae[106] (Figure 18.8.) as opposed to ova, which are rarely evident. The diagnosis should not depend on the finding of peripheral blood eosinophilia. Rather, strongyloidiasis must be considered in any patient with compromised cell-mediated immunity, in particular those with unexplained gram-negative meningitis, bacteremia, or pulmonary infiltrates. For the 25% of patients with negative stool examinations, endoscopy and aspiration of duodenal contents for larvae may be necessary when other tests do not reveal organisms. If endoscopy is contraindicated, a simple string examination may be performed. A capsule with a nylon line is swallowed and retrieved after four hours; adherent mucus is examined for larvae.[107] CSF findings are nonspecific and will likely only refect coexistent bacillary meningitis. Neither eosinophils nor larvae are usually present.[103,108]

In the nonimmunocompromised patient with strongyloidiasis 25 mg/kg of thiabendazole orally, twice daily for 2 days, cures most infection.[109] For compromised patients, immunosuppression must be reversed and therapy must be prolonged for a week or more until stools have been clear of larvae for several days.[102] Damaged intestinal lymphatics, edema of bowel, malabsorption, or ileus may hinder oral therapy. To prevent disseminated strongyliodiasis, all potentially immunocompromised patients should be screened by stool examination for the presence of strongyloides larvae, particularly if a serum antibody test indicates prior infection with *S steroralis.*

Eosinophilic Meningitis

Eosinophils may be found in the CSF during many diseases, including parasitic infections, granulomatous or viral meningitis, CNS syphilis, drug allergy,

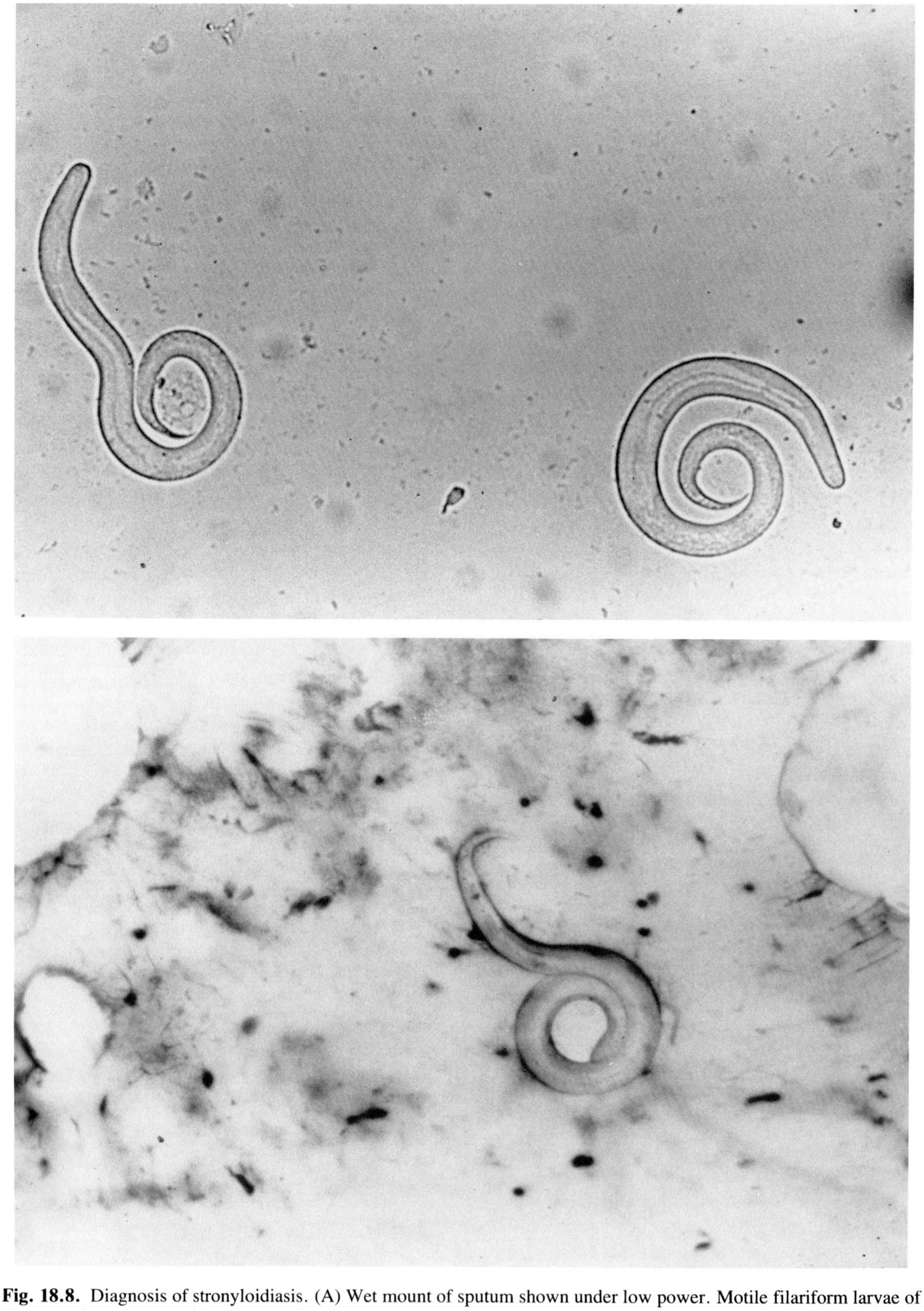

A

B

Fig. 18.8. Diagnosis of stronyloidiasis. (A) Wet mount of sputum shown under low power. Motile filariform larvae of *S stercoralis* are present. (B) Gram stain of sputum shown under low power. *Strongyloides* filariform larvae are noted. Organism was no longer motile and displays Gram-variable staining along its outer margin. (Reprinted with permission from Berenson CS, Dobuler KJ, Bia FJ. Fever, petechiae and pulmonary infiltrates in an immunocompromised Peruvian man. *Yale J Biol Med* 1987;60:437–445.)

neoplasms such as lymphoma or leukemia, and multiple sclerosis.[110] Parasites causing CSF eosinophilia include *Angiostrongylus cantonensis, Gnathostoma spinigerum,* and, rarely, *Cysticercus cellulosae, Toxocara canis,* or *Trichuris trichiuria*.[110,111,112] The term eosinophilic meningitis usually refers to CNS infection in which the CSF eosinophilia is out of proportion to peripheral blood eosinophilia; these infections are caused by *A cantonensis,* the rat lungworm, or *G spinigerum,* a tissue nematode of cats and dogs. *A cantonensis* is a small roundworm whose definitive host is the domestic rat. Freshwater crustaceans such as snails, slugs, prawns, and crabs are intermediate hosts. Human infection occurs after the ingestion of infected intermediate hosts that have not been properly cooked. Larvae migrate to the CNS after ingestion by the rat or by an incidental human host. In rats, the nematode matures in the CNS and migrates to the lung, where it deposits ova and completes the cycle. In humans, extensive tissue damage is produced during the CNS migration.[113] Marked lymphocytic and eosinophilic infiltration, hemorrhagic worm tracts, and granuloma formation characterize the pathologic changes in this disease.[114] Most cases of human infection have been found in Thailand, Vietnam, Cambodia, Indonesia, the Philippines, Taiwan, the Pacific Islands, and Hawaii.[115] Estimates of the rates of rat infection in endemic areas range from 1.2%[116] to 40.5% in urban Bangkok.[117]

The nematode *G spinigerum* is also found in these Southeast Asia countries. Humans may become infected at two different stages in the life cycle. Infection may occur after the ingestion of poorly cooked intermediate hosts such as freshwater fish, frogs, and snakes, or after ingestion of poorly cooked paratenic hosts, such as chicken and ducks, that have eaten the intermediate hosts. The most important source of human infection is probably the ingestion of undercooked poultry.[116]

The average incubation period after ingestion of these parasites is two to three weeks. Frank meningitis is the most common manifestation, but cranial-nerve palsies, particularly of the sixth and seventh nerves, are also seen. Radiculitis and radiculomyelitis have been observed with both infections, but were more common during gnathostomiasis in one series.[111] Subarachnoid hemorrhage, with the typical sudden onset of symptoms, was noted to be particularly common in gnathostomiasis; intracranial hemorrhage and obstructive hydrocephalus may also occur in this disease.[111] The CSF eosinophilic pleocytosis may range from 10 to 90%; peripheral eosinophilia is common but is not always seen.[113] The CSF protein concentration is usually slightly elevated and glucose concentrations are normal to low.

In angiostrongyliasis, neurologic sequelae are rare, and spontaneous recovery is the usual outcome. In CNS gnathostomiasis, however, up to 45% of patients may incur neurologic deficits.[111] The differential diagnosis is based on suggestive clinical findings in a patient with the characteristic CSF eosinophilic pleocytosis and a history of parasite exposure in an endemic area. The diagnosis may be missed unless a Wright or Giemsa stain of the CSF sediment is done to identify eosinophils; this is critical in patients from an endemic area. Serologic studies may differentiate between *A cantonensis* and *G spinigerum* infection if the clinical presentation does not. There is no effective antihelminthic therapy currently available, although thiabendazole has been used. Steroids may decrease inflammation but no clear efficacy has been demonstrated for any drug regimen.[118] Disease prevention depends on avoidance of exposure to and proper cooking or freezing (at –15°C for 2 hours) of crustaceans, freshwater fish, and poultry from endemic areas.

Visceral and Ocular Larva Migrans

Toxocariasis is largely responsible for visceral larva migrans (VLM) and ocular larva migrans (OLM). The dog ascarid *Toxocara canis* is the most common etiology of these syndromes in the United States. OLM is often mistaken for retinoblastoma.[119] *Toxocara* ova are deposited in soil by their hosts, infected puppies in particular, and are usually ingested by young children with pica. The larvae can migrate to many tissues, including the eyes and brain;[119] however, CNS infection is usually subclinical. Patients with OLM are generally asymptomatic, but they develop peripheral blood eosinophilia and circulating *Toxocara* antibodies. If larvae migrate to ocular structures, an inflammatory mass that resembles retinoblastoma develops in the fundus.[119] In one series, 25% of cases referred for evaluation of retinoblastoma were actually ocular toxocariasis.[119] Fragments of *Toxocara* larvae have been found in eyes enucleated for retinoblastoma.

Fever, hepatomegaly, eosinophilia, and hypergammaglobulinemia characterize the VLM syndrome. Pulmonary symptoms and infiltrates may also be seen. A recent review suggests that toxocariasis may be the cause of unexplained nonspecific symptoms, such as abdominal pain in children who are seropositive. Eosinophilia may not be necessary to make a diagnosis.[120]

Although *Toxocara* species most commonly cause VLM, in his original description of the disease, Beaver and colleagues[121] predicted that other roundworm species might cause the syndrome. Indeed, fatal eosinophilic meningoencephalitis in a child was caused by raccoon ascarid, *Baylisascaric procyonis.*[122] The mode of infection appeared to be ingestion of larvae after chewing on wood bark contaminated with raccoon feces. *B procyonis* CNS infection is a well-recognized veterinary syndrome, but had not been described previously in humans. The CSF eosinophilia was pronounced in this *B procyonis* infection. It is reported, but distinctly rare, that *Toxocara* invades the CNS.

Tissue biopsy is not usually required to diagnose VLM or OLM. Pica, exposure to puppies, and an otherwise unexplained eosinophilia suggest the diagnosis. Ocular findings are present in OLM. A diagnosis of VLM can be confirmed by a rise in serum anti-A and anti-B isohemagglutinin titers. OLM is more insidious and difficult to diagnose serologically because of the low serum antibody levels, and yet it must be distinguished from retinoblastoma. Aqueous and vitreous humors may have higher *Toxocara* antibody levels than those in serum.[119]

Either diethylcarbamazine or thiabendazole is recommended therapy.[123] Some authors suggest that only symptomatic children be treated.[124] Control of inflammation is important and includes the use of steroids, particularly in ocular disease.[119] Treating puppy roundworm infection, screening adult pet dogs for roundworm, and preventing canine fecal contamination in children's play areas will aid in the prevention of this disease.

Neurologic Manifestations of Schistosomiasis

Schistosomiasis (bilharziasis) remains a serious and widespread parasitic infection affecting more than 200 million people on three continents. Over 400,000 infected persons currently live in the continental United States.[125] The major trematodes causing this disease are the blood flukes *Schistosoma hematobium, Schistosoma mansoni,* and *Schistosoma japonicum.* Snails are intermediate hosts and humans are the definitive hosts who are exposed to the microscopic infective forms (cercairiae) of schistosomiasis in freshwater streams or lakes where the snail resides. Cercariae released by snails penetrate human skin and migrate to the venous system. As mating adult worms, they may live for as long as 20–30 years, releasing hundreds of thousands of eggs daily into the circulation. For the most part, *S japonicum* lives in the venules of the mesenteric veins, *S hematobium* in the vesical plexus, and *S mansoni* in the inferior mesenteric veins (Figure 18.9).

There are three stages of schistosomal infection, which correlate with this life cycle: (1) cercarial dermatitis, or "swimmers itch," caused by penetration of cercariae; (2) Katayma fever, a syndrome of eosinophilia, fever, lymphadenopathy, and diarrhea occurring during oviposition, 6–8 weeks after heavy infection; and (3) chronic fibrosis resulting from the human immune response to egg deposition, usually beginning with early granuloma formation and followed by late fibrotic reactions.[125]

CNS schistosomiasis results from the immunologic and pathologic reactions to ova in the brain or spinal cord. There are also rare reports of ecotopic adult worms living within the CNS vasculature.[126] Depending on the species of parasitic and the pattern of egg deposition, various neurologic syndromes are described (Figure 18.9).[127] Cerebral infection is more likely to be caused by *S japonicum* infection and myelopathy is associated with both *S mansoni* and *S hematobium* infections. The pathologic response in the CNS is not predictable. It depends largely on the intensity of infection, the host immunity, and the allergic response to ova.[128]

S hematobium

Adult worms of this species reside in the vesical venous plexus, depositing their ova in the urinary bladder and ureter. Hematuria, obstructive uropathy, and ultimately calcification of bladder and lower ureters result. Rarely, schistosome-associated bladder cancer will follow. *S hematobium* ova are likely carried from the vesical plexus, through the valveless venous plexus of Batson, to the spinal cord.[129] Scrimgeour and Gadjusek[129] reviewed reports of cerebral schistosomiasis and emphasized that *S hematobium* ova reach the brain more often than do those of *S mansoni*. Silent lesions are usual but occasionally ova cause epilepsy, encephalitis, or focal symptoms. The prevalence of clinically silent

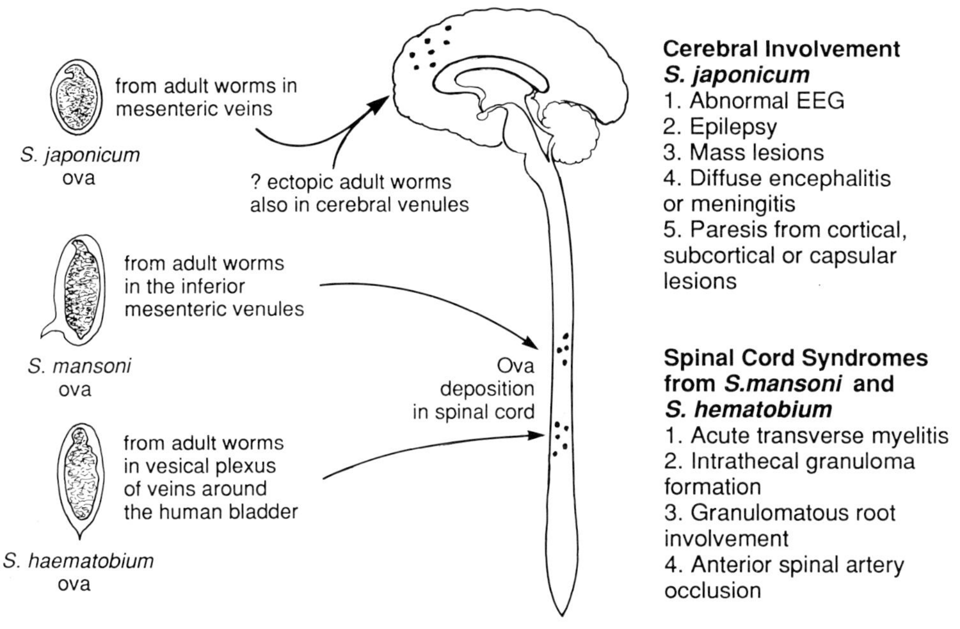

Fig. 18.9. The neurologic syndromes associated with schistosomiasis vary with the species of infecting organisms. *S japonicum* is associated with cerebral involvement whereas *S mansoni* and *S haematobium* are more likely to cause ova deposition in the spinal cord. [Adapted with permission from Bia FJ Barry M: Parasitic infections of the central nervous system. *Neurol Clin* 1986;4(1):196.]

ova deposition was assessed in Zimbabwe by Gelfand, who examined 50 cadavers both with *S hematobium* infection of the bladder and concomittant *S mansoni* infection. *S hematobium* ova were identified in 28 brains (56%). No cerebral *S mansoni* ova were found.[130]

The usual neurologic presentation for *S hematobium* infection is myelopathy. In 75% of cases with neurologic involvement reviewed by Scrimgeour and Gajduske[129] an intramedullary granuloma of the conus medullaris was identified, with extension to the cauda equina in some cases. The usual clinical presentation was a flaccid areflexic paraplegia with sphincter dysfunction and sensory disturbances. Spastic paraplegia has also been reported.[131]

S mansoni

The adult worms of this species reside in the inferior mesenteric veins. Egg deposition occurs in the liver and colon, and occassionally lungs, via portosystemic collateral circulation as a result of portal hypertension. CNS lesions predominately affect the spinal cord. Large granulomatous masses in cerebral cortex and rare episodes of cerebral and subarachnoid hemorrhage have been associated with *S mansoni* ova.[129] Locke[128] recently summarized four spinal-cord syndromes that occur with *S mansoni*, as well as with *S hematobium* infections. The syndromes include rare occlusion of the anterior spinal artery, a granulomatous multiple-root syndrome, intrathecal granuloma formation, and myelitis attributable to ova deposition and immunologic reactions within the spinal cord.[128] The damage caused by myelitis may be quite severe, as showed by the autopsy of a 19-year-old Brazilian woman that demonstrated total myelonecrosis (Figure 18.10).[132]

S japonicum

This species of schistosome is most likely to cause cerebral complications. It is estimated that over 30 million people from endemic areas of China, the Philippines, Indonesia, Laos, Thailand, and Cambodia are infected with *S japonicum*.[133] Although severe hepatosplenic and pulmonary disease occur with *S japonicum* infections, cerebral involvement is more frequent than with *S mansoni* or *S hematobium* infection.[134] The acute Katayama fever stage is occasionally associated with diffuse encephalitis, headache, speech impairment, visual disturbances, and even focal findings. Two percent of 1,200 military personnel infected on Leyte Island in the Philip-

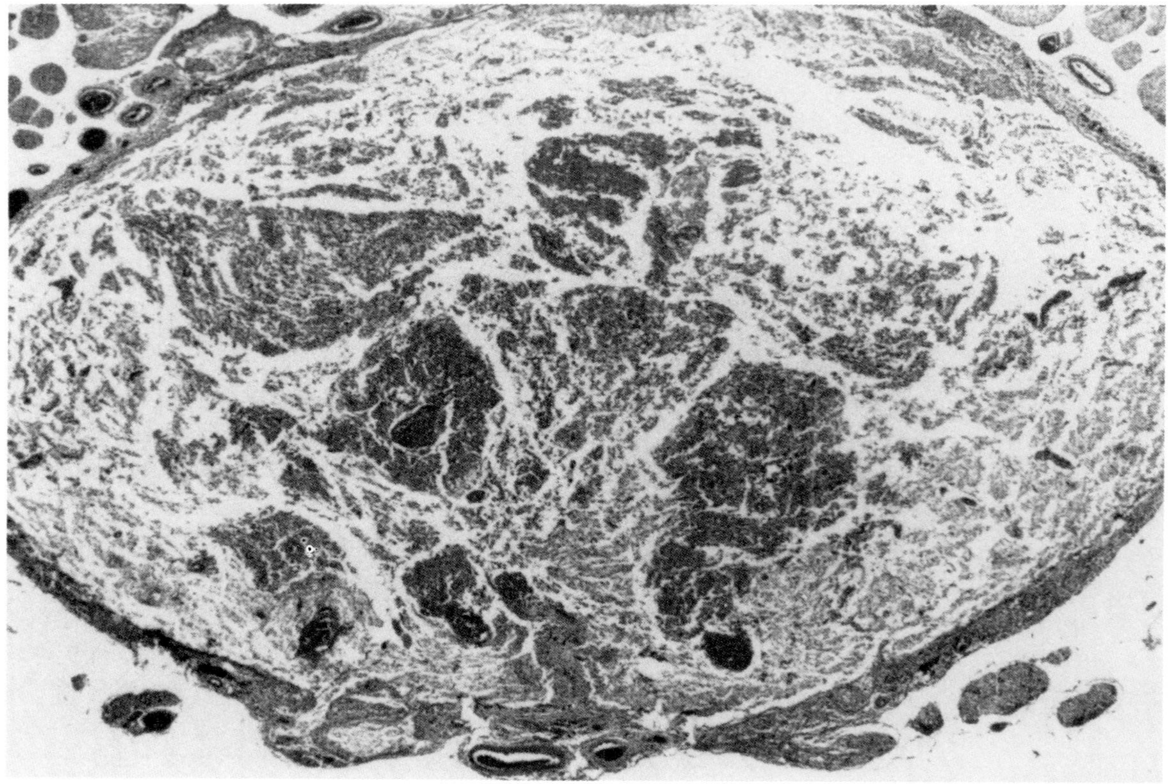

A

Fig. 18.10. Massive spinal-cord necrosis in a 19-year-old Brazilian woman with transverse myelitis caused by *S mansoni*. (A) Transverse section of cord showing widespread necrosis (hematoxylin-eosin X 15). (B) At left, thickening of pia mater with infiltrate and degenerated schistosomal egg are shown (arrow). Shells of ova are visible (double arrows), with necrosis at right (X100). Inset (300X) shows severe proliferative endarteritis in spinal leptomeninges. (Reprinted with permission from Querioz, L de S, Nucci, A, Facure, NO, et al: Massive spinal cord necrosis in schistosomiasis. *Arch Neurol* 1979;36:517–519. Copyright 1979. American Medical Assocation.)

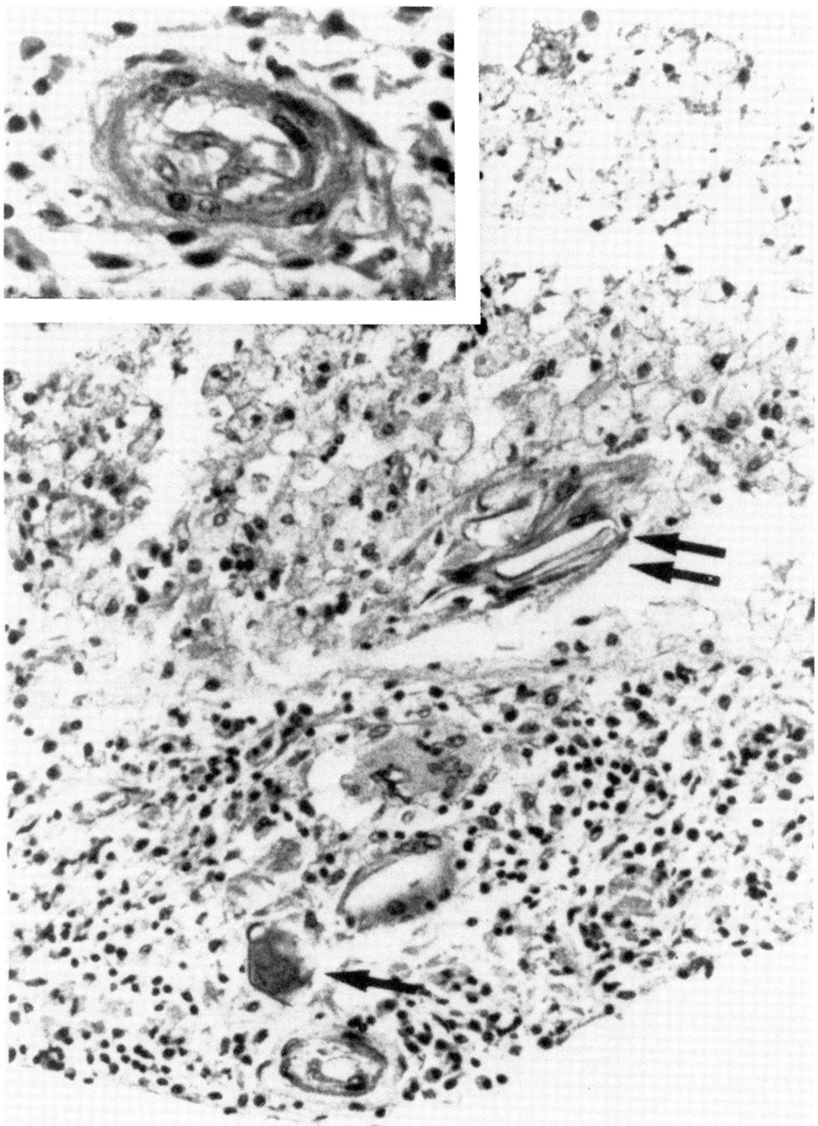

B

Fig. 18.10. *(Continued)*

pines during World War II had acute CNS findings.[134,135] Untreated chronic *S japonicum* CNS infection can result in monoplegias, hemiplegias, or quadriplegias. Epilepsy is a common presentation, and syndromes simulating brain tumors have been observed.[136] Spinal-cord lesions have also been described, but much less frequently than with other species.[136]

Diagnosis

Stool or urine examinations for ova and demonstration of ova in tissues such as rectum remain the basis for diagnosis. Yield from these areas may be low with CNS involvement. Serologic tests for antibodies are problematic in patients from endemic areas where positive serology may be ubiquitous. For *S mansoni* or *S hematobium* endemic areas, the CDC[137] suggests a presumptive diagnosis and initiation of therapy for schistosomal transverse myelitis if:

1. Low thoracic or upper lumbar spinal-cord neurologic symptoms are present.
2. Exposure to schistosomes, either serologically or parasitologically, can be demonstrated.
3. Other causes for transverse myelitis are excluded.

In contrast to schistosomal transverse myelitis, which affects the upper lumbar and low thoracic cord, other causes of transverse myelitis commonly affect the midthoracic cord. Eosinophilis in the CSF suggest schistosomiasis, but they are not commonly observed. Peripheral eosinophilia is also an inconstant finding. CSF usually shows a mild lymphocytic pleocytosis, a mild protein elevation, and a normal glucose concentration.[129] Ova of these parasites have never been found in the CSF.[129] Myelography is a valuable diagnostic aid in schistosomal myelophathy, revealing partial or complete block extending the length of a vertebral body. "Trifid" edges (cleft in three parts) or abrupt intramedullary cord swelling, usually at the T12 to L1 level, are observed.[129] A normal myelogram does not exclude the diagnosis, and a CT scan may demonstrate spinal-cord swelling despite a normal myelogram.[137] A CT scan can also demonstrate intracerebral schistosomal granulomas.[135]

Therapy

Praziquantel results in a 80% rate of parasitologic cure after a single administration, with relatively few side effects. Clinicians are justified in treating quickly when CNS manifestations of schistosomiasis seem apparent. The currently recommended treatment regimens are shown in Table 18.2. Because inflammatory edema around ova in the cord or brain may contribute to tissue necrosis, many clinicians favor the use of corticosteroids as an adjunct to chemotherapy.[137] Surgical decompression may be necessary if a surgically correctable mass lesion is noted on CT scan or myelography and other measures do not produce rapid improvement.

Prevention of schistosomal disease involves avoidance of freshwater swimming in endemic areas. Heating, filtering, or halogenating bathing water may be effective.[137] The efficacy of antischistosomal drugs as chemoprophylactic agents has not been evaluated.

Cerebral Paragonimiasis

In Europe and North America, paragonimiasis is an uncommonly encountered pulmonary and CNS infection caused by the oriental lung fluke *Paragoni-*

Table 18.2. Treatment of schistosomiasis.

		Adult dosage	Pediatric dosage
S hematobium			
Drug of Choice:	Praziquantel	40 mg/kg/d in 2 doses × 1 d	40 mg/kg/d in 2 doses × 1 d
S japonicum			
Drug of Choice:	Praziquantel	60 mg/kg/d in 3 doses × 1 d	60 mg/kg/d in 3 doses × 1 d
S mansoni			
Drug of Choice:	Praziquantel	40 mg/kg/d in 2 doses × 1 d	40 mg/kg/d in 2 doses × 1 d
Alternative:	Oxamniquine	15 mg/kg once[a]	20 mg/kg/d in 2 doses × 1 d
S mekongi			
Drug of Choice:	Praziquantel	60 mg/kg/d in 3 doses × 1 d	60 mg/kg/d in 3 doses × 1 d

[a]In East Africa, the dose should be increased to 30 mg/kg/d, and in Egypt and South Africa, 30 mg/kg/d × 2d for *S. mansoni* infections (adapted with permission from *Med Lett*. 1990;32:23–32, Ref. 138)]. (Neuropsychiatric disturbances and seizures have been reported in some patients.) Praziquantel is effective against all schistosomes. Oxamniquine is only effective against *S. mansoni*. Steroids are used in neurological disease, along with antiparastic agents, to suppress the immune response around ova. Myelography may identify mass lesions amendable to surgical removal.

mus westermani or other related species from Africa and Central and South America.[139] Pulmonary disease can be cured relatively quickly and easily by antiparasitic therapy, particularly if detected prior to CNS dissemination. Unfortunately, ectopic cerebral infections are common in young children, as most cerebral infections occur before the age of ten.[140] For clinicians, the presentation of paragonimiasis may easily be confused with that of pulmonary or CNS tuberculosis, which it most closely mimics. Although several organ systems may be infected, the CNS is actually the most common site of extrapulmonary paragonimiasis.[141]

The life cycle of paragonimus is complex (Figure 18.11), but is the key to prevention. Humans become infected after eating raw freshwater crabs or crayfish (the intermediate hosts containing infective metacercaria) or drinking water containing the juices of these crustaceans. Following their penetration of the human intestine, young flukes ultimately migrate through the diaphragm and into lungs. There they mature into adults, about the size of coffee beans, while residing in pulmonary abscess cavities. Chronic hemoptysis may be present for many years as the next generation of ova is excreted in both sputum and feces. The life cycle of the parasite continues when these ova hatch; intermediate snail hosts, and ultimately crustaceans, again become infected.

The diagnosis of paragonimiasis is suggested by a history of ingesting raw crustaceans or their juices. The picture is often one of chronic hemoptysis, which suggests a diagnosis of tuberculosis. Both diseases may actually occur simultaneously. The chest radiograph often suggests cavitary tuberculosis, with which paragonimiasis can easily be confused, particularly in a population with a high prevalence of positive tuberculin test reactions. When the brain harbors adult flukes, skull films may demonstrate punctate or nodular calcifications, and occasionally charcteristic advanced lesions with a "soap bubble" appearance[142] (Figure 18.12). Such lesions are caused by the degeneration of ectopic adult flukes rather than by reactions to ova.

By 1966, there were an estimated 5,000 active cases of cerebral paragonimiasis in South Korea.[143] In 62 patients from South Korea with CNS infections, the most common neurologic symptoms reported by Oh were seizure disorders, headache, visual disturbances, hemiplegia, nausea, and vomiting. Seventy-five percent of Oh's patients presented with clinical illness prior to age 20. In two thirds, the onset was insidious, but most did have significant cough or hemoptysis. The acute neurologic event was often a symptomatic seizure disorder, as seen in two thirds of his patients. Meningitis may also herald an acute onset. Other syndromes included subacute progressive encephalopahty, chron-

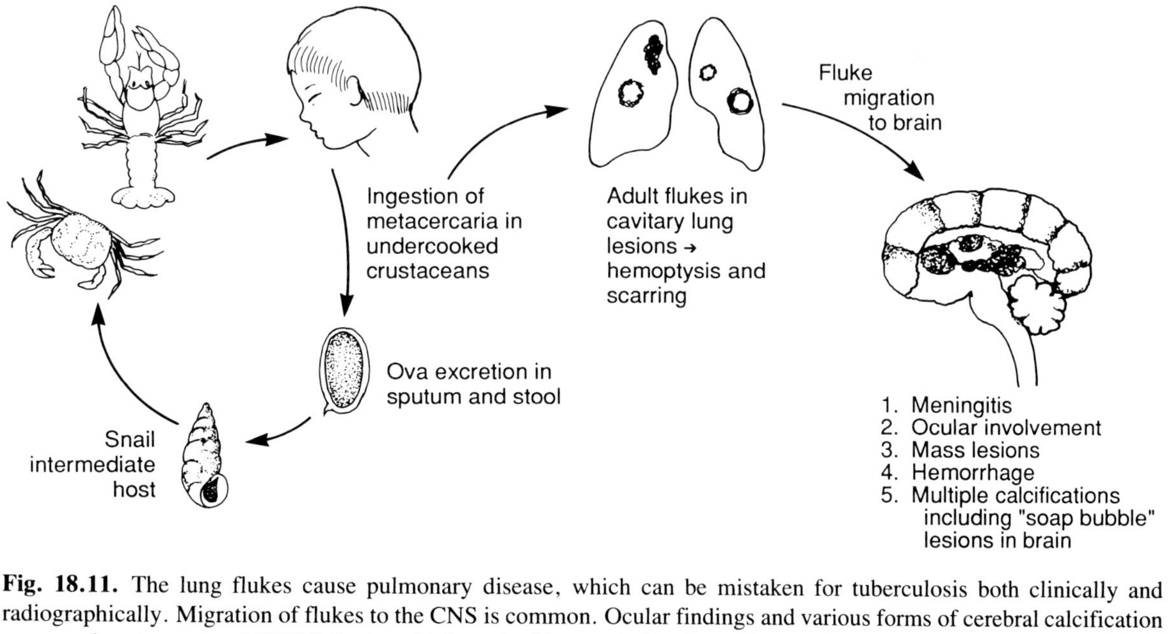

Fig. 18.11. The lung flukes cause pulmonary disease, which can be mistaken for tuberculosis both clinically and radiographically. Migration of flukes to the CNS is common. Ocular findings and various forms of cerebral calcification are prominant aspects of CNS infection. [Adapted with permission from Bia FJ, Barry M: Parasitic infections of the central nervous system. *Neurol Clin* 1986;4(1):200.]

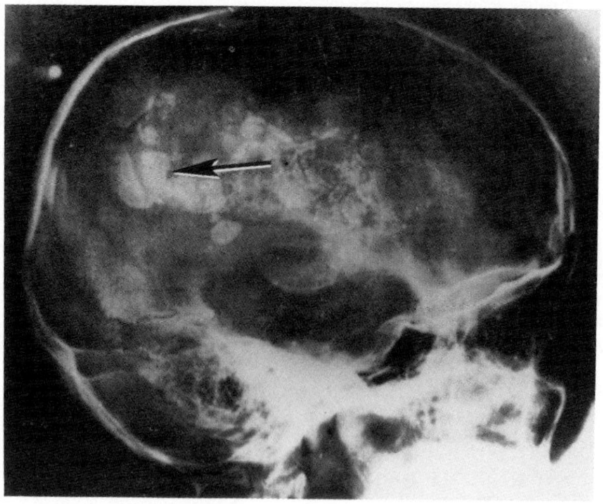

Fig. 18.12. Skull x-ray film from an 18-year-old Korean man thought originally to have a brain tumor. Sputum showed *P westermani* ova. This lateral view shows typical "soap bubble" appearance of intracranial calcifications (arrow) in cerebral paragonimiasis. (Reprinted with permission from Oh SJ: Ophthalmological signs in cerebral paragonimiasis. *Trop Geogr Med* 1968;20:13–20.)

ic brain syndrome, a tumorlike presentation, and one of cerebral infarction. Occipital, temporal, and parietal lobe lesions have variably predominated in different reported series. Cord compression may occur with spinal involvement.

A majority of Oh's cases of cerebral paragonimiasis had abnormal eye findings, emphasizing that cerebral involvement is characterized by ocular abnormalities. Nearly half complained of blurring or impairment of vision. Frequent findings included impaired visual acuity, homonymous hemianopsia, optic atrophy, papilledema, nystagmus, and pupillary abnormalities.[142]

For a diagnosis of CNS paragonimiasis, the evaluation of serum or CSF for the presence of specific antibodies is particularly useful in geographic areas where the disease is not endemic. Paragonimus ova may be found in sputum, feces, pleural and peritoneal fluid, or biopsy tissue. Lung or brain tissue may demonstrate sectioned parts of the adult fluke. CSF findings also mimic tuberculosis, showing a mononuclear pleocytosis and elevated CSF protein concentration, including gamma globulins. Oh found only 5 of 62 patients had eosinophils present in CSF. Intradermal skin testing is being gradually replaced by more specific and sensitive serologic techniques. Skin tests may remain positive for years, and cannot be used to confirm the presence of an active infection.

CT findings in cerebral paragonimiasis were reported by Yoshida and associates[144] in a 48-year-old man with hemiparesis and dysarthria. Findings included dilated ventricles and multiple dense calcifications, including soap-bubble calcifications. In three cases of *Paragonimiasis mexicanus* infection from Costa Rica, hemorrhagic brain lesions predominated.[139]

The dichlorophenol, bithionol, was introduced in 1961 for the treatment of pulmonary paragonimiasis, but subsequently failures were reported.[145] Praziquantel has replaced this agent, in a dose of 25 mg/kg three times a day for two days, resulting in virtually 100% cure rates for both adults and children. It is still unclear what praziquantel will offer in addition to surgery for more advanced cerebral lesions.

As observed regarding the treatment of neurocysticercosis, therapy may cause worsened symptoms because of the death of adult parasites, and corticosteroids are indicated during treatment. The prevention of cerebral paragonimiasis will depend on the early detection and treatment of pulmonary disease in children and changes in food preparation, which interrupt the fluke's life cycle.

References

1. McCabe RE, Remington JS: Toxoplasmosis, in Warren KS, Mahmoud AAF (eds): *Tropical and Geographical Medicine*. New York, McGraw-Hill Book Co., 1984, pp 281–292.
2. Navia BA, Petito CK, Gold JWM, et al: Cerebral toxoplasmosis complicating the acquired immune deficiency syndrome: clinical and neuropathological findings in 27 patients. *Ann Neurol* 1986;19:224–238.
3. Israelski DM, Remington JS: Toxoplasmic encephalitis in patients with AIDS. *Infect Dis Clin North Am* 1988;2:429–445.
4. Krick JA, Remington JS: Toxoplasmosis in the adult—an overview. *N Engl J Med* 1978;298:550–553.
5. Anderson SE, Remington JS: The diagnosis of toxoplasmosis. *South Med J* 1975;68:1433–1443.
6. Hooper DC, Pruitt AA, Rubin RH: Central nervous system infection in the chronically immunosuppressed. *Medicine* 1982;61:166–188.
7. Carey RM, Kimball AC, Armstrong D, et al: Toxoplasmosis. Clinical experiences in a cancer hospital. *Am J Med* 1973;54:30–38.
8. Conti DJ, Rubin RH: Infection of the central nervous system in organ transplant recipients. *Neurol Clin* 1988;6:241–260.
9. Luft BJ, Naot Y, Araujo FG, et al: Primary and reactivated toxoplasma infection in patients with cardiac transplants. *Ann Intern Med* 1983;99:27–31.
10. Lowenberg B, van Gijn J, Prins E, et al: Fatal cerebral toxoplasmosis in a bone marrow transplant recipient with leukemia. *Transplantation* 1983; 35:30–34.
11. Gottesdiener KM: Transplanted infections: donor-to-host transmission with the allograft. *Ann Intern Med* 1989;110:1001–1006.
12. Reynolds ES, Walls KW, Pfeiffer RI: Generalized toxoplasmosis following renal transplantation. *Arch Intern Med* 1966;118:401–405.
13. Hakes TB, Armstrong D: Toxoplamosis. Problems in diagnosis and treatment. *Cancer* 1983;52:1535–1540.
14. Townsend JJ, Wolinsky JS, Baringer JR, et al: Acquired toxoplasmosis. A neglected cause of treatable nervous system disease. *Arch Neurol* 1975;32:335–343.
15. Ryning FW, McLeod R, Maddox JC, et al: Probable transmission of *Toxoplasma gondii* by organ transplantation. *Ann Intern Med* 1979;90:47–49.
16. Hotson JR, Enzmann DR: Neurologic complications of cardiac transplantation. *Neurol Clin* 1988;6:349–365.
17. Britt RH, Enzmann DR, Remington JS: Intracranial infection in cardiac transplant recipients. *Ann Neurol* 1981;9:107–119.
18. Hofflin JM, Potasman I, Baldwin JC, et al: Infectious complications in heart transplant recipients receiving cyclosporine and corticosteroids. *Ann Intern Med* 1987;106:209–216.
19. Frenkel JK, Nelson BM, Arias-Stella J: Immunosuppression and toxoplasmic encephalitis. Clinical and experimental aspects. *Hum Pathol* 1975;6:97–110.
20. Bia FJ, Barry M: Parasitic infections of the central nervous system. *Neurol Clin* 1986;4:171–206.
21. Luft BJ, Brooks RG, Conley RK, et al: Toxoplasmic encephalitis in patients with acquired immune deficiency syndrome. *JAMA* 1984;252:913–917.
22. Snider WD, Simpson DM, Nielsen S, et al: Neurological complications of acquired immune deficiency syndrome: analysis of 50 patients. *Ann Neurol* 1983;14:403–418.
23. Levy RM, Bredesen DE, Rosenblum ML: Neurological manifestations of the acquired immunodeficiency syndrome (AIDS): experience at UCSF and review of the literature. *J Neurosurg* 1985;62:475–495.
24. Levy RM, Bredesen DE, Roseblum, ML: Opportunistic central nervous system pathology in patients with AIDS. *Ann Neurol* 1988;23(suppl):S7–S12.
25. Wong G, Gold JWM, Brown AE, et al: Central-nervous-system toxoplasmosis in homosexual men and parenteral drug abusers. *Ann Intern Med* 1984;100:36–42.
26. Pitchenik AE, Fischl MA, Walls KW: Evaluation of cerebral-mass lesions in acquired immunodeficiency syndrome. *N Engl J Med* 1983;308:1099.
27. Horowitz SL, Bentson JR, Benson F, et al: CNS toxoplasmosis in acqured immunodeficiency syndrome. *Arch Neurol* 1983;40:649–652.
28. Potasman I, Resnick L, Luft BJ, et al: Intrathecal production of antibodies against *Toxoplasma gondii* in patients with toxoplasmic encephalitis and the acquired immunodeficiency syndrome (AIDS). *Ann Intern Med* 1988;108:49–51.
29. Levy RM, Rosenbloom S, Perrett LV: Neuroradiologic findings in AIDS: a review of 200 cases. *AJR* 1986;147:977–983.
30. Mehren M, Burns PJ, Mamani F, et al: Toxoplasmic myelitis mimicking intramedullary spinal cord tumor. *Neurology* 1988;38:1648–1650.
31. Cohn JA, McMeeking A, Cohen W, et al: Evaluation of the policy of empiric treatment of suspected *Toxoplasma* encephalitis in patients with the acquired immunodficiency syndrome. *Am J Med* 1989;86:521–532.
32. Leport C, Raffi F, Matheron S, et al: Treatment of central nervous system toxoplasmosis with pyrimethamine/sulfadiazine combination in patients with the acquired immunodeficiency syndrome. Efficacy of long-term continuous therapy. *An J Med* 1988;84:94–100.

33. Rolston KVI, Hoy J: Role of clindamycin in the treatment of central nervous system toxoplasmosis. *Am J Med* 1987;83:551–554.
34. Maegraith B: Malaria, in Adams ARD, Maegraith B (eds): *Clinical Tropical Diseases*. Oxford, Blackwell Scientific Publications, Alden Press, 1980, pp 240–291.
35. Wyler DJ: Malaria: resurgence, resistance and research. *N Engl J Med* 1983;308:875–878.
36. Luse SA, Miller LH: Plasmodium falciparum malaria. Ultrastructure of parasitized erythrocytes in cardiac vessels. *Am J Trop Med Hyg* 1971;20:655–660.
37. Grau GE, Fajardo LF, Piguet PF, et al: Tumor necrosis factor (cachectin) as an essential mediator in murine cerebral malaria. *Science* 1987;237:1210–1211.
38. MacPherson GG, Warrell MJ, White NJ, et al: Human cerebral malaria, A quantitative ultrastructural analysis of parasitized erythrocyte sequestration. *Am J Pathol* 1985;119:385–401.
39. Daroff RB, Deller JJ Jr., Kastl, AJ Jr, et al: Cerebral malaria. *JAMA* 1967;202:679–682.
40. Anderson WK: *Malarial Psychosis and Neurosis*. Edinburgh, Oxford University Press, 1927, p 395.
41. Jong E: *The Travel and Tropical Medicine Manual*. Philadelphia, WB Saunders Co, 1987, pp 79–89.
42. Centers for Disease Control: Recommendations for the prevention of malaria in travelers. *MMWR* 1990;39:1–10.
43. Phillips RE, Warrell DA, White NJ, et al: Intravenous quinidine for the treatment of severe falciparum malaria. *N Engl J Med* 1985;312:1273–1278.
44. Warrel DA, Looareesuwan S, Warrell MJ, et al: Dexamethasone proves deleterious in cerebral malaria. *N Engl J Med* 1982;306:313–319.
45. Fowler M, Carter RF: Acute pyongenic meningitis probably due to *Acanthamoeba* sp.: a preliminary report. *Br Med J* 1965;2:740–742.
46. Carter R: Primary amoebic meningo-encephalitis: an appraisal of present knowledge. *Trans R Soc Trop Med Hyg* 1972;66:193–213.
47. Cleland PG, Lawande RV, Geoffrey-Onyemelukwe MB, et al: Chronic amebic meningoencephalitis. *Arch Neurol* 1982;39:56–57.
48. Robert V, Rorke L: Primary amoebic encephalitis probably from Acanthamoeba. *Ann Intern Med* 1983;79:174–179.
49. Martinez AJ, Janitschke K: Acanthamoeba, an opportunistic microorganism: a review. *Infection* 1985;13:251–256.
50. John DT: Primary amebic meningoencephalitis and the biology of *Naegleria fowleri*. *Ann Rev Microbiol* 1982;36:101–123.
51. Bia FJ, Barry M: Parasitic infections of the central nervous system. *Neurol Clin* 1986;4:171–206.
52. Seidel JS, Harmatz P, Visvesvara GS, et al: Successful treatment of primary amebic meningoencephalitis. *N Engl J Med* 1982;306:346–348.
53. Nelson JD, McCracken GH: Amebae in swimming pools. *Ped Infect Dis J Newslet* 1988;14:3–4.
54. Barry M, Bia FJ: Acanthamoeba meningoencephalitis, in Goldsmith R, Heyneman D (eds): *Tropical Medicine and Parasitology*. Norwalk, Conn, Appleton & Lange, 1989, pp 253–254.
55. Gray F, Gherardi R, Scaravilli F: Then neuropathology of the acquired immunne deficiency syndrome (AIDS). *Brain* 1988;111:245–266.
56. Rowan-Kelly B, Ferrante A, Thong YH: The chemotherapeutic value of sulphadiazine in treatment of *Acathamoeba* meningoencephalitis in mice. *Trans R Soc Trop Med Hyg* 1982;76:636–638.
57. Lombardo L, Alonso P, Arroyo LS, et al: Cerebral amebiasis. Report of 17 cases. *J Neurosurg* 1964; 21:704–708.
58. Hughes FB, Faehnle ST, Simon JL: Multiple cerebral abscesses complicating hepatopulmonary amebiasis. *J Pedratr* 1975;86:95–96.
59. Bia FJ, Barry M: Brain abscess due to *Entamoeba histolytica,* in Goldsmith R, Heyneman D (eds): *Tropical Medicine and Parasitology*. Norwalk, Conn: Appleton & Lange, 1989, p 255.
60. Nash TE, Neva FA: Recent advances in the diagnosis and treatment of cerebral cysticercosis. *N Engl J Med* 1984;311:1492–1496.
61. Pawlowsi ZS: Cestodiasis: Taeniasis diphyllobothriasis, hymenolepsiasis and others, in Warren KS, Mahmoud AAF (eds): *Tropical Geographical Medicine*. New York, McGraw-Hill, 1984, pp 471–479.
62. Del Brutto OH, Sotelo J: Neurocysticercosis: an update. *Rev Infect Dis* 1988;10:1075–1087.
63. Shanley JD, Jordan MC: Clinical aspects of CNS cysticercosis. *Arch Intern Med* 1980;140:1309–1313.
64. Keane JR: Death from cysticercosis. Seven patients with unrecognized obstructive hydrocephalus. *West J Med* 1984;140:787–789.
65. McCormick GF, Chi-Shing Zee, Heiden J: Cysticercosis cerebri. *Arch Neurol* 1982;39:534–539.
66. McCormick GF, Giannotta S, Chi-shing Zee, et al: Carotid occulsion in cysticercosis. *Neurology (Clevland)* 1983;33:1078–1080.
67. Byrd SE, Locke GE, Biggers S, et al: The computed tomographic appearance of cerebral cysticercosis in adults and children. *Radiology* 1982;144:819–823.
68. Minguetti G, Ferreira, MVC: Computed tomography in neurocysticercosis. *J Neurol Neurosurg Psychiatry* 1983;46:936–942.
69. Sotelo J, Escobedo, F, Rodriguez-Carbajal J, et al: Therapy of parenchymal brain cysticercosis with praziquantel. *N Engl J Med* 1984;310:1001–1007.
70. DeGhetaldi LD, Norman RM, Douville AW Jr: Cerebral cysticercosis treated biphasically with dex-

amethasone and praziquantel. *Ann Intern Med* 1983;99:179–181.
71. Sotelo J, Torres B, Rubio-Donnadieu F, et al: Praziquantel in the treatment of neurocysticercosis: Long-term follow-up. *Neurology* 1985;35:752–755.
72. Apuzzo MLJ, Dobkin WR, Chi-Shing Zee, et al: Surgical considerations in treatment of intraventricular cysticercosis. *J Neurosurg* 1984;60:400–407.
73. Sotelo J, Penagos P, Escobedo F, et al: Short course of albendazole therapy for neurocysticercosis. *Arch Neurol* 1988;45:1130–1133.
74. Vazquez, ML, Jung H, Sotelo J: Plasma levels of praziquantel decrease when dexamethasone is given simultaneously. *Neurology* 1987;37:1561–1562.
75. Agapegev S, Meira, DA, Barraviera B: Neurocysticercosis: treatment with albendazole and dextrochlorpheniramine. *Trans R Soc Trop Med Hyg* 1989;83:377–383.
76. Richards F Jr, Schantz PM: Cysticercosis and taeniasis. *N Engl J Med* 1985;312:787–788.
77. Schantz PM: Echinococcosis (hydatidosis), in Warren, KS, Mahmoud AAF (eds): *Tropical and Geographical Medicine*. New York, McGraw-Hill, 1984, pp 487–497.
78. Rausch RL, Wilson JF, McMahon BJ, et al: Consequences of continuous mebendazaole therapy in alveolar hydatid disease—with a summary of a ten-year clinical trail. *Ann Trop Med Parasitol* 1986; 80:403–419.
79. Honma K, Sasano N, Andoh N, et al: Hepatic alveolar echinococcosis invading pancreas vertebrae and spinal cord. *Hum Pathol* 1982;13:944–946.
80. Katz AM, Pan CT: Echinococcus disease in the United States. *Am J Med* 1958;25:759–770.
81. Slim MS, Khayat G, Nasr AT, et al: Hydatid disease in childhood. *J Pediatr Surg* 1971;6:440–448.
82. Arana-Iniguez R, Lopez-Fernandez JR: Parasitosis of the nervous system with special reference to echinococcosis. *Clin Neurosurg* 1967;14:123–144.
83. Pamir MN, Akalan N, Ozgen T, et al: Spinal hydatid cysts. *Surg Neurol* 1984;21:53–57.
84. Tiberin P, Heibronn YD, Hirsch M, et al: Giant cerebral *echinococcus* cyst with galactorrhea and amenorrhea. *Surg Neurol* 1984;21:505–506.
85. Mikhael MA, Ciric IS, Tarkington JA: MR imaging in spinal echinococcus. *J Comput Assist Tomogr* 1985;9:398–400.
86. Massachusetts General Hospital: *Case Records of the Massachusetts Gen Hosp* (case no. 45-1987). *N Engl J Med* 1987;317,1209–1217.
87. Saidi F, Nazarian I: Surgical treatment of hydatid cysts by freezing of cysts wall and instillation of 0.5 per cent silver nitrate solution. *N Engl J Med* 1971;284:1346–1350.
88. Morris DL, Lamont G: Suction curettage in the management of hydatid cysts. *Br J Surg* 1987; 74:323.
89. Teres J, Gomez-Moli J, Bruguera M, et al: Sclerosing cholangitis after surgical treatment of hepatic echinococcal cysts. Report of 3 cases. *Am J Surg* 1984;148:694–697.
90. Morris DL, Dykes PW, Marriner S, et al: Albendazole—objective evidence of response in human hydatid disease. *JAMA* 1985;253:2053–2057.
91. Thompson RCA, Reynoldson JA, Riddler CR: Praziquantel adversely affects protoscolices of *Echinococcus granulosus in vitro*. *J Helminth* 1986;60: 279–286.
92. Morris DL, Chinnery JB, Hardcastle JD: Can albendazole reduce the risk of implantation of spilled protoscoleces? An animal study. *Trans R Soc Trop Med Hyg* 1986;80:481–484.
93. Most H, Abeles MM: Trichiniasis involving the nervous system. *Arch Neurol Psychiatry* 1937; 37:589–616.
94. Van Cott JM, Lintz W: Trichinosis. *JAMA* 1914; 62:680–684.
95. Kazura JW: Trichinosis, in Warren KS, Mahmoud AAF. (eds): *Tropical and Geographical Medicine*. New York, McGraw-Hill, 1984, pp 427–430.
96. Gay T, Pankey GA, Beckman EN, et al: Fatal CNS trichinosis. *JAMA* 1982;247:1024–1025.
97. Ellrodt A, Halfon P, LeBras P, et al: Multifocal central nervous system lesions in three patients with trichinosis. *Arch Neurol* 1987;44:432–434.
98. Drugs for parasitic infections. *Med Lett* 1990;32:23–32.
99. Scowden EB, Schaffner W, Stone WJ: Overwhelming strongyloidiasis. *Medicine* 1978;57:527–544.
100. Pelletier LL Jr: Chronic strongylodiasis in World War II Far East ex-prisoners of war. *Am J Trop Med Hyg* 1984;33:55–61.
101. Faust EC, DeGroat A: Internal autoinfection in human strongyloidiasis. *Am J Trop Med* 1940;20:359–375.
102. Purtilo DT, Myers WM, Connor DH: Fatal strongyloidiasis in immunosuppressed patients. *Am J Med* 1974;56:488–493.
103. Neefe LI, Pinilla O, Garagusl VF., et al: Disseminated strongyloidiasis with cerebral involvement. A complication of corticosteroid therapy. *Am J Med* 1973;55:832–838.
104. Masdeu JC, Tantulavanich S, Gorelick PP, et al: Brain abscess caused by *Strongyloides stercoralis*. *Arch Neurol* 1982;39:62–63.
105. Wachter RM, Burke AM, MacGregor RR: *Strongyloides stercoralis* hyperinfection masquerading as cerebral vasculitis. *Arch Neurol* 1984;41:1213–1216.
106. Berenson CS, Dobuler KJ, Bia FJ: Fever, petechiae and pulmonary infiltrates in an immunocompromised Peruvian man. *Yale J Biol Med* 1987;60:437–445.

107. Grove DI, Warren KS, Mahmoud AAF: Algorithms in the diagnosis and management of exotic diseases. III. Strongyloidiasis. *J Infect Dis* 1975;131:755–758.
108. Owor R, Wamukota WM: A fatal case of strongyloidiasis with Strongyloides larvae in the meninges. *Trans R Soc Trop Med Hyg* 1976;70:497–499.
109. Grove DI: Treatment of strongyloidiasis with thiabendazole. An analysis of toxity and effectiveness. *Trans R Soc Trop Med Hyg* 1982;76:114–118.
110. Bosch I, Oehmichen M: Eosinophilic granulocytes in cerebrospinal fluid: analysis of 94 cerebrospinal fluid specimens and review of the literature. *J Neurol* 1978;219:93–105.
111. Schmutzhard E, Boongird P, Vejjajiva A: Eosinophilic meningitis and radiculomyelitis in Thailand caused by CNS invasion of *Gnathostoma spinigerum* and *Angiostrongylus cantonensis*. *J Neurol Neurosurg Psychiatry* 1988;51:80–87.
112. Gould IM, Newell S, Green SH, et al: Toxocariasis and eosinophilic meningitis. *Br Med J* 1985; 291:1239–1240.
113. Kuberski T, Wallace GD: Clinical manifestations of eosinophilic meningitis due to *Angiostrongylus cantonensis*. *Neurology* 1979;29:1566–1570.
114. Nye SW, Tangchai P, Sundarakiti S., et al: Lesions of the brain in eosinophilic meningitis. *Arch Pathol* 1970;89:9.
115. Smit AM: Eosinophilic meningitis. *Trop Geog Med* 1963;15:225–232.
116. Punyagupta S, Bunnag T, Juttijudata P, et al: Eosinophilic meningitis in Thailand: epidemiologic studies of 484 typical cases and the etiologic role of *Angiostrongylus cantonensis*. *Am J Trop Med Hyg* 1970;19:950–958.
117. Hinz E: Angiostrongylus Belfall bei Wanderratten in Bangkok, Thailand. *Mitt Osterr Ges Tropenmed Parasitol* 1986;8:83–88.
118. Punyagupta S, Bunnag T, Juttijudata P: Eosinophilic meningitis in Thailand: clinical studies of 484 typical cases probably caused by *Angiostrongylus cantonensis*. *Am J Trop Med Hyg* 1975;24:921–931.
119. Glickman LT: Toxocariasis, in Warren KS, Mahmoud AAF (eds): *Tropical and Geographical Medicine*. New York, McGraw-Hill, 1984; pp 431–437.
120. Taylor MRH, Keane CT, O'Connor P, et al: The expanded spectrum of toxocaral disease. *Lancet* 1988;1(8587):692–695.
121. Beaver PC, Snyder CH, Carerra GM, et al: Chronic eosinophilia due to visceral larva migrans; report of three cases. *Pediatrics* 1952;9:7–19.
122. Fox AS, Kazacos KR, Gould NS, et al: Fatal eosinophilic meningoencephalitis and visceral larva migrans caused by the racoon ascarid *Baylisascaris procyonis*. *N Engl J Med* 1985;312:1619–1622.
123. Drugs for parasitic infections. *Med Lett* 1990;32:23–32.
124. Gill D, Dunne K, Kenny V: Toxocariasis in children. *Lancet* 1988;1:1172.
125. Mahmoud AA: Schistosomiasis. *N Engl J Med.* 1977;297:1329–1331.
126. Chitiyo ME: Schistosomal involvement of the choroid plexus. *Central African J Med* 1972;18:45–47.
127. Bia FJ, Barry M: Parasitic infections of the central nervous system. *Neurol Clin* 1986;4:171–206.
128. Massachusetts General Hospital: Case records of the Massachusetts General Hospital (case no. 21-1985). *N Engl J Med* 1985;312:1376–1383.
129. Scrimgeour EM, Gajdusek DC: Involvement of the central nervous system in *Schistosoma mansoni* and *S haematobium* infection. *Brain* 1985;108:1023–1038.
130. Gelfand M: Schistosomiasis in south central Africa. The postgraduate Pross-Juba and Co. Ltd Capetown and Johannesburg 1950. Cited in Marcial-Rojas RA, Fiol RE: Neurological complications of schistosomiasis. *Ann Intern Med* 1963;59:215–230.
131. Odeku EL, Lucas AO, Richard DR: Intramedullary spinal cord schistosomiasis: case report. *J Neurosurg* 29:417–423.
132. Querioz L de S, Nucci A, Facure NO. et al: Massive spinal cord necrosis in schistosmiasis. *Arch Neurol* 1979;36:517–519.
133. Warren KS: Schistosomiasis Japonica. *Clin Gastroenterol* 1978;7:77–85.
134. Pesigan TP, Hairston NG, Jauregui JJ, et al: Studies on *Schistosoma japonicum* infection in the Philippines I. general considerations and epidemiology. *Bull WHO* 1958;18:481–578.
135. Kirchoff LV, Nash TE: A case of schistosomiasis japonica: resolution of CAT-scan detected abnormalities without specific therapy. *Am J Trop Med Hyg* 1984;33:1155–1158.
136. Marcial-Rojas RA, Fiol RE: Neurological complications of schistosomiasis. *Ann Intern Med* 1963;59:215–230.
137. Centers for Disease Control: Acute schistosomiasis with transverse myelitis in American students returning from Kenya. MMWR 1984;33:445–447.
138. Drugs for parasitic infections: *Med Lett* 1990;32:23–32.
139. Brenes Madrigal R, Rodriquez-Ortiz B, Vargas Solano G, et al: Cerebral hemorrhagic lesions produced by *Paragonimus mexicanus*. *Am J Trop Med Hyg* 1982;31:522–526.
140. Bunnag D, Harinasuta T: Opisthorchiasis, clonorchiasis, paragonimiasis, in Warren KS, Mahmoud

AAF. (eds): *Tropical and Geographical Medicine*. New York, McGraw-Hill, 1984, pp 461–469.
141. Higashi K, Aoki H, Tatebayashi K, et al: Cerebral paragonimiasis. *J Neurosurg* 1971;34:515–527.
142. Oh SJ: Ophthalmological signs in cerebral paragonimiasis. *Trop Geogr Med* 1968;20:13–20.
143. Oh SJ: Cerebral paragonimiasis. *Trans Am Neurol Assoc* 1967;92:275–277.
144. Yoshida M, Moritaka K, Kuga S, et al: CT findings of cerebral paragonimiasis in the chronic state. *J Comput Assist Tomogr* 1982;6:195–196.
145. Coleman D, Barry M: Relapse of *Paragonimiasis westermani* lung infection after bithional therapy. *Am J Trop Hyg* 1982;3:71–74.

19
Neurosyphilis

Nicholas J. Fiumara

Syphilis is an infectious disease caused by *Treponema pallidum*. Except for congenital syphilis, it is acquired principally through sexual exposure and sex play during the infectious period. In acquired syphilis, the disease passes through the primary stage, which is manifested by a chancre, an ulceration at the point of inoculation; a secondary stage, with systemic symptoms, adenopathy, and rash; a latent stage, which is an asymptomatic period of variable duration with reactive serologic tests; and, finally, a late stage with mucocutaneous, osseous, visceral, cardiovascular, and neural involvement. Infectious syphilis consists of the primary and secondary stages and an early latent phase of less than 1 year in duration: it is during these stages that syphilis may be spread sexually. During pregnancy, however, syphilis in all stages—and particularly early syphilis—is infectious to the developing fetus.

The invasion of the central nervous system (CNS) occurs early during the course of infection when there is a generalized dissemination of spirochetes. About 13% of untreated primary syphilis[1] and 20–30% of untreated secondary syphilis[2,3] will manifest abnormalities in the spinal fluid, such as an increase in lymphocytes of greater than five per cubic millimeter, a rise in total protein greater than 35 mg/dl, and even a reactive VDRL test. These abnormalities will continue or progress during the years when relapsing secondary syphilis may occur. About 25% of cases of untreated or inadequately treated secondary syphilis will relapse. Of these, about 90% will take place during the first year, about 95% within 2 years, and none at all after the fourth year. Thus, if the spinal-fluid VDRL is nonreactive 4 years or more after infection, one can postulate that neurosyphilis will not occur, barring a reinfection.

Symptomatic neurosyphilis, other than acute meningitis, does not appear for at least 2 years after the initial infection. Neurosyphilis may be divided into the following stages: asymptomatic neurosyphilis, acute meningitis, chronic meningovascular neurosyphilis, general paresis, tabes dorsalis, and combinations such as meningomyelitis and taboparesis.

Asymptomatic Neurosyphilis

Asymptomatic neurosyphilis is defined as the presence of syphilis characterized by repeated reactive blood reagin and treponemal tests and a reactive spinal-fluid reagin test such as the VDRL. (The fluorescent treponemal antibody absorption (FTA-ABS) test for spinal-fluid examination is not recommended at this time.) There is also an absence of clinical signs and symptoms of CNS disease. In addition to the reactive spinal-fluid VDRL test, if infection is active, the spinal fluid will show an increase in lymphocytes (five cells/mm^3 or more) and total protein (35 mg/dl or more).

Patients with asymptomatic neurosyphilis are at risk of developing symptomatic neurosyphilis, and the degree of risk correlates directly with the extent of spinal-fluid abnormality. Thus, patients with minimal spinal-fluid changes are more likely to go into a spontaneous remission.[4] In an Oslo study of untreated syphilis, 6.5% of the infected patients developed symptomatic neurosyphilis.[5]

On the other hand, asymptomatic neurosyphilis is uncommon among the elderly. Merritt and associates[6] found only 9 patients (4.5%) out of 200 with asymptomatic neurosyphilis who were older than 61. However, patients with asymptomatic neurosyphilis, regardless of age or degree of activity in the spinal fluid, need treatment.

Acute Meningitis

Acute meningitis may appear within the first 2 years of infection, and is usually associated with the secondary stage of syphilis or a relapsing secondary process—with most cases occurring during the first 6 months of the disease. Acute syphilitic meningitis essentially presents the clinical picture of any acute meningitis, except that there is a greater variability in the extent and intensity of the symptoms because of the constant absorption and reformation of the exudate. It is principally a basilar meningitis with headache appearing either continuously or in paroxysms, which are usually worse at night. Attacks of vertigo, nausea, and vomiting are frequent. The convulsions are usually generalized. The patient may become stuporous but may have periods of alertness and greater activity, often merging into delirium. There are cervical rigidity and positive Kernig's and Brudzinski's signs. The fever is irregular and moderately high.

Depending on the location of the exudate, which is usually most intense at the base, various cranial nerves are involved by a perineuritis. The third cranial nerve is most frequently implicated, in whole or in part. Various ocular palsies and gradations of external and internal ophthalmoplegia may be seen. Nystagmus, facial palsies, deafness, and facial pain are likely to appear. The spinal fluid will have an elevated pressure, increased lymphocytes (25–100 mm^3 or more), an elevated protein of 50 mg/dl, normal glucose, and a reactive VDRL.

Chronic Meningovascular Neurosyphilis

In 2–5 years, but not later than 10 years, after the initial infection, meningovascular syphilis occurs as a result of no treatment, inadequate treatment, or a reinfection. The signs and symptoms will vary according to the degree of involvement of the cerebral blood vessels and cranial nerves. There is a proliferative endarteritis and a perivascular infiltration with lymphocytes and plasma cells.

Perivascular cuffing is particularly marked around the blood vessels of the pia-arachnoid. Because of swelling of the endothelial cells of the small and middle-sized vessels and diminution of blood supply, vascular thrombosis results in infarction of the nerve tissue, followed by gradual intellectual and emotional deterioration. Any of the cerebral blood vessels may be involved, but, most commonly, the middle and posterior cerebral arteries and their branches are affected. Therefore, the patient may suffer from a weakening of one side of the body, progressing to hemiplegia. However, hemiplegia is rarely complete and there is rapid recovery with treatment.

The meningeal involvement will cause the patient to complain of headaches, tenderness of the head on percussion, irritability, and double vision. With increased intracranial pressure, nausea and vomiting occur. The cranial nerves may be completely or incompletely involved. Argyll Robertson pupils frequently are found. There may be papilledema and secondary optic atrophy. The third, fourth, and sixth cranial nerves are frequently affected. Less often, there are vertigo and deafness resulting from impairment of the eighth cranial nerve. With all of this, the spinal-fluid examination will show increased pressure, a marked increase in lymphocytes, elevated total protein, and positive serologic findings.

General Paresis

About 5% of patients with untreated syphilis develop general paresis. This condition usually appears 20 or more years after the original infection. In general paresis, both the blood and spinal fluid will have reactive reagin and treponemal tests. Both neurologic and psychiatric symptoms are present in varying proportions. These may be summarized by the following acrostic schema:

P Personality changes: deterioration of social habits, exaggeration of basic personality—neurosis with organic symptoms, euphoria, depression, overactivity, paranoid reactive state, follows crowd, commits moral offenses.
A Affect: quantitative term to express patient's capacity and degree of reaction, which is not consistent with or appropriate to the problem. Mood encompasses mood shifts, irritability, and emotional reactions of an "all-out" type, such as those seen in childhood, which are not regulated in intensity to fit the situation.
R Reflexes: hyperactive.
E Eyes: Argyll Robertson pupils.
S Sensorium: delusions, illusions, hallucinations, and paranoid ideas.
I Intellect: reduction in mental capacity, orientation, memory, retention and recall, calcula-

tions, general information, judgment, and insight.

S Speech: slurred speech, s and l consonants pronounced slowly, coarse tremors of lips and tongue, omission of words and phrases, repetition of last few words, face often smooth and masklike.

Stages of Paresis

General paresis can be classified into the following forms.

Early Stage

The early symptoms of general paresis are usually a change in personality, irritability, outbursts of temper, and an inability to concentrate. Slovenliness of the person or dress may become apparent in individuals previously not showing such characteristics. Insomnia, anxiety states, headache, and ease of fatigue may provide reasons for the patient's consulting a doctor. Loss of weight is often marked. Lack of judgment in a formerly astute businessperson may be striking. With progression of the disease, loss of memory becomes prominent, a lowering of ethical and moral standards takes place, and loss of the ability to make simple calculations appears. Because of the clouding of consciousness, the patient loses rapport with the environment and, as a result, has difficulty in comprehending the details of business and family life. As this condition increases, the patient becomes more and more disoriented, eventually becoming unaware of time, place, or person, and seeming to live in an individual dreamlike state. Hallucinations are not common, but delusional states frequently occur.

Simple Dementia

The most common type of paresis is the simple dementing form, in which a simple organic deterioration takes place without excitement or emotional changes. There is a rapid and profound lowering of ethical and moral standards. Patients quickly lose interest in their environment and rapidly pass through a phase of forgetfulness into a state of dullness and apathy, with little insight into their condition. These patients eventually become entirely demented and bedridden. They lose weight, soil themselves, and die in a state of general paralysis.

Euphoric or Expansive Paretic

This is the type of paretic who has delusions of grandeur. The course of this form of the disease is longer and beset with remissions. Aside from the delusions of power, position, and wealth, the patients are cheerful and euphoric. Like the manic individual, they are in a constant state of psychomotor activity. At the same time, mental deterioration gradually progresses.

Agitated Paretic

This is the dangerous individual, especially since this type of psychosis is so frequently and suddenly precipitated. Mental deterioration may be quickly succeeded by an impulsive manic state in which the patient becomes violently excited and destructive. Homicide is not infrequently the result of such outbursts in the noninstitutionalized patient.

Depressed Paretic

This is the depressed patient of the ward, one who is melancholy and has somatic hypochondriacal delusions. There is a marked psychomotor slowing and other physiologic disturbances. Typical depressive guilt feelings with self-condemnation, self-accusation, and self-punishing tendencies are present. At times, the negativism and catatonic state of a schizophrenic are seen.

Tabes Dorsalis

This disease becomes evident 5 to 20 years after the primary or secondary stages. About 5% of patients with untreated syphilis develop tabes. Tabes is divided into three stages of development: preataxic, ataxic, and paralytic.

Pain is characteristically the earliest symptom of tabes. The patient has what appears to be rheumatic or muscular pain for years before other symptoms develop. The pain is often likened to lightning because of its characteristic sudden appearance, rapid spread, and then disappearance. It is often described as radiating from the gluteal region to the heel or foot, although it may be limited to the leg and, less commonly, to the arm. The pain may simulate a constricting band about the trunk, and under such circumstances it is called girdle pain. In addition to the pain, there may be marked paresthesia and hypesthesia. The paresthesia is most commonly referred to the soles of the feet and is described as a sensation of walking on a thick, soft carpet or walking on wool. The patient develops a loss of sense of position and passive motion, and may be able to recognize only imperfectly, if at all, the movement of toes or feet. As a result, the patient has poor control of the extremities. The vibratory sensibility is usually affected to the same degree as is the position sense.

Because of a deep sensory loss, such patients are ataxic. They at first notice a slight difficulty in maintaining balance, tending to sway back and forth when shutting their eyes while washing. They are less sure of their gait at night and have to be observant of even visible landmarks. They gradually unconsciously assume a broad base while walking, and, when not moving, they tend to take hold of nearby fixed objects. These patients can keep a sense of balance as long as their eyes are open, but upon closing them, will begin to sway from side to side. Normal equilibrium in humans is maintained by three systems: the somatic afferents, principally from the muscles and joints; the labyrinthine afferents; and the visual system. Any two of these may compensate, even though imperfectly, for the loss of one of them. Tabes patients use gravity as a supplemental control of movement. Holding the body stiffly and groping for position by continual muscle stimulation, they consciously watch their movements and position in efforts to control them. They attempt to obtain the maximum effect of their proprioceptive sense when, while walking, they overflex their knees to be sure that their feet have cleared the ground and bring their extremities down forcibly to stimulate any remaining deep sensibility. Later, the tabetic must use one or even two canes.

Treatment of Neurosyphilis

The drug of choice for the treatment of neurosyphilis is penicillin. Effective therapy requires that the patient have a serum spirochetal level of 0.03 units/mm [7] or higher and maintain it for 3–4 weeks. This can be achieved with the following regimens [8,9]:

1. Benzathine penicillin G, 2.4 million units intramuscularly (IM) weekly for three to four doses.
2. Procaine penicillin G, aqueous, 2.4 million units IM daily for 15–20 days.
3. Procaine penicillin G, aqueous, 2.4 million units IM daily for 10 days followed by benzathine penicillin G, 2.4 million units weekly for 3 weeks.
4. Aqueous crystalline penicillin G, 12–24 units intravenously (IV) daily (2–4 million units IV every 4 hours) for 10 days followed by benzathine penicillin G, 2.4 million units weekly for three doses.

For patients allergic to penicillin, suggested drugs are:

1. Doxycycline, 100 mg twice a day for 20–30 days.
2. Minocycline, 100 mg twice a day for 20–30 days.
3. Tetracycline, 500 mg four times daily for 20–30 days.

It must be emphasized that benzathine penicillin G will achieve spirochetal levels in serum, but there may be little or none detected in spinal fluid.[10] However, spinal fluid is not a simple filtrate from the capillaries but a choroid secretion. Thus, its concentration of sodium is 7% higher than the concentration in extracellular fluid, its glucose concentration is 30% less, and potassium is 40% less. More important, the essential pathology of neurosyphilis stems from the middle and small blood vessels where the spirochetal blood levels of penicillin are adequate.

Posttreatment Results

In evaluating the effectiveness of treatment, the physician is guided by:

1. The clinical response of the patient.
2. The decreasing titer of the quantitative VDRL in the blood.
3. The number of lymphocytes in the spinal fluid, five or more lymphocytes per cubic millimeter, and its decrease after treatment.
4. Elevated protein in spinal fluid, 35 mg/dl or more, and its decrease after treatment.
5. The quantitative spinal-fluid VDRL and its decrease after treatment.

Asymptomatic Neurosyphilis

The patient by definition is symptomless. If the disease is less than 2 years old, there are usually elevations in cell count and total protein. The VDRL in spinal fluid is reactive and should be quantitated.

About 3 months after treatment, the cell count should be normal and the elevated protein should be less, and at 12 months be normal or near normal. The quantitative spinal-fluid VDRL should be decreasing at the third month and normal or near normal in 12 months. The quantitative blood RPR should exhibit a fourfold decrease in titer in six months; 95% of the patients should have a nonreactive reagin blood test in 2 years—and all should be seronegative in 4 years.

Acute Meningitis

The clinical response during treatment is dramatic and very few or no residual effects appear after treatment. The quantitative blood VDRL will have a fourfold or greater decrease in 6 months and be nonreactive in 2 years. The spinal-cell count is always elevated and should be normal in 3 months, at which time the spinal-fluid protein is decreased, as is the titer of the spinal-fluid VDRL. At 1 year, cell count, total protein, and VDRL should be normal.

Chronic Meningovascular Syphilis

This condition generally is markedly improved after treatment, but some patients will have residual neurologic weakness. The cell count and protein should behave as in acute meningitis, but the spinal-fluid VDRL may not be normal after 1 year.

General Paresis

While patients may show marked clinical improvement, they will still have some neurologic and psychiatric residual effects.

Tabes Dorsalis

Unhappily, here the physician can expect little or no improvement. Progression to a charcot joint is common. Tabetic crises do not respond to any known therapy. One must turn to a good brace manufacturer or to joint replacement to help these patients. Wasserman fastness of blood and spinal fluid is common. Patients with active spinal fluid seem to do better.

Since 1985 and continuing through the calendar year 1989, infectious syphilis—primary, secondary, and early latent syphilis—increased in the United States. The rise was not in the homosexual community, but in heterosexual males and females, with the tragic increase of congenital syphilis in the newborn. It is in patients with infectious syphilis and those with relapses where most of our cases of neurosyphilis will be seen. Late symptomatic neurosyphilis occurs in about 8–10% of untreated syphilitic patients. The prevalence of these cases is so low that the Centers for Disease Control includes them under late and late latent syphilis. Since 1983, these reported cases have been decreasing, but in 1989 reported cases went from 18,501 to 21,418, a 12% increase.

The relative rarity of late symptomatic syphilis should not blind us to its possible presence when dealing with a patient with neurologic and psychiatric problems. However, the antibiotic era has reduced late symptomatic syphilis, particularly tabes and paresis, to a relatively rare disease. The effective treatment of infectious syphilis will speed its eradication.

Neurosyphilis and AIDS

In the more recent literature, there are reports that human immunodeficiency virus (HIV) infection may modify the clinical manifestations, serologic responses, and efficacy of treatment of primary and secondary syphilis with the development of acute meningitis, as well as meningovascular syphilis.[11–14] HIV infects not only the T4 lymphocytes, but also monocytes, macrophages, and colorectal cells, as well as the B lymphocytes. Thus, both cellular and humoral responses may be altered. If the circulating T4 cells fall by roughly 90%, the potential for initiation of new immune responses of the cell-mediated or antibody type appears to be lost.[15]

The clinical manifestations of syphilis in patients with the acquired immune deficiency syndrome (AIDS) tend to vary from more florid skin lesions to few atypical ones. The RPR titers also vary from 1:1 to 1:2 in secondary syphilis to 1:4056 in a recent case. The treponemal tests—Microhemagglutination or FTA-ABS—have so far been reactive, although there is a report of a nonreactive VDRL and FTA-ABS in a patient with secondary syphilis.[13] However, most of our patients follow the predictable serologic patterns seen in patients without coexisting AIDS infection.

In the author's opinion, adequate penicillin therapy for early infectious syphilis requires a minimum of two doses of 2.4 million units of benzathine penicillin G IM weekly for two consecutive weeks for a total of 4.8 million units. Unfortunately, some patients with primary and secondary syphilis treated only with a single dose of benzathine penicillin G 2.4 million units IM, may have a clinical relapse with or without neural involvement, as in two reports.[11,12] The physician in these situations is hard pressed to distinguish a true relapse resulting from inadequate therapy from one caused by impaired cellular or humoral immunity.

Fortunately, most patients have a normal serologic response in primary and secondary syphilis.[16] However, in the very few patients with secondary syphilis and AIDS with nonreactive reagin and treponemal tests, a biopsy should confirm the clinical diagnosis. Patients with primary and secondary syphilis should then have a posttreatment serologic examination with the quantitative reagin test monthly during the first year and quarterly during the second year.

If this is the patient's first attack of primary or secondary syphilis, a predictable serologic pattern should appear if the treatment was adequate. At the third and sixth month, a fourfold and eightfold drop, respectively, should be observed.[17] In 12 months, all patients treated for primary syphilis should be nonreactive and those treated for secondary syphilis must have a nonreactive RPR or VDRL test by the 24th month.[18,19] But in patients with reinfection primary and secondary syphilis, the initial titer is always higher than the previous infection, and the posttreatment serologic responses are much slower, and some may be still reactive in low titers five years after treatment.[20]

Some patients with AIDS may require the high-dose aqueous crystalline penicillin regimen listed earlier, although neurosyphilis has been treated with doxycycline in an HIV-infected patient. Regardless of the regimen employed, careful follow-up of clinical status, serologic titers, and CSF is essential.

References

1. Hahn RD, Clerk EF: Asymptomatic neurosyphilis: a review of the literature. *Am J Syph Gon Vener Dis* 1946;30:305.
2. Merritt HH: Early clinical and laboratory manifestations of syphilis of the central nervous system. *N Engl J Med* 1940;223:446.
3. Moschella SL, Hurley HJ: Dermatology, in *The Treponematoses*. Philadelphia, WB Saunders Co, 1985.
4. Moore JE, Hopkins HH: Asymptomatic neurosyphilis—the prognosis of early and late asymptomatic neurosyphilis. *JAMA* 1930;95:1037–1040.
5. Gjestland T: The Oslo study of untreated syphilis. *Acta Derm Venerol* 1955;35(supp 34):1–368.
6. Merritt HH, Adams RD, Solomon HC: *Neurosyphilis*. New York, Oxford University Press, 1946, pp. 72–73.
7. Idsoe O et al: Penicillin, the treatment of syphilis. *Bull WHO* 1972;47 (suppl).
8. Centers for Disease Control: *STD Treatment Guidelines 1985*, vol 34, no. 4S, pp. 755–1085.
9. Rudolph AH, Duncan WC, Kettles HH: The treponematoses. *J Am Acad Dermatol* 1988;18:1121–1129.
10. Mohr JA. et al: Neurosyphilis and penicillin levels in cerebrospinal fluids. *JAMA* 1976;236:2208.
11. Johns DR, Tierney M, Felsenstein D: Alteration in the natural history of neurosyphilis by concurrent infection with the human immunodeficiency virus. *N Engl J Med* 1987; 316:1569–1572.
12. Berry CD, Hooton TM, Collier AC, Lukehart SA: Neurologic relapse after benzathine penicillin therapy for secondary syphilis in a patient with HIV infection. *N Engl J Med* 1987;316:1587–1589.
13. Hicks CB, Benson PM, Lupton GP, et al: Seronegative secondary syphilis in a patient infested with the immunodeficiency virus (HIV) with Kaposi sarcoma. *Ann Intern Med* 1987;107:492–495.
14. Tramont EC: Syphilis in the AIDS era. *N Engl J Med* 1987;316:1600–1601.
15. Weissman I: Approaches to an understanding of pathogenetic mechanisms in AIDS. *Rev Infect Dis* 1988;10:385–398.
16. Centers for Disease Control: Recommendations for diagnosing and treating syphilis in HIV infected patients. *MMWR* 1988;37:600–608.
17. Brown ST, Zaidi A, Larsen SA et al: Serologic response to syphilis treatment. *JAMA* 1985;253:1296–1299.
18. Fiumara NJ: The treatment of primary and secondary syphilis: the serologic response. *J Am Acad Dermatol* 1986;14:487–491.
19. Fiumara NJ. Human immunodeficiency virus infection and syphilis *J Am Acad Dermatol* 1989;21:141–142.
20. Fiumara NJ: Reinfection primary and secondary syphilis: the serologic response after treatment. *Sex Trans Dis* 1980;7:111–115.

20
AIDS and Other Immunocompromised States

JOSEPH R. BERGER, ROBERT M. LEVY, AND RICHARD DIX

Alterations in host defense mechanisms that predispose to infection can be broadly classified into three major categories: abnormalities of cell-mediated immunity (T-lymphocytes and macrophages), abnormalities of humoral immunity (immunoglobulins), and abnormal neutrophils. Currently, the most common cause of abnormalities in the cell-mediated arm of immunity is the acquired immunodeficiency syndrome (AIDS), but among other causes, abnormalities in this system are also associated with lymphoma, particularly Hodgkin's disease, corticosteroid and antineoplastic therapy, organ transplantation, and malnutrition.

Abnormalities in humoral immunity may be congenital or acquired. The latter includes defects in humoral immunity resulting from multiple myeloma, chronic lymphocytic leukemia, and combined radiation and multidrug chemotherapy for advanced malignancies or bone-marrow transplantation. Splenectomy is associated with a range of infections similar to those resulting from defects in humoral immunity. Quantitative or qualitative defects in neutrophils are associated with a different spectrum of nervous-system infections than that which attends abnormalities in cellular or humoral immunity. Absolute neutropenia may occur as a congenital condition or be acquired. The etiologies of the latter include aplastic anemia, acute leukemia, certain infections, malnutrition, and drugs. Defects of neutrophil function may be congenital, such as chronic granulomatous disease, or acquired, such as those related to diabetes mellitus and corticosteroid therapy. Because of the increasing prevalence of AIDS and its role as the prototype of an immunlogical disorder that frequently involves neurological disease, most of this chapter will be devoted to that illness.

This work was supported in part by grant PO1 NS 25569-01 from the National Institute of Neurological Disease and Stroke.

HIV Infection and Defects in Cell-Mediated Immunity

HIV-1

Retroviruses are a family of RNA viruses that are unique because of the presence of RNA-dependent DNA polymerase (reverse transcriptase), an enzyme enabling these RNA viruses to produce DNA, which may then be incorporated into the host genome. This family of viruses, widely distributed in the vertebrate species, has been divided into three subfamilies: lentivirus ("lente" = slow), oncovirus ("onco" = tumor), and spumivirus ("spuma" = foam). To date, only the last subfamily has not been associated with disease in humans.

The human immunodeficiency virus type 1 (HIV-1)—the virus that causes (AIDS),[1] formerly referred to as human T-lymphotropic virus type 3 (HTLV-3)/the AIDS associated virus (ARV), the lymphadenopathy-associated virus (LAV), and the human immunodeficiency virus type 2 (HIV-2), a virus also capable of causing an AIDS-like illness in humans, belong to the lentivirus subfamily. The prototypical lentivirus is visna, a virus known to produce a demyelinating disorder in sheep. All known lentiviruses, including visna, caprine arthritis encephalopathy virus (CAEV), bovine visna, feline immunodeficiency virus, and simian immunodeficiency virus, are capable of causing neurologic disease.[2]

Human T-lymphotropic virus type I HTLV-1 belongs to the largest retroviral subfamily, the oncoviruses. Though initially demonstrated to be capable of causing T-cell leukemia and lymphomas,[3] seroepidemiologic investigations have subsequently demonstrated an association with between it and a progressive myelopathy.[4] This progressive myelopathy has been referred to as tropical spastic paraparesis (TSP) or HTLV-I–associated myelopathy (HAM), but other neurologic conditions may result as a consequence of HTLV-I infection.

In 1981, an immunodeficiency state occurring in homosexual males characterized by such illnesses as *Pneumocystis carinii* pneumonia[5,6] and chronic ulcerative genitoanal herpes simplex virus (HSV) infection[7] was described. Shortly thereafter, it became apparent that neurologic disease was also a frequent complication of this immunodeficient state, subsequently referred to as the acquired immunodeficiency syndrome, or AIDS. Clinically evident neurologic disease occurs in approximately 50% of all HIV-infected individuals and may be the presenting manifestation of AIDS. In retrospective studies from San Francisco[8] and New York,[9] the incidences of neurologic complications occurring in association with AIDS were 39% and 41% respectively. Another combined retrospective and prospective study detected neurologic illness in 63% of 132 patients with AIDS.[10] In 10%[11] to 20%[10] of HIV-1 infected patients, neurologic disease heralds the HIV-1 infection. During a six-month follow-up period, 30% of patients with AIDS and AIDS-related complex (ARC) developed neurologic symptoms or signs.

The incidence of neurologic abnormality in AIDS patients exceeds that of clinically recognized neurologic disease. The frequency with which the nervous system is involved in such patients examined postmortem averages approximately 75%[12] and is remarkably diverse.[13] The frequency with which neuropathologic abnormalities are observed depends, in large measure, on the diligence with which they are sought.[14] Nielsen and associates[15] demonstrated neuropathologic abnormalities in 31 of 40 patients with AIDS. Similarly, Moskowitz and colleagues[16] found neuropathologic lesions in 38 of 52 unselected AIDS cases at autopsy. The most common neuropathologic finding in patients dying from AIDS appears to be microglial nodules, which occasionally occur in association with multinucleated giant cells.[13,17]

The spectrum of neurologic disease that complicates HIV is extremely broad. These illnesses can be classified into those that result from a direct involvement of the nervous system by HIV and those that result either directly or indirectly from the concomitant immunosuppression (Table 20.1). Infectious complications are the most common but not the sole cause of neurologic disability in the latter category. Among other causes of neurologic disease seen in association with HIV-1 infection are neoplasms, metabolic-nutritional disorders, and vascular complications.

Neurological complications of HIV infection should not be surprising. Though HIV can be demonstrated in virtually all body fluids, the concentration of free, non-cell–associated virus is particularly high in the cerebrospinal fluid (CSF).[18] Furthermore, HIV-1 has been recovered from the brain,[18,19] spinal cord,[19,20] and peripheral nerves of infected individuals.[19] By electron microscopy, the virus can be demonstrated in central-nervous-system (CNS) tissue.[21] Also, by in situ hybridization and Southern blot analysis, Shaw and co-workers[22] were able to demonstrate the presence of HIV-1 DNA, and RNA in the brains of patients with AIDS. Resnick and associates[23] demonstrated the intrablood–brain-barrier synthesis of antibody directed to HIV, suggesting the presence of a localized infection. The brain tissue of humans with AIDS is infectious when injected either intracerebrally or intravenously into chimpanzees.[24] Human glial cell lines have been demonstrated to be permissive for HIV-1.[25] Lastly,

Table 20.1. Spectrum of neurologic diseases occurring with HIV-1 infection.

DIRECT
HIV meningitis
acute, subacute, chronic
HIV encephalopathy (AIDS dementia complex)
HIV myelopathy
HIV peripheral neuropathy
HIV myopathy
INDIRECT
Opportunistic infections[a]
Cytomegalovirus
Progressive multifocal leukoencephalopathy (JC virus)
Tuberculous meningitis
Cryptococcal meningitis
Toxoplasmosis
CNS neoplasms
Primary brain lymphoma
Metastatic disease
Metabolic-nutritional disease
Cerebrovascular disease

[a]Only the most common opportunistic infections are listed.

sequence homology and viral morphology indicate a strong evolutionary relationship between HIV-1 and the Lentivirinae subfamily,[26] and all lentiviruses have been demonstrated to be capable of causing neurologic disease.[2]

HIV Meningitis and Meningoencephalitis

Acute infection with HIV may result in neurologic disease, with the incubation time from infection to acute manifestations is estimated at 3 to 6 weeks. An illness resembling infectious mononucleosis frequently, though not invariably, develops. Symptoms include sweats, rigors, arthralgias, myalgias, nausea and vomiting, sore throat, abdominal cramps, and diarrhea. The physical examination may reveal fever, generalized lymphadenopathy, pharyngeal injection, splenomegaly and splenic tenderness, maculopapular rash, and urticaria.[27,28] Laboratory studies, even in this early phase of the illness, may show thrombocytopenia and lymphopenia with an inversion of the T4/T8 (helper/suppressor) CD4 lymphocyte ratio. However, seropositivity for HIV-1 antibodies generally does not become apparent until 8–12 weeks after exposure. Indeed, recent studies indicate that some patients may not seroconvert for many months after having been exposed.[29,30] Transient HIV antigenemia that precedes the development of HIV antibody seroconversion by 6–8 weeks may be seen with acute infection.[31] The HIV antigenemia typically lasts 3 to 4 months[31] and subsides until advanced stages of the illness. In addition to measuring HIV p24 antigen, the use of polymerase chain reaction (PCR) may be helpful in detecting HIV provirus before HIV seroconversion.[32]

During this acute illness, a meningitis[27,33] or meningoencephalitis[34] may supervene. These disorders are characterized by headache, meningismus, photophobia, generalized seizures, and altered mental state. Rarely, acute myelopathy[35] or brachial plexitis[36] has been described as accompanying acute HIV-1 infection. CSF examination typically reveals an increased protein (less than 100 mg%), mononuclear pleocytosis (200 cells/mm^3 or less), and normal glucose.[33] HIV can be isolated from the CSF, but requires special virologic laboratories equipped to perform the cultures. HIV-1-specific antibody production is not detected in this early stage of infection; however, intrathecal synthesis of HIV-1-specific antibody can be demonstrated within months of primary infection.[24] Therefore, antibody studies will need to be repeated in 2–3 months in a patient with a suspected acute HIV-1 infection. Alternatively, viral cultures or viral antigen studies may provide the diagnosis before the establishment of an antibody response. Conversely, even in neurologically asymptomatic HIV-infected individuals, CSF studies reveal that more than 80% will exhibit HIV-1 in their CSF and/or evidence of intrathecal synthesis of HIV-1-specific antibody production once the latency period for an antibody response to develop has elapsed, which is indicative of early penetration of the blood–brain barrier and the establishment of local CNS infection.[24] To illustrate the last point, the CSF of 52 HIV-1-seropositive patients (29 with and 23 without neurologic disease) was studied.[24] HIV was recovered from the CSF of 17% of those with neurologic disease and 22% of those without such disease.[24] All patients with positive CSF cultures had CSF antibodies directed against HIV p24 and gp41 antigens had an elevated intrablood–brain barrier total IgG and HIV-specific IgG synthesis rates. The frequency of CSF isolation from the group of seropositive patients without AIDS (28%) exceeded that of patients with AIDS (5%).[24] Similarly, Elovaara and colleagues[37] have demonstrated intrathecal HIV-specific IgG synthesis in patients with early infection and in individuals who are symptom-free. They attribute the poor correlation with HIV-1-specific IgG synthesis and the presence of neurologic symptoms to infection of neurologically "silent" areas of the brain's white matter.[37] Viral recovery from the CSF can be demonstrated in 28% or more HIV-1-infected individuals, often apparently early in the infection.[23]

A small percentage of people with HIV-1 meningitis will present in subacute fashion and have features of the illness persist for months. Among 14 patients with HIV-1 infection and relatively preserved immune function studied by Hollander and Stringari,[33] an unexplained CSF lymphocytic pleocytosis was associated with two patterns of illness. In seven patients, an acute, self-limited meningitis occurred. In the other seven patients, chronic headaches with or without meningeal signs accompanied the pleocytosis. CSF findings were less striking in this latter group. In four of five CSF specimens studied, HIV-1 was recovered. The authors concluded that in addition to the acute HIV-1 meningitis associated with recent seroconversion, sporadic episodes of acute and chronic meningitis may complicate prior HIV-1 infection. Abnormal CSF findings are extraordinarily common in HIV-1-infected individuals, even in the absence of any symptoms. Marshall and associates[38] found some CSF abnormality in 63% of HIV-1-infected U.S. Air Force personnel, 80% of whom were entirely asymptomatic. These CSF abnormalities are diverse in nature and do not appear to be predictive of the subsequent development of clinically manifest neurologic disease.[38]

HIV Encephalopathy

Shortly after the initial description of AIDS, an unusual, slowly progressive, dementing illness was recognized in association with this disorder.[8,39] At first it was referred to as a "subacute viral encephalitis," though the specific etiology was uncertain and many investigators considered cytomegalovirus (CMV) the likely etiology.[8,15,39] Subsequently, compelling evidence accumulated to link HIV-1 directly to this encephalopathy. Currently, it is widely referred to as the AIDS dementia complex, but other appelations have included AIDS dementia, AIDS encephalopathy, and HIV-1 encephalopathy. Perhaps the last term is most correct in designating this illness as it may be the initial manifestation of HIV infection, before the infected individual exhibits any other illnesses characteristic of impaired immunity.[40] However, by Centers for Disease Control (CDC) criteria, this dementing syndrome is an AIDS-defining condition, as are other neurologic disorders (Table 20.2).

The exact incidence of this disorder in HIV-infected patients is uncertain. Studies by Navia, Jordan, and Price[41] suggest that as many as two thirds of autopsied AIDS patients have this encephalopathy,[41] but it is likely that its incidence is even

Table 20.2. Centers for Disease Control (CDC) classification system.

Group	Description
I	Acute infection
II	Asymptomatic infection
III	Persistent generalized lymphadenopathy
IV	Other diseases
Subgroup A	Constitutional disease
Subgroup B	Neurologic disease
Subgroup C	Secondary infectious diseases
Category C-1	Specified secondary infectious diseases listed in the CDC surveillance definition for AIDS
Category C-2	Other specified secondary infectious diseases
Group D	Secondary cancers
Group E	Other conditions

higher and depends on the duration of HIV infection. In a study of patients entered into drug trials for ARC or early AIDS, more than 80% displayed subtle evidence of neurologic disease and CSF abnormalities, including intrathecal HIV-1-specific antibody synthesis compatible with the diagnosis of HIV-1 encephalopathy.[42] Similarly, Grant and coworkers[43] demonstrated a high prevalence of early CNS involvement with neurologically asymptomatic HIV-1 infection using a detailed neuropsychologic battery and magnetic-resonance imaging (MRI).[43] Neuropsychologic evaluation revealed abnormalities in 13 of 15 patients with AIDS, 7 of 16 with ARC, and 7 of 13 with HIV seropositivity alone. The abnormalities in the first group included impaired abstract reasoning, learning difficulties, and slowed speed of information processing.[43] Abnormalities on MRI were noted in 9 of 13 AIDS patients and 5 of 10 ARC patients.[43] Wilkie and colleagues[44] have found significant slowing of information processing in otherwise asymptomatic, HIV-seropositive homosexual men. Other investigators have reported a decline in performance on a number of tests of neuropsychometric function in asymptomatic HIV-1-seropositive homosexual men when compared with seronegative controls,[45,46] and progression to ARC and AIDS appears to be associated with an even greater degree of cognitive decline.[47]

The presence of early cognitive dysfunction with HIV-1 infection, however, has been refuted by others.[48,49] The explanation for this discrepancy is unknown. Possible factors include differences in the populations studied, differences in the duration of the disease, absence of a suitable control population, cofactors for the expression of neurologic disease, and differences in the test batteries used and the techniques by which they were performed. Furthermore, whether the presence of early intellectual problems signals the onset of a progressive HIV-1 encephalopathy (AIDS dementia complex) or they exist in a static, isolated form is unclear at present. Despite these caveats, the clinical recognition of HIV-1 encephalopathy underestimates its true incidence. At autopsy, De la Monte and colleagues[50] demonstrated pathologic evidence of a subacute encephalitis in 27 of 30 (90%) patients with AIDS or ARC. Even in the absence of pathologic evidence of encephalitis, HIV-1 can be recovered from the CSF.[50] Other neuropathologic postmortem studies demonstrate evidence of a viral encephalitis characterized by microglial nodules and multinucleated giant cells in a smaller percentage of cases.[14,16,17]

Price and colleagues[51] have postulated that the brain pathogenicity of the HIV-1 increases with the degree of immunosuppression. These investigators suggest "that asymptomatic CNS infection on the one hand indicates that the virus is 'neurotropic' by virtue of its predilection to infect the leptomeninges early and frequently, and, on the other hand, provides evidence of the low neurovirulence of HIV-1 despite its persistence, at least as long as immune defenses restrict its replication and spread."[51] In their clinical experience, overt dementia was detected in one third of the patients at the time of diagnosis of AIDS and an additional one quarter had subclinical dementia. Preterminally, they estimated the prevalence of overt dementia to be approximately 66% and subclinical dementia to be 25%. Subclinical dementia is best detected by neuropsychologic tests that measure performance under time constraints, problem solving, visual scanning, visual-motor integration, and alternation between two or more performance rules or sets.[52,53] Though rare, instances of classic HIV encephalopathy occurring in the absence of significant immunosuppression have also been observed.[54] In fact, the illness may the presenting manifestation of AIDS.[55]

Clinically, the encephalopathy is characterized by an insidious onset of a disturbance in intellect. Fatigue and malaise, headaches, increasing social isolation, and loss of sexual drive are noted. Rarely, the disorder may begin abruptly and progress rapidly. Patients often complain of increasing forgetfulness and a slowness in their thinking. Their business acumen begins to wane and jobs at which they were formerly successful they are no longer capable of performing. Eventually, self-care becomes a problem. A diagnosis of depression is frequently considered; however, dysphoria is typically absent.[51] Language skills suffer as well, and word-finding difficulties are common. Some patients complain of imbalance and gait disturbances, as well as tremor. Painful peripheral dyesthesias may occur and are probably the result of a superimposed HIV-1-related peripheral neuropathy.

In perhaps 10–15% of the affected individuals, the illness may present as a frank psychosis. In fact, HIV-1 encephalopathy may mimic diverse psychiatric illnesses. Among the other psychiatric manifestations also recognized are delusions, hallucinations, mania, paranoia, and depression,[56–60] each of which may occur in isolation. As observed with other HIV neurologic complications, the psychoses may be the presenting manifestation of HIV infection and be seen in the absence of immune-system compromise.[61] A triad of mood disturbance, thought disorder with grandiose delusions, and severe memory deficits has been described.[62]

The dementia that these patients exhibit has the hallmarks of a "subcortical dementia.[63] Bradyphrenia, forgetfulness, an inability to attend to tasks, and poor sequential processing are typical. Examination reveals not only abnormalities of cognitive function, but also other disturbances—among them a sustension tremor of the outstretched upper extremities, which is usually fine and fast in frequency, but may be coarse. A resting tremor is not observed, though features reminiscent of parkinsonism—namely, bradykinesia, postural instability, cogwheel rigidity, hypomimetic facies, and eye-movement disorders—may be observed. In this context, there is a striking sensitivity to dopamine-receptor blocking agents, even with drugs that have a low potential for the development of parkinsonism, such as prochlorperazine and metoclopropamide.[64,65] Dystonia has been reported in the absence of antipsychiatric exposure.[66] Frontal release signs, including a positive snout, grasps, Myerson sign, and palmomental reflex, are common. Slowed rapid alternating eye movements,[51] impaired pursuit movements,[67] and convergence may be noted. Other disorders of ocular motility resulting from CNS dysfunction have been described.[68] These eye findings may be an early sign of HIV encephalopathy.[67,68] Lower-extremity weakness, paratonia of the limbs, gait unsteadiness, poor tandem gait, and brisk muscle stretch reflexes and jaw jerk are also commonly observed.[69] On rare occasion, generalized or focal seizures may be experienced, and may even herald the illness. Myoclonus is also observed, but typically in the late stages of the illness. Preterminally, like other dementing illnesses, the patient is bedridden, and is mute, with a vacuous facial expression and fetal body posture.

Children infected with HIV also develop a progressive encephalopathy.[70,71] As in adults, the neurologic manifestations may be seen before any signs of immunodeficiency, as exemplified by the infant, described by Davis and co-workers,[72] who—at the age of 6 months—developed progressive spastic diplegia and dementia resulting from HIV infection in the absence of any evidence of immunosuppression. A progressive infantile encephalopathy caused by HIV-1 has also been described by enzyme-linked immunosorbent assay (ELISA) in an HIV-antibody-negative child.[73] However, generally, the neurologic disease progresses in tandem with the degree of immunodeficiency.[74] The incubation period from initial infection in the perinatal period to the development of the encephalopathy varied from 2 months to 5 years in one study of 36 infected children.[74] This encephalopathy is characterized by a developmental delay or the loss of motor milestones and intellectual abilities that had been previously acquired.[74,75] Examination may reveal weakness, with pyramidal-tract signs, extrapyramidal signs, pseudobulbar palsy, ataxia, and secondary microcephaly. Myoclonus and seizures have also been observed.

The gross pathology of HIV encephalopathy is characterized by brain atrophy with sulcal widening and ventricular dilatation. Meningeal fibrosis may occasionally be observed. Histologically, the most common and distinctive feature of this illness is white-matter pallor.[41] This pallor largely appears to be the result of paravascular demyelination and is located chiefly in the periventricular and central white matter and accompanied by an astrocytic reaction. Rarefaction of the white matter and, in severe cases, diffuse or focal microvacuolation may be detected. In the series of Kato and co-workers,[17] true demyelination appeared to be rare, being found in only one of 53 AIDS brains. Multinucleate giant cells (Figure 20.1) are believed by some investigators to be a pathologic hallmark of the disease. Others observe these morphologic correlates of HIV-1 encephalopathy only rarely.[76–78] The multinucleate giant cell appears to result from direct virus-induced cell fusion.[51] This phenomenon is identical to that which has been demonstrated by Popovic and colleagues[79] to occur in vitro in HIV-1-infected cell cultures. These multinucleate giant cells appear to cluster around the microvasculature. They are also present in normal neuropil, gliomesenchymal cell nodules and in cavitating lesions.[13] Other microscopic features include a microglial nodules (Figure 20.2), diffuse astrocytosis, and perivascular mononuclear inflammation.

The presence of microglial nodules is believed by investigators to correlate with the presence of CMV

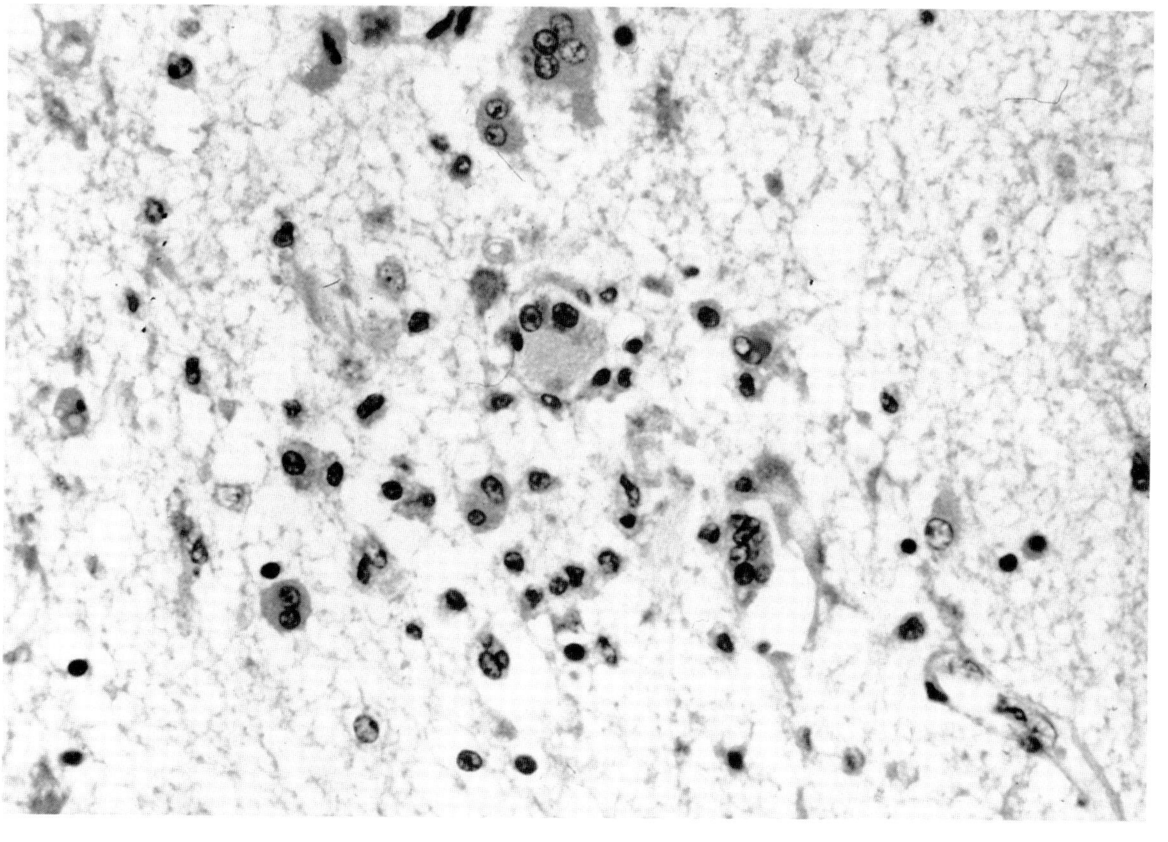

Fig. 20.1. Multinucleate giant cells observed in a patient with HIV-1 encephalopathy. (Hematoxylin & eosin.)

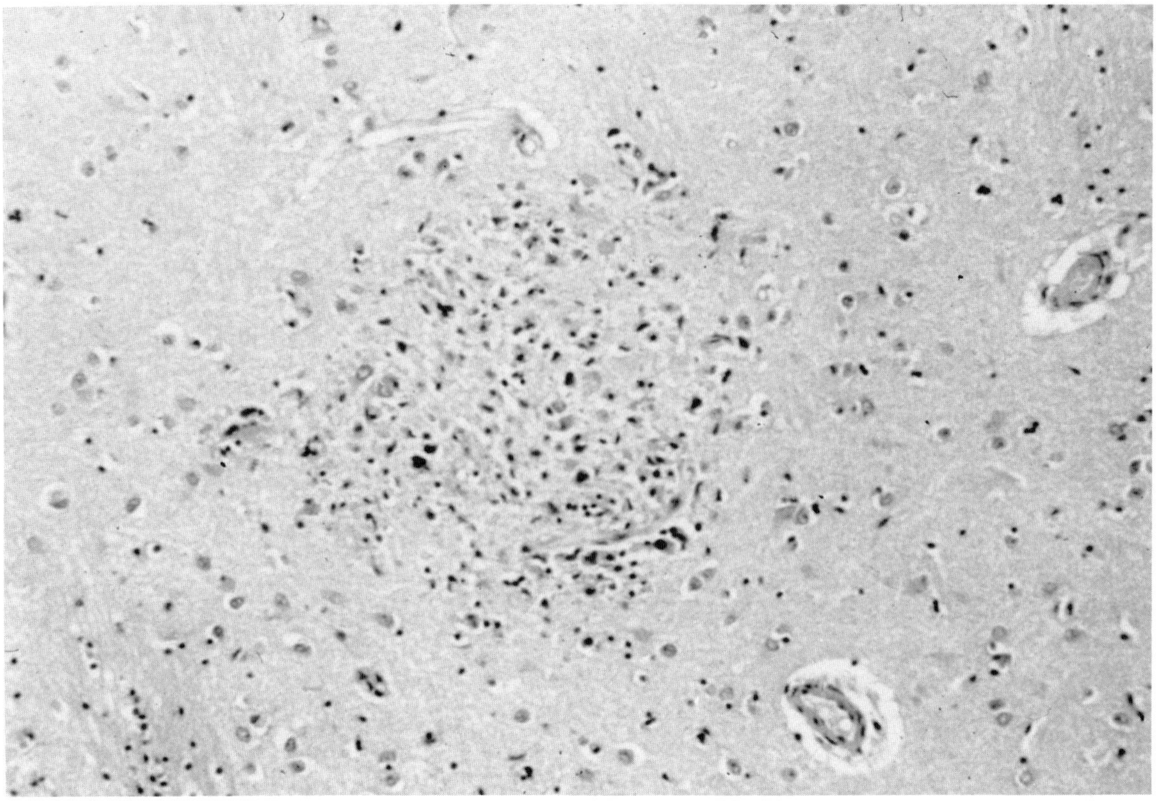

Fig. 20.2. Microglial nodule observed in a patient with HIV-1 encephalopathy. Multinucleate giant cells are also present within the lesion. (Hematoxylin & eosin.) Reprinted with permission from Broder S (ed): *AIDS: Modern Concepts and Therapeutic Challenges*. 1986. Marcel Dekker, Inc. New York, p. 174.

infection.[76] However, in the study by Kato and colleagues,[79] of 53 brains with AIDS patients, microglial nodules in varying frequency were detected in 24 (45%), and of these 24, only 11 (46%) were accompanied by CMV infection. The mononuclear inflammation may be particularly prominent in the brain stem.[13] Ependymal lesions are also frequently observed in the brains of both adults and infants with HIV-1 encephalopathy.[13] Rarely, other forms of pathology have been associated with HIV encephalopathy. Schwenk and collaborators[80] describe a 28-year-old homosexual man with AIDS complicated by toxoplasmosis and plastmacytoma and a dementing illness characterized by disorientation, lassitude, and somnolence at onset, whose brain at autopsy revealed histologic and ultrastructural changes of subacute spongiform encephalopathy. Though they were unable to demonstrate HIV-1 specific antigens by monoclonal antibodies, their failure to do so was attributed to the paraffin embedding of the brain material. Multinucleate cells were not observed. An alternative consideration, however, is the presence of concomitant infection with the Creutzfeld-Jakob agent. In children, the pathologic features of HIV encephalopathy arise as a unique constellation characterized by diminished brain weight, inflammatory cell infiltrates, multinucleated giant cells, vascular calcifications, perivascular inflammation, and white-matter changes.[81] The calcification of the basal ganglia is unique to childhood HIV encephalopathy.[81,82] As in adult cases, the genome of HIV can be demonstrated in the brains of these patients with in situ hybridization techniques.[73,81]

At present, uncertainty surrounds the exact cellular localization of the HIV-1 infection in the CNS. As previously noted, the virus can be detected in the CNS by a variety of methods. A consensus exists among most investigators that the brain macrophage is infected. The multinucleate giant cells observed result from fusion of these macrophages. Some, but not all, investigators have found evidence of the virus in endothelial cells,[83] glia, and neurons.[84,85]

According to Pumarola-Sune and colleagues,[85] the distribution of HIV-1 in the brain parallels the distribution of the pathologic changes, though the findings of Gabuzda and co-workers[86] indicate that infected monocyte/macrophage cells are most often located in the cortex of the frontal, temporal, and parietal lobes.

The exact mechanism by which HIV infection results in CNS dysfunction remains intriguingly enigmatic. Of considerable importance has been the demonstration by autoradiographic techniques of CD4 receptors in monkey and rat brain.[87] Hill and collaborators[87] detected particularly high rates of T4 binding in the hippocampus, amygdala, and many regions of the neocortex. The specific cell types to which the T4 binding occurred were not identified in this study. However, other investigators have demonstrated the presence of CD4 molecules or mRNA for CD4 in neurons and glial cells from various areas of the brain.[88–90] Despite the demonstration of CD4 receptors on neurons and glial, most investigators have found little or no evidence of viral infection in these cells at postmortem. Alternatively, the monocyte/microglial cell is clearly infected. Using cocultivation for virus isolation, in situ hybridization, immunocytochemistry, and transmission electron microscopy, Koenig and colleagues[91] detected HIV-1 in the brain macrophages of two patients with AIDS and a subacute encephalopathy. Likewise, Gartner and associates[92] were able to detect reverse transcriptase activity in monocytoid cells from a brain biopsy of an HIV-1-seropositive individual with progressive dementia. Electron microscopy revealed the presence of HIV in these cells and, when subcultured, they were demonstrated to be nonspecific esterase positive (suggestive of macrophages), unlike the subcultured cell lines that did not express virus.[92] Immunoperoxidase staining with goat anti-HIV-1 serum on frozen brain sections revealed HIV-1 antigen in 5 of 13 specimens.[93] Morphologically, the cells infected appeared to be in monocyte/macrophages and were most frequently observed in association with capillaries or near microglial nodules in the cortex of the frontal, temporal, and parietal lobes.[93]

Occasionally, HIV-1 may be detected in other cell lines within the CNS. Using in situ hybridization to detect HIV-1 nucleic-acid sequences and immunocytochemistry to identify viral and cellular proteins on the brains of 12 AIDS patients, Wiley and colleagues[83] detected HIV in mononuclear inflammatory cells, capillary endothelial cells, and giant cells. These investigators noted the white matter to be more involved than the gray matter. In one patient with severe neurologic dysfunction, a low-level infection was seen in astrocytes and neurons. A fascinating discovery by Koyanagi and colleagues[94] of genetically distinct but related HIV-1 in the CSF and brain tissue of a patient with HIV encephalopathy suggests possible cellular tropism. Both of these viruses were able to replicate in peripheral blood lymphycytes, but only the virus from brain tissue was able efficiently to infect macrophage/monocytes.[94] The authors suggest that certain strains of HIV-1 could exhibit glial-cell tropism and be pathogenetically responsible for some of the neurologic disorders observed with AIDS. Similarly, Anand and co-workers[95] found that five HIV-1 isolates from four AIDS patients with primary CNS involvement had replication equivalence to viral isolates from lymphadenopathy syndrome, but unlike the latter, four of these five isolates did not kill T4 cells. Cheng-Mayer and Levy[96] also argue that brain isolates may represent a distinct subtype of HIV-1 based on the ability of viral isolates from the brain and lymph node of one patient to infect established human cell lines and their sensitivity to serum neutralization. Another study that seems to confirm the observation of neurotropic HIV-1 subtypes is that by Von Briesen and colleagues.[97] In the majority of their AIDS cases with neurologic symptoms, HIV-1 from the peripheral blood grew well on fresh peripheral human lymphocytes, while all but two isolates from the CSF of the same patients grew slowly and at low titers.

The relative absence of HIV-1 from CNS neurons, the often poor correlation of degree of cognitive disturbance with the neuropathologic findings at autopsy, and the anecdotal observations of improvement in mental capacities following the use of zidovudine,[98] an inhibitor of HIV replication, suggest that neuronal death from HIV-1 infection is not the primary or sole cause of HIV-1 encephalopathy. Other potential factors are listed in Table 20.3. Provocative evidence of the role of humoral factors in the etiopathogenesis of HIV-1 encephalopathy includes the association of intramuscular administration of alpha-interferon with the development of transient fatigue, a loss of interest, an inability to concentrate, anxiety, and depression, as well as phobias and paranoid ideation.[99] These changes are especially prominent in HIV-seropositive individuals.[99] The presence of brain-reactive antibodies directed at a 45-kilodalton pro-

Table 20.3. Potential mechanisms by which HIV-1 results in encephalopathy

1. HIV-1 infects neurons and results in cell death.
2. HIV-1 infects neurons and results in cellular dysfunction without cell death.
3. HIV-1 alters levels of trophic factors, e.g., nerve-growth factor, responsible for neuronal survival.
4. HIV-1 alters neurotransmitter production and release.
5. HIV-1 binds to neurotransmitter receptor site, e.g., that of vasoactive intestinal peptide (VIP) or neuroleukin, resulting in cellular dysfunction or death.
6. HIV-1 infects macrophages and microglia in the brain and results in the elaboration of humoral immunomodulators that are toxic to the nervous system.

tein has been demonstrated in these patients by Kumar,[100] and may be of clinical consequence. An interesting and potentially important observation of Pert and colleagues[101] suggests that there is a potentially pathogenically important homology between a portion of the HIV-1 envelope protein and the neurotransmitter vasopressin. CD4-receptor activity appears to be primarily specified by N-terminal (vasoactive intestinal peptide 1–12) amino acids.[102] In a similar vein, the HIV-1 envelope protein gp120 inhibited the growth of neurons in the presence of neuroleukin, but not in the presence of nerve-growth factor.[103] This inhibition suggests a partial sequence homology between gp120 and neuroleukin. A comprehensive discussion of the cellular localization of HIV-1 and the pathogenesis of HIV-1-related neurologic manifestations is outside the scope of this chapter, but can be found in the excellent review by Michaels and associates.[104]

Preliminary studies with positron emission tomography (PET) using ({18-F} fluorodeoxyglucose (FDG) have defined the functional pathology of HIV-1 encephalopathy in nine patients.[105] The FDG/PET scans of these cognitively impaired individuals were analyzed by a mathematical model of regional metabolic interactions referred to as the Subprofile Scaling Model.[106] Assessment of the regional cerebral metabolic rate for glucose demonstrated relative subcortical (thalamus and basal ganglia) hypermetabolism in early HIV encephalopathy and cortical and subcortical gray-matter hypometabolism in advanced stages of the disease.[105] The alterations in subcortical metabolism appear to correlate with impairment of fine motor control and that of cortical metabolism with impairments in verbal fluency and problem solving. Investigators have suggested that FDG/PET may be a useful objective means of demonstrating the onset of HIV-1 encephalopathy and also of following the response to antiviral therapy.[105] A study of cerebral blood flow using single-photon emission tomography with 99mTc-hexmethylpropyleneamineoxime (HMPAO) in two AIDS patients with cognitive disturbances revealed bilateral cerebral-blood-flow loss in the temporal lobes in one and in the temporal and parietal lobes in the other.[107]

The diagnosis of HIV-1 encephalopathy still remains one of exclusion. Computed tomography (CT) of the brain usually reveals brain atrophy characterized by sulcal widening and hydrocephalus ex vacuo.[108–110] In children, calcification of the basal ganglia is frequently detected.[82] MRI reveals not only the brain atrophy, but also the demyelinative lesion in the periventricular white matter and centrum semiovale.[110,111] The latter is characterized by focal or diffuse high-intensity signal abnormalities on T2-weighted images (Figure 20.3). Futhermore, MRI is quite sensitive in detecting other cerebral lesions that accompany HIV infection. In that context, it is an extraordinarily useful tool in excluding other possible etiologies of CNS disturbance.[112] But despite the relative sensitivity of MRI, both it and CT may be relatively insensitive early in the disease.[108,110]

CSF studies show an increased protein in two thirds and a mononuclear pleocytosis in one fifth of people with HIV encephalitis.[113] In our experience, the protein seldom exceeds 100 mg% and is frequently accompanied by an increase in immunoglobulins. Intrathecal synthesis of HIV-1-specific antibody can be demonstrated in virtually all, and HIV-1 isolation in the CSF or its detection by tests for HIV-1 antigens is also frequently positive. According to Goudsmit and collaborators,[31] the persistence of HIV-1 antigen in the CSF appears to be pathognomonic of progressive encephalopathy, particularly in children. The mononuclear pleocytosis observed may be as high as 200 cell/mm^3. The CSF glucose is normal or borderline. Antibody in the serum should be positive by the time the patient presents with HIV encephalopathy, but Price and Navia[113] have observed one patient who presented with the encephalopathy before seroconversion.

Initial anecdotal reports[98] regarding improvement in HIV encephalopathy in adults following the use of zidovudine have been confirmed by more comprehensive studies.[114] Further studies to confirm its value in this condition may be difficult to perform because of its use early in the course of infection. In

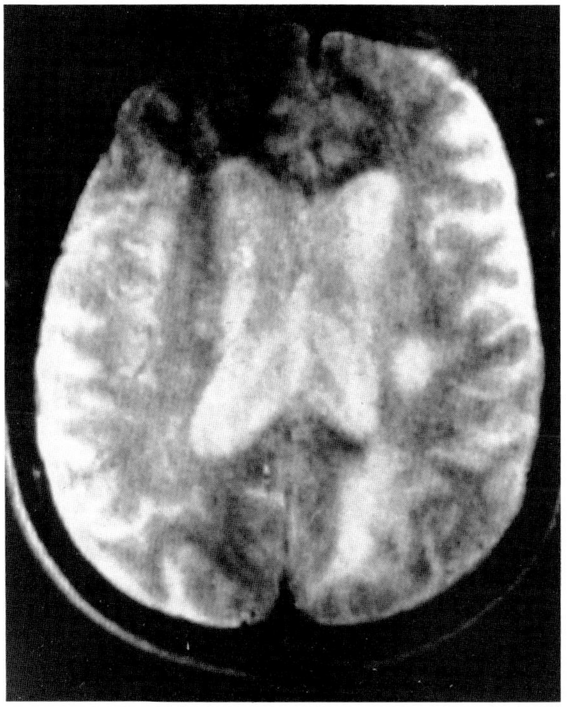

Fig. 20.3. A T2 weighted magnetic resonance image of the brain of a patient with HIV-1 encephalopathy. Two large confluent hyperintense lesions are present in the left cerebral hemisphere. Several smaller discrete hyperintense lesions are noted in the contralateral hemisphere.

children, a similar, and perhaps more dramatic, improvement in encephalopathy was demonstrated by Pizzo and colleagues[115] with continuous-infusion zidovudine.

HIV Myelopathy

A unique degeneration of the spinal cord is commonly seen in association with HIV-1 infection.[8,116,117] Petito and colleagues[116] observed this myelopathy in 20 of 89 consecutively autopsied AIDS patients. Though the clinical presentation of this myeloopathy may overlap with that of other myelopathies related to HIV-1 infection, the pathologic appearance is quite distinct. Clinically, these patients complain of leg weakness, unsteadiness, and gait impairment. Incontinence of bladder and bowel often supervenes. In one study, incontinence was observed in 60% of patients.[116] Patients with this disorder often complain of paresthesias and vague discomfort in their legs. Frequently, these complaints are attributed to the general debilitation of the patient and the true nature of the illness remains undiagnosed until pathologic examination of the spinal cord at the time of autopsy. On physical examination, a spastic paraparesis is detected, with the degree of weakness exceeding that of spasticity. Rarely, marked asymmetry of the leg weakness, a monoparesis or quadriparesis, may be found. Gait ataxia is seen and the heel-to-knee-to-toe test may reveal dysmetria and dyssynergy. On occasion, weakness is slight or absent on confrontation testing, but hyperreflexia of the lower extremities and extensor plantar responses are noted. However, muscle stretch reflexes may also be diminished or absent in this disorder as a result of concomitant peripheral neuropathy.

Sensory examination reveals that vibratory and position senses are disproportionately affected in comparison with pinprick, temperature, or light touch. A significant impairment of these modalities suggests the presence of a concomitant peripheral neuropathy. Electrophysiologic studies may reveal a prolonged latency of cortical evoked responses following tibial nerve stimulation.[118] Typically, this myelopathy is seen late in the course of HIV-1 infection; however, it also has been described as the presenting manifestation of this viral infection.[119]

Gross examination of the spinal cord and dura is generally normal in this condition unless the myelopathy is particularly severe.[116] The striking finding on histologic examination is myelin loss and spongy degeneration, with the lateral and posterior columns more severely affected than the anterior columns. A microvacuolization of the white matter of the spinal cord (Figure 20.4) associated with lipid-laden macrophages bears an uncanny resemblance to the pathology of subacute combined degeneration of the spinal cord. The vacuolization appears to result from intramyelin swelling. Axons are preserved, except in areas of marked vacuolization. Microglial nodules may be detected in the spinal-cord gray matter, and 20% of the patients in one series also exhibited central chromatolysis of the anterior horn motor cells.[116] Inflammation and intranuclear viral inclusions are generally not seen.[116]

Although HIV-1 has been cultured from the spinal cord,[14] its specific role in the causation of this illness is uncertain. The spinal-cord pathology is most prominent in the middle and lower thoracic regions.

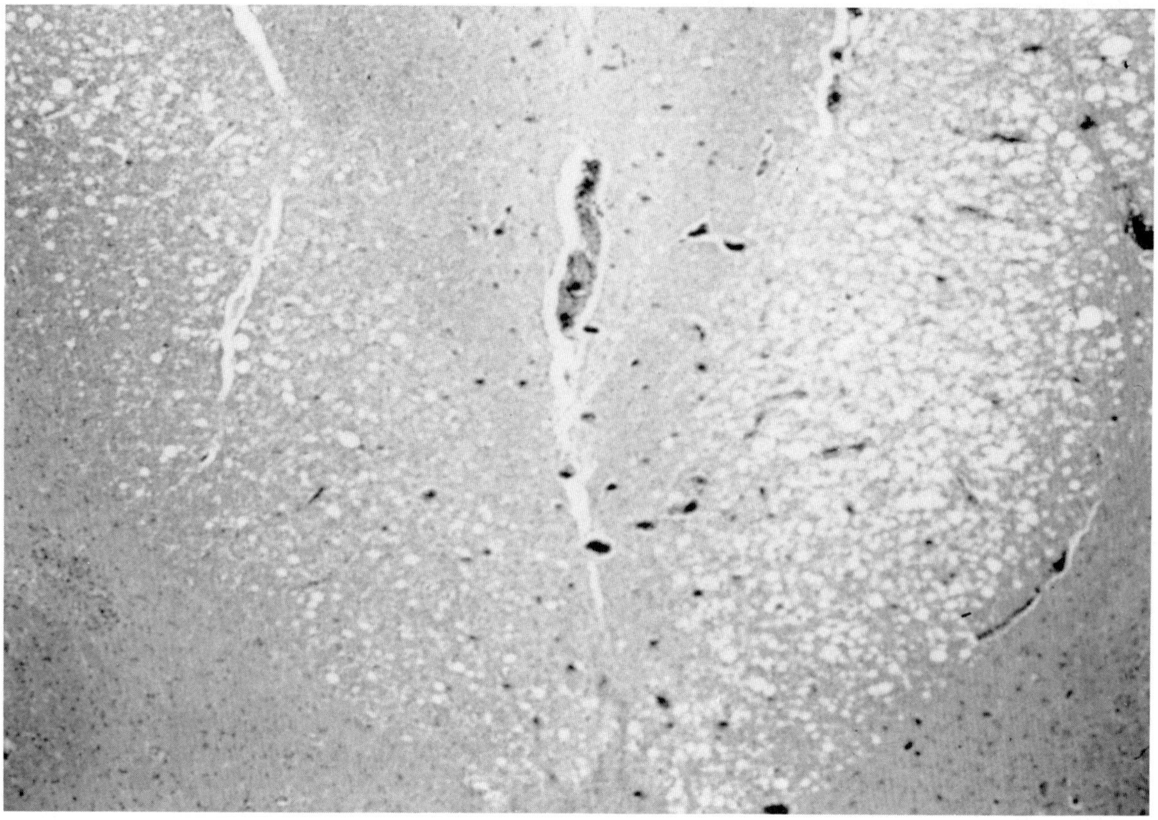

Fig. 20.4. Microvacuolar changes in the posterior columns of the thoracic spinal cord of a patient with HIV-1-associated vacuolar myelopathy. (Hematoxylin & eosin.)

The cord involvement may be asymmetric and does not appear to be confined to particular tracts.[116] However, Goldstick and colleagues[117] have described involvement of the posterior columns as increasing in intensity with rostral progression, whereas pyramidal-tract involvement increased caudally. Petito and associates[116] were able to correlate the frequency and severity of symptoms with the degree of spinal-cord pathology in their series. They classified the patients into three groups based on the severity of the illness quantified neuropathologically. All patients with severe involvement of the spinal cord displayed clinical features of spinal-cord disease, but only five of seven with moderate changes and two of eight with mild changes did. Features of HIV encephalopathy are often observed in patients with HIV myelopathy. In one instance, lesions resembling Marchiafava-Bignami disease were seen in the brain of a patient with HIV myelopathy.[120] The authors suggested the potential role of nutritional deficiency in the causation of the brain and spinal-cord pathology. In young children with AIDS, vacuolar myelopathy is not observed, however, pathologic abnormalities of the spinal cord are frequently seen at autopsy.[121] The most common abnormality appears to be a loss of both myelin and axons in the corticospinal tracts.[121]

The diagnosis of this illness is, like that of HIV encephalopathy, one of exclusion. A number of other myelopathies have been observed in association with HIV-1 infection. An acute myelopathy of uncertain pathogenesis has been noted at the time of seroconversion.[122] Other infectious etiologies of the myelopathies occurring in association with HIV-1 include CMV,[123] HSV type 2,[124] Varicella-zoster virus (VZV), HTLV-1,[126], mycobacteria,[127] *Treponema pallidum,*[13] and epidural abcesses.[128] Additionally, myelopathy may complicate vascular disease, tumor,[8,129,130] or a peculiar relapsing and remitting neurologic disorder resembling multiple sclerosis.[131]

The most useful study is MRI of the spinal cord.

Our practice has been, generally, to forgo myelography if MRI of the spinal cord reveals no evidence of mass lesion. The presence of unusual features such as back pain or radicular findings may dictate a more aggressive diagnostic approach. If the MRI is negative, the CSF is examined for the presence of HIV and other pathogens, including viral cultures with specific emphasis on CMV and HSV types 1 and 2. Additionally, routine bacterial and fungal cultures and cryptococcal antigen are obtained. No treatment is known to be effective for this condition.

HIV Peripheral Neuropathy

A diverse group of peripheral neuropathies (Table 20.4) have been described in association with various stages of HIV-1 infection. The exact role of HIV in the etiopathogenesis of these neuropathies remains obscure, though HIV can be isolated from the peripheral nerve in many instances.[14] Multiple factors, such as nutritional deficiencies, concomitant metabolic disorders, and drug side effects, may be responsible for these neuropathies. An indication of the frequency with which peripheral-nerve disorders are observed in HIV-seropositive patients is provided by the study of Janssen and colleagues.[132] In this study, 39 homosexual/bisexual men with the lymphadenopathy syndrome were examined for the presence of neurologic disease. Eighteen of the 39 had symptoms or signs of peripheral neuropathy. The most common neuropathic features were complaints of numbness, tingling, or burning sensations or loss of temperature sense in a distal symmetric distribution in the lower extremities. The existence of a mononeuropathy was suggested in six (two with Bell's palsy, two with bilateral carpal-tunnel syndrome, and two with ulnar neuropathy). Not unexpectedly, nine patients had a history of VZV radiculitis.

Table 20.4. Spectrum of peripheral neuropathies occurring with HIV-1 infection.[144]

Neuropathy associated with HIV seroconversion
Acute inflammatory demyelinating polyneuropathy
Ganglioneuropathy
Neuropathy associated with asymptomatic HIV infection
Acute inflammatory demyelinating polyneuropathy
Chronic inflammatory demyelinating polyneuropathy
Polyradiculopathy
Neuropathy associated with AIDS-related complex
Acute inflammatory demyelinating polyneuropathy
Chronic inflammatory demyelinating polyneuropathy
Distal symmetric polyneuropathy
Polyradiculopathy
Mononeuritis multiplex
Neuropathy associated with AIDS
Distal symmetric polyneuropathy
Acute inflammatory demyelinating polyneuropathy
Chronic inflammatory demyelinating polyneuropathy
Mononeuritis multiplex
Autonomic neuropathy

The peripheral neuropathies that attend HIV-1 infection can be characteristically divided into three groups: a distal, symmetric, peripheral neuropathy; inflammatory demyelinating peripheral neuropathy; and mononeuritis multiplex. The most common peripheral neuropathy observed with HIV-1 infection is a symmetric, distal, sensorimotor neuropathy. This neuropathy may be the first manifestation of the infection, but more often appears in later stages of the illness. Typically, the patient complains of dysesthesias of the toes and soles of the feet and associated numbness in a similar distribution. Occasionally, the dysesthesias may begin in the hands. Though usually described as a "pins and needle" sensation, several of our patients have complained of other peculiar sensations, such as a sense of being splashed with cold water, a feeling of burning, or shooting electric-like pains. These discomforts are seldom debilitating and sensory symptoms and signs predominate. Weakness is generally slight, but often evident on the physical examination. Confrontation testing may reveal weakness of the distal-lower-extremity musculature and the patient may find it difficult to walk on the toes or heels. Muscle stretch reflexes, particularly the ankle jerks, are depressed or absent. Sensory loss is greatest for vibratory perception, but decreased pinprick sensation in a distal symmetric "stocking–glove" distribution is also noted. Temperature and, to a lesser extent, light touch are similarly impaired. Position-sense loss in the later phases of this illness may contribute to the ataxic gait, but is seldom severe. Electromyographic (EMG) and nerve-conduction studies confirm the presence of a mixed sensorimotor peripheral neuropathy. Nerve-conduction velocities are usually slightly decreased and sensory potentials are either absent or of low potential suggestive of an axonal neuropathy, although features of demyelination may also be seen.[133] Nerve biopsy has demonstrated epineural and endoneural perivascular inflammation with axonal degeneration or demyelination.[134]

In four homosexual men with AIDS and these neuropathic features, postmortem examination of the spinal cord revealed a striking loss of both axons and myelin sheaths of the rostral fasciculus gracilis, particularly in the upper thoracic and cervical regions.[135] A "dying-back" process of the dorsal-root ganglion neurons was suggested by the combination of distal sensory neuropathy and gracile-tract degeneration.[135] The CSF may be normal or demonstrate a modest elevation of the protein concentration with a mononuclear pleocytosis. This neuropathy is slowly progressive and seldom markedly debilitating. Preliminary observations suggest that zidovudine is helpful in halting the progression or reversing this condition.[98] Plasmapheresis does not appear to be useful,[136] but symptomatic therapy may be extremely helpful. Carbamazepine, diphenylhydantoin, tricyclic antidepressants, and topical capsaicin are often helpful in managing the dysesthetic component of the illness.

A peripheral neuropathy identical to Guillain-Barré syndrome has been described in HIV-1 infection.[137,138] This neuropathy typically presents as an ascending lower-extremity weakness, but may present with greater proximal weakness or facial weakness. The motor deficit progresses over 5 to 21 days. Muscle stretch reflexes are diminished or absent. A minimal distal sensory deficit may be detected. Respiratory paralysis is rare. Nerve-conduction studies are compatible with a demyelinating neuropathy. CSF examination reveals a normal to increased protein (less than 200 mg%) with a mononuclear pleocytosis (less than 50 cells/mm^3) or, more rarely, a normal cell count. Therefore, in contrast to the typical Guillain-Barré syndrome, a CSF albuminocytologic dissociation is seen in a minority of affected individuals. Plasmapheresis is recommended for these patients,[137] though total recovery may ensue spontaneously without it.[139]

Similarly, a chronic, progressive demyelinating peripheral neuropathy may be observed in association with HIV infection.[137] This neuropathy is identical to that referred to as chronic Guillain-Barré syndrome or chronic relapsing inflammatory demyelinating polyneuropathy (CRIP), with a subacute onset, elevated CSF protein, and segmental demyelination on nerve biopsy.[140] If this neuropathy proves unresponsibe to plasmapheresis, a short course of steroids may be of value.

Mononeuritis multiplex also has been observed as complicating HIV infection. The mononeuropathy may affect cranial, peripheral, or spinal nerves.[140,141] Mononeuritis multiplex may precede the development of a generalized inflammatory neuropathy.[134] In some instances, this neuropathy appears to be the result of immune complex deposition with an associated necrotizing vasculitis. Etiologies other than HIV, such as VZV, CMV, and lymphomatous-nerve-root infiltration have also been implicated. Mononeuritis multiplex appears to be less common in association with HIV-1 infection than inflammatory demyelinating polyradiculoneuropathy. CSF findings are nonspecific, but typically reflect inflammatory changes with mononuclear pleocytosis and oligoclonal bands.[134] EMG and nerve-conduction studies suggest combined axonal loss and demyelination. Sural-nerve biopsies may be normal or demonstrate axonal degeneration, segmental demyelination, endoneural edema, and endoneural and epineural inflammation. Unexpectedly, vasculitis is rarely observed.[133,134] Plasmapheresis may afford improvement.[133,134]

The therapeutic value of plasmapheresis in many of these peripheral neuropathies associated with HIV-1 infection should not be surprising. Circulating antibodies to normal sural nerve were consistently demonstrated in 30 patients with AIDS or ARC and peripheral neuropathy by Kiprov and Miller.[133] Further studies by Stricker and colleagues[142] have characterized these antibodies as cross-reacting with antigens of HIV-1.

A wide variety of other neuropathic conditions have also been described with HIV-1 infection. A progressive polyradiculopathy that may also be associated with a myelopathy has been described in patients with AIDS.[133,143,144] This condition generally begins with asymmetric leg weakness and then, over several weeks, progresses cephalad. Sensory loss is observed, but tends to be less severe than the degree of motor weakness. Urinary retention is characteristic. The CSF typically shows a mononuclear pleocytosis, elevated protein, and hypoglycorrhachia. Early in the course of the illness, nerve-conduction studies may be normal, though the EMG shows a reduced recruitment pattern. Ultimately, compound muscle action potentials are reduced and the EMG shows abnormal spontaneous activity.[133,143] CMV and other herpesviruses have been cultured from the CSF,[123] and the former has been chiefly implicated as the etiologic agent.[144] Though herpesviruses have been isolated in this condition, the value of antiviral therapy remains in question. In one patient, no improvement of the radiculomyelopathy with acyclovir, ganciclovir, or plasmapheresis was noted, despite an arrest of a concomitant CMV retinitis.[133]

Other forms of peripheral and cranial neuropathy have been observed in association with HIV-1 infection. A severe ataxic neuropathy secondary to ganglioneuritis has been described.[145] A high incidence of subclinical dorsal ganglion and adjacent spinal-nerve-root inflammation has been observed in a consecutive autopsy study of AIDS patients (S. Tarras, personal communication). Completely or partially reversible, multiple cranial neuropathies have also been seen in AIDS.[146] Isolated or recurrent Bell's palsy has been noted with HIV-1 infection.[132,147] Indeed, here, the facial paresis may be the presenting manifestation, and may return in the ipsilateral or contralateral face. Cranial and peripheral neuropathies with HIV-1 infection may be the result of VZV infection,[148,149] meningovascular syphilis,[150] mycobacterial and fungal meningitis, or lymphomatous meningitis. Transient brachial plexopathy has also been noted with HIV-1 infection,[133] and autonomic neuropathy may be observed in AIDS.[144] Lastly, another form of polyneuropathy to be expected in AIDS patients has been referred to as "critical illness polyneuropathy," which has been described in individuals with sepsis and multiple-organ failure.[151] This neuropathy varies in severity from mild to marked. Nerve-conduction studies and pathologic examination reveal evidence of axonal neuropathy. Denervation atrophy of the limbs and respiratory muscles is also observed. Commonly, the illness is manifested by weakness, atrophy, and impaired tendon reflexes.[151]

HIV Myopathy

Several forms of myopathy have been recognized in association with HIV infection, including a subacute, predominantly proximal muscle weakness with myalgias, excessive fatiguability, and an increase in creatine kinase (CK).[140,141,152] EMG features may be identical to those of polymyositis. Though laboratory evidence of immunologic impairment is usually present at the time of presentation, this myopathy may herald HIV-1 infection before any clinical evidence of cellular immunosuppression arises.[140,141] In the muscle-biopsy specimen of one AIDS patient with myositis, multinucleated giant cells, the hallmark of HIV infection of the CNS, were a prominent histopathologic feature.[153] Polymyositis with immunodeficiency has been induced in monkeys with a type D retrovirus, providing an animal model of this disease.[154] Eleven of 25 rhesus monkeys with simian AIDS had muscle weakness and atrophy and elevated levels of muscle enzymes.[155] The characteristic features of polymyositis were apparent on light microscopy and by enzyme histochemistry of biopsied muscle.[155] The former included fibrous-tissue proliferation, necrosis, and phagocytosis of muscle fibers accompanied by an intense inflammatory infiltrate.[155] A polymyositis-like syndrome has been reported with the use of zidovudine therapy of AIDS and ARC in patients receiving 1,200 mg daily for 6.5 to 17 months.[156] The occurrence of this myopathy may depend on the total dose of zidovudine received. Though controversial,[157] some investigators believe that a distinguishable muscle histopathology exists with zidovudine myopathy characterized by the presence of ragged red fibers,[158] the presence of which suggests that an impairment of mitochondiral function is responsible for this myopathy.

Nemaline rod myopathy as a cause of muscle weakness and wasting has been described in association with HIV-1 infection,[159] as has muscle weakness without CK elevation.[152] Muscle biopsy in such patients generally reveals type II muscle-fiber atrophy.[152] Potential etiologies of this weakness include impaired nutrition and excessive weight loss, immobility, and the remote effects of the malignancy that often attends HIV infection. As with peripheral nerves, a high incidence of subclinical muscle disease is suggested by autopsy studies. Among other forms of muscle disease observed with HIV-1 infection are toxoplasmosis myositis, pyomyositis,[160] paralysis of an isolated muscle,[161] and heterotopic calcification of muscle (myositis ossificans) in association with CNS disease.[162]

Opportunistic Infections of the Nervous System in AIDS

A discussion of the various opportunistic infections of the nervous system that accompany HIV-1 infection is beyond the scope of this chapter. Only the most common of these infections will be described. The majority of these illnesses result from the recrudescence of a latent infection in the immunosuppressed individual.

Viruses

Cytomegalovirus

Human CMV is a ubiquitous, enveloped, DNA-containing herpesvirus that infects peripheral blood leukocytes during primary infection of healthy young adults. Nearly 50% of adults in the United

States have antibody to CMV by the age of 50.[163] Active virus infection may be cleared by humoral and cell-mediated immune responses, but the virus becomes latent in leukocytes and can be reactivated during immune suppression induced by either chemotherapy or HIV-1 infection. Hundreds of different strains of CMV have been identified by restriction analysis of DNA purified from clinical isolates;[164,165] a single patient may harbor multiple strains of the virus.[166]

Although considered a lymphotropic herpesvirus, CMV has been associated with several neurologic disorders in newborns and adults without HIV infection.[167] Congenital CMV infection of the CNS may result in motor deficits, seizures, chorioretinitis, deafness, and mental retardation. Similarly, acquired CMV infection has been linked with chorioretinitis, inflammatory polyradiculoneuropathy, and an adult encephalitis that may be slowly progressive. Prior to 1978, at least nine reports described a total of 31 patients with encephalitis of suspected or culture-proved CMV origin.[168–174] Of these, 26 patients had immune suppression related to organ transplantation. Thus, the neurotropic potential of this virus in immunodeficient patients had been previously documented.

That CMV is one of the major opportunistic infections associated with AIDS was recognized early.[177] Indeed, high antibody titers to CMV may be an independent predictor for the development of AIDS in HIV-1-infected individuals.[178] Virus can be isolated from peripheral blood leukocytes and urine during progressive HIV-1-induced immune suppression. Ultimately, the virus will disseminate to produce retinitis, pneumonitis, gastroenteritis, or hepatitis.[163] Initial evidence that CMV was involved in the etiology of subacute encephalitis was provided by Snider and co-workers,[8] who examined 50 AIDS patients with the neurologic disorder. Based on neuropathologic findings (i.e., microglial nodules, cytomegaly, and inclusions), disseminated CMV infection, or serologic evidence of prior CMV infection, these workers suggested that 18 of the 50 patients suffered from a subacute encephalopathy due to CMV. However, attempts to detect CMV-specific antigens in neural tissues by immunoperoxidase staining yielded inconclusive results and CMV was never recovered from the brain or CSF of these patients. Additional reports continued to implicate CMV as a cause of AIDS-associated subacute encephalopathy,[15,16,70,179–183] but again relied on indirect neuropathologic or serologic findings to support this claim.

In 1983, Hawley and colleagues[184] examined the brain of a homosexual man with culture-proved CMV pancolitis and pneumonitis who died suddenly of a subarachnoid hemorrhage. Numerous giant cells containing characteristic CMV inclusions were found in and around the lateral ventricles. More important, CMV-specific antigens were detected within neural cells of this patient by immunoperoxidase staining, a finding that provided direct evidence for CMV encephalitis. Subsequent reports have demonstrated CMV infection of the CNS or AIDS patients by immunoperoxidase staining[123,185–188] or in situ hybridization[184] analysis.

Direct recovery of infectious CMV from neurologic tissues[123,189] and CSF[123,191] of AIDS patients has also been reported. Tucker and colleagues[123] described a homosexual man with AIDS who had progressive ascending myelitis of six weeks' duration that was associated with concomitant CMV and HSV type 2 infection. At the time of autopsy, infectious CMV was recovered from cultures of pons, medulla, hypothalamus, third cranial nerve, spinal cord, and CSF. Cytomegalic inclusions were found throughout the brain and spinal cord, and these stained positive for CMV-specific antigens.[123]

While histopathologic and virologic evidence has clearly implicated CMV in the etiology of sole encephalitides that arise during AIDS, the clinical features of CMV encephalitis in this patient population remains poorly characterized, making definitive clinical diagnosis of this neurologic disorder difficult. The overall spectrum of CMV-related microscopic lesions has been summarized by Morgello and co-workers,[192] who reported microglial nodules and inclusions in the brain tissues of 30 AIDS patients with CMV encephalitis. Microglial nodules predominated in the subcortical gray matter while virus inclusions were present in capillary endothelia, astrocytes, and neurons. Dissemination of virus infection through the CSF was suggested by the detection of diffuse ependymal and subpial distribution of pathology of some patients. Ventriculofugal spread of CMV has been suggested by others.[187] More recently, Vinters and his associates[193] examined the histopathologic features of the brains of 31 AIDS patients at the time of autopsy. The neuropathology was extremely variable, ranging from rare isolated CMV inclusions without inflammation or necrosis to severe necrotizing ependymitis and meningoencephalitis. These authors concluded that CMV may localize to CNS tissues without significant clinical sequelae, a finding shared by others.[194] While imaging studies and analysis of CSF may reveal abnormalities in many patients, none have been specific enough to allow a definitive diagnosis of CMV encephalitis.

Furthermore, frequent coinfection with HIV[185,189,193] makes identification of the precise contribution of each virus to neurologic disease impossible at the present time. Moreover, at least in culture, CMV and HIV may synergistically infect the same cell.[195]

Attempts to manage dissemination of CMV during AIDS have met with mixed results. Ganciclovir (DHPG), a selective guanosine analog, has shown extreme potency against CMV replication in vitro.[196] This antiviral appears to function by limiting virus-specific DNA synthesis. Clinical trials have shown ganciclovir to be effective in the management of CMV retinitis[197,198] and CMV gastroenteritis[199] in AIDS patients. Ganciclovir may be associated with significant neutropenia.[199] Clinical trials are currently under way to assess the therapeutic efficacy of foscarnet in the treatment of AIDS-related retinitis.[200,201] Whether these drugs or others will modify the clinical course of CMV-associated subacute encephalopathy or encephalitis remains to be determined, but depends in part on their ability to cross an intact blood–brain barrier and clear infectious virus with minimal toxicity to neural tissue.

Varicella-Zoster Virus

VZV is an enveloped DNA-containing virus belonging to the family Herpesviridae. The DNA of individual VZV clinical isolates may yield unique restriction enzyme profiles, a finding that was proved useful in molecular epidemiologic studies[202,203] However, because of its extreme lability, in vitro infection is inefficient, making recovery of infectious virus from clinical specimens difficult.

VZV is the etiologic agent of two distinct clinical syndromes: varicella (chicken pox) and herpes zoster (shingles).[204] Varicella usually occurs in children as a consequence of primary VZV infection. Following viremia and the appearance of focal cutaneous and mucosal lesions characteristic of the disease, the virus spreads centripetally by neural route to corresponding sensory ganglia, where it becomes latent within neuronal cells.[209] Upon reactivation later in life, the virus may travel centrifugally down the sensory nerves to the skin and produce the clusters of vesicles along the dermatome that are the hallmark of herpes zoster. Common to most patients with herpes zoster is an underlying decline in immune competence; it and more severe disseminated infections are most notable in organ-transplant patients who have received immunosuppressive therapy and in patients with lymphoma or AIDS. Indeed, herpes zoster may be a predictor of HIV-1-induced immune suppression during the evolution of AIDS.[205]

Being a neurotropic herpesvirus, it is not surprising that VZV infection has been associated with a wide spectrum of neurologic disease,[206] including transverse myelitis, ascending myelitis, encephalitis, leukoencephalopathy, and a contralateral hemiplegia attributable to cerebral vasculitis that may accompany herpes-zoster ophthalmicus. Of these, herpes-zoster encephalitis has received the most attention. Jensek and colleagues[207] reviewed the clinical, pathologic, and virologic features of 39 patients without HIV-1 infection who developed herpes-zoster encephalitis. Most exhibited underlying immune deficiencies resulting from Hodgkin's disease, non-Hodgkin's lymphoma, chronic lymphocytic leukemia, or corticosteroid therapy. While clinical features of herpes-zoster encephalitis include headache, fever, hallucinations, delerium, mild confusion, and signs of meningeal irritation, rarely are focal neurologic signs, deep alterations in consciousness, or seizures associated with the disease. Moreover, the disease is usually not life threatening in this patient population. Of the 39 patients reviewed by Jemsek and associates,[207] only seven died; with few exceptions, survivors experienced no neurologic deficits following recovery.

Surprisingly, few neurologic complications associated with VZV infection have been reported in patients with AIDS, although most are temporally associated with episodes of herpes zoster. Levy and associates[9] reported several neurologic syndromes temporally related to outbreaks of cutaneous herpes zoster during AIDS. These included three cases of encephalitis, two cases of cerebral angiitis, four cases of radiculomyelitis, and two cases of multiple neuropathies. However, diagnosis of these cases was based on indirect evidence.

Ryder and colleagues[208] were the first to provide direct evidence for VZV-associated neurologic disease during AIDS. These workers described the progression of a fatal neurologic illness in a patient 12 weeks after the resolution of cutaneous herpes zoster. At the time of autopsy, numerous areas of necrosis and demyelination associated with prominent Cowdry A type intranuclear inclusions were observed throughout the brain. While infectious virus could not be recovered from cultured brain (or CSF prior to death), VZV-specific antigens were detected in brain tissue by immunoperoxidase staining. In addition, DNA extracted from frozen brain hybridized with VZV-specific DNA fragments by Southern blot analysis.

Similarly, Gilden and colleagues[209] reported the slow progression of mental impairment and neurologic deterioration in an AIDS patient who had a history of recurrent genital herpes and herpes zoster. Histopathology of brain tisues taken at the time of atuopsy revealed a diffuse ventriculitis and encephalitis containing numerous Cowdry A type intranuclear inclusions. More important, however, were the results of hybridization studies using DNA extracted from brain tissues. When reacted with RNA probes of VZV, HSV, CMV, and HIV-1 origin, VZV was identified as the cause of this patient's neurologic illness.

Additional evidence for direct VZV involvement in the progression of neurologic disease during AIDS has been provided by direct recovery of infectious virus from CSF.[189,190]

Progressive Multifocal Leukoencephalopathy

Progressive multifocal leukoencephalopathy (PML) is the result of a papovavirus infection, typically the JC virus. The virus exerts a cytopathic effect on oligodendrocytes and results in demyelination. PML is characterized pathologically by demyelination; giant astrocytes with pleomorphic, hyperchromatic nuclei; and altered oligodendrocytes containing enlarged nuclei that stain abnormally densely with hematoxylin. These nuclei may contain ill-defined inclusion bodies. PML is almost always associated with impaired immunity, specifically, an altered cell-mediated immunity. Previously, it had been most often associated with lymphoproliferative disorders, but also with antineoplastic therapy, organ transplantation, autoimmune diseases, sarcoidosis, tuberculosis, Whipple disease, and nontropical sprue. In 1982, AIDS was added to the list of diseases that can lead to PML.[210] PML is seen in as many as 3.8% of all cases of AIDS.[211] In some institutions, PML occurring in the setting of the immunodeficiency of HIV infection far outnumbers that with other disorders.

In 29% of cases in which PML complicated HIV infection, the neurologic illness was the presenting manifestation of AIDS.[211] The clinical picture of PML with AIDS varies little from that observed with other disorders. Limb weakness is the most common initial manifestation, followed (in descending order of frequency) by cognitive dysfunction, visual loss, gait disturbance, limb incoordination, speech or language disturbance, and headache. All patients exhibit some evidence of immunologic impairment. A CT scan of the brain typically, although not invariably, reveals nonenhancing, hypodense white-matter lesions without mass effect located in the centrum semiovale, predominantly in the parieto-occipital region, and the cerebellum. MRI on T2-weighted spin-echo images is highly sensitive in detecting these lesions. The CSF is usually normal, though an elevated opening pressure, increased protein (range 57–72 mg/dl), the presence of basic myelin protein, an increase in IgG, and pleocytosis (9–25 mononuclear cells/mm^3) have all been reported.[211] Brain biopsy is diagnostic. Additionally, by in situ hybridization, JC-virus infection of bone-marrow lymphocytes can be demonstrated.[212]

In a large series of PML and AIDS, the mean survival was 4 months, ranging from 0.3 to 18 months.[211] However, two patients have been personally followed in excess of 30 months from the time of diagnosis and have exhibited some degree of neurologic improvement.[213] Both had a significant inflammatory component in their biopsies, but their courses appear to be unrelated to immune function. To date, no therapy appears to be beneficial.

Bacteria

Mycobacterial Infections

Mycobacterium tuberculosis, Mycobacterium avium-intracellulare, (MAI) and, rarely, other atypical mycobacteria occur frequently in AIDS, and are often extrapulmonary in nature.[85] In one study, MAI was the most common bacteremia observed in patients with AIDS.[214] Despite the frequency of mycobacterial infection, involvement of the CNS is not as common as may be expected, and it is almost always due to *M tuberculosis,* though atypical mycobacterial infection of the CNS in AIDS has been reported.[8–10,215–217] The frequency with which mycobacterial infection of the CNS is observed in AIDS patients depends on the nature of the population studied. For instance, in an early review of AIDS patients with neurologic disease in San Francisco,[8] none had mycobacterial CNS infection. However, in Miami, which has the highest case rate of tuberculosis and where 31% of all patients with tuberculosis are HIV-1 positive,[218] 2.4% of HIV-1-infected patients with CNS disease had CNS tuberculosis.[10] Haitians, American blacks, and intravenous-drug abusers[219] appear to be the risk groups with the highest incidences of mycobacteria infection.

The clinical spectrum of CNS tuberculosis with HIV infection includes meningitis, cerebral abscesses, and tuberculomas.[220] Amoung the most common clinical manifestations are seizures, altered mental status, and fever with meningismus.[220] In patients with MAI, single or multiple mass lesions were more than twice as common as meningitis. CT characteristics are diverse and include ring-enhancing lesions and hypodense areas. The CSF may, on occasion, be normal,[220] further emphasizing the value of brain biopsy in establishing the diagnosis in some patients. Mycobacterial spinal-cord abscess has also been reported in AIDS.[221]

All HIV-seropositive patients should be skin tested for tuberculosis, and, if positive, should be treated. In those with active tuberculosis, a regimen of three or more drugs is required for a minimum of 9 months. The response of *M tuberculosis* in patients with AIDS is generally favorable.[219] Atypical mycobacterial infection requires a four-drug regimen and may include experimental antimicrobials such as rifabutyn and clofazimine.[222]

Other Bacterial Infections

In a study of 49 episodes of bacteremia and fungemia occurring in 38 of 336 patients with AIDS, Whimbey and colleagues[214] classified five types of infection. Those infections commonly associated with T-cell deficiency occurred in 16 cases and included *Salmonella, Listeria monocytogenes, Cryptococcus neoformans,* and *Histoplasma capsulatum*.[214] Infections commonly associated with B-cell immunodeficiency occurred in three and included *Streptococcus pneumonia* and *Hemophilus influenza*. Infections commonly associated with neutropenia (*Pseudomonas aeruginosa, Staphylococcus epidermis,* and *Streptococcus fecalis*) were observed in three. Other in-hospital infections and infections occurring outside the hospital setting made up the other two major groups.[214]

Listeria monocytogenes

The low incidence of *L monocytogenes* in AIDS patients is surprising in view of its extraordinarily high frequency in patients with other causes of impaired cell-mediated immunity. Pons and associates[223] report on three others, two with meningitis and one with a brain abscess. Ampicillin or high-dose penicillin is curative.

Nocardia Asteroides

Nocardia asteroides, a gram-positive, weakly acid-fast bacillus, may occasionally be seen in the setting of HIV infection. Isolated case descriptions can be found in the literature.[224,225] The incidence of nocardial infection in AIDS has been estimated to be approximately 0.3%.[226] In one series, three of 34 AIDS patients with primary nocardial lung involvement had lesions of the CNS [R. Umchatandrani, personal communication]. Fever, headache, and focal neurologic findings occur with active nocardial pulmonary disease. The brain abscesses are often multiple. Although successful treatment of nocardial brain abscesses with antibiotics alone has been reported,[227,228] it is unusual in patients with AIDS.

Treponema pallidum

Neurosyphilis always must be considered in the differential diagnosis of the HIV-1-seropositive individual presenting with neurologic disease. The frequency of positive syphilis serologies in AIDS patients approaches 50% in some institutions.[229] Some investigators believe that syphilis occurring in association with HIV-1 infection can present in a peculiar and florid fashion. An acute, symptomatic, syphilitic meningitis during the course of secondary syphilis appears to be more common than otherwise anticipated, with frequent eye involvement.[230]

Neurosyphilitic manifestations that generally arise years after the initial infection, such as meningovascular syphilis and general paresis, may occur after much shorter periods. Johns and colleagues[231] noted the development of meningovascular syphilis within 4 months of primary infection in a patient who had received "adequate" penicillin therapy prior to the development of the syphilitic neurologic manifestations. Neurologic relapse of syphilis in HIV-1-infected individuals after appropriate benzathine penicillin doses for secondary syphilis has also been noted by other investigators.[232] Other unusual manifestations of syphilis that have been reported in this regard include unexplained fever,[233] bilateral optic neuritis with blindness,[234] Bell's palsy, and severe bilateral sensorineural hearing loss.[235]

Though still controversial, concomitant HIV-1 infection appears to alter the natural course of syphilis. Furthermore, the serodiagnosis of syphilis may require repeated testing of the patient[236] or be artifactually negative.[237] Seronegative secondary syphilis developed in a HIV-1-infected patient with Kaposi sarcoma.[238] Both the serum VDRL and fluorescent treponamal antibody-absorption test were negative and the diagnosis was established by demonstrating the treponemes on skin biopsy.[238]

Fungi

Cryptococcal Meningitis

Cryptococcal infection is not uncommonly associated with AIDS, with the estimated incidence varying between 1.9%[239] and 11%.[8] In the United Kingdom, the reported frequency is 3.2%.[239] Of nearly 3,000 patients with AIDS registered by the New York City Department of Health, 6% had cryptococcosis,[240] and the CDC estimates that it is found in 7% of AIDS patients in the United States.[241] Geography and the varying susceptibility to acquiring cryptococcal infection may account, in part, for the difference in rates. Blacks and intravenous-drug abusers have higher rates of this illness than others. Like other opportunistic infections, cryptococcal meningitis is rare in children with AIDS.[241]

Cryptococcosis may be the initial manifestation of HIV infection or occur simultaneously with other opportunistic infections.[10,243,244] Indeed, 7 of 27 patients with cryptococcosis and AIDS in one series, cryptococcosis was the initial manifestation of the immunodeficiency.[243] In some communities, cryptococcal meningitis is more commonly the presenting neurologic illness associated with HIV infection than is toxoplasmosis.[223]

The chief clinical consequence of cryptococcal infection in AIDS patients is cryptococcal meningitis.[243] Extraneural sites of infection include the blood, bone marrow, lungs, pericardium, myocardium, skin, mucous membranes, peritoneum, stomach, intestines, adrenal gland, and urinary tract. These extraneural sites, particularly the blood and lungs,[245] may be concomitantly infected at the time of cryptococcal meningitis. With rare exceptions,[246,247] in patients with AIDS, cryptococcal meningitis, is the result of infection with *Cryptococcus neoformans,* an encapsulated yeast 4–6 μm in diameter that reproduces budding. In tissues, *C neoformans* develops a large capsule. This extracellular polysaccharide capsule exerts a significant influence on the pathogenicity of the organism. *C neoformans* is present throughout the world, and has a particularly high incidence in pigeon habitats. Infection takes place through the inhalation of organisms from environmental sources, resulting in a primary pulmonary focus of infection. In most individuals with intact immunity, the infection is contained. However, before the AIDS epidemic, 50% of those with cryptococcal meningitis in a general population had no known predisposing cause for the infection. Among the situations where immunologic impairment predisposed patients to cryptococcal meningitis were steroid treatment, lymphoproliferative disorders, sarcoidosis, and organ transplantation. Even in people with no known immunologic dysfunction, testing often revealed abnormalities of cell-mediated immunity, particularly decreased lymphocyte response to cryptococcal antigen.[248] In patients with AIDS, a predisposition to cryptococcal infection may not only be the result of impairment of cell-mediated immunity, but also a defect in the synthesis of anti–*C neoformans* capsular polysaccharide antibodies.[249] Generally, cryptococcal meningitis appears to result from reactivation of primary disease, in a fashion analogous to that at secondary, extrapulmonary tuberculosis.[250] *C neoformans* elaborates no toxins and usually evokes minimal inflammatory reaction.

Symptomatically, headache is almost universally noted in patients with cryptococcal meningitis. Other frequently observed clinical features include nausea and vomiting, photophobia, blurred vision, fever, mental-status changes, and meningismus. On rare occasions, psychiatric disturbances may be the initial manifestation.[251] Cranial-nerve palsies, hemiparesis, language disturbances, seizures, and cerebellar findings are less frequent. In a series of 25 patients with AIDS and cryptococcal meningitis studied by Chernoff and colleagues[223] at the University of California at San Francisco, headache was present in 88%, fever in 84%, meningeal signs in 36%, mental-status changes in 12%, and other neurologic findings (cranial-nerve palsies, papilledema, ataxia, and seizures) in 10%.[223] Focal findings are unusual with cryptococcus, but are observed, both with and without the presence of meningitis.[9,240,252] Pathologic examination reveals a basilar, chronic meningitis. Typically, the meningitis is not particularly thick or exudative. Diffuse or focal opacifications of the leptomeninges and brain edema may be noted on gross examination. Small nodules (2–3 mm) studding the leptomeninges may be observed, particularly in the interpeduncular fossa and in the sulci. Cystic lesions consisting of clusters of budding yeast are seen throughout the brain but cheifly affect the superficial layers of the cerebral cortex. Typically, they exhibit little surrounding inflammation or reactive gliosis and can sometimes reach a size that can be detected macroscopically (cryptococcomas).

CSF examination often reveals an elevated opening pressure, increased protein, and depressed glucose. A CSF pleocytosis is not invariable. In approximately 70% of patients, the CSF white blood cells (WBC) number less than 20 cells/mm.[3] In one study, 11 of 17 patients with cryptococcal meningitis and AIDS had CSF white blood cells below five cells per cubic millimeter.[223] The pleocytosis is always mononuclear. In the setting of AIDS, routine studies may be completely unremarkable. Two or three standard CSF parameters (glucose, protein, white-cell count) may be normal in up to 50% of these individuals.[223] The India-ink test was positive in 72% in one study[240] and 79% in another,[245] somewhat higher than the 50% incidence reported with large general series of cryptococcal meningitis. The frequency with which CSF cryptococcal antigen, CSF culture, and serum cryptococcal antigen were positive all exceeded 90% in one study.[240] In 24 AIDS patients with cryptococcal meningitis studied by Gal and colleagues,[245] all initial CSF cultures were positive. Cryptococcal-antigen studies have a high degree of sensitivity. The average CSF cryptococcal antigen titer in the spinal fluid in Chernoff's study was 1:4,096.[223] However, two patients have been reported by Pons and associates[223] and two by Zuger and associates[240] who had negative CSF cryptococcal-antigen studies, but positive cultures. The former investigators suggest that this phenomenon may be the result of an early infection with too little production of cryptococcal antigen, a difference in the serotypes between the infecting and test strains of cryptococcus, or a cryptococcal infection with strains deficient in their capsular polysaccharides.[223] When cryptococcal meningitis is suspected, blood should be cultured and serum assayed for the presence of cryptococcal antigen. The serum frequently exhibits a positive cryptococcal antigen and the blood cultures are often positive.[243,245] In one study,[245] 100% of the blood cultures were positive in the face of cryptococcal meningitis. Cultures of other extraneural sites, such as bronchoalveolar lavage fluid, may also be particularly rewarding.[245]

As had been noted, prior to the appearance of AIDS, CT scans of the brain were generally normal.[253] They were negative in 8 of 10 patients in one series,[51] and in the other, two patients were positive as the result of a superimposed disease process. These findings mirror those of radiologic investigators.[254-256]

In a review of cryptococcal infection and AIDS, 7 of 22 patients with cryptococcal meningitis and AIDS died during treatment.[240] In one study, a high titer of cryptococcal antigen (>1 : 10,000) and a positive India-ink test correlated with increased mortality.[240] However, other investigators have found extremely variable levels of initial CSF and serum-cryptococcal-antigen titers and no apparent correlation between these levels and prognosis.[245] A positive serum-cryptococcal-antigen titer greater than 1 : 8 suggests disseminated infection.[245] Half of the patients who were not treated with maintenance amphotericin following the completion of their initial therapy relapsed,[240] indicating the need for secondary prophylaxis (maintenance therapy). Persistence of *C neoformans* in the prostate following treatment of cryptococcal meningitis may explain the high frequency of relapse. Twenty percent of AIDS patients who had completed treatment for cryptococcal meningitis had positive urine cultures for *C neoformans,* and the percentage increased to 29% with prostatic massage.[257] Routinely, the treatment of cryptococcal meningitis consists of intravenous amphotericin B (0.6–1 mg/kg/day) for a minimum of six weeks. Controversy surrounds the routine use of additional antifungal agents such as ketoconazole. The combination of amphotericin and 5-flucytosine has been demonstrated to be superior to the use of amphotericin alone[258] and has been recommended in the patient with AIDS-associated cryptococcal meningitis. Pons and collaborators[223] suggest the use of amphotericin B (0.6 mg/kg/day) and 5-fluocytosine (75–100 mg/day in four divided doses). Toxicity with amphotericin includes hypokalemia and hypomagnesemia, as well as renal failure, though it is generally well tolerated. Toxicity with 5-flucytosine includes leukopenia, thrombocytopenia, and abnormal liver-function studies and is seen in as many as 35% of patients.[240,243] Therapy should be continued for a minimum of 6 weeks. The use of shorter durations of therapy in some patients as recently reported by Dismukes and colleagues[259] has not been studied in this disorder.

Intraventricular administration of amphotericin B is necessary for those patients for whom parenteral administration fails to clear the meningitis. In vitro susceptibility testing of *C neoformans* isolates from patients with AIDS suggests that the minimum fungicidal concentrations of amphotericin B, flucytosine, ketoconazole, and miconazole nitrate exceeded obtainable CSF concentrations, despite inhibition of 90% of the isolates at drug concentrations within achievable serum levels.[260] Once therapy is completed, the India-ink mounts demonstrate 84% sensitivity and 53% specificity with respect to culture outcome.[245] A negative CSF culture during therapy does not necessarily indicate the eradication of the infection.[245] Furthermore, a decline in the serum or CSF cryptococcal-antigen titer during treatment does not appear to be useful in predicting outcome.[243] Relapse is observed in over half the patients,[223] therefore, weekly prophylactic anticryptococcal therapy is warranted. A suggested regimen consists of the parenteral administration of 100 mg of amphotericin B weekly after therapy is completed.[223]

Despite maintenance therapy, patients may relapse, as demonstrated in 2 of 14 patients in Zuger and colleagues' study.[240] Ketoconazole may not be sufficiently protective as a prophylactic agent.[223] However, preliminary studies suggest that oral fluconazole is an effective prophylactic antifungal.[261] Twenty patients treated with amphotericin B with or without flucytosine were given fluconazole, 50–200 mg/day, as maintenance therapy; only one relapsed and only 2 of 7 had demonstrable *C neoformans* infection at autopsy.[261] Fluconazole has also proved to be an effective primary therapy in a patient with AIDS who failed amphotericin B treatment.[262]

Predicting the prognosis of cryptococcal meningitis in AIDS is difficult. Recurrent cryptococcal meningitis over 7 years in one Haitian patient with AIDS was observed by one of us (J.R.B.). Many of the factors that predict a poor prognosis of cryptococcal meningitis are present in AIDS. As enumerated by Diamond and Bennett,[263] these factors are a positive India-ink test, a low CSF leukocyte count, a positive blood culture, the presence of *C neoformans* at extraneural sites, a high CSF cryptococcal-antigen titer, CSF hypoglycorrhachia, and an increased CSF opening pressure.

Other Fungal Infections

Candida

Although 40–60% of patients with AIDS develop oropharyngeal or esophageal candidiasis, it is infrequently found in the brains of patients with AIDS. Six cases with *Candida* encephalopathy and AIDS have been reported.[223] The pathology is classically that of microabscesses and few patients exhibit focal features or meningitis.

Mucormycosis

Cuadrado and colleagues[264] have reported two intravenous-drug abusers with AIDS who developed mucormycosis of the brain. Neither had the classical triad of ophthalmoplegia, necrotic nares, and diabetes insipidus. Extensive intracerebral lesions with vascular involvement were noted pathologically and the course was fatal in both.[264] Another case was described by Micozzi and Wetli[265] in an individual who used intravenous amphetamines.

Aspergillus

Several cases of *Aspergillus fumigatus* affecting the CNS in patients with AIDS have been reported.[179,243,254] Typically, the patients had brain abscesses requiring surgical excision, but occasionally fungal meningitis ensued.

Miscellaneous

Among other fungal illnesses that have also been reported infrequently with HIV infection are histoplasmosis and coccidiomycosis. As noted by Pons and colleagues,[223] their relationship to AIDS is uncertain.

Parasites

Toxoplasma gondii

Toxoplasma gondii is among the most common of the neurologic complications occurring in patients with HIV infection. In a study from San Francisco, cerebral toxoplasmosis was seen in 28% of patients with AIDS,[9] and in another combined clinicopathologic series from Miami,[10] it accounted for 40% of all identified neurologic illnesses. In one autopsy review from New York of AIDS patients, 10% were found to have CNS toxoplasmosis.[266] Another autopsy series from Miami[16] found a rate of 30%. The risk of developing toxoplasmosis is 6–12% in HIV-1-infected individuals who have IgG toxoplasma antibody.[267] Clearly, toxoplasmosis is the most common cause of intracerebral mass lesion occurring in association with HIV infection.[125,268]

T gondii is an obligate intracellular parasite that is found worldwide in mammals. Humans typically become infected after the ingestion of raw or undercooked meat that contains tissue cysts of the organisms. Alternatively, cats, the normal host for this parasite, may infect humans by passing oocysts that, if ingested, release infective organisms into the gastrointestinal tract.[269] Adult-acquired toxoplasma infection is asymptomatic in all but approximately 5% of cases in which a "mononucleosis" syndrome characterized by fever, lymphadenopathy, splenomegaly, and hepatitis may arise.[269] After acute infection, whether symptomatic or asymptomatic, the parasite assumes a latent form (tissue cysts containing bradyzoites). Any tissue previously infected may harbor these cysts. A decline in cell-mediated immunity, as occurs with HIV infection, can result in rupture of these cysts and release of invasive trophozoites (tachyzoites). The tachyzoites result in the release of adjacent host cells. The fact that toxoplasma encephalitis in the AIDS patient represents a recrudescence of infection rather than a newly acquired infection probably accounts for its increased incidence in certain populations, such as Haitians. These populations demonstrate serologic evidence of high rates of latent infection.

Generally, the presenting neurologic symptoms and signs in HIV-infected individuals with toxoplasma encephalitis are focal in nature, often superimposed on a global encephalopathy. A prodrome of fever and malaise for several days to weeks before the onset of the neurologic illness was observed in 15 of 27 patients in one series,[270] but in only 1 of 15 in another.[125] In 27 patients studied by Navia and colleagues,[270] 24 had focal findings, of which mild hemiparesis, noted in 14 patients, was the most common. Brain stem and cerebellar involvement was noted in eight patients and seizures developed in four. Confusion and lethargy were observed in 63% of these patients and headache in 55%. However, in McArthur's[125] series, confusion and headache were present in only a minority of patients. The appearance of chorea in AIDS patients is believed to be virtually pathognomonic of toxoplasmosis.[271] The course of the illness is typically subacute, with symptoms arising over the course of 1–2 weeks. Similar features have been noted by other investigators,[272] as well as ourselves. Fever is not invariably present, occurring in approximately 50% of AIDS-associated toxoplasma encephalitis. Occasionally, toxoplasma chorioretinitis may coexist. Ocular toxoplasmosis in patients with AIDS differs both clinically and histopathologically from that in the immunocompetent individual.[273] The disease does not originate in preexisting retinochoriodal scars and probably results from dissemination of organisms from nonocular sites of disease or newly acquired infection.[273] Toxoplasma has been known to involve other organ sites,[274] such as the heart,[274] lung,[275] peritoneum,[276] testes,[277] and skin.[278] Death may result from toxoplasmic myocarditis.[274]

CT scan of the brain usually reveals multiple nodular or ring-enhancing lesions with edema and mass effect.[270,272,279] In some instances, the CT scan may simply show a hypodense lesion that fails to contrast enhance or may fail to demonstrate any lesions. Most lesions occur in the basal ganglia[125,279] and the crebral hemispheres, particularly the frontoparietal lobes.[270] Rarely, the CT scan may reveal hydrocephalus resulting from aqueductal occlusion.[280] Axial and coronal thin-section, double-dose, contrast CT is the most useful neurodiagnostic study, but it is not diagnostically pathognomonic. CT scans are most helpful in identifying lesions for biopsy or following the progression of the disease or response to therapy. MRI of the brain appears to be more sensitive than CT scans in this setting, but is less specific.[281,282] MRI reveals discrete areas of increased signal intensity on T2-weighted images.[283] The MRI is inadequate in gauging the activity of a lesion and in distinguishing those lesions in close proximity to one another.[112]

CSF findings in these patients are nonspecific, but are generally abnormal. Most show an elevation of CSF protein (50–200) and one third show a mononuclear pleocytosis (less than 100 cells/mm^3). Cell counts in excess of 100 cells/mm^3 suggest the presence of another disease. Rarely, mild hypoglychorrhachia is noted. Serologic studies (immunofluorescent antibody, Sabin-Feldman dye test, ELISA titer) for toxoplasmosis are typically elevated,[284] but not invariably.[285] Navia and colleagues[270] found that all patients were positive for IgG antibody against *T gondii* in blood, both before the onset of the illness and at the time of presentation. Western-blot analysis of the antibody response to *Toxoplasma* of patients with AIDS failed to distinguish between acute and chronic *Toxoplasma* infection.[286] However, the CSF antibody studies may be negative in the presence of toxoplasmic encephalitis.[284] Wong and associates[267] have suggested measuring local CSF *Toxoplasma* IgG antibody production to support the diagnosis.

In another study, 37 patients with AIDS and toxoplasmic encephalitis were compared with 11 patients with AIDS alone.[287] Twenty-three of the former group and none of the latter had CSF *Toxoplasma* antibody.[287] Eleven of 16 patients with toxoplasmic encephalitis had intrathecal production of *Toxoplasma* antibody.[287] In one instance, *Toxoplasma* was isolated in tissue culture from the blood.[288] Other investigators have been able to identify free tachyzoites in the CSF.[289,290] Routine CSF staining for tachyzoites has been advocated,[290] but they also may be seen in individuals with inactive disease. Brain biopsy is the only unequivocal means to establish the diagnosis. Excisional biopsies usually show tachyzoites on routine histology, particularly in the periphery of the necrotic lesion.[268] Needle biopsies are often negative unless mouse inoculation or immunoperoxidase staining is employed.[268] Pathologic study in toxoplasmic encephalitis reveals multifocal necrotic and inflammatory abscesses. The organism may exist in several forms and be present both intracellularly and extracellularly.[291] It may have a predeliction for cerebral arterial walls and adjacent brain tissue at hyperemic rims of centrally necrotic lesions.[292] Before resorting to brain biopsy, we recommend a trial of antitoxoplasmosis therapy of 2 weeks' duration in those patients with suspected toxoplasmic encephalitis, during which they are monitored clinically and by radiographic criteria for resolution of their lesions. When the antitoxoplasmosis regimen fails to effect clinical and radiographic improvement, brain biopsy should then be performed. The use of corticosteroids may confuse the interpretation of this therapeutic trial and their use should be avoided in this context.

The therapy of toxoplasmic encephalitis is oral pyrimethamine (an initial loading dose of 50–100 mg followed by 25 mg/day) and 6–8 g of sulfadiazine per day divided into four equal doses. Both drugs cross the blood–brain barrier.[293] Folinic acid, 5–10 mg/day, is generally used to diminish bone-marrow suppression. Side effects of these medications are common, being found in as many as 60% of patients.[294] Pyrimethamine can cause leukopenia and thrombocytopenia and the chief side effect of sulfadiazine is rash; however, it may result in crystalluria,[295] particularly in the presence of dehydration or preexisting renal disease. In published series, the use of corticosteroids has shown no demonstrable effect, either beneficial or harmful.[294] Therapy needs to be continued weeks after the resolution of the lesions by CT scan. As the frequency of relapse following successful treatment is more than 30%, a suppressive dose of medication must be administered lifelong.[296] Patients who cannot tolerate sulfadiazine may be treated with pyrimethamine alone.

Clinical trials with clindamycin and spiramycin[272] have generally proved disappointing. However, in one study of three patients with CNS toxoplasmosis who developed a hypersensitivity to sulfadiazine, clindamycin plus pyrimethamine demonstrated efficacy by both clinical and radiographic criteria.[297] A similar study using intravenous clindamycin either along or in combination with pyrimethamine in 11 patients who experienced adverse reactions to sulfonamides suggested that it was an effective alternative therapy.[298] An additional patient who had failed to respond to the standard regimen of sulfadiazine plus pyrimethamine improved after clindamycin was added.[297] Trimetrexate and other experimental folate antagonists may be useful in the treatment of toxoplasmic encephalitis.[285] The prognosis for AIDS-associated toxoplasmic encephalitis is poor; the average survival is 4 months and appears to correlate directly with mental function at the time treatment is instituted.[294]

Other Parasitic Infections

Acanthamoeba

An isolated case of fatal *Acanthamoeba* meningoencephalitis in a 34-year-old homosexual Mexican man has been reported.[299] The organism was identified postmortem as *Acanthamoeba culbertsoni*. An acute necrotizing meningoencephalitis was found at autopsy.

Other Neurologic Conditions

Other neurologic conditions associated with HIV-1 infection (brain tumors, cerebrovascular disease, metabolic and nutritional disturbances, and drug side effects) are beyond the scope of this chapter.

HIV-2

In 1985, a virus that was related to but distinct from the well-characterized AIDS virus was isolated from asymptomatic West African prostitutes,[300] and the following year, it was reported in two West Africans with AIDS.[301,302] This virus has been designated as human immunodeficiency virus type 2 (HIV-2) and differs antigenically from standard HIV isolates, particularly in the envelope glycoprotein, which more closely resembles that of the simian immunodeficiency virus.[302] This virus is chiefly confined to West Africa, though it has been occasionally detected in Europe and North America.[303] In late 1987, it was first reported in a West African woman living in the United States,[304] and as of September 1989, there have been eight confirmed and five suspected cases of HIV-2 in the United States.[305] In all documented instances, the infected individuals were of West African origin.[305]

Because HIV-1 and HIV-2 are closely related, cross-reactivity with antibody directed to the other virus may be observed.[306] As ELISA tests for HIV-1 may detect anitbody to HIV-2 in 60% to more than 90%,[307] confirmation of HIV-2 infection requires HIV-1 and HIV-2 Western-blot testing,[303] viral cultures,[308] or PCR procedures.[309]

People infected with HIV-2 may be asymptomatic or exhibit laboratory and clinical features of immunodeficiency identical to those caused by HIV-1.[302] The incubation period is estimated to be 11–19 years, substantially longer than that of HIV-1 infection.[310] Not unexpectedly, encephalopathy,[302,311,312] spastic paraplegia,[311] and peripheral neuropathy[311] may occur as a consequence of HIV-2 infection. Furthermore, the neurologic illness may be the presenting manifestation of the infection.[311,312]

Neurologic illnesses resulting from the immunodeficiency that attends HIV-2 infection have been observed, in addition to those that are a direct consequence of the viral infection. Two HIV-2–infected patients with toxoplasmic encephalitis[305,313] and another with brain lymphoma[302] have been described.

Other Defects in Cell-Mediated Immunity

Bacterial

Listeria monocytogenes

L monocytogenes is the most common cause of bacterial meningitis in patients with altered cellular immunity, despite its relative rarity in patients with AIDS. This infection appears to be particularly common with renal transplantation and lymphoreticular malignancy,[314-317] and is the leading cause of bacterial meningitis in patients with cancer. *L monocytogenes* is a Gram-positive motile aerobic bacillus that is widely disseminated in nature. The most likely portal of entry in humans is believed to be the gastrointestinal tract.[318] Meningitis follows a septicemic phase.

In renal-transplant patients, CNS invasion appears in 75% of infected patients.[317] The clinical picture is typically one of meningitis, though focal CNS disturbances, resulting cerebritis, brain abscesses, or brain-stem infection (rhomboencephalitis) may also occur.[319,320] The lumbar puncture reveals an increased opening pressure, a mononuclear or polymorphonuclear pleocytosis, increased protein, and hypoglychorrhachia.[319,321] Occasionally, the CSF cell count is normal. The organism can be cultured from blood and CSF; however, recovery from the CSF is improved by the prompt delivery to the laboratory of at least 10 ml as the organism may be present in only small numbers.[322] Although treatment failures with both penicillin and ampicillin have been reported,[322] these antibiotics remain the mainstay of therapy for listeriosis. Because of relapse of infection following two weeks of therapy in immunosuppressed patients,[323] 3–6 weeks of therapy is currently recommended.

Nocardia asteroides

CNS infection with *N asteroides,* a soil-borne, aerobic actinomycete, is not infrequently observed in immunosuppressed patients, particularly those receiving corticosteroids or cytotoxic therapy.[324,325] Generally, the primary infection is pulmonary, though on occasion the origin may be the skin. The CNS is involved in approximately one third of all nocardial infections, being more common in patients with immunosuppression. Dissemination to the CNS is hematogenous, with the exception of the rare instances in which extradural abscesses arise from osteomyelitis of the skull or vertebral bodies. Brain abscess, usually multiloculated, resulting in an expanding mass lesion with focal neurologic findings, is the most common CNS presentation, but meningitis and venticulitis associated with a ventriculoperitoneal shunt have been reported.[326,327] Treatment with sulfa preparations (sulfadiazine, sulfisoxasole, or triple sulfaonamide combinations) for 6 weeks is recommended in conjunction with surgical drainage of large (greater than 3 cm in diameter) or nonresponding abscesses. The latter can be adquately gauged by CT scan or MRI.

Mycobacterium tuberculosis

See the discussion above.

Fungi

C neoformans, Coccidiodes immitis, and *H capsulatum* all occur with increased frequency in patients with impaired cellular immunity.

Parasites

Toxoplasma gondi

See the discussion above.

Strongyloides stercoralis

The nematode *Strongyloides stercoralis* may cause an overwhelming autoinfection in the immunosuppressed host, particularly in the patient being treated with high doses of corticosteroids.[328,329] Massive invasion of the lungs and other tissues follows larval disruption of the bowel wall. CNS complications are rare and include meningitis, diffuse microinfarcts, and brain abscesses.[330]

Defects of Humoral Immunity

CNS infections in patients with immunoglobulin deficiency or splenectomy is chiefly bacterial meningitis resulting from encapsulated bacteria, *S pneumoniae, H influenza,* or *Neisseria meningitidis*. Discussions of these infections can be found elsewhere in this book.

Defects in Neutrophils

Bacteria

The infectious neurologic consequences of neutropenia or abnormalities in neutrophil function include bacterial meningitis with *P aeruginosa,* other Gram-negative bacilli, or *Staphylococcus aureus*.[331] Blood cultures are typically positive, indicating the dissemination of the infection to the CNS from other sites. The absence of fever and headache and the often bland nature of the CSF may be diagnostically confusing. However, CSF cultures and Gram stains are positive in over 90% of patients.

Fungi

Fungal CNS infections in these patients include candidiasis, aspergillosis, and mucormycosis. Descriptions of these infections can be found elsewhere in this text.

Acknowledgment. This work was supported in part by grant PO1 NS 25569-01 from the National Institute of Neurological Disease and Stroke.

References

1. Gallo RC, Salahuddin SZ, Popovic M, et al: Frequent detection and isolation of cytopathic retroviruses (HTLV-III) from patients with AIDS and at risk for AIDS. *Science* 1984;224:500–503.
2. Johnson RT, McArthur JC, Narayan O: The neurology of human immunodeficiency virus infections. *FASEB J* 1988;2:2970–2981.
3. Gallo RC, Kalyanaraman VS, Sarngadharan MG, et al: Assoccation of the human type-C retrovirus with a subset of adult T-cell cancers. *Cancer Res* 1983;43:3892–3899.
4. deThe G: HTLV-I and chronic progressive encephalomyelopathies: an immunolovirological perspective, in Roman GC, Vernant J-C, Osame M (eds): *HTLV-I and the Nervous System*. New York, Alan R. Liss, 1989, pp 3–8.
5. Gottlieb MS, Schroff R, Schranker HM, et al: *Pneumocystis carinii* pneumonia and mucosal candidiasis in previously healthy homosexual men. *N Engl J Med* 1981;305:1425–1431.
6. Masur H, Michelis MA, Greene JB, et al: An outbreak of community-acquired *Pneumocystis carinii* pneumonia: initial manifestation of cellular immune dysfunction. *N Engl J Med* 1981;305:1431–1438.
7. Siegal FP, Lopez C, Hammer GS, et al: Severe acquired immunodeficiency in male homosexuals manifested by chronic perianal ulcerative Herpes simplex lesions. *N Engl J Med* 1981;305:1439–1444.
8. Snider WD, Simpson DM, Nielsen S, et al: Neurological complications of the acquired immunodeficiency syndrome: analysis of 50 patients. *Ann Neurol* 1983;14:403–418.
9. Levy RM, Bredesen DE, Rosenblum ML: Neurological manifestations of the acquired immunodeficiency syndrome (AIDS): experience at UCSF and

review of the literature. *J Neurosurg* 1985;62:475–495.
10. Berger JR, Moskowitz L, Fischl M, Kelley RE: Neurologic disease as the presenting manifestation of acquired immunodeficiency syndrome. *South Med J* 1987;80:683–686.
11. Bredesen DE, Messing R: Neurological syndromes heralding the acquired immunodeficiency syndrome (abstract). *Ann Neurol* 1983;14:141.
12. Gray F, Gherardi R, Scaravilli F: The neuropathology of the acquired immune deficiency syndrome (AIDS). *Brain* 1988;111:245–266.
13. Rhodes R: Histopathology of the central nervous system in the acquired immunodeficiency syndrome. *Hum Pathol* 1987;18:636–643.
14. Ho DD, Bredesen DE, Vinters, Daar ES: The acquired immunodeficiency syndrome (AIDS) dementia complex. *Ann Intern Med* 1989;111:400–410.
15. Nielsen SL, Petito CK, Urmacher CS, Posner JB: Subacute encephalitis in acquired immune deficiency syndrome: a postmortem study. *Am J Clin Pathol* 1984;82:678–682.
16. Moskowitz LB, Hensley GT, Chan JC, et al: The neuropathology of acquired immunodeficiency syndrome. *Arch Pathol Lab Med* 1984;108:867–872.
17. Kato T, Hirano A, Llena JF, Dembitzer HM: Neuropathology of acquired immune deficiency syndrome (AIDS) in 53 autopsy cases with particular emphasis on microglial nodules and multinucleated giant cells. *Acta Neuropathol (Berl)* 1987;73:287–294.
18. Levy JA, Shimabukuro J, Hollander H, et al: Isolation of AIDS assocated retroviruses from cerebrospinal fluid and brain of patients with neurological symptoms. *Lancet* 1985;2:586–588.
19. Ho DD, Rota TR, Schooley RT, et al: Isolation of HTLV-III from cerebrospinal fluid and neural *N Engl J Med* 1985;313:1493–1497.
20. De la Monte SM, Moore T, Hedley-Whyte ET: Vacuolar encephalopathy of AIDS (letter). *N Engl J Med* 1986;315:1549–1550.
21. Epstein LG, Sharer LR, Cho E-S, et al: HTLV-III/LAV-like retrovirus particles in the brains of patients with AIDS encephalopathy. *AIDS Res* 1985; 1:447–454.
22. Shaw GM, Harper ME, Hahn BH, et al: HTLV-III infection in brains of children and adults with AIDS encephalopathy. *Science* 1985;227:177–182.
23. Resnick L, Berger JR, Shapshak P. Tourtellotte WW: Early penetration of the blood-brain-barrier by HIV. *Neurology* 1988;38:9–14.
24. Gajdusek DC, Amyx HL, Gibbs CJ, et al: Infection of chimpanzees by human T-lymphotropic retroviruses in brain and other tissues from AIDS patients. *Lancet* 1985;1:55–56.
25. Cheng-Mayer C, Rutka JK, Rosenblum ML, et al: HIV can productively infect cultured human glial cells. *PNAS (USA)* 1987;84:3526–3530.
26. Gonda MA, Wong-Stall F, Gallo RV, et al: Sequence homology and morphologic similarity of HITLV-III and visna virus, a pathogenic lentivirus. *Science* 1985;227:173–177.
27. Ho DD, Sarngadharan MG, Resnick L, et al: Primary human T-lymphotropic virus type III infection. *Ann Intern Med* 1985;103:880–883.
28. Cooper DA, Gold J, Maclean P, et al: Acute AIDS retrovirus infection: definition of a clinical illness associated with seroconversion. *Lancet* 1985;1:537–540.
29. Ranki A, Vallf SL, Krohn M, et al: Long latency precedes overt seroconversion in sexually transmitted immunodeficiency-virus infection. *Lancet* 1987; 2:589–593.
30. Imagawa DT, Lee MH, Wolinsky SM, et al: Human immunodeficiency virus type 1 infection in homosexual men who remain seronegative for prolonged periods. *N Engl J Med* 1989;320:1458–1462.
31. Goudsmit J, Lange JM, Krone WJ, et al: Pathogenesis of HIV and its implications for serodiagnosis and monitoring of antiviral therapy. *J Virol Meth* 1987; 17:19–34.
32. Wolinsky S, Rinaldo C, Farzedegan H, et al: Polymerase chain reaction (PCR) detection of HIV provirus before HIV seroconversion. Presented at the Fourth International Conference on AIDS. Stockholm, June 12–16, 1988 (abstract).
33. Hollander H, Stringari S: Human immunodeficiency virus-associated meningitis. Clinical course and correlations. *Am J Med* 1987;83:813–816.
34. Carne CA, Tedder RS, Smith A, et al: Acute encephalopathy coincident with seroconversion for anti-HTLV-III. *Lancet* 1985;1206–1208.
35. Denning DW, Anderson J, Rudge P, Smith H: Acute myelopathy associated with primary infection with human immunodeficiency virus. *Br Med J (Clin Res)* 1987;294:143–144.
36. Calabrese LH, Profitt MR, Levin KH, et al: Acute infection with human immunodeficiency virus (HIV) associated with acute brachial neuritis and exanthematous rash. *Ann Intern Med* 1987;107:849–851.
37. Elovaara I, Iivanainen M, Valle SL, et al: CSF protein and cellular profiles in various stages of HIV infection related to neurological manifestations. *J Neurol Sci* 1987;78:331–342.
38. Marshall DW, Brey RL, Cahill WT, et al: Spectrum of cerebrospinal fluid findings in various stages of human immunodeficiency virus infection. *Arch Neurol* 1988;45:954–958.
39. Britton CB, Miller JR: Neurologic complications in acquired immunodeficiency syndrome. *Neurol Clin* 1984;2:315–339.
40. Navia BA, Price RW: AIDS dementia complex as

the presenting or sole manifestation of HIV infection. *Arch Neurol* 1987;44:65–72.
41. Navia BA, Price RW: AIDS dementia complex: *Ann Neurol* 1986;19:525–535.
42. Berger JR, Fischl M, Resnick L, et al: Evidence of human immunodeficiency virus encephalopathy in the absence of overt neurological disease (abstract). *Proc Int Conf AIDS* 1987;3:85.
43. Grant I, Atkinson JH, Hesselink JR, et al: Evidence for early central nervous system involvement in the acquired immunodeficiency syndrome (AIDS) and other human immunodeficiency virus (HIV) infections: studies with neuropsychologic testing and magnetic resonance imaging. *Ann Intern Med* 1987;107:828–836.
44. Wilkie FL, Eisdorfer C, Morgan R, et al: Cognition in early HIV infection. *Arch Neurol* 1990;47:433–440.
45. Stern Y, Sano M, Goldtein S, et al: Neuropsychological manifestations of HIV infection in gay men (abstract). Fifth International Conference on AIDS, Montreal, 1988, p 383.
46. Clifford D, Miller JP, Deyfried E, et al: Neuropsychometric function in early HIV positive patients compared with a matched HIV negative population. Fifth International Conference on AIDS, Montreal, 1988, p 460.
47. Woo S, Hunter J, Wang P, et al: A brief screening test battery for cognitive deficits in HIV infection (abstract). Fifth International Conference on AIDS, Montreal, 1988, p 384.
48. Becky-Barr D, Perry S, Swanda R, et al: Neuropsychological function in physically asymptomatic HIV seropositive and seronegative gay/bisexual men (abstract). Fifth International Conference on AIDS, Montreal, 1988, p 381.
40. Perdices M, Cooper DA: Simple and choice reaction time in patients with human immunodeficiency virus infection. *Ann Neurol* 1989;25:460–467.
50. De la Monte SM, Ho DD, Schooley RT, et al: Subacute encephalomyelitis of AIDS and its relation to HTLV-III infection. *Neurology* 1987;37:562–569.
51. Price RW, Brew B, Sidtis J, et al: The brain in AIDS: central nervous system HIV-1 infection and AIDS dementia complex. *Science* 1988;239:586–592.
52. Tross S, Price RW, Navia B, et al: Neuropsychological characterization of the AIDS dementia complex: a preliminary report. *AIDS* 1988;2:81–88.
53. Sidtis J, Amitai H, Ornitz D, Price RW: The brief neuropsychological examination for AIDS dementia complex correlations with functional status scales and other neuropsychological tests. *Proceedings of Third Interational Conference on AIDS*, Washington, DC, June 1987, p 55.
54. Beckett A, Manschreck T, Vitagliano H, et al: Symptomatic HIV infection of the CNS in a patient without clinical evidence of immune deficiency. *Am J Psychiatry* 1987;44:1342–1344.
55. Navia BA, Price RW: The acquired immunodeficiency syndrome dementia complex as the presenting or sole manifestation of human immunodeficiency virus infection. *Arch Neurol* 1987;44:64–69.
56. Faulstich ME: Acquired immune deficiency syndrome: an overview of central nervous system complications and neuropsychological sequelae. *Int J Neurosci* 1986;30:249–254.
57. Commings MA, Cummings KL, Rapaport MH, et al: Acquired immunodeficiency syndrome presenting as schizophrenia. *West J Med* 1987;146:615–618.
58. Nurnberg HG, Prudic J, Fiori M, et al: Psychopathology complicating acquired immune deficiency syndrome (AIDS). *Am J Psychiatry* 1985; 141:95–96.
59. Thomas CS, Toone BK, El Komy A, et al: HTLV III and psychiatric disturbance (letter). *Lancet* 1985;1:395–396.
60. Kermani EJ, Borod JC, Brown P, et al: New psychopathologic findings in AIDS: case report. *J Clin Psychiatry* 1985;46:240–241.
61. Beckett A, Summergrad P, Manschreck T, et al: Symptomatic HIV infection of the CNS in a patient without clinical evidence of immune deficiency. *Am J Psychiatry* 1987;144:1342–1344.
62. Kermani E, Drob S, Alpert M: Organic brain syndrome in three cases of acquired immune deficiency syndrome. *Compr Psychiatry* 1984;25:294–297.
63. McHugh PR, Folstein MF: Psychiatric syndromes of Huntingtons chorea: a clinical and phenomenologic study, in Benson F, Blumer D (eds): *Psychiatric Aspects of Neurological Disease*. New York, Grune & Stratton, 1975.
64. Hollander H, Golden J, Mendelson T, et al: Extrapyramidal symptoms in AIDS patients given low-dose metoclopropamide or chlorpromazine (letter). *Lancet* 1985;2:1186.
65. Edelstein H, Knight RT: Severe parkinsonism in two AIDS patients taking prochlorperazine (letter). *Lancet* 1987;2:341–342.
66. Metzer WS: Movement disorders with AIDS encephalopathy: case report. *Neurology* 1987;37: 1438.
67. Currie J, Benson E, Ramsden B, et al: Eye movement abnormalities as a predictor of the acquired immunodeficiency syndrome dementia complex. *Arch Neurol* 1988;45:949–953.
68. Tervo T, Elovaara H, Karli SL, et al: Ocular motility abnormalities as an early sign of CNS involvement in HIV infection (letter). *Lancet* 1986;2:512.
69. Navia BA, Jordan BD, Price RW: The AIDS dementia complex: I Clinical features. *Ann Neurol* 1986;19:517–524.

70. Epstein LG, Sharer LR, Joshi VV, et al: Progressive encephalopathy in children with acquired immune deficiency syndrome. *Ann Neurol* 1985;17:488–496.
71. Belman AL, Ultmann MH, Horoupian D, et al: Neurological complications in infants and children with acquired immune deficiency syndrome *Ann Neurol* 1985;18:560–566.
72. Davis SL, Halsted CC, Levy N, Ellis W: Acquired immune deficiency syndrome presenting as progressive infantile encephalopathy. *J Pediatr* 1987; 110:884–888.
73. Ragni MV, Urbach AH, Taylor S, et al: Isolation of human immunodeficiency virus and detection deficiency syndrome and progressive encephalopathy. *J Pediatr* 1987;110:892–894.
74. Epstein LG, Sharer LR, Oleske JM, et al: Neurologic manifestations of human immunodeficiency virus infection in children. *Pediatrics* 1986;78:678–687.
75. Ultmann MH, Belman AL, Ruff HA, et al: Developmental abnormalities in infants and children with acquired immune deficiency syndrome (AIDS) and AIDS-related complex. *Dev Med Child Neurol* 1985;27:563–571.
76. Vinters HV: The AIDS dementia complex (letter). *Ann Neurol* 1987;21:612.
77. Anders KH, Guerra WF, Tomiyasu U, et al: The neuropathology of AIDS, UCLA experience and review. *Am J Pathol* 1986;124:537–558.
78. Anders K, Steinsapir KD, Iverson DJ, et al: Neuropathologic findings in the acquired immunodeficiency syndrome (AIDS) *Clin Neuropathol* 1986;5:1–20.
79. Popovic M, Sarngadharan MG, Read E, Gallo RC: Detection, isolation, and continuous production of cytopathic retroviruses (HTLV-III) from patients with AIDS and pre-AIDS. *Science* 1984;224:497–500.
80. Schwenk J, Cruz-Sanchez F, Gosztonyi G, Cervos-Navarro J: Spongiform encephalopathy in a patient with the acquired immune deficiency syndrome (AIDS). *Acta Neuropathol* 1987;74:389–392.
81. Sharer LR, Epstein LG, Cho E-S, et al: Pathologic features of AIDS encephalopathy in children: evidence for LAV/HTLV-III infection of brain. *Hum Pathol* 1986;17:271–284.
82. Belman AL, Lantos G, Horoupian D, et al: AIDS: Calcification of the basal ganglia in infants and children. *Neurology* 1986;36:1192–1199.
83. Wiley CA, Schrier RD, Nelson JA, et al: Cellular localization of human immunodeficiency virus infection within the brains of acquired immune deficiency patients. *Proc Natl Acad Sci* 1986;83:7089–7093.
84. Stoler MH, Eskin TA, Benn S, et al: Human T-cell lymphotropic virus type III infection of the central nervous system—a preliminary in situ analysis. *JAMA* 1986;256:2360–2364.
85. Pumarola-Sune T, Navia BA, Cardon-Cardo C, et al: HIV antigen in the brains of patients with AIDS dementia complex. *Ann Neurol* 1987;21:490–496.
86. Gabuzda DH, Ho DD, de la Monte SM, et al: Immunohistochemical identification of HTLV-III antigen in brains of patients with AIDS. *Ann Neurol* 1986;20:289–295.
87. Hill JM, Farrar WL, Pert CB: Localization of the T4 antigen/AIDS virus receptor in monkey and rat brain: prominence in cortical regions. *Psychopharmacol Bull* 1986;22:689–694.
88. Fauci AS: The immunopathogenesis of AIDS, in Gottlieb MS, et al (eds): *Current Topics in AIDS,* Vol 1. New York, Wiley, 1987, pp 119–232.
89. Moargolick JB, Lane HC, Fauci AS: Immunopathogenesis of HTLV-III/LAV infection, in Gallo RC, Haseltine W, Klein G, zur Hausen H, (eds): *Viruses and Brain Cancer,* Vol 1. New York, Alan Liss, 1987, pp 59–79.
90. Funke I, Hahn A, Rieber EP, et al: The cellular receptor (CD 4) of the human immunodeficiency virus is expressed on neurons and glial cells of human brain. *J Exp Med* 1987;165:1230–1235.
91. Koenig S, Gendelman HE, Orenstein JM, et al: Detection of AIDS virus in macrophages in brain tissue from AIDS patients with encephalopathy. *Science* 1986;233:1089–1093.
92. Gartner S, Markovits P, Markovits DM, et al: Virus isolation from and identification of HTLV-III/LAV-producing cells in brain tissue from a patient with AIDS. *JAMA* 1986;256:2365–2371.
93. Gabuzda DH, Ho DD, de la Monte SM, et al: Immunohistochemical identification of HTLV-III antigen in brains of patients with AIDS. *Ann Neurol* 1986;20:289–295.
94. Koyanagi Y, Miles S, Mitsuyasu RT, et al: Dual infection of the central nervous system by AIDS viruses with distinct cellular tropisms. *Science* 1987;236:819–822.
95. Anand R, Siegal F, Reed C, et al: Non-cytocidal natural variants of human immunodeficiency virus isolated from AIDS patients with neurological disorders. *Lancet* 1987;2:234–238.
96. Cheng-Mayer C, Levy JA: Distinct biological and serological properties of human immunodeficiency viruses from the brain. *Ann Neurol* 1988;23 (suppl):S58–S61.
97. Von Briesen H, Becker WB, Henco K, et al: Isolation frequency and growth properties of HIV-variants: multiple simultaneous variants in a patient demonstrated by molecular cloning. *J Med Virol* 1987;23:51–66.
98. Yarchoan R, Weinhold KJ, Lyerly HK, et al: Administration of 3'-azido-3'-deoxythymidine, and inhibitor of HTLV III/LAV replication, to patients

with AIDS or AIDS-related complex. *Lancet* 1986;1:570–580.

99. McDonald EM, Mann AH, Thomas HC: Interferons as mediators of psychiatric morbidity. *Lancet* 1987; 2:1175–1178.
100. Kumar M, Resnick L, Berger JR, et al: AIDS dementia complex associated with brain reactive antibodies. *J AIDS* 1989;2:469–471.
101. Pert CB, Hill JH, Ruff MR, et al: Octapeptides deduced from the neuropeptide receptor-like pattern of antigen T4 in brain potently inhibits human immunodeficiency virus receptor binding and T-cell infectivity. *Proc Natl Acad Sci USA* 1986;83:9254–9258.
102. Sacerdote P, Ruff MR, Pert CB: Vasocactive intestinal peptide 1-12: a ligand for the CD4 (T4) human immunodeficiency virus receptor. *J Neurosci Res* 1987;18:102–107.
103. Lee MR, Ho DD, Gurney ME. Functional interaction and partial homology between human immunodeficiency virus and neuroleukin. *Science* 1987;237:1047–1051.
104. Michaels J, Sharer LR, Epstein LG: Human immunodeficiency virus type 1 (HIV-1) infection of the nervous system: a review. *Immunodeficiency Rev* 1988;1:71–104.
105. Rottenberg DA, Moeller JR, Strother SC, et al: The metabolic pathology of the AIDS dementia complex. *Ann Neurol* 1987;22:700–706.
106. Moeller JR, Strother SC, Sidtis JJ, Rottenberg DA: The scaled subprofile model: a statistical approach to the analysis of functional patterns in positron emission tomographic data. *J Cereb Blood Flow Metab* 1987;7:649–658.
107. Ell PJ, Costa DC, Harrison M: Imaging cerebral damage in HIV infection. *Lancet* 1987;2:569–570.
108. Brun B, Boesen F, Gerstoft J, et al: Crebral computed tomography in men with acquired immunodeficiency syndrome. *Acta Radiol Diagn* 1986; 27:385–387.
109. Post MJD, Tate LG, Quencer R, et al: HIV encephalitis and meningitis. *AJNR* (in press).
110. Post MJD, Berger JR, Hensley GT: The radiology of central nervous system disease in acquired immunodeficiency syndrome, in Taveras JM, Ferrucci JT (eds): *Radiology: Diagnosis-Imaging-Intervention*. Philadelphia, J.B. Lippincott, 1988, pp 1–26.
111. Olesen WL, Longo FM, Mills CM, Norman D: White matter disease in AIDS: findings at MR imaging. *Radiology* 1988;169:445–448.
112. Post MJD, Sheldon JJ, Hensley GT, et al: Central nervous system disease in acquired immunodeficiency syndrome: prospective correlation using CT, MR imaging and pathologic studies. *Radiology* 1986;158:141–148.
113. Price RW, Navia BA: Infections in AIDS and in other immunosuppressed patients, in Kennedy PGE, Johnson RT (eds). *Infections of the Nervous System*, London, Butterworth, 1987, pp 248–273.
114. Schmitt FA, Bigley JW, McKinnis R, et al: Neuropsychological outcome of zidovudine (AZT) treatment of patients with AIDS and AIDS-related complex. *N Engl J Med* 1988;319:1573–1578.
115. Pizzo PA, Eddy J, Falloon J, et al: Effect of continuous intravenous infusion of zidovudine (AZT) in children with symptomatic HIV infection. *N Engl J Med* 1988;319:889–896.
116. Petito CK, Navia BA, Cho ES, et al: Vacuolar myelopathy pathologically resembling subacute combined degeneration in patients with the acquired immunodeficiency syndrome. *N Engl J Med* 1985; 312:874–879.
117. Goldstick L, Mandybur TI, Bode R: Spinal cord degeneration in AIDS. *Neurology* 1985;35:103.
118. Helweg-Larsen S, Jakobsen J, Boesen F, et al: Myelopathy in AIDS. A clinical and electrophysiological study of 23 Danish patients. *Acta Neurol Scand* 1988;77:64–73.
119. Honig LS, Vogel H, Horoupian DS: Chronic myelopathy as a presenting symptom in HIV infection (abstract). *Neurology* 1989;39(suppl 1):419.
120. Signh BM, Levine S, Yarrish RL, et al: Spinal cord syndromes in the acquired immune deficiency syndrome. *Acta Neurol Scand* 1986;73:590–598.
121. Dickson DW, Belman AL, Km TS, et al: Spinal cord pathology in pediatric acquired immunodeficiency syndrome. *Neurology* 1989;39:227–235.
122. Denning DW, Anderson J, Rudge P, Smith H: Acute myelopathy associated with primary infection with human immunodeficiency virus. *Br Med J* 1987;294:143–144.
123. Tucker T, Dix RD, Katzen C, et al: Cytomegalovirus and herpes simplex virus ascending myelitis in a patient with acquired immune deficiency syndrome. *Ann Neurol* 1985;18:74–79.
124. Britton CB, Mesa-Tejada R, Fenoglio CM, et al: A new complication of AIDS: thoracic myelitis caused by herpes simplex virus. *Neurology* 1985;35:1071–1074.
125. McArthur JC: Neurologic manifestations of AIDS. *Medicine* 1987;66:407–437.
126. McArthur JC, Griffin JW, Cornblath DR, Farzadegan H: Progressive HTLV-1-associated myeloneuropathy in a patient with HIV-1 (abstract). *Neurology* 1989;39(suppl 1):419.
127. Woolsey RM, Chanmbers TJ, Chung HK, McGarry JD: Mycobacterial meningomyelitis associated with human immunodeficiency virus infection. *Arch Neurol* 1988;45:691–693.
128. Doll DC, Yarbro JW, Phillips K, Klott C: Mycobacterial spinal cord abscess with an ascending polyneuropathy (letter). *Ann Intern Med* 1987; 106:333–334.
129. Jordan BD, Navia BA, Petito C, et al: Neurological

syndromes complicating AIDS. *Front Radiat Ther Oncol* 1985;19:82–87.
130. Weill O, Finaud M, Bille F, et al: Gliome malin medullaire: une nouvelle complication de l'infection par le HIV? (letter). *Presse Med* 1987;16:1977.
131. Berger JR, Sheremata WA, Resnick L, et al: Multiple sclerosis-like illness occurring with human immunodeficiency virus infection. *Neurology* 1989; 39:324–328.
132. Janssen RS, Saykin AJ, Kaplan JE, et al: Neurological complications of human immunodeficiency virus infection in patients with lymphadenopathy syndrome. *Ann Neurol* 1988;23:49–55.
133. Miller RG, Kiprov DD, Parry G, Bredesen DE: Peripheral nervous system dysfunction in acquired immunodeficiency syndrome, in Rosenblum ML, Levy RM, Bredesen DE (eds): *Aids and the Nervous System*. New York, Raven Press, 1988, pp 65–78.
134. Lipkin WI, Parry G, Kiprov D, et al: Inflammatory neuropathy in homosexual men with lymphadenopathy. *Neurology* 1985;35:1479–1483.
135. Rance NE, McArthur JC, Cornblath DR, et al: Gracile tract degeneration in patients with sensory neuropathy and AIDS. *Neurology* 1988;38:265–271.
136. Miller RG, Parry G, Lang W, et al: AIDS-related inflammatory polyradiculopathy: prediction of response to plasma exchange with electrophysiologic testing. *Muscle Nerve* 1985;8:626.
137. Cornblath DR, McArthur JC, Kennedy PGE, et al: Inflammatory demyelinating peripheral neuropathies associated with human T-cell lymphotropic virus type III infection. *Ann Neurol* 1987;21:32–40.
138. Mishra BB, Sommers W, Koski CK, Greenstein JI: Acute inflammatory demyelinatig polyneuropathy in the acquired immune deficiency syndrome. *Ann Neurol* 1985;131–132.
139. Berger JR, Difini JA, Swerdloff MA, Ayyar DR: HIV seropositivity in Guillain-Barré syndrome (letter). *Ann Neurol* 1987;22:393–394.
140. Cornblath DR, McArthur JC, Griffin JW: The spectrum of peripheral neuropathies in HTLV-III infection. *Muscle Nerve* 1986;9:76.
141. Dalakas MC: Neuromuscular complications of AIDS. *Muscle Nerve* 1986;9:92.
142. Stricker RB, Bredesen DE, Wesley AM, et al: Autoantibodies in HIV-related peripheral neuropathy. Presented at the Neurological and Neuropsychological Complications of HIV Infection Satellite Symposia to the Fifth International Conference on AIDS, Quebec City, 1989, p 30.
143. Eidelberg D, Sotrel A, Vogel H, et al: Progressive polyradiculopathy in acquired immunie deficiency syndrome. *Neurology* 1986;36:912–916.
144. Parry GJ: Peripheral neuropathies associated with human immunodeficiency virus infection. *Ann Neurol* 1988;23(suppl):S49–S53.
145. Elder G, Dalakas M, Pezeshkpour G, et al: Ataxic neuropathy due to ganglioneuritis after probable acute human immunodeficiency virus infection. *Lancet* 1986;ii:1275–1276.
146. Pialoux G, Dupont B, Sansonetti P, et al: Polyradiculonevrite des nerfs craniens au cous du syndrome d'immunodeficit acquis. *Pressè Med* 1987;16:967.
147. Brown MA, Thompson A, Goh BT, et al: Bell's palsy and HIV infection. *J Neurol Neurosurg Psychiatry* 1988;51:424–426.
148. Cole EL, Meisler DM, Calabrese LH, et al: Herpes zoster ophthalmicus and acquired immune deficiency syndrome. *Arch Ophthalmol* 1984;102: 1027.
149. Graham SH, Bredesen DE: Neurologic complications of herpes zoster in patients with HGIV infection. *Neurology* (in press).
150. Lanska MJ, Lanska DJ, Schmidley JW: Syphilitic polyradiculopathy in an HIV-positive man. *Neurology* 1988;38:1297–1301.
151. Zochodne DW, Bolton CF, Wells GA, et al: Critical illness polyneuropathy: a complication of sepsis and multiple organ failure. *Brain* 1987;110:819–842.
152. Dalakas MC, Pezeshkpour GH, Gravell M, et al: Polymyositis associated with AIDS retrovirus. *JAMA* 1986;256:2381–2383.
153. Bailey RO, Turok DI, Jaufman BP, Singh JK: Myositis and acquired immunodeficiency syndrome. *Hum Pathol* 1987;18:749–751.
154. Dalakas MC, London WT, Gravell M, et al: Polymyositis in an immunodeficiency disease in monkeys induced by a type D retrovirus. *Neurology* 1986;36:569–572.
155. Dalakas MC, Gravell M, London WT, et al: Morphological changes of an inflammatory myopathy in rhesus monkeys with simian acquired immunodeficiency syndrome. *Proc Soc Exp Biol Med* 1987; 185:368–376.
156. Bessen LJ, Greene JB, Louie E: Severe polymyositis-like syndrome associated with zidovudinee therapy of AIDS and ARC (letter). *N Engl J Med* 1988;318:708.
157. Simpson D, Wolfe D, Farraye J, Bender A: HIV associated myopathy: features in 21 patients and role of AZT (abstract). Fifth International Conference on AIDS, Montreal, 1989, p 276.
158. Dalakas M, Peseahkpoor GH, Illa I, Nath A: Destructive inflammatory myopathy with abnormal mitochondria (DIM-Mi) in nine HIV-positive patients treated with zidovudine. Presented at the Neurological and Neuropsychological Complications of HIV Satellite Symposium to the Fifth International Conference on AIDS, Quebec City, 1989, p 120.
159. Dalakas MC, Pezeshkpour GH, Flaherty M: Progressive nemaline (rod) myopathy associated with

HIV infection (letter). *N Engl J Med* 1987;317: 1602–1603.
160. Watts RA, Hoffbrand BI, Paton DF, Davis JC: Pyomyositis associated with human immunodeficiency virus infection. *Br Med J* 1987;294:1524–1525.
161. Uldry PA, Steck AJ, Regli F: Paralysis of the trapezius muscle in HIV infection (letter). *Presse Med* 1987;16:1654.
162. Drane WE, Tipler BM: Heterotopic ossification (myositis ossificans) in acquired immunodeficiency syndrome. Detection by gallium scintigraphy. *Clin Nucl Med* 1987;12:433–435.
163. Drew WL: Cytomegalovirus infection in patients with AIDS. *J Infect Dis* 1988;158:449–456.
164. Huang ES, Alford CA, Reynolds DW, et al: Molecular epidemiology of cytomegalovirus infections in women and their infants. *N Engl J Med* 1980;303:958–962.
165. Hutto C, Ricks R, Garvie M, et al: Epidemiology of cytomegalovirus infections in young children: day care vs. home care. *Pediatr Infect Dis* 1985;4:149–152.
166. Spector SA, Hirata KK, Neuman TR: Identification of multiple cytomegalovirus strains in homosexual men with acquired immunodeficiency syndrome. *J Infect Dis* 1984;150:953–956.
167. Bale JF Jr: Human cytomegalovirus infection and disorders of the nervous system. *Arch Neurol* 1984;41:310–320.
168. Dorfman LJ: Cytomegalovirus encephalitis in adults. *Neurology* 1973;23:136–143.
169. Chin W, Magoffin R, Frierson G, Lennette EH: Cytomegalovirus infection. A case of meningoencephalitis. *JAMA* 1973;225:740–741.
170. Duchowny M, Caplan L, Siber G: Cytomegalovirus infection of the adult nervous system. *Ann Neurol* 1979;5:458–461.
171. Linneman CC Jr, Dunn CR, First MR, et al: Late onset of fatal cytomegalovirus infection after renal transplantation. Primary or reactivation infection? *Arch Intern Med* 1978;138:1247–1250.
172. Perham TGM, Caul EO, Clarke SKR, Gibson AGF: Cytomegalovirus meningoencephalitis. *Br Med J* 1971;2:50.
173. Philips CA, Fanning WL, Gump DW, Phillips CF: Cytomegalovirus encephalitis in immunologically normal adults. Successful treatments with vidarabine. *JAMA* 1977;21:2299–2300.
174. Schneck SA: Neuropathological features of human organ transplantation. *J Neuropathol Exp Neurol* 1965;24:415–429.
175. Schober R, Herman MM: Neuropathology of cardiac transplantation. *Lancet* 1973;1:962–967.
176. Yanagisaw N, Toyokura Y, Shiraki B: Double encephalitis with herpes simplex virus and cytomegalovirus in an adult. *Acta Neuropathol (Berl)* 1975;33:153–164.
177. Reichert CM, O'Leary TJ, Levens DL, et al: Autopsy pathology in the acquired immune deficiency syndrome. *Am J Pathol* 1983;112:357–382.
178. Detels R, Visscher BR, Fahey JL, et al: Predictors of clinical AIDS in young homosexual men in a high risk area. *Int J Epidemiol* 1987;16:271–276.
179. Koppel BS, Wormser GP, Tuchman AJ, et al: Central nervous system involvement in patients with acquired immune deficiency syndrome (AIDS). *Acta Neurol Scand* 1985;71:337–353.
180. Moskovitz LB, Gregorios JB, Hensley GT, Berger JR: Cytomegalovirus-induced demyelination associated with acquired immune deficiency syndrome. *Arch Pathol Lab Med* 1984;108:873–877.
181. Reichert CM, O'Leary TJ, Levens, DL: Autopsy pathology in the acquired immune deficiency syndrome. *Am J Pathol* 1983;112:357–382.
182. Vital C, Vital A, Vignoly B, et al: Cytomegalovirus encephalitis in a patient with acquired immunodeficiency syndrome. *Arch Pathol Lab Med* 1985; 109:105–106.
183. Welsh K, Finkbeiner W, Alpers CE, et al: Autopsy findings in the acquired immune deficiency syndrome. *JAMA* 1984;252:1152–1159.
184. Hawley DA, Schaefer JF, Schulz DM, Muller J: Cytomegalovirus encephalitis in acquired immunodeficiency syndrome. *Am J Clin Pathol* 1983; 80:874–877.
185. Wiley CA, Nelson JA: Role of human immunodeficiency virus and cytomegalovirus in AIDS encephalitis. *Am J Pathol* 1988;33:73–81.
186. Pepose JS, Hilborne LH, Cancilla PA, Foos RY: Concurrent herpes simplex and cytomegalovirus retinitis and encephalitis in the acquired immune deficiency syndrome (AIDS). *Ophthalmology* 1984; 91:1669–1677.
187. Wiley CA, Schrier RD, Denaro FJ, et al: Localization of cytomegalovirus proteins and genome during fulminant central nervous system infection in an AIDS patient. *J Neuropathol Exp Neurol* 1986; 45:127–139.
188. Grafe MR, Wiley CA: Spinal cord and peripheral nerve pathology in AIDS: the roles of cytomegalovirus and human immunodeficiency virus. *Ann Neurol* 1989;25:561–566.
189. Dix RD, Bredesen DE: Opportunistic viral infections in acquired immunodeficiency syndrome, in ML Rosenblum, RM Levy, DE Bredesen (eds): *AIDS and the Nervous System*. New York, Raven Press, 1988, pp 221–261.
190. Dix RD, Bredesen DE, Erlich KS, Mills J: Recovery of herpesviruses from cerebrospinal fluid of immunodeficient homosexual men. *Ann Neurol* 1985;18:611–614.
191. Edwards RH, Messing R, McKendall RR: Cytomegalovirus meningoencephalitis in a homosexual

man with Kaposi's sarcoma: isolation of CMV from CSF cells. *Neurology* 1985;35:560–562.
192. Morgello S, Cho ES, Nielsen S, et al: Cytomegalovirus encephalitis in patients with acquired immunodeficiency syndrome: an autopsy study of 30 cases and a review of the literature. *Hum Pathol* 1987;18:289–297.
193. Vinters HV, Kwok MK, Ho HW, et al: Cytomegalovirus in the nervous system of patients with the acquired immune deficiency syndrome. *Brain* 1989;112:245–268.
194. Post MJ, Hensley GT, Moskowitz LB, et al: Cytomegalic inclusion virus encephalitis in patients with AIDS: CT, clinical, and pathologic correlation. *AJR* 1986;146:1229–1234.
195. Skolnik PR, Kosloff BR, Hirsch MS: Bidirectional interactions between human immunodeficiency virus type 1 and cytomegalovirus. *J Infect Dis* 1988;157:508–514.
196. Mar EC, Cheng YC, Huang ES: Effect of 9-(1,3-dihydroxy-2-propoxymethyl) guanine on human cytomegalovirus in vitro. *Antimicrob Agents Chemother* 1983;24:518–521.
197. Pepose JS, Newman C, Bach MC, et al: Pathologic features of cytomegalovirus retinopathy after treatment with the antiviral agent ganciclovir. *Ophthalmology* 1987;94:414–424.
198. Felsenstein D, D'Amico DJ, Hirsch MS, et al: Treatment of cytomegalovirus retinitis with 9-(2-hydroxymethyl) ethoxymethyl)guanine. *Ann Intern Med* 1985;103:377–380.
199. Laskin OL, Cederberg DM, Mills J, et al: Ganciclovir for the treatment and suppression of serious infections caused by cytomegalovirus. *Am J Med* 1987;83:201–207.
200. Walmsley SL, Chew E, Read SE, et al: Treatment of cytomegalovirus retinitis with trisodium phosphonoformate hexahydrate (Foscarnet). *J Infect Dis* 1988;157:569–572.
201. Le Hoang P, Girard B, Robinet M, et al: Foscarnet in the treatment of cytomegalovirus retinitis in acquired immune deficiency syndrome. *Ophthalmology* 1989;96:865–874.
202. Martin JH, Dohner DE, Wellinghoff WJ, Gelb LD: Restriction endonuclease analysis of varicella-zoster vaccine virus and wild-type DNAs. *J Med Virol* 1982;9:69–76.
203. Straus SE, Hay J, Smith H, Owens J: Genome differences among varicella-zoster virus isolates. *J Gen Virol* 1983;64:1031–1041.
204. Gelb LD: Varicella-zoster virus, in Fields BN, Knipe DM, Chanock RM, et al (eds): *Virology*. New York, Raven Press, 1985, pp 591–627.
205. Kestelyn P, Stevens AM, Bakkers E, et al: Sever hepes zoster ophthalmicus in young African adults: a marker for HTLV-III seropositivity. *Br J Ophthalmol* 1987;71:806–809.
206. McKendall RR, Klawans HL: Nervous system complications of varicella-zoster virus, in Vinken PJ, Bruyn GW (eds): *Handbook of Clinical Neurology*, Vol 34. New York, North-Holland, 1978, pp 161–183.
207. Jemsek J, Greenberg SB, Taber L, et al: Herpes zoster-associated encephalitis: clinicopathologic report of 12 cases and review of the literature. *Medicine* 1983;62:81–97.
208. Ryder JW, Croen D, Kleinschmidt-DeMasters BK, et al: Progressive encephalitis 3 months after resolution of cutaneous zoster in a patient with AIDS. *Ann Neurol* 1986;19:182–188.
209. Gilden DH, Murray RS, Wellish BS, et al: Chronic progressive varicella-zoster virus encephalitis in an AIDS patient. *Neurology* 1988;38:1150–1153.
210. Miller JR, Barrett RE, Britton CB, et al: Progressive multifocal leukoencephalopathy in a male homosexual with T-cell immune deficiency syndrome. *N Engl J Med* 1982;307:1436–1438.
211. Berger JR, Kaszovitz B, Post MJD, et al: Progressive multifocal leukoencephalopathy associated with human immunodeficiency virus infection: a review of the literature with a report of 16 cases. *Ann Intern Med* 1987;107:78–87.
212. Houff SA, Major EO, Katz DA, et al: Involvement of JC virus-infected mononuclear cells from the bone marrow and spleen in the pathogenesis of progressive multifocal leukoencephalopathy. *N Engl J Med* 1988;318:301–305.
213. Berger JR, Mucke L: Prolonged survival and partial recovery in AIDS-associated progressive multifocal leukoencephalopathy. *Neurology* 1988;38:1060–1064.
214. Whimbey E, Gold JWM, Polsky B, et al: Bacteremia and fungemia in patients with the acquired immunodeficiency syndrome. *Ann Intern Med* 1986;10:511–514.
215. Levy RM, Pons VG, Rosenblum ML: Central nervous system mass lesions in the acquired immunodeficiency syndrome (AIDS). *J Nerosurg* 1984; 61:9–16.
216. Kelly WM, Brant-Zawadzki M: Acquired immunodeficiency syndrome: neuroradiologic findings. *Radiology* 1983;149:485–491.
217. Henin D, Duycaerts C, Chaunu MP, et al: Etude neuropathologique de 31 cas de syndrome d'immuno-depression acquise. *Rev Neurol* 1987;143: 631–642.
218. Pitchenik AE, Burr J, Fertel D, et al: Human T-cell lymphotropic virus III (HTLV III) seropositivity and related disease among 71 consecutive patients in whom tuberculosis was diagnosed. A prospective study. *Am Rev Resp Dis* 1987;135:875–879.
219. Chaisson RE, Schecter GF, Theuer CP, et al: Tuberculosis in patients with the acquired immunodeficiency syndrome. Clinical features, response to

therapy, and survival. *Am Rev Resp Dis* 1987; 136:570–574.

220. Bishburg E, Sunderam G, Reichman LB, et al: Central nervous system tuberculosis with the acquired immunodeficiency syndrome and its related complex. *Ann Intern Med* 1986;105:210–213.
221. Doll DC, Yarbro JW: Mycobacterial spinal cord abscess with an ascending polyneuropathy (letter). *Ann Intern Med* 1987;106:333–334.
222. Centers for Disease Control: Diagnosis and management of mycobacterial infection and disease in persons with human immunodeficiency virus infection. *Ann Intern Med* 1987;106:204–206.
223. Pons VG, Jacobs RA, Hollander H: Nonviral infections of the central nervous system in patients with acquired immunodeficiency syndrome, in Rosenblum ML, Levy RM, Bredesen DE (eds): *AIDS and the Central Nervous System*. New York, Raven Press, 1988, pp 263–283.
224. Sharer LR, Kapila R: Neuropathologic observations in the acquired immunodeficiency syndrome. *Acta Neuropathol* 1985;66:188–198.
225. Adair JC, Beck AC, Apfelbaum RI, Baringer JR: Nocardial cerebral abscess in the acquired immunodeficiency syndrome. *Arch Neurol* 1987;44: 548–50.
226. Holtz HA, Lavery DP, Kapila R: Actinomcetales infection in the acquired immunodeficiency syndrome. *Acta Neuropathol* 1985;66:203–205.
227. Viroslav J, Williams T: Nocardial infection of the pulmonary and central nervous system: successful treatment with medical therapy. *South Med J* 1971;64:1382–1385.
228. Byrne E, Brophy BP, Perrett LV: Nocardia cerebral abscess: new concepts in diagnosis, management, and prognosis. *J Neurol Neurosurg Psychiatry* 1979;42:1038–1045.
229. Berger JR, McCarthy M, Resnick L, et al: History of syphilis as a cofactor for the expression of HIV infection (abstract). Fifth International Conference on AIDS, Montreal, 1989, p 93.
230. Katz D, Berger JR: Neurosyphilis in AIDS. *Arch Neurol* 1989;46:895–901.
231. Johns DR, Tierney M, Felsenstein D: Alteration in the natural history of neurosyphilis by concurrent infection with the human immunodeficiency virus. *N Engl J Med* 1987;316:1569–1572.
232. Berry CD, Hooton TM, Collier AC, et al: Neurologic relapse after benzathine penicillin therapy for secondary syphilis in a patient with HIV infection. *N Engl J Med* 1987;316:1587–1589.
233. Chung WM, Pien FD, Grekin JL: Syphilis: a cause of fever of unknown origin. *Cutis* 1983;31:537–540.
234. Zambrano W, Perez GM, Smith JL: Acute syphilitic blindness in AIDS. *J Clin Neurol Opthalmol* 1987;7:1–5.
235. Fernandez-Guerrero ML, Miranda C, Cenjor C, Sanabria F: The treatment of neurosyphilis in patients with HIV infection (letter). *JAMA* 1988; 259:1495–1496.
236. Spence MR, Abrutyn E: Syphilis and infection with the human immunodeficiency virus. *Ann Intern Med* 1987;107:587.
237. Haas JS, Bolan G, Larsen S, et al: "Seroreversion" of treponemal tests during HIV infection. Fifth International Conference on AIDS, Montreal, June 1989, p 360 (abstract).
238. Hicks CB, Benson PM, Lupton GP, Tramont EC: Seronegative secondary syphilis in a patient infected with the human immunodeficiency virus (HIV) with Kaposi sarcoma. *Ann Intern Med* 1987;107:492–495.
239. Editorial: Cryptococcus in AIDS. *Lancet* 1988; 25:1434–1436.
240. Zuger A, Louie E, Holzman RS, et al: Cryptococcal disease in patients with the acquired immunodeficiency syndrome. *Ann Intern Med* 1986;104: 234–240.
241. Centers for Disease Control: Update: Acquired immunodeficiency syndrome—United States. *MMWR* 1986;35:542.
242. Pizzo PA, Eddy J, Faloon J: Acquired immune deficiency syndrome in children. Current problems and therapeutic considerations. *Am J Med* 1988; 85:195–202.
243. Kovacs JA, Kovacs AA, Polis M, et al: Cryptococcosis in the acquired immunodeficiency syndrome. *Ann Intern Med* 1985;103:533–538.
244. Giberson TP, Kalyan-Raman K: Cryptococcal meningitis: initial presentation of acquired immunodeficiency syndrome. *Ann Emerg Med* 1987; 16:802–804.
245. Gal AA, Evans S, Meyer PR: The clinical laboratory evaluation of cryptococcal infections in the acquired immunodeficiency syndrome. *Diagn Microbiol Infect Dis* 1987;7:249–254.
246. Kapend K, Komichelo K, Swinne D, et al: Meningitis due to *Cryptococcus neoformans* biovar gattii in a Zairian AIDS patient. *Eur J Clin Microbiol Infect Dis* 1987;6:320–321.
247. St-Germain G, Noel G, Chung KJ: Disseminated cryptococcosis due to *Cryptococcus neoformans* variety gattii in a Canadian patient with AIDS (letter). *Eur J Clin Microbiol Infect Dis* 1988;7:587–588.
248. Schimpff SC, Bennett JE: Abnormalities in cell-mediated immunity in patients with *Cryptococcus neoformans* infection. *J Allerg Clin Immunol* 1975;55:430–441.
249. Dromer F, Aucouturier P, Clauvel JP, et al: *Cryptococcus neoformans* anitbody levels in patients with AIDS. *Scand J Infect Dis* 1988;20:283–285.
250. Sabetta JR, Andriole VT: Cryptococcal infection of

the central nervous system. *Med Clin North Am* 1985;69:333–344.
251. Johannessen DJ, Wilson LG: Mania with cryptococcal meningitis in two AIDS patients. *J Clin Psychiatr* 1988;49:200–201.
252. Maayan S, Wormser GP, Hewlett D, et al: Acquired immunodeficiency syndrome (AIDS) in an economically disadvantaged population. *Arch Intern Med* 1985;145:1607–1612.
253. Diamond RD, Bennett JE: Prognostic factors in cryptococcal meningitis. A study of 111 cases. *Ann Intern Med* 1974;80:176–181.
254. Kelly WM, Brant-Zawadzki M: Acquired immunodeficiency syndrome: neuroradiologic findings. *Radiology* 1983;149:485–491.
255. Post MJD, Kursunoglu SJ, Hensley GT, et al: Cranial CT in acquired immunodeficiency syndrome: spectrum of diseases and optimal contrast enhancement technique. *AJR* 1985;145:929–940.
256. Whelan MA, Kricheff II, Handler M, et al: Acquired immunodeficiency syndrome: cerebral computed tomographic manifestations. *Radiology* 1983;149:477–484.
257. Larsen RA, Bozetta S, McCutchan JA, et al: California Collaborative Treatment Group: persistence of *Cryptococcus neoformans* infection of the prostate after successful treatment of meningitis. *Ann Intern Med* 1989;111:125–128
258. Stern JJ, Hartman BJ, Sharkey P, et al: Oral fluconazole therapy for patients with acquired immunodeficiency syndrome and cryptococcosis: experience with 22 patients. *Am J Med* 1988;85:477–480.
259. Dismukes WE, Cloud G, Gallis HA, et al: Treatment of cryptococcal meningitis with combination amphotericin and flucytosine for four as compared to six weeks. *N Engl J Med* 1987;317:334–341.
260. Poon M, Cronin DC, Wormser GP, Bottone EJ: In vitro susceptibility of *Cryptococcus neoformans* isolates from patient with acquired immunodeficiency syndrome. *Arch Pathol Lab Med* 1988;112:161–162.
261. Sugar AM, Saunders C: Oral fluconazole as suppressive therapy of disseminated cryptococcosis in patients with acquired immunodeficiency syndrome. *Am J Med* 1988;85:481–489.
262. Byrne WR, Wajszczuk CP: Cryptococcal meningitis in the acquired immunodeficiency syndrome (AIDS): successful treatment with fluconazole after failure of amphotericin B (letter). *Ann Intern Med* 1988;108:384–385.
263. Diamond RD, Bennett JE: Prognostic factors in cryptococcal meningitis. *Ann Intern Med* 1974;80:176–181.
264. Cuadrado LM, Guerrero A, Lopez Garcia Asenjo JA, et al: Cerebral mucormycosis in two cases of the acquired immunodeficiency syndrome. *Arch Neurol* 1988;45:109–111.
265. Micozzi MS, Wetli CV: Intravenous amphetamine abuse, primary cerebral mucormycosis, and acquired immunodeficiency. *J Forensic Sci* 1985;30:504–510.
266. Petito CK, Cho ES, Lemann W, et al: Neuropathology of acquired immunodeficiency syndrome (AIDS): an autopsy review. *J Neuropathol Exp Neurol* 1986;45:635–646.
267. Wong B, Gold JWM, Brown AE, et al: Central nervous system toxoplasmosis in homosexual men and parenteral drug abusers. *Ann Intern Med* 1984;100:36–42.
268. Wanke C, Tuazon CU, Kovacs A, et al: Toxoplasma encephalitis in patients with acquired immunodeficiency syndrome: diagnosis and response to therapy. *Am J Trop Med Hyg* 1987;36:509–516.
269. Bia FJ, Barry M: Parasitic infections of the central nervous system. *Neurol Clin* 1986;171–206.
270. Navia BA, Petito CK, Gold JW, et al: Cerebral toxoplasmosis complicating the acquired immune deficiency syndrome: clinical and neuropathological findings in 27 patients. *Ann Neurol* 1986;19:224–238.
271. Nath A, Jankovic J, Pettigrew LC: Movement disorders and AIDS. *Neurology* 1987;37:37–41.
272. Leport C, Vilde JL, Katlama C, et al: Toxoplasmose cerebrale de l'immunodeprime: diagnostic et traitement. *Ann Med Interne* 1987;138:30–33.
273. Holland GN, Enstrom RE Jr, Glasgow BJ, et al: Ocular toxoplasmosis in patients with the acquired immunodeficiency syndrome. *Am J Ophthalmol* 1988;106:653–667.
274. Tschihart D, Klatt EC: Disseminated toxoplasmosis in the acquire immunodeficiency syndrome. *Arch Pathol Lab Med* 1988;112:1237–1241.
275. Touboul JL, Salmon D, Lancastre F, et al: Toxoplasma gondii pneumopathy in a patient with the acquired immunodeficiency syndrome: demonstration of the parasite by bronchioalveolar lavage. *Rev Pneumol Clin* 1986;42:150–152.
276. Israelski DM, Skowron G, Leventhal JP, et al: Toxoplasma peritonitis in a patient with acquired immunodeficiency syndrome. *Arch Intern Med* 1988;148:1655–1657.
277. Nistal M, Santana A, Paniaqua L, et al: Testicular toxoplasmosis in two men with acquired immunodeficiency syndrome (AIDS). *Arch Pathol Lab Med* 1986;110:744–746.
278. Hirschmann JV, Chu AC: Skin lesions with disseminated toxoplasmosis in patient with the acquired immunodeficiency syndrome (letter). *Arch Dermatol* 1988;124:1446–1447.
279. Post MJD, Chan JC, Hensley GT, et al: Toxoplasma encephalitis in Haitian adults with acquired immunodeficiency syndrome: a clinical-pathologic-CT correlation. *AJNR* 1983;4:155–162.

280. Nolla-Salas J, Ricart C, D'Olhaberriague L, et al: Hydrocephalus: an unusual CT presentation of cerebral toxoplasmosis in a patient with acquired immunodeficiency syndrome. *Eur Neurol* 1987;27: 130–132.
281. Krol G, Becker R, Zimmerman R, et al: Contribution of MRI to the diagnosis of intracranial complications of acquired immune deficiency syndrome. *Neuroradiology* 1986;?:99–104.
282. Levy RM, Rosenbloom S, Perrett LV: Neuroradiologic findings in AIDS: a review of 200 cases. *AJR* 1986;147:977–983.
283. Jarvik JG, Hesselink JR, Kennedy C, et al: Acquired immunodeficiency syndrome. Magnetic resonance patterns of brain involvement with pathologic correlation. *Arch Neurol* 1988;45:731–736.
284. Farkash AE, Maccabee PJ, Sher JH, et al: CNS toxoplasmosis in acquired immunodeficiency syndrome: a clinical-pathological-radiological review of 12 cases. *J Neurol Neurosurg Psychiatry* 1986; 49:744–748.
285. Luft BJ, Brooks RG, Conley FK, et al: Toxoplasmic encephalitis in patients with acquired immune deficiency syndrome. *JAMA* 1984;252:913–917.
286. Weiss LM, Udem SA, Tanowitz H, Wittner M: Western blot analysis of the antibody response of patients with AIDS and toxoplasma encephalitis: antigenic diversity among *Toxoplasma* strains. *J Infect Dis* 1988;157:7–13.
287. Potasman I, Resnick L, Luft BJ, Remington JS: Intrathecal production of antibodies against *Toxoplasma gondii* in patients with toxoplasmic encephalitis and the acquired immunodeficiency syndrome (AIDS). *Ann Intern Med* 1988;108:49–51.
288. Hofflin JM, Remington JS: Tissue culture isolation of *Toxoplasma* from blood of a patient with AIDS. *Arch Intern Med* 1985;145:925–926.
289. DeMent SH, Cox M, Gupta PK: Diagnosis of central nervous system *Toxoplasma gondii* from the cerebrospinal fluid in a patient with acquired immunodeficiency syndrome. *Diagn Cytopathol* 1987; 3:148–151.
290. Threlkeld MG, Graves AH, Cobbs CG: Cerebrospinal fluid staining for the diagnosis of toxoplasmosis in patients with the acquired immune deficiency syndrome (letter). *Am J Med* 1987;83:599–600.
291. Horowitz S, Bentson JR, Benson DF, et al: CNS toxoplasmosis in acquired immunodeficiency syndrome. *Arch Neurol* 1983;40:649–652.
292. Huang TE, Chou SM: Occlusive hypertrophic arteritis as the cause of discrete necrosis in CNS toxoplasmosis in the acquired immunodeficiency syndrome. *Hum Pathol* 1988;19:1210–1214.
293. Ruskin J, Remington JS: Toxoplasmosis in the compromised host. *Ann Intern Med* 1976;84:193–199.
294. Haverkos HW: Assessment of therapy for toxoplasma encephalitis. The TE study group. *Am J Med* 1987;82:907–914.
295. Sahai J, Heimberger T, Collins K, et al: Sulfadiazine-induced crystalluria in a patient with acquired immunodeficiency syndrome: a reminder. *Am J Med* 1988;84:791–792.
296. Leport C, Raffi F, Matheron B, et al: Treatment of central nervous system toxoplasmosis with pyrimethamine/sulfadiazine combination in 35 patients with the acquired immunodeficiency syndrome: efficacy of long term continuous therapy. *Am J Med* 1988;84:94–100.
297. Rolston KV, Hoy J: Role of clindamycin in the treatment of central nervous system toxoplasmosis. *Am J Med* 1987;83:551–554.
298. Danneman BR, Israelski DM, Remington JS: Treatment of toxoplasmic encephalitis with intravenous clindamycin. *Arch Intern Med* 1988;148:2477–2482.
299. Wiley CA, Safrin RE, Davis CE, et al: Acanthamoeba meningoencephalitis in a patient with AIDS. *J Infect Dis* 1987;155:130–133.
300. Barin F, M'Boup S, Denis F, et al: Serological evidence for cirus related to simian T-lymphotropic retrovirus III in residents of West Africa. *Lancet* 1985;2:1387–1389.
301. Clavel F, Guetard D, Brun-Vezinet F, et al: Isolation of a new human retrovirus from West African patients with AIDS. *Science* 1986;233:343–346.
302. Clavel F, Mansinho K, Chamaret S, et al: Human immunodeficiency virus type 2 infection associated with AIDS in West Africa. *N Engl J Med* 1986; 316:1180–1185.
303. Editorial: HIV-2 in perspective. *Lancet* 1988;1: 1027–1028.
304. Centers for Disease Control: AIDS due to HIV-2 infection—New Jersey. *MMWR* 1987;37:33–35.
305. Centers for Disease Control: Update: HIV-2 infection—United States. *MMWR* 1989;38:572–580.
306. Clavel F: Editorial review: HIV-2, the West African AIDS virus. *AIDS* 1987;1:35–40.
307. Denis F, Leonard G, Sangare A, et al: Comparison of 10 enzyme immunoassays for detection of antibody to human immunodeficiency virus type 2 in West African sera. *J Clin Microbiol* 1988;26:1000–1004.
308. Jackson JB, Balfour HH Jr: Practical diagnostic testing for human immunodeficiency virus. *Clin Microbiol Rev* 1988;1:124–138.
309. Schochetman G, Ou C-Y, Jones WK: Polymerase chain reaction. *J Infect Dis* 1988;158:1154–1157.
310. Ancelle R, Bletry O, Baglin AG, et al: Long incubation period for HIV-2 infection. *Lancet* 1987;1:688–689.
311. Klemm E, Schneweis KE, Horn R, et al: HIV-II

infection with initial neurological manifestation. *J Neurol* 1988;235:304–307.
312. Belec L, Martin PM, Georges-Courbot MC, et al: Dementia as the primary manifestation of HIV-2 infection in a Central African patient. *Ann Inst Pasteur Virol* 1988;139:291–294.
313. Brun-Vesinet F, Katlama C, Roulot D, et al: Lymphadenopathy-associated virus type 2 in AIDS and AIDS-related complex. *Lancet* 1987,1:128–132.
314. Simpson JF: Listeria monocytogenes meningitis: an opportunistic infection. *J Neurol Neurosurg Psychiatry* 1971;34:657–663.
315. Gantz NM, Myerowitz RL, Medeiros AA, et al: Listerosis in immunosuppressed patients. A cluster of eight cases. *Am J Med* 1975;58:627–643.
316. Chernik NL, Armstrong D, Posner JV: Central nervous system infections in patients with cancer: changing patterns. *Cancer* 1977;40:268–274.
317. Hooper DC, Pruitt AA, Rubin RH: Central nervous system infection in the chronically immunosuppressed. *Medicine* 1982;61:166–188.
318. Gray ML, Killinger AH: *Listeria monocytogenes* and listeric infections. *Bacteriol Rev* 1966;30:573.
319. Neiman RE, Lorber B: Listeriosis in adults: a changing pattern. Report of eight cases and review of the literature, 1968–1978. *Rev Infect Dis* 1980;2:207–227.
320. Weinstein AJ, Schiavone WA, Furlan AJ: Listeria rhomboencephalitis—report of a case. *Arch Neurol* 1982;39:514–516.
321. Lavetter A, Leedom JM, Mathies AW, et al: Meningitis due to Listeria monocytogenes. A review of 25 cases. *N Engl J Med* 1971;285:598–603.
322. Armstrong D: Listeria monocytogenes, in Mandell GL, Douglas RG Jr, Bennett JE (eds): *Principles and Practice of Infectious Diseases,* 2nd ed, New York, John Wiley & Sons, 1985, pp 1179–1182.
323. Watson GW, Fuller TJ, Elms J, Kluge RM: Listeria cerebritis: relapse of infection in renal transplant patients. *Arch Intern Med* 1978;138:83–87.
324. Fetter BF, Klintworth GK, Hendry WS: *Mycosis of the Central Nervous System,* Baltimore, Williams & Wilkins, 1967.
325. Causey WA, Lee R: Nocardia, in Vinken PJ, Bruyn GW (eds): *Handbook of the Clinical Neurology,* Vol 35, Amsterdam, North Holland Publishing Co, 1978, pp 517–530.
326. Law BJ, Marks MI: Pediatric nocardiosis. *Pediatrics* 1975;55:135.
327. Byrne E, Brophy BP, Pettett LV: Nocardia cerebral abscess: new concepts in diagnosis, management, and prognosis. *J Neurol Neurosurg Psychiatry* 1979;42:1038.
328. Scowden EB, Schaffner W, Stone WJ: Overwhelming strongyloidiasis: an unappreciated opportunistic infection. *Medicine* 1978;57:527–544.
329. Purtilo DT, Meyers WM, Connor DH: Fatal strongyloidiasis in immunosuppressed patients. *Am J Med* 1974;56:488.
330. Price RW, Navia BA: Infections in AIDS and in other immunosuppressed patients, in Kennedy PGE, Johnson RT (eds): *Infections of the Nervous System.* London, Butterworths, 1987, pp 247–273.
331. Lukes SA, Posner JB, Nielsen S, Armstrong D: Bacterial infection of the CNS in neutropenic patients. *Neurology* 1984;34:269–275.

21
Neurologic Manifestations of Lyme Disease

JOHN J. HALPERIN

The identification of *Borrelia burgdorferi* as the tick-borne pathogen responsible for Lyme disease[1–3] has rekindled interest in spirochetal diseases of the nervous system for the first time since penicillin threatened to relegate neurosyphilis to obscurity. Anecdotal reports have suggested that this novel organism might be responsible for neurologic disorders affecting the cerebral cortex, skeletal muscle, and all points in between. Reports in the lay press have implied that this is a health menace of plaguelike proportions. However, the true spectrum of problems caused by this infection remains to be defined.

Even before *B burgdorferi* was first isolated in 1982, it was apparent that several seemingly disparate clinical phenomena tended to occur together following bites by *Ixodes* ticks. In 1909, Afzelius recognized what has come to be considered the pathognomic rash, erythema chronicum migrans (ECM). This large, erythematous lesion, which develops at the site of a tick bite, is typically quite large (5–10 cm in diameter or more). It persists for days to weeks, typically continuing to enlarge, often clearing centrally as it grows. Nonspecific signs of a systemic infection, such as low-grade fever, lymphadenopathy, and malaise, are often present as well. In a significant proportion of patients, the rash becomes multicentric, representing dissemination of infection. There is some evidence (E. Asbrink, personal communication) that this dissemination is often also accompanied by meningeal seeding—a significant proportion of patients with multifocal ECM may have a cerebrospinal-fluid (CSF) pleocytosis. As more and more patients with *B burgdorferi* infection have been recognized, it has become clear that the cutaneous manifestations may be even more pleomorphic and more evanescent; therefore, it is now becoming customary to refer to the rash as erythema migrans (EM) instead of ECM.

Once the infection disseminates, other organ systems frequently become involved. Joint pain, and subsequently large-joint oligoarticular arthritis, are quite common. Heart block of varying degrees (rarely, accompanied by myocarditis) is not infrequent. Some patients develop evidence of a mild hepatitis. Particularly common is involvement of the nervous system, producing a wide variety of different signs and symptoms. Almost 70 years ago, it was first recognized that aseptic meningitis, radicular pain, and a patchy but severe neuropathy could develop following tick bites.[4] Subsequent European reports elaborated considerably on this,[5,6] and once it was recognized that the same infection occurred in North America, it became clear that aseptic meningitis, painful radiculoneuritis, and cranial neuritis were extremely common concomitants in North America as well.[7,8] Then, with the identification of *B burgdorferi* as the causative organism, and the subsequent rapid development of serologic tests to demonstrate exposure to it, there followed a large number of anecdotal reports trying to define the range of clinical phenomena attributable to this infection. The problem with this approach has been threefold. First, there has been little standardization of techniques used to assess serologic evidence of exposure, with different laboratories using completely different reagents, different definitions of normality, and different methods of dealing with potential false positives and false negatives. Second, in most reports, patients have had a single positive serology, without evidence of a rising or falling titer, something that at best can be taken as evidence of exposure to an antigen and not as proof of ongoing infection. There are few data indicating what proportion of patients spontaneously clear the infectious agent—that is, how many will have a positive serology because of prior exposure, but will no longer have an active infection and will have no potential for subsequent complications. Third, in highly endemic areas, anywhere between 5 and 50% of the population may have serologic evidence of exposure to *B burgdorferi*, making interpretation of a single positive serology particularly difficult.[9,10]

The reason that serodiagnosis has so dominated this field is that there are few alternatives available. The spirochetes are few and far between. Even in biopsies of the expanding edge of an EM where the organisms are known to be present, it takes a long and diligent search of meticulously prepared tissue to visualize them. Although easier to grow in vitro than their biologic cousins *Treponema pallidum*, borrelia are technically difficult to culture. This, combined with the fact that not many organisms are present circulating in accessible body fluids, makes it virtually impossible to rely on culture techniques to confirm a diagnosis. Efforts to find evidence of fragments of borrelia in either blood, CSF, or urine are at a very preliminary stage and considerable additional work will be necessary before they can be considered reliable.

Establishing causal relationships between particular neurologic disorders and this infection obviously is difficult. Sufficient epidemiologic data exist to establish some relationships but many others remain conjectural. Since biopsies have generally proved to be of limited utility, other, more indirect methods have been used to try to establish causality. One paradigm has been to apply quantitative techniques to the assessment of specific neurologic problems, treat with antimicrobials, and then requantitate to see if the abnormality consistently resolves.[11] The other, of particular use in assessment of the central nervous system (CNS), has been to seek evidence of intrathecal synthesis of anti–*B burgorderi* antibody. For this to be meaningful, it is necessary to determine simultaneously the amount of specific antibody present in both the CSF and serum, taking into account the differences in total amount of immunoglobulin present in these two fluids, and then determining if there is proportionately more specific antibody in the CSF. This technique has been validated in numerous other CNS infections, and has been shown to be quite useful in Lyme neuroborreliosis as well.[12–14] Although there undoubtedly are patients who have CNS infection without evidence of intrathecal antibody synthesis, this does seem to be a useful "gold standard" to apply to determine if particular classes of CNS process are attributable to CNS infection.

In considering the different neurologic phenomena that have been reported to occur in Lyme neuroborreliosis, it is useful to divide them in two different ways. For purposes of clinical consideration, it is most useful to separate them on an anatomic basis, considering the peripheral nervous system, central nervous system, and cranial nerves individually. For purposes of understanding pathophysiology, though, it is far more interesting to consider the biologic processes underlying the different clinical entities.

Peripheral Nervous System

The peripheral nervous system (PNS) appears to be the most common site of neurologic involvement in Lyme disease. Although peripheral nerves are protected by a blood–nerve barrier, this is generally considerably less impregnable than the blood–brain barrier, making the PNS more susceptible to insults than the CNS. Involvement of the PNS can take many clinical forms, but these probably are less dissimilar than initially meets the eye—probably, more than anything else, they reflect differences in the particular nerve bundles involved, and the severity of the infection and the immune response to it. Pathophysiologically, these "protean manifestations" are probably closely interrelated. (See Table 21.1.)

Since the initial report by Garin and Boujadoux,[4] it has been clear that a particularly common phenomenon is the development of radicular-type pain, often with associated motor weakness in the corresponding nerve-root distribution. This sciatica-like pain may occur in a limb or the trunk, and tends to arise in the limb that is the site of the tick bite. Many patients with this picture have a CSF lymphocytic pleocytosis. This, combined with the radicular char-

Table 21.1. Peripheral nervous system.

1. Presumed PNS infection:
   - Painful radiculoneuritis
   - Mononeuropathy multiplex
   - Milder disseminated neuropathy
   - Brachial and lumbosacral plexopathies
   - "Guillain-Barré–like" neuropathies
2. Neuropathy + entrapment neuropathies
3. Myositis

acter and distribution of the pain, has led to the impression that the syndrome is due primarily to a "radiculitis"—an inflammation of the nerve roots. Interestingly, though, all published pathologic studies of nerve biopsies of these patients have demonstrated prominent perivascular inflammatory infiltrates and axonal loss in peripherally located sensory nerves.[15,16] Such findings would not be expected in a process limited to the nerve roots. Similarly, neurophysiologic studies of patients with "Lyme radiculitis" have usually demonstrated more disseminated abnormalities.[17,18] The bulk of evidence to date suggests that this painful radiculitis, rather than being a process limited to the nerve roots in the subarachnoid space, is part of a disseminated multifocal neuropathy. The pathophysiology remains to be determined. Although nerve biopsies consistently demonstrate axonal loss and prominent perivascular inflammatory infiltrates, they have generally not provided evidence of vessel-wall necrosis or of deposition of complement, antibodies, or antigen, to allow further conclusions as to the underlying mechanism.

More recent work has emphasized the frequent occurrence of a much milder disseminated, neuropathy in patients with otherwise typical *B burgdorferi* infection.[19] In one study of 76 patients presenting to a Lyme Disease Clinic with primarily rheumatologic and systemic symptoms, more than a third had neurophysiologic evidence of a disseminated neuropathy.[18] Sural-nerve biopsies in several of these patients have been quite similar to those described in the more fulminant, painful radiculoneuritis, and in fact, neurophysiologic findings in these two populations are virtually identical, indicating that these two rather disparate clinical presentations are closely related pathophysiologically.[18,19] Interestingly, by analogy to syphilis, there has been a tendency to suggest that different manifestations of Lyme disease occur in separate, distinguishable stages, and, in particular, that Lyme radiculitis takes place early in the disease, whereas the more indolent neuropathies and CNS processes occur later. A detailed analysis of a large number of such patients suggests that this perception is somewhat artifactual. Patients with painful radiculitis do present to their physicians earlier in the course of their illness; however, their symptoms probably develop at about the same latency following initial infection as do the milder neuropathies. The principal difference is that patients with milder symptoms are more likely to defer seeking medical attention.[18]

Several case reports of a "Guillain-Barré–like" neuropathy have appeared, describing patients with Lyme and an acute ascending peripheral neuropathy[20–22]. In fact, in the first case described by Garin and Bujadoux, the patient had a rapidly progressive paralytic illness with loss of reflexes. These patients have generally been likened to the Guillain-Barré syndrome (GBS); however, most have differed from typical GBS in two important ways. First, in GBS, the process is, by definition, demyelinating. In none of the Lyme-associated cases where sufficient data have been presented has there been unequivocal evidence of a primarily demyelinating neuropathy. Second, in GBS, the CSF is typically acellular despite an elevated protein ("albuminocytologic dissociation"). In most of the reported cases in association with neuroborreliosis, there has been a vigorous pleocytosis. Although a few case reports remain describing typical GBS in patients with positive Lyme serologies, causality cannot be considered clearly established. If Lyme does cause a primarily demyelinating neuropathy, it would appear to be very infrequent.

Individual reports have also described the occurrence of "brachial neuritis" in patients with Lyme. Detailed analysis of a small number of such cases suggests that this actually is just a subset of patients with painful radiculitis. If the radiculoneuritis affects the distribution of the midcervical nerve roots, the clinical presentation will resemble brachial neuritis, a clinically defined entity in which there are pain and denervation in the shoulder region, suggesting an inflammation of the upper brachial plexus. Brachial neuritis is generally considered a parainfectious phenomenon, meaning that it occurs following a nonspecific infection; in patients with Lyme, it appears to be more directly related to active infection. Isolated reports of lumbosacral plexopathy can probably be explained in a similar fashion. Other studies have emphasized instances of "mononeuritis multiplex," a clinical term indicating a process involving multiple different unrelated nerves in a patchy fashion. This is precisely what is seen neurophysiologically in patients with Lyme radiculoneuritis, with the more indolent neuropathy, with the Guillain-Barré-like illness, and with brachial neuritis; that is, it appears that all of these clinically diverse phenomena are in fact slightly different presentations of the same pathophysiologic process.

Recently, considerable attention has focused on a possible association between *B burgdorferi* infection and motor-neuron disease.(MND)[23–26] Although this subject remains extremely controversial, there is some epidemiologic evidence to suggest that in hyperendemic areas, a disproportionate number of patients with MND (particularly those with a primarily lower motor-neuron–type presentation) have serologic evidence of exposure to this infection.[26] Whether these patients actually have a Lyme-related motor polyradiculitis rather than typical MND, or there is some other explanation for this observation, remains to be determined.

Finally, several case reports have appeared indicating a polymyositis-like picture in patients with Lyme.[27–29] In view of the pathology seen in other organ systems in patients with *B burgdorferi* infection, these pathologic findings would not be surprising. However, the inconsistent response to antimicrobial therapy described in these reports would appear to necessitate further work to establish a clear causal relationship between this infection and clinically significant myositis.

Cranial Nerves

It has long been recognized that *B burgdorferi* infection is commonly associated with Bell's palsy[7,8] (facial-nerve paralysis), and, in fact, Lyme disease is one of the few entities frequently associated with bilateral Bell's palsies (the others being GBS, sarcoidosis, and other basilar meningitides). As more and more patients have been seen, it has become apparent that other cranial nerves are frequently involved as well. Most Lyme patients with these other cranial neuropathies have also had a lymphocytic meningitis. In this setting, it should not be surprising that cranial nerves might become involved—these nerves must cross through the subarachnoid space, a site in which they are often damaged in other types of infectious meningitis. Particularly common is involvement of the nerves controlling extraocular movements.[30] These nerves have particularly long courses through the subarachnoid space and are prone to injury in many other disorders. According to the European literature, the eighth (acoustic/vestibular) nerve also appears to be involved frequently, as indicated in numerous descriptions of vertigo and/or deafness. This has been reported less frequently in the North American literature, but almost certainly is seen in this population too. Interestingly, very few reported series have described abnormalities of the lowest cranial nerves (IX–XII). These nerves, which control the bulbar musculature, appear to be spared, for reasons that are completely unclear.

It is quite clear that the seventh (facial) cranial nerve is the one most comonly involved. Several different factors probably contribute to this. First, as with the other cranial nerves, it is at risk of being damaged as it passes through the subarachnoid space. In addition, its long peripheral processes are commonly damaged in other types of mononeuropathy multiplex. Neurophysiologic studies in patients with Lyme-associated Bell's palsy suggest that, in many instances, the facial weakness is part of a disseminated multifocal neuropathy, rather than a result of meningitis.[18] Thus, this nerve appears to be doubly susceptible to injury in this disease that is capable of causing both meningitis and peripheral neuropathies.

Involvement of the optic nerve (II) has also been reported in patients with *B burgdorferi* infection.[31] This must be viewed with some caution, and in a somewhat different light, for several reasons. First, it must be remembered that the optic nerve is actually a CNS tract rather than a true cranial nerve. As such, its structure and environment are quite different from those of the other cranial nerves. Second, this nerve is less likely to be involved in other meningeal inflammatory processes than are other cranial nerves. Third, the meningeal processes that damage this nerve tend to produce visual-field restrictions without significantly affecting visual acuity. Thus, cases of true optic neuritis, with striking loss of visual acuity, must be due to a different pathophysiologic process, and must be considered in a different context, perhaps more closely related to the focal encephalitis that is known to occur in Lyme. For now, an association between *B burgdorferi* infection and optic neuritis must be considered possible but unproved.

Central Nervous System

Since the earliest case reports, it has been obvious that *B burgdorferi* infection causes an aseptic meningitis-like picture, with a predominantly lymphocytic pleocytosis, mild elevation of CSF protein, and ususally normal CSF glucose. Patients typically present with a severe headache, photophobia, and stiff neck, or they may have a deceptively benign clinical picture, without significant meningismus, despite a CSF pleocytosis. Often the headache can be quite chronic (weeks in duration) before the diagnosis is finally made. Symptoms may be self-limited, resolving spontaneously, but probably improve more rapidly when antimicrobials are used. This meningitis may occur in isolation, or in combination with radiculoneuritis, cranial neuritis, or encephalitis. (See Table 21.2.)

Although much less common, it is also quite clear that *B burgdorferi* infection can cause a unifocal or multifocal encephalitis. This occasionally involves gray matter, but in most instances it is the white matter that appears to be primarily involved[11]; therefore, the term "leukoencephalitis" might well be applied to this disorder. This anatomic predilection may well explain why this brain infection virtually never causes seizures. Clinically, this disorder may take one of several forms. In the European literature, there are many reports of a chronically progresive disorder, primarily manifest as a chronic spastic paraparesis that progresses over months or years, with or without additional CNS abnormalities.[32] Antimicrobial therapy may arrest the progression of this disorder, but generally recovery from acquired deficits is minimal. Examination of the CSF in these patients often provides evidence of a chronic meningoencephalitis, with a lymphocytic pleocytosis, elevation of protein, increased synthesis of immunoglobulins in the CSF, and oligoclonal bands. The last can be shown to be specific to *B burgdorferi*.[33] Moreover, it has been demonstrated that many of the lymphocytes present in these patients' CSF are B cells similarly specific for *B burgdorferi*.[34]

Other patients may present with a more fulminant encephalitis, with alteration of consciousness in addition to focal CNS abnormalities. As in patients with the more chronic form of encephalitis, brain magnetic-resonance imaging (MRI) scans may demonstrate multifocal abnormalities in the cerebral white matter;[11,35] these may resolve following antimicrobial therapy.[11] CSF again tends to be quite active with a lymphocytic pleocytosis and normal glucose, although these patients are less likely to have nonspecific increase in intrathecal immunoglobulin production, or CSF oligoclonal bands. Yet other patients may present at the other end of the spectrum, with an even more indolent progressive CNS disorder. This may present with focal abnormalities on examination and/or brain MRI, or in its mildest form, as progressive but mild cognitive decline.[11,14] (Since gray matter seems to be involved only infrequently, a direct effect on intellectual function would be expected to be inherently uncommon and mild.)

Table 21.2. Central nervous system.

1. Presumed CNS infection:
Lymphocytic meningitis
Cranial neuritis
Multifocal encephalitis
2. Without apparent CNS infection
Encephalopathy (presumed toxic/metabolic)
3. Unclear relationship
CNS vasculitis
Motor-neuron disease
4. Probably no relationship
Dementia
Multiple sclerosis

The pathophysiologic mechanisms underlying this multifocal inflammatory process remain undetermined. Brain biopsies have been performed rarely, and have generally been unhelpful. Rarely, cerebral angiography has demonstrated a large-vessel vasculitis.[36,37] Such a process might be associated with a multifocal leukoencephalitis, but the number of well-documented cases remains so small that, for now, its potential role is very unclear, at least as it pertains to most cases of neuroborreliosis.

The predilection of Lyme encephalitis for the cerebral white matter has led to repeated allusions in the literature to the similarities between this disorder and multiple sclerosis (MS). This is probably misleading and unfortunate; although it is possible to confuse this illness with a severe first episode of MS, generally neuroborreliosis does not cause a relapsing remitting illness analogous to the most common form of MS.[14] Epidemiologic studies have provided evidence that *B burgdorferi* infection is no more common among MS patients than among controls.[38] Of considerable clinical utility is the observation that most patients with CNS *B burgdorferi* infection have evidence of intrathecal synthesis of specific antibody; MS patients do not.[14] Since patients with neuroborreliosis may temporarily improve with immunosuppressive therapy, only to be more difficult to treat subsequently, it is worth looking for evidence of intrathecal synthesis of anti–*B burgdorferi* antibody in patients with a first episode of a leukoencephalitis to exclude the possibility of this infectious illness at a time when it is still potentially treatable.

Probably completely unrelated to this encephalitic process, but quite frequent in patients with Lyme disease, is a mild impairment of memory and cognition in patients with other systemic evidence of *B burgdorferi* infection (i.e., arthritis, fever, etc.).[11,39] These patients not uncommonly describe difficulty with day-to-day intellectual functioning—difficulties that can be quantitated using neuropsychologic testing and that can be shown to resolve following antimicrobial therapy. In a small proportion of these patients, this may be due to active CNS infection; in the overwhelming majority, it almost certainly represents a "toxic-metabolic" encephalopathy no different from that in numerous other systemic, non–nervous-system infections.

Finally, numerous anecdotal reports have appeared attempting to link Lyme disease with other neuropsychiatric illnesses. Since patients with Lyme commonly describe some confusion and memory difficulty, several reports have considered a possible association with dementia and Alzheimer's disease. Since it is well known that patients with early dementia may appear much worse clinically when ill with other systemic processes (pneumonia, sepsis, etc.), it certainly would not be surprising if Lyme disease might make such a patient appear worse, and perhaps even bring the patient to medical attention earlier than might have been true otherwise. However, at this point there is no evidence to suggest that this infection can cause a severe and irreversible dementing illness. Similarly, questions have been raised about a possible association between the infection and depression or other psychiatric disorders. The only systematic studies performed to date indicate, first, that seropositive patients with psychiatric illness are unlikely to have evidence (by clinical examination, CSF studies, or brain MRI scan) of CNS infection,[14] and second, that depression and other psychiatric disorders are no more prevalent among patients with *B burgdorferi* infection than among patients with other chronic medical illnesses.[39]

Therapy

The optimal treatment regimen for this infectious disease remains to be determined. When the CNS is involved, penetration of the blood–brain barrier becomes very important. Early studies used intravenous penicillin in meningeal doses, for 10–14 days.[40] In view of the relatively poor CNS penetration of this agent in the absence of substantial inflammation, it is not surprising that treatment failures occurred with some frequency. In view of this, more recent studies have focused on third-generation cephalosporins. Ceftriaxone (2 g intravenously or intramuscularly, once a day for 2 weeks) appears to be effective in many patients.[41] There is no evidence that higher doses are any more useful,[41] and, in fact, the complication rate seems to increase significantly. Patients with focal encephalitis (as evidenced by abnormal brain MRI scans, focally abnormal neurologic examinations, a CSF pleocytosis, and intrathecal synthesis of anti–*B burgdorferi* antibody) may need a longer course (4 to 6 weeks); however, these cases are so uncommon that definitive data are not yet available. Prelimary data suggest that the efficacy of cefotaxime may prove comparable. In penicillin-allergic patients, chloramphenicol has been used successfully.[42] In patients with cranial neuropathies or peripheral neuropathies (without a CSF pleocytosis or any other evidence of CNS infection), oral regimens may provide a useful alternative. Doxycycline is generally well tolerated at doses of 200–300 mg/day, and at 400 mg/day, may even achieve therapeutic levels in the CSF.[43] Amoxicillin (500–1,000 mg 3–4 times per day), with probenecid (500 mg 3 times per day), has also been used. Both regimens are often effective, and usually well tolerated. Whether or not corticosteroids should be used in combination with antibiotics remains to be determined. When used alone, they appear to increase the likelihood that patients will respond incompletely to subsequent antimicrobials, and they may increase the risk of long-term complications. Whether they may play a role in treating patients with severe CNS inflammation that either does not improve, or even worsens in the presence of appropriate antibiotics, is yet to be determined.

Conclusions

Lyme disease is a recently recognized spirochetal infection with a particular propensity for affecting the nervous system. Clinical symptoms may be quite protean; this probably represents variability in the particular structures involved and severity of infection, but not differences in the underlying pathophysiologic processes. In both the CNS and the PNS, this illness produces patchy multifocal inflammatory lesions, but the underlying mechanisms remain to be elucidated. Particularly common syndromes are a radiculoneuropathy that may be painful and focal, or mild, less symptomatic, and disseminated. Similarly, meningitis occurs frequently;

this may be mild or severe, and may be accompanied by involvement of the cranial nerves, particularly the VIIth. A multifocal leukoencephalitis also appears, and may be mild or severe. In general, CNS infection is best diagnosed by determining whether or not there is intrathecal synthesis of anti–*B burgdorferi* antibody. In the next several years, as diagnostic tools are further refined, it should become possible both to define better the range of clinical phenomena actually caused by this infection and to begin to understand the underlying pathophysiologic mechanisms.

References

1. Burgdorfer W, Barbour AG, Hayes SF, et al: Lyme disease: a tick borne spirochetosis? *Science* 1982; 216:1317–1319.
2. Benach JL, Bosler EM, Hanrahan JP, et al: Spirochetes isolated from the blood of two patients with Lyme disease. *N Engl J Med* 1983;308:740–742.
3. Steere AC, Grodzicki RL, Kornblatt AN, et al: The spirochetal etiology of Lyme disease. *N Engl J Med* 1983;308:733–740.
4. Garin, Bujadoux. Paralysie par les tiques. *J Med Lyon* 1922;71:765–767.
5. Bannwarth A. Chronische lymphcytare meningitis, entzundliche polyneuritis und "rheumtismus." *Arch Psychiatr Nervenkr* 1941;113:284–376.
6. Hellerstrom S: Erythema chronicum migrans afzelius with meningitis. *Acta Derm Venerol* 1951;31:227–234.
7. Reik L, Steere AC, Bartenhagen NH, et al: Neurologic abnormalities of Lyme disease. *Medicine* 1979; 58:281–294.
8. Pachner AR, Steere AC: The triad of neurologic manifestations of Lyme disease. *Neurology* 1985;35:47–53.
9. Hanrahan JP, Benach JL, Coleman JL, et al: Incidence and cumulative frequency of endemic Lyme disease in a community. *J Infect Dis* 1984;150:489–496.
10. Lastavica CC, Wilson ML, Beradi VP, et al: Rapid emergence of a focal epidemic of Lyme disease in coastal Massachusetts. *N Engl J Med* 1989;320:133–137.
11. Halperin JJ, Pass HL, Anand AK, et al: Nervous system abnormalities in Lyme disease. *Ann NY Acad Sci* 1988;539:24–34.
12. Wilske B, Scierz G, Preac-Mursic V, et al: Intrathecal production of specific antibodies against *Borrelia burgdorferi* in patients with lymphocytic meningoradiculitis. *J Infect Dis* 1986;153:304–314.
13. Stiernstedt GT, Granstrom M, Hederstedt B, Skoldenberg B: Diagnosis of spirochetal meningitis by enzyme linked immunosorbent assay and indirect immunofluorescense assay in serum and cerebrospinal fluid. *J Clin Microbiol* 1985;21:819–825.
14. Halperin JJ, Luft BJ, Vokman DJ, Dattwyler RJ: Lyme neuroborreliosis—central nervous system manifestations. *Neurology* 1989;39:753–759.
15. Camponovo F, Meier C: Neuropathy of vasculitic origin in a case of Garin-Bujadoux-Bannwarth syndrome with positive borrelia antibody response. *J Neurol* 1986;233:69–72.
16. Vallat JM, Hugon J, Lubeau M, et al: Tick bite meningoradiculoneuritis. *Neurology* 1987;37:749–753.
17. Graf M, Kristoferitsch W, Baumhackl U, Zeithofer J: Electrophysiologic findings in meningopolyneuritis of Garin-Bujadoux-Bannwarth. *Zbl Bakt Hyg A* 1986;263:324–327.
18. Halperin JJ, Luft BJ, Volkman DJ, Dattwyler RJ: Lyme neuroborreliosis—peripheral nervous system manifestations. *Brain* (in press).
19. Halperin JJ, Little BW, Coyle PK, Dattwyler RJ: Lyme disease—a treatable cause of peripheral neuropathy. *Neurology* 1987;37:1700–1706.
20. Sterman AB, Nelson S, Barclay P: Demyelinating neuropathy accompanying Lyme disease. *Neurology* 1982;32:1302–1305.
21. Clavelou P, Beytout J, Vernay D, et al: Neurologic manifestations of Lyme disease in the northern part of the Auvergne. *Neurology* 1989;39 (suppl 1):350.
22. Bouma PD, Carpay HA, Rijpkema SGT: Antibodies to *Borrelia burgdorferi* in Guillain-Barré syndrome. *Lancet* 1989;11:739.
23. Waisbren, BA, Cashmen N. Schell RF, Jonson R: *Borrelia burgdorfeir* antibodies and amyotrophic lateral sclerosis. *Lancet* 1987;11:332–333.
24. Fredrikson S, Link H: CNS borreliosis selectively affecting central motor neurons. *Acta Neurol Scand* 1988;78:181–184.
25. Mandell H, Steere AC, Reinhardt BN, et al: Lack of antibodies to *Borrelia burgdorferi* in patients with amyotrophic lateral sclerosis. *N Engl J Med* 1984; 320:255–256.
26. Halperin JJ, Kaplan GP, Brazinsky S, et al: Immunologic reactivity against *Borrelia burgdorferi* in patients with motor neuron disease. *Arch Neurol* 1990;47:586–594.
27. Schmutzhard E, Willeit J, Gerstenbrand F: Meningopolyneuritis Bannwarth with focal nodular myositis. *Klin Wochenschr* 1986;64:1204–1208.
28. Wokke JHJ, de Koning J, Stanek G, Jennekens FGI: Chronic muscle weakness caused by *Borrelia burgdorferi* meningoradiculitis. *Ann Neurol* 1987;22:389–392.
29. Atlas E, Novak SN, Duray PH, Steere AC: Lyme myositis: muscle invasion by *Borrelia burgdorferi*. *Ann Int Med* 1988;109:245–246.

30. Stiernstedt G, Gustafsson R, Karlsson M, et al: Clinical manifestations and diagnosis of neuroborreliosis. *Ann NY Acad Sci* 1988;539:46–55.
31. Steere AC, Duray PH, Danny JH, et al: Unilateral blindness caused by infection with Lyme disease spirochete *Borrelia burgdorferi*. *Ann Int Med* 1985; 103:382–384.
32. Ackermann R, Gollmer E, Rehse, B Kupper: Progressive borrelia encephalomyelitis. Chronic manifestation of erythema chronicum migrans disease of the nervous system. *Dtsch Med Wochenschr* 1985;110:1039–1042.
33. Martin R, Martens U, Sticht-Groh V, et al: Persistent intrathecal secretion of oligoclonal, *Borrelia burgdorferi* specific IgG in chronic meningoradiculomyelitis. *J Neurol* 1988;235:229–233.
34. Baig S, Olsson T, Link H: Predominance of *Borrelia burgdorferi* specific B cells in CSF in neuroborreliosis. *Lancet* 1989; 11:71–74.
35. Sindic CJM, Depre A, Bigaignon G, et al: Lymphocytic meningoradiculitis and encephalomyelitis due to *Borellia burgdorferi*. *J Neurol Neurosurg Psychiatry* 1987;50:1565–1571.
36. Uldry PA, Regli F, Bogousslavsky J: Cerebral angiopathy and recurrent strokes following *Borrelia burgdorferi* infection. *J Neurol Neurosurg Psychiatry* 1987;50:1703–1704.
37. Veenedaal-Hilbers JA, Perquin WVM, Hoogland PG, Doornbos L: Basal meningovasculitis and occlusion of the basilar artery in two cases of *Borrelia burgdorferi* infection. *Neurology* 1988;38:1317–1319.
38. Schmutzhard E, Pohl P, Stanek P: *Borrelia burgdorferi* antibodies in patients with relapsing-remitting form and chronic progressive form of multiple sclerosis. *J Neurol Neurosurg Psychiatry* 1988;51:1215–1218.
39. Krupp LB, LaRocca NG, Luft BJ, Halperin JJ: Comparison of neurologic and psychologic findings in patients with Lyme disease and chronic fatigue syndrome. *Neurology* 1989;39(suppl 1):144.
40. Steere AC, Pachner AR, Malawista SE: Neurologic abnormalities of Lyme disease: successful treatment with high-dose intravenous penicillin. *Ann Int Med* 1983;99:767–772.
41. Dattwyler RJ, Halperin JJ, Volkman DJ, Luft BJ: Treatment of late Lyme disease. *Lancet* 1988; 1:1191–193.
42. Diringer, MN, Halperin JJ, Dattwyler RJ: Lyme meningoencephalitis—report of a severe, penicillin-resistant case. *Arthritis Rheum* 1987;30:705–708.
43. Dotevall L, Hagberg L: Penetration of doxycycline into CSF in patients treatee for suspected Lyme neuroborreliosis. *Antimicrob Agents Chemother* 1989;33:1078–1080.

Part V
Diagnosis

22
Diagnostic Imaging of CNS Infection and Inflammation

BRIAN C. BOWEN AND M. JUDITH DONOVAN POST

When intracranial or spinal infection is suspected clinically, the primary imaging studies that are most often requested to help in diagnosis and treatment are computed tomography (CT) and magnetic resonance (MR). While the choice of one modality over the other as the initial study is sometimes determined by the type of infection suspected, it often depends on the patient's clinical condition (critically or not, requiring life-support systems or not), availability (whether MR imaging (MRI) available, or whether MRI or CT is available sooner), and medical economics (a routine CT examination is currently about one half to one third as expensive as an unenhanced MRI study).

As will be evident from this chapter, MRI is, in general, the preferred modality for imaging central-nervous-system (CNS) infection and inflammation. Intracranially, when one or a few space-occupying lesions are present, both CT and MRI may be equally sensitive. However, in the detection of subtle, non–mass-producing lesions (especially white-matter lesions), multifocal or diffuse processes, and complications such as ischemia/infarction, hemorrhage, hydrocephalus, and extra-axial fluid collections, MRI is proving to be more sensitive than CT. Similarly, MRI is usually more sensitive than CT in the detection of intraspinal soft-tissue masses and abnormalities of the spinal cord.

The greater sensitivity of MRI is due in part to its direct multiplanar capability, without the image degradation in sagittal and coronal planes that occurs with reconstructed CT images, and in part to the relative absence of signal from bone, which, because it is dense, causes x-ray CT attenuation artifacts that often limit evaluation of intracranial soft tissues (in the posterior fossa, middle cranial fossa, and near the vetex) and intraspinal soft tissues (cord, epidural space).

However, MRI is more sensitive primarily because it images water protons, which are present in great abundance and are often markedly altered as to local amount and physical state when there is CNS infection with associated inflammation, edema, and/or demyelination. In general, it is the long TR (recovery time)/long TE (echo delay time) (T2-weighted) images that have more contrast resolution and better detect pathology, while it is the short TR/short TE (T1-weighted) images that have better spatial resolution and better delineate morphology.*

Although the long TR/long TE images are more sensitive, short TR/short TE images obtained after intravenous (IV) gadolinium administration are more specific, because areas of enhancement indicate sites of blood–brain-barrier breakdown, associated with an active process, as they do on contrast-enhanced CT.

When comparing CT with unenhanced MR images, it may be helpful to remember that an area of inflammation and edema that is hypodense on CT

---

*Statements regarding MRI refer to spin-echo proton MRI performed at approximately 0.5–1.5 Tesla, unless otherwise stated. For simplicity, spin-echo MR images are described as long TR/long TE, long TR/short TE, or short TR/short TE, rather than as T2-weighted, proton-density-weighted, or T1-weighted images, respectively, although the terms may be used interchangeably in general. Long TR refers to TR = 1,500–3,000 ms and short TR to TR = 300–800 ms, approximately. Long TE refers to TE = 80–120 ms and short TE to TE = 10–30 ms, approximately. The MRI intravenous contrast agent used routinely for CNS imaging is gadopentetate dimeglumine (Berlex Laboratories, Inc., Wayne, N.J.), referred to as gadolinium-DTPA, or simply gadolinium.

will usually appear as hypointense on short TR/short TE MRI and as hyperintense on long TR/long TE MRI relative to normal surrounding brain, and that contrast-enhanced CT and contrast-enhanced, short TR/short TE MRI will have similar enhancement patterns (e.g., nodular or ring).

If a patient is unable to cooperate or to remain still for intervals of a few minutes, then CT is preferable to spin-echo MRI because there is less motion artifact. Individual slices on cranial CT scans can be obtained in a few seconds, while long TR/long TE spin-echo MRI requires approximately 5 minutes per slice, although multiple slices are acquired almost simultaneously. However, gradient-echo slices, which may have satisfactory spatial resolution and yet are not strictly T1- or T2-weighted, can be acquired in a few seconds, and thus can sometimes allow MRI with less severe motion artifacts.

As discussed in the chapter, cases of CNS infection in which hemorrhage is suspected are often better imaged by MRI, as long as one is aware that the appearance of hemorrhage varies with time (acute, subacute, chronic), and that the evolution of signal abnormalities for extracerebral hemorrhage does not follow the same time course as that of intracerebral hemorrhage.

Where CT has proved superior to spin-echo MRI is in the detection of calcification, which can improve sensitivity and specificity in the detection of suspected granulomatous and parasitic infection. The sensitivity of MRI can be improved by using gradient-echo sequences. In cases of posttraumatic infection, CT can demostrate the site of fracture (e.g., cranial vault or base of skull) at which the infection develops.

CT plays an important role in diagnostic needle-aspiration biopsy of spinal infection and stereotactic aspiration of intracranial inflammatory masses. Yet the recent commercial availability of MRI-compatible needles should result in more diagnostic aspirations being done with MR guidance.

Angiography no longer plays a primary role in the workup of CNS infection and inflammation; however, it is often necessary in those cases where vasculitis and aneurysm formation are suspected complications. A modality that is not used in the initial workup, but is a valuable adjunct to treatment, is intraoperative ultrasonography, which facilitates the identification and treatment of both intracranial and spinal/paraspinal cystic and solid masses.

New developments in MRI and CT are already contributing to the evaluation of patients with CNS infection. For example, in cases of communicating versus obstructive hydrocephalus secondary to infection, cardiac-gated, sagittal MRI may be used to assess cerebrospinal-fluid (CSF) flow dynamics in the third and fourth ventricles and through the aqueduct. MR angiography is rapidly being developed and has the potential to show vascular complications associated with infection. Three-dimensional reconstructions from MR or CT cross-sectional images are being used to facilitate surgical treatment of intracranial and spinal lesions. Combined with the exquisite sensitivity of routine MRI, these new developments should add further to the significant advance in imaging of CNS infection and inflammation that began with the application of x-ray CT.

Intracranial Infection

Pyogenic Bacterial Infection

The most commonly encountered forms of bacterial infection of the CNS are meningitis, cerebritis/abscess, and extra-axial (subdural/epidural) empyema.

Meningitis

Leptomeningitis may be acute, subacute, or chronic, and it may be suppurative or nonsuppurative, depending on the pathogen (Figure 22.1).[1] In acute suppurative meningitis, pyogenic organisms reach the pia-arachnoid by hematogenous spread, by direct spread from an adjacent infection (such as otorhinologic infection), or by direct inoculation accompanying penetrating injury. Hematogenous spread is the most common route, and most of these cases in immune-competent patients are due to one of three organisms: *Hemophilus influenzae, Streptococcus pneumoniae,* or *Neisseria meningitis.*[1,2] In neonates, *Streptococcus agalactias* (group B streptococci and gram-negative rods, especially *Escherichia coli* and *Citrobacter* strains) are the principal pathogens.[3]

Pathologically, there is acute inflammation of the pia-arachnoid, with accompanying vascular engorgement and dilatation, and the subarachnoid space becomes distended by the inflammatory exudate. Several complications may ensure. The subpial cortex and the ependymal lining of the ventricles may become involved in the inflammatory process,

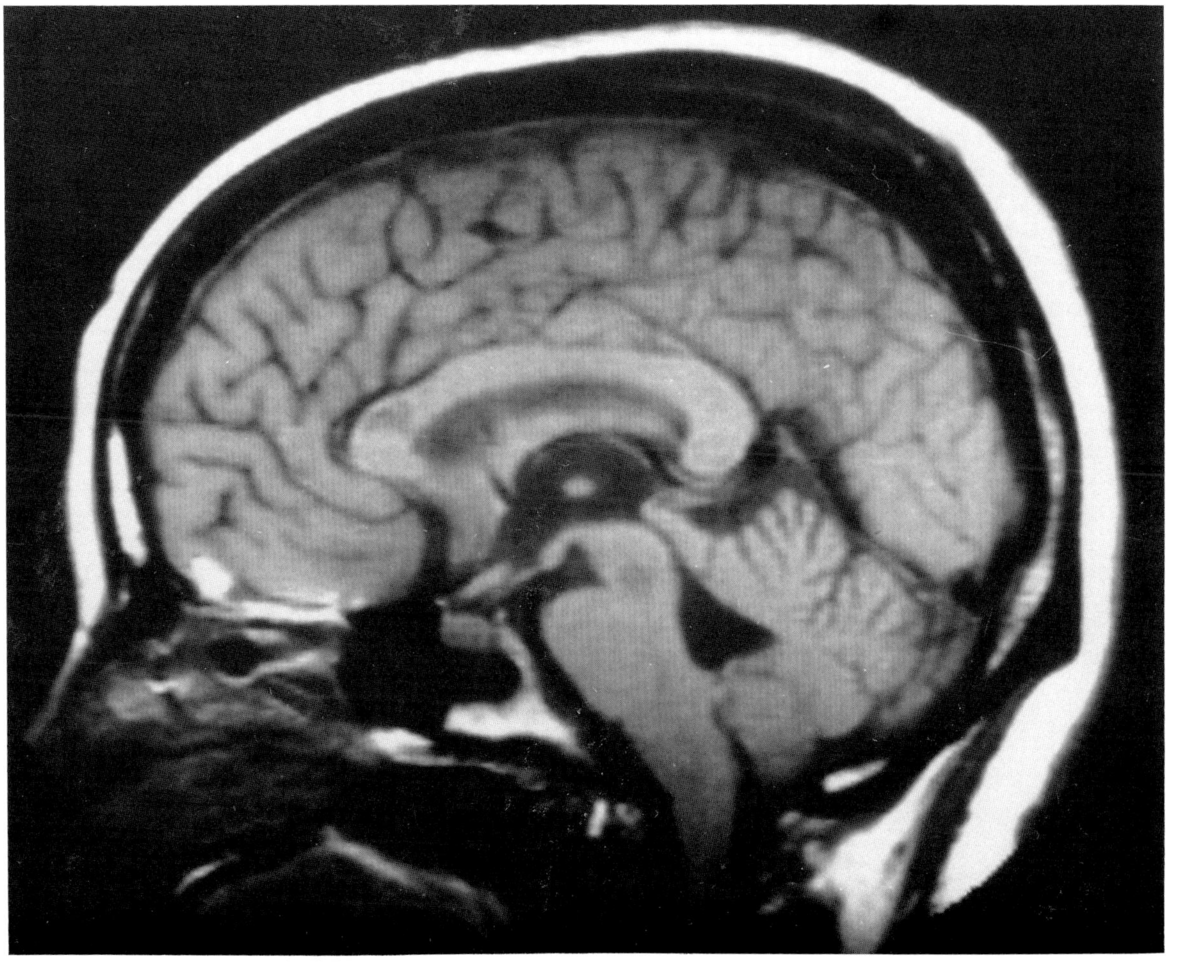

A

Fig. 22.1. Chronic meningitis with communicating hydrocephalus and brain stem infarct. (A) Pregadolinium short TR/short TE (800 msc/20 msc) sagittal scan shows focal hypointensity at pontomesencephalic junction. No abnormal signal intensity is evident in the basal cisterns. (B) Postgadolinium short TR/short TE (800/20) sagittal scan shows abnormal enhancement (arrowheads) of meninges anterior to pons and medulla, within the guadrigeminal cistern, and at the outlet of the fourth ventricle. Normal enhancement of the vein of Galen and dural venous sinuses is noted. There is no enhancement of the pontomesencephalic hypointense focus. (C) Postgadolinium short TR/short TE (800/20) axial scan shows enhancement (arrowheads) in the basal cisterns anterior and to the left of the upper pons. As in (B), there is no enhancement of the infarct. There is mild ventricular enlargement.

resulting in cerebritis and/or ventriculitis. Blood vessels exposed to the subarachnoid inflammatory exudate may undergo spasm and/or thrombosis leading to infarction, either arterial or venous, and sometimes hemorrhagic. Cortical infarction, with accompanying disruption of the pia, facilitates the spread of infection into the brain parenchyma, which is normally protected by the pial barrier. Depending on the extent of involvement and complications, there can be diffuse or localized cerebral edema with marked mass effect. Necrosis and breakdown of the arachnoid permit formation of a subdural collection that may or may not be infected, depending on the success of treatment.[4] Hydrocephalus attributable to blockage of CSF pathways by the subarachnoid exudate may occur at any time, but usually develops in the subacute or chronic phase of infection.

In the patient with suspected acute bacterial meningitis, CT or MRI is used to detect the complications described above. Uncomplicated acute meningitis usually produces no abnormal CT find-

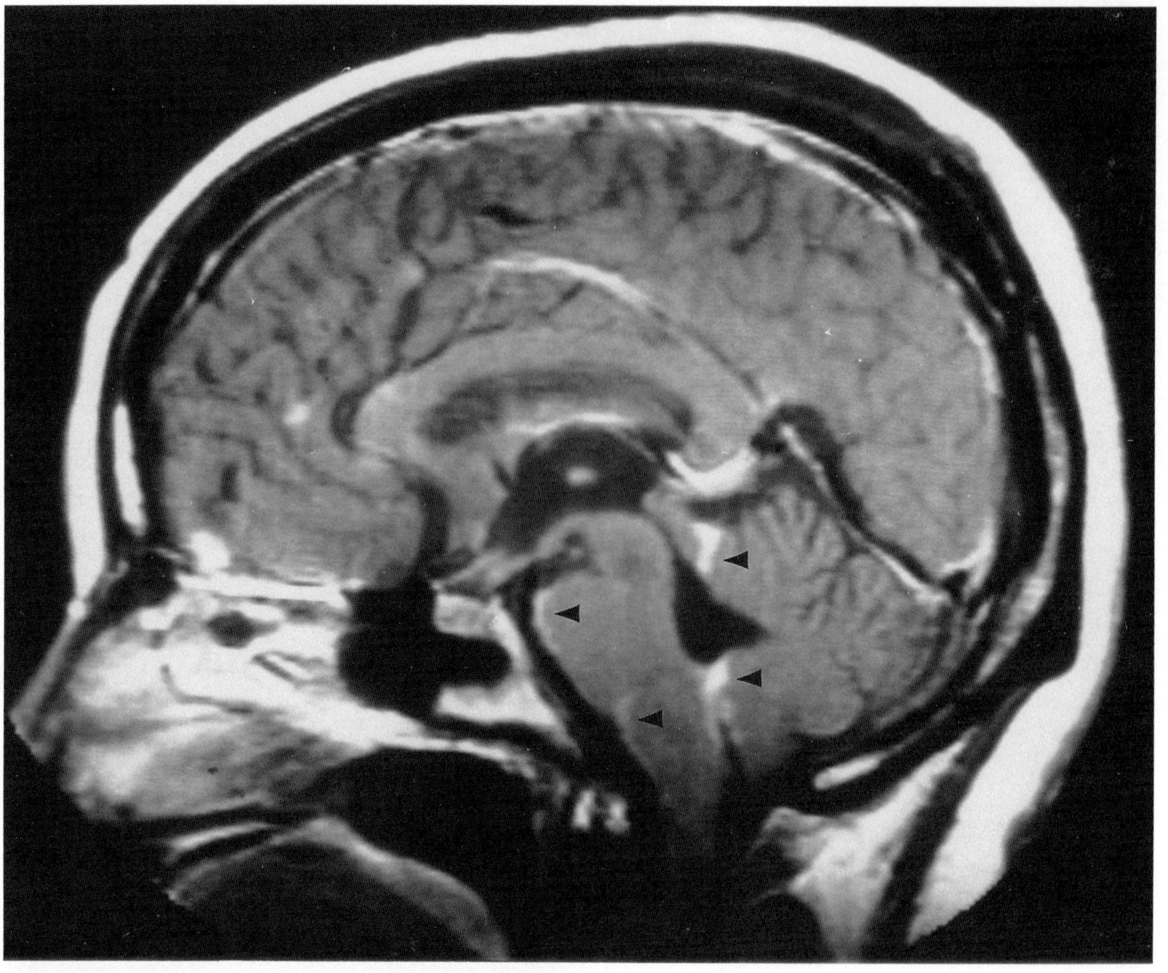

B

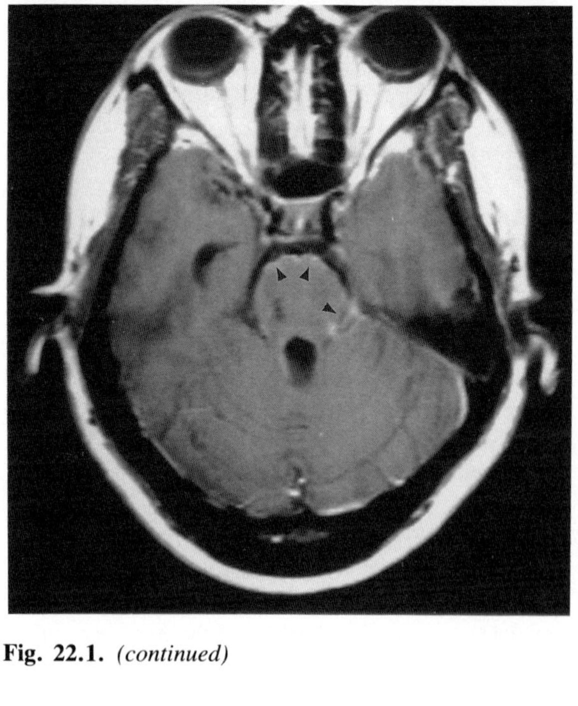

C

Fig. 22.1. *(continued)*

ings.[5,6] With severe meningitis, the earliest finding is reported to be the distention of the subarachnoid space, often best seen along the interhemispheric fissure.[4] Later, CT without IV contrast may show increased density in basal cisterns and interhemispheric fissures, and loss of definition of the sulci over the convexities.[7] The combination of cortical vascular congestion and white-matter edema may accentuate the attenuation differences between cortical gray matter and subcortical white matter. If there is marked diffuse brain swelling, the lateral and third ventricles are compressed and very small.[7] With IV contrast, there is prominent meningeal enhancement with a bandlike or gyral pattern. This enhancement is attributed to the meningeal hyperemia and vascular congestion, as well as to the breakdown of leptomeningeal capillaries (blood–meningeal barrier) and leakage of contrast from newly formed capillaries into the subarachnoid space.[8-10]

CT demonstrates the pattern and degree of ventricular enlargement. Hydrocephalus may be either communicating or obstructive, and is a complication seen more frequently in children than in adults. Diffuse or localized areas of low attenuation within the brain parenchyma on noncontrast CT scans of patients with acute meningitis are most likely to represent one or more of the following complications: edema, arterial or venous occlusion, cerebritis.[11] Occlusion of small perforating arteries results in focal infarcts in the basal ganglia, while spasm of anterior or middle cerebral arteries can lead to massive infarctions. Cortical venous occlusions, with or without dural venous thrombosis, result in low-density areas, which do not conform to an expected arterial distribution, in the subpial cortex and the underlying white matter, sometimes with irregular hyperdensities representing acute hemorrhage. A favored site for this complication is near the vertex secondary to superior sagittal sinus thrombosis.[12] Cerebritis frequently appears as a cortical and subcortical, poorly demarcated zone of low density, indistinguishable from edema (see discussion below). On contrast-enhanced CT scans, an area of cerebritis may show heterogeneous enhancement; however, so may subacute infarction.[13] Hydrocephalus is a complication seen more frequently in children than in adults.[2] It may be either communicating or obstructive, and CT helps to differentiate these two types because it demonstrates the pattern and degree of ventricular enlargement. When ventriculitis accompanies meningitis, there is either regional or diffuse contrast enhancement of thickened ependyma, appearing as a thin line of marked enhancement conforming to the ventricular border (Figure 22.2).[14] This is usually associated with a decrease in density of the adjacent periventricular white matter, representing edema[4] or possibly cerebritis. Irregularity in contour of the ventricular margins is another reported CT finding in patients with ventriculitis.[15] Obstructive hydrocephalus and intraventricular- or periventricular-cyst formation, resulting from ependymal inflammation with associated adhesions and septations, are well demonstrated by CT (Figure 22.2).[16,17] "Trapping" or a portion of the ventricles, such as the temporal horn or fourth ventricle, may appear as an expanding low-density mass.[18]

Subdural fluid collection as a complication of acute meningitis is usually seen as a crescentric zone of low density in the extra-axial space. When the collection is an effusion, such as in association with *H influenzae* meningitis in children, its density will be equivalent to CSF, and it will not have an enhancing membrane. Subdural effusions can be bilateral and are usually adjacent to the frontal and parietal lobes.[11] As a late result, the wall of an effusion may demonstrate calcification.[19] If the collection is an empyema, its shape may be elliptical and its density may be slightly greater than CSF. With IV contrast, CT shows an enhancing membrane bordering the collection (see discussion below).[20]

As with CT, MRI of patients with uncomplicated acute bacterial meningitis usually produces no abnormal findings.[5,21] However, recent experimental studies of *Staphylococcus aureus* meningitis in dogs showed that gadolinium-enhanced, short TR/short TE MRI demonstrates abnormal leptomeningeal enhancement that more closely approximates the extent of inflammatory cell infiltration than does CT.[22] Enhancement with gadolinium more likely is due to blood–meningeal abnormalities than to the presence of contrast agent in vessels. Spin-echo MRI is probably better than CT in displaying the early finding of distended subarachnoid space because of MR's direct multiplanar imaging capability.[4]

Unenhanced MRI and gadolinium-enhanced MRI are also proving better at detecting or depicting the complications of meningitis—hydrocephalus, infarction, cerebritis/abscess, ventriculitis, subdural empyema/effusion.[22] Obstructive hydrocephalus is demonstrated equally well by CT and axial MRI, however, short TR/short TE sagittal MR images with or without gadolinium enhancement allow direct evaluation of midline structures for such abnormalities as aqueduct narrowing and occlusion. CSF dynamics can be displayed cinematographically.[23] Long TR (short or long TE) images are the most sensitive for detecting periventricular CSF accumulation secondary to ventricular obstruction and demonstrate bilateral areas of hyperintensity. Similar periventricular hyperintense areas may be seen in cases of ependymitis without ventricular obstruction; however, in these cases, gadolinium-enhanced short TR/short TE images would show ependymal enhancement.

Cortical and subcortical ischemic infarctions, appearing as areas of increased signal intensity, are detected earlier and better by MRI than by CT.[24] Hemorrhagic infarctions have a characteristic appearance on long TR/long TE images depending on their age, with the areas of hemorrhage being decreased in intensity acutely and increased sub-

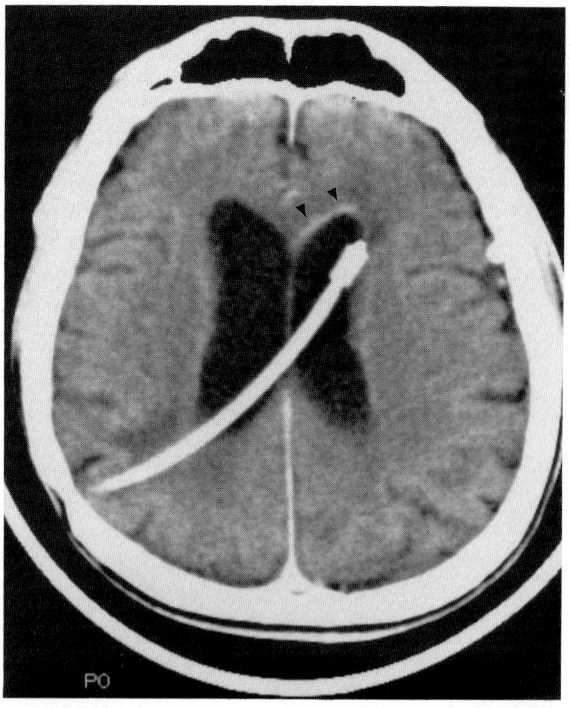

A

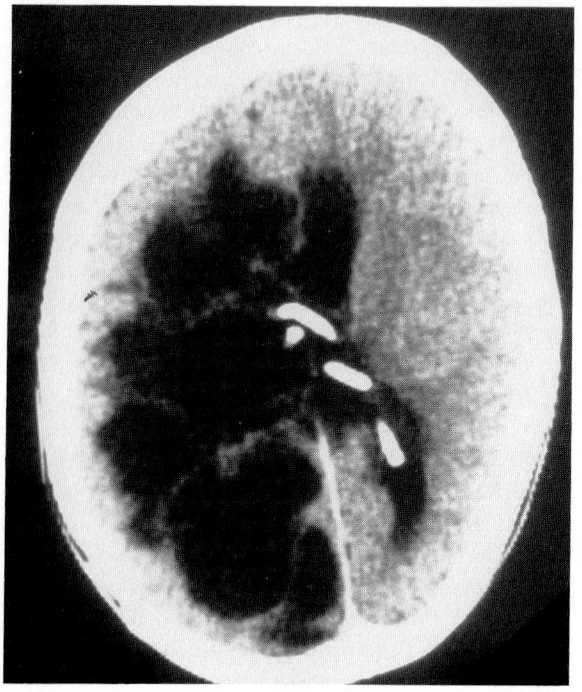

C

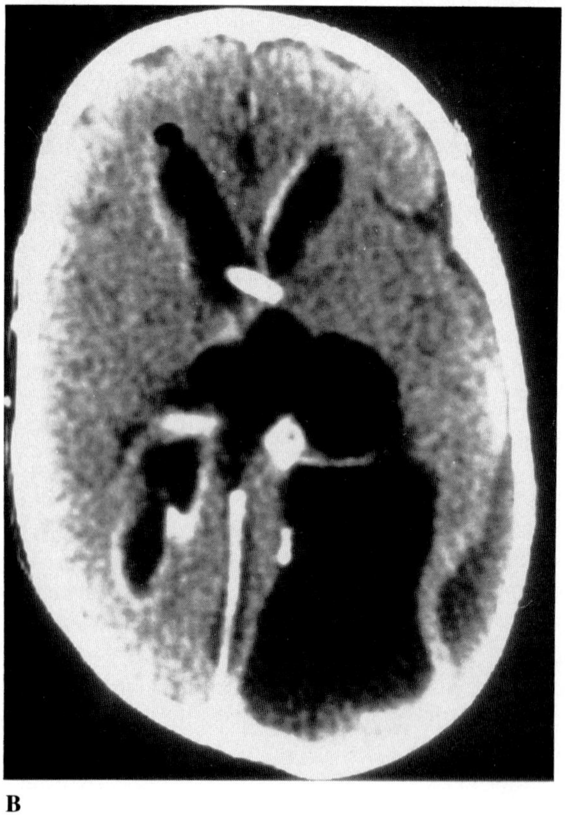

B

Fig. 22.2. Ventriculitis (ependymitis) with associated complications. (A) Shunt-related infection. A 74-year-old man, with a ventriculoperitoneal shunt for six years, presented with fever and confusion, and was found to have an *Enterobacter* bacteremia. Postcontrast CT shows a thin enhancing band (arrowheads) along the anterior margin of the left lateral ventricle (adjacent to the tip of the shunt catheter) compatible with ventriculitis and hydrocephalus. (B) Ventriculitis with periventricular-cyst formation. A three-month-old girl with gram-negative bacterial meningitis developed hydrocephalus. Postcontrast CT shows diffuse enhancement of the ventricular margins and enlarged ventricles. The area with CSF density located posteriorly in the left hemisphere is a large periventricular cyst. Several shunt catheters were placed. Also note the extra-axial collection along the left temporal convexity. (C) Periventricular-cyst formation. A six-year-old boy with *E coli* meningitis/ventriculitis. Precontrast CT shows enlargement of lateral ventricles with periventricular cystic spaces in the right hemisphere. Multiple shunt catheters are present. (Cases B. and C. are courtesy of Dr. Tom Naidich, Baptist Hospital, Miami, Fla.)

acutely, whereas on short TR/short TE images, intensity increases with evolution from the acute to the subacute phase.[24,26] Gadolinium enhancement of subacute infarcts in MRI mimics iodinated contrast enhancement in CT. Major vessels that are narrowed or occluded may be identified by either spin-echo[27] or gradient-recalled-echo[28] MRI when there is an absence or alteration of expected flow-related phenomena.

Long TR/long TE MR images very sensitively depict edema and cerebritis as poorly defined areas of increased intensity. As tissue necrosis develops, the area of cerebritis develops a central zone with a lower intensity than the surrounding edema (see below).[5]

Subdural collections are detected sooner and their extent is better demonstrated by MRI than by CT because the multiplanar imaging and the lack of signal from bone. By nonenhanced MRI, effusion should sometimes be distinguishable from empyema since effusion will have signal characteristics identical to CSF while empyema with high protein content will not (see below).[29] Also, long TR/long TE images may show areas of hyperintensity in the cortex, representing inflammatory changes, adjacent to an empyema.

Extra-axial Empyemas

Pyogenic infection may involve either the epidural or, more frequently, the subdural space, or both together, resulting in a fluid collection containing pus. Collectively, these extra-axial empyemas are not very common, occurring one half[30] to one fourth as often as intracerebral abscesses.[29,32] Otorhinologic infection is the most common cause, accounting for 65–90% of cases.[30,32,33] The mechanism of spread is either by retrograde thromboplebitis via bridging emissary veins or by direct spread of osteomyelitis.[34,35] Alternatively, extra-axial empyema may develop as a result of previous trauma (penetrating injury or infection of subdural hematoma) or infection of a craniotomy site. Less commonly, empyemas occur as complications of meningitis or bacteremia.[32]

While empyemas arising secondary to previous surgery or trauma are often indolent clinically, those resulting from sinusitis or mastoiditis frequently have a rapid course, with seizures, focal deficits, and obtundation, progressing to coma.[5,20,36] Subdural empyema should be considered a neurosurgical emergency, and CT or MRI is essential to early diagnosis. Mortality associated with subdural empyema, which was approximately 40% in the pre-CT era,[19,20] now approaches 10%,[5] although some series report 25%[33] and 25–40%[37] mortality since the advent of CT.

Epidural empyema or abscess is typically an illdefined, lentiform extra-axial area of low or intermediate density on unenhanced CT scans. Subdural empyema appears as a lentiform or crescentric area of low density slightly greater than or equal to CSF density. Sometimes it may be difficult to distin-

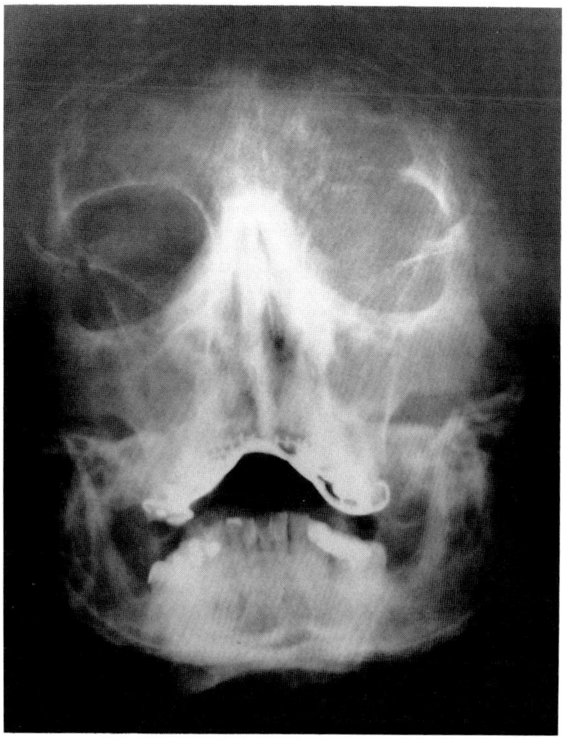

A

Fig. 22.3. Bilateral frontal sinus mucopyoceles and epidural abscesses. An 81-year-old man with a history of sinusitis and left periorbital cellulitis. (A) Conventional Water's view shows opacified paranasal sinuses. The margins and midline septum of the frontal sinuses are unsharp and in some places are disrupted. There is also poor delineation of the left orbital roof. These findings indicate bone erosion. (B) Postcontrast CT demonstrates opacified fronal sinuses with focal destruction of the posterior wall of the right frontal sinus (bilateral posterior wall dehiscence was found a surgery) with bilateral, isodense, rim-enhancing, lentiform extra-axial masses (arrows). Cultures of the purulent fluid removed at surgery grew *Pseudomonas aeruginosa*. The bilateral periventricular white-matter hypodense areas, with focal infarcts, represent unrelated vascular disease.

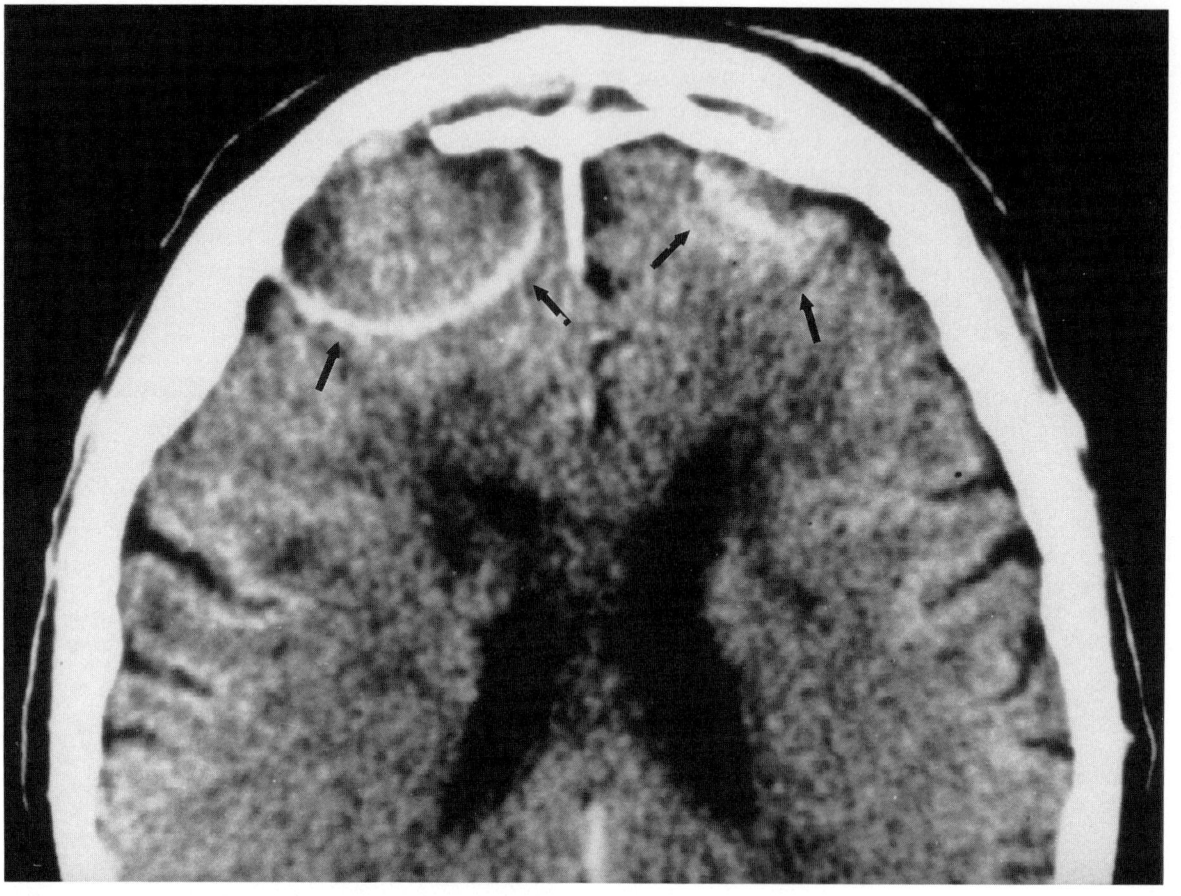

B

Fig. 22.3. *(continued)*

guish the two. If the extra-axial collection is continuous across the midline, displacing the falx inward, or across the tentorium, then the collection is epidural. Subdural empyema is most commonly located over the cerebral convexity and is frequently bilateral.[20,38] The next more common location is the interhemispheric and parafalcine subdural space, often resulting from extension from a convexity collection.[20] A paratentorial location is the least common.[7,39] Subdural empyema may be isodense by noncontrast CT and suspected only because of diffuse mass effect with compression of underlying cerebral ventricular structures.[36] An important CT finding in cases of extra-axial empyema is prominent enhancement of its margin (Figures 22.3 and 22.4). For convexity collections, enhancement of the medial margin is seen.[20] In subdural empyema, marked enhancement is due to formation of a membrane of granulomatous tissue on the leptomeninges and inflammation in the subjacent cerebral cortex.[39] The enhancing zone is typically thin and uniform, but may be thicker in chronic subdural empyema. Interhemispheric subdural empyema demonstrates marked enhancement of its margin continuous with the falx, which appears thickened, and less prominent enhancement of the margin along the cerebral cortex (Figure 22.4).[20,32] The marked degree of enhancement seen with empyema rarely occurs with subdural hematoma, and is a key differential finding.[20] However, chronic subdural hematoma that has undergone several episodes of rehemorrhage may show prominent rim enhancement.

CT often demonstrates additional findings important to the diagnosis and management of extra-axial empyema. Opacification of paranasal sinuses and/or mastoid air cells, periorbital and intraorbital inflammatory changes, calvarial destruction attributable to osteomyelitis, and subgaleal abscess are

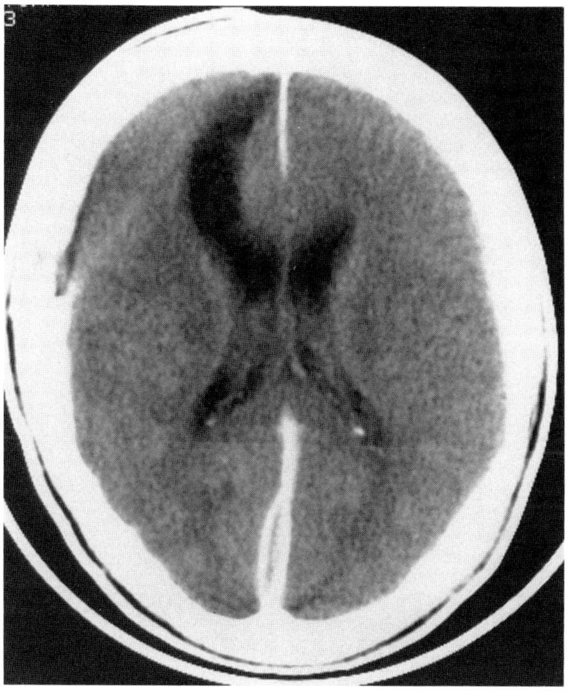

Fig. 22.4. Chronic subdural empyema. A 22-year-old man had surgery for a right frontal subdural empyema and right frontal-lobe abscess, secondary to frontal sinusitis, four weeks prior to this CT scan. Cultures of abscess fluid grew *Streptococcus milleri*. The postcontrast CT scan, obtained while the patient was receiving IV antibiotics, shows a posterior interhemispheric fissure collection with marked enhancement of its margins and apparent thickening of the falx. There is postoperative encephalomalacia/porencephaly in the right frontal lobe.

clues to be sought (Figure 22.3).[14] Abnormalities demonstrated by plain CT in the brain parenchyma underlying subdural empyema (SDE) result from retrograde thrombophlebitis and may appear early. They include slightly increased density and thickening of the cortex caused by hyperemia and low density of the white matter due to edema, with resultant swelling and diffuse mass effect.[20] With IV contrast, diffuse gyral enhancement often occurs, facilitating differentiation from subdural hematoma.[20] When the underlying cortex has predominantly low attenuation with mass effect, this may represent infarction or cerebritis (Figure 22.5).

The value of CT in the early diagnosis of SDE has been controversial.[33,36,37,40,41] MRI is now preferred because the presence and extent of extra-axial collections are better detected.[29] The increased sensitivity and specificity are due to direct multiplanar imaging, increased contrast resolution between brain and CSF, and the fact that bone has negligible signal intensity because of a paucity of mobile protons. Furthermore, subdural and epidural empyema may be differentiated because only the later has a hypointense rim, representing displaced dura, at the interface between the collection and the brain on both short and long TR images.[29] On short TR images, convexity and interhemispheric collection appear hypointense relative to brain and hyperintense relative to CSF. On long TR sequences, the collections characteristically become hyperintense to brain, while remaining hyperintense to or approaching isointensity with CSF. These signal characteristics are typical of a proteinaceous fluid with T1 and T2 values intermediate between gray matter/white matter and CSF. The signal intensity of the collection may not be markedly different from underlying brain if significant edema is present, secondary to ischemia/infarction and/or early cerebritis. In the early stages of SDE, long TR MRI can demonstrate a thin hyperintense convexity and interhemispheric collection not visible by CT.[5] Paratentorial and subtemporal extensions are well demonstrated in coronal images. MRI is superior to CT in demonstrating the sulcal effacement and parenchymal abnormalities that can develop.[29] Long TR images, which are very sensitive in detecting abnormal amounts of tissue water, may show cortical hyperintensities that are reversible and are thought to represent edema caused by reversible ischemia produced by inflammatory vasospasm and venous stasis.[5,29] Since MRI detects edema resulting from ischemia/infarction within the first few hours of its onset,[24] edema associated with cerebritis should be detected much earlier by MRI than by CT. Gradient-recalled MRI and spin-echo MRI have the ability to display cortical vein and/or dural sinus thrombosis,[28,42,43] and also demonstrate the characteristic signal properities of acute and subacute hemorrhagic infarctions (see earlier discussion).[25,65]

Chronic subdural hematoma (weeks to months old) may be differentiated from SDE since the former is usually hyerintense relative to the latter on both short and long TR images, owing to the presence of extracellular methemoglobin and iron.[26]

Finally, MRI is highly sensitive in identifying inflammatory changes in the paranasal sinuses and mastoid air cells, usually as areas of high signal

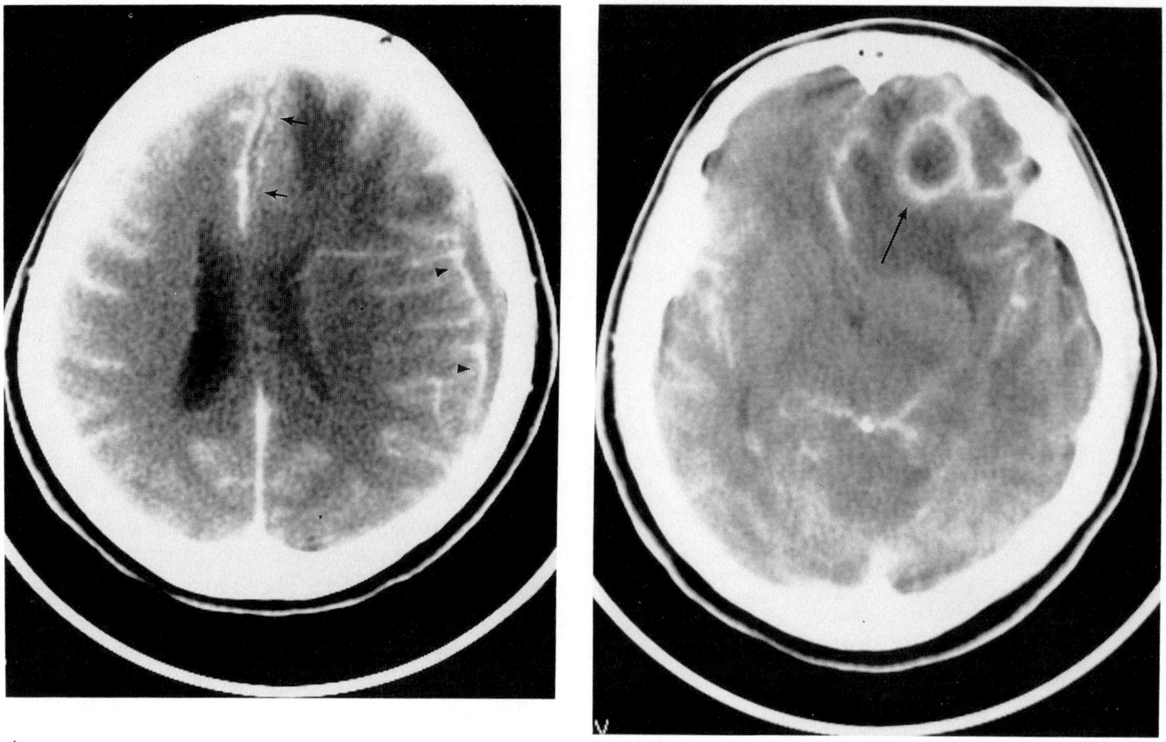

A B

Fig. 22.5. Subdural empyema and left-frontal-lobe abscess. A 40-year-old woman with left frontal sinusitis and periodontal disease presented with a right hemiparesis and the inability to speak. (A) Post contrast CT scan shows an isodense to hypodense, crescentic extra-axial collection along the left parietal convexity and a thinner collection in the anterior interhemispheric fissure. There is prominent enhancement (arrowheads) along the medial margin of the convexity collection and along the anterior falx, with less prominent enhancement of the left lateral margin (short arrows) of the interhemispheric collection. (B) Postcontrast CT scan, at a level 3 cm inferior to (A), shows a ring-enhancing mass (long arrow) with central low density, representing an abscess, in the left frontal lobe. An anterolateral, adjacent hypodense area with peripheral irregular enhancement, representing abscess or cerebritis, extends to the inner table of the frontal bone. Diffuse hypodensity in the left frontal deep white matter represents vasogenic edema. Gram stain of the abscess fluid revealed a mixture of gram-positive cocci and gram-negative rods, although no organisms were cultured.

intensity on long TR/long TE images,[45,46] and as peripheral, prominent enhancement on gadolinium-enhanced short TR/short TE images.[46]

Cerebritis/Abscess

Cerebritis represents the earliest stage of localized infection of the brain parenchyma with pyogenic organisms. Pathologically, there is a poorly demarcated area of parenchymal softening with scattered necrosis, vascular congestion, edema, and perivascular inflammatory infiltrates and petechial hemorrhages.[1,47] Cerebritis, if unsuccessfully treated medically, can progress to mature abscess formation. Commonly, cerebritis results from hematogenous spread of infection from an extracranial source or direct spread of infection, either otorhinologic infection or meningitis, that may involve retrograde septic thrombophlebitis.

CT findings are nonspecific. A poorly circumscribed zone of low attenuation with mass effect is identified by plain CT and may show minimal heterogeneous enhancement.[48] Because of its greater sensitivity to alterations in tissue water, MRI with long TR/long TE spin-echo sequences is better able to detect early cerebritis, which is seen as an area of hyperintensity.[4] On short TR/short TE images, the same area is isointense or slightly hypointense to adjacent normal brain parenchyma. If multiple areas are involved, they are better demonstrated by multiplanar long TR/long TE sequences. Mass effect, manifested as sulcal effacement or ventricular distortion, is better demonstrated using short TR/short TE or long TR/short TE sequences. These sequences also show areas of subacute hemorrhage as hyperintense relative to normal and edematous brain. On long TR images, the focus of early cerebritis may be indistinguishable from surrounding edema or may be seen as a central area of slightly lower signal intensity.[5] The results of gadolinium enhancement have not yet been reported in detail.

An abscess results when the central zone of necrosis within an area of cerebritis becomes liquefied, better defined, and encircled by a collagen capsule, which itself is surrounded by a prominent zone of gliosis.[1,47] The evolutionary process, described by Enzmann and colleagues[47] in studies on dogs, produces histologic and CT-scan changes that are continuous over a 14-day period, yet can be divided into four stages: early cerebritis, late cerebritis, early capsule formation, and late capsule formation. During the progression from early cerebritis to late cerebritis, the poorly marginated area of acute inflammation surrounding a necrotic center increases in size, yet becomes better defined. Neovascularization occurs at the edge of the necrotic center, and near these blood vessels, there is reticulin plus minimal amounts of collagen derived from endothelial cells. However, fibrous collagen bridging between vessels is not prominent until the stage of early capsule formation, when there is a well-defined margin to the liquified necrotic center, as well as a decrease in size of the surrounding area of cerebritis and edema. Gliosis in the adjacent parenchyma becomes more apparent in proceeding from the early to late capsule-formation stages. In the late capsule-formation stage, the collagen capsule becomes more complete (about 1 mm thick in the experimental studies), yet is less well developed on the ventricular side than on the cortical side. The asymmetry in development is attributed to fewer vessels being present on the ventricular (white-matter) side, thus reducing potential collagen production and available bridging sites.[47] The necrotic center decreases in size and the area of cerebritis extends only minimally beyond the capsule in this final stage. There are decreased edema and mass effect with prominent gliosis outside the capsule. Also, daughter abscesses become apparent during this stage.

CT findings corresponding to the histologic changes described above are characteristic,[47] and have been shown to correlate well with findings for human-brain abscesses.[49-52] Ring enhancement is seen in the late cerebritis stage, as well as in the early and late capsule-formation stages. In the late cerebritis stage, immediate postcontrast scans show ring enhancement, which correlates with the annular area of cerebritis, with delayed filling in the lucent center. In the capsule-formation stages, as the abscess matures, the enhancing ring has a progressively smaller diameter and maximal enhancement occurs earlier following contrast injection, with no filling of the lucent center in delayed scans.[47,52] Also, as the abscess matures, both the size of the surrounding area of edema and the degree of mass effect decrease.

Brain abscesses in humans likely go through the same evolutionary stages, although the time varies from 2 weeks to months.[1,6,47,53] The mature abscess has an inner layer of granulation tissue, a middle layer of collagen, and an outer layer of reactive astrogliosis.[6,54] Abscesses arising from hematogenous spread are most often caused by anaerobic, or a mixture of anaerobic and aerobic, bacteria.[1,53,55,56] Abscesses in patients with previous trauma or who have undergone a neurosurgical procedure are usually due to *S aureus*.[1,53] In children, staphylococci, streptococci, and pneumococci are the most common pathogens.[1,4,53]

Most patients present in the late cerebritis or mature-abscess stage.[5] In more than 50% of cases of hematogenously disseminated infection, a solitary abscess is found, which is usually located at the gray-matter/white-matter junction in the distribution of the anterior or middle cerebral arteries, that is, most commonly in the frontal and parietal lobes.[1] Cerebellar abscesses constitute 2–14% of all brain ascesses, and CT scanning identifies the presence of hydrocephalus, an important prognostic factor (Figure 22.6).[57,58]

By plain CT, an abscess appears as a circumscribed area of low density, occasionally with a surrounding, slightly hyperdense rim.[50,51,59] Corresponding to the experimental model, a contrast-enhancing peripheral ring is seen.[31,60,61] It is usually smooth and thin walled (on the order of 5 mm in thickness), and often is thinner along the medial margin.[6,13,47,48] The differential diagnosis for a ring-enhancing lesion includes high-grade astrocytoma (glioblastoma), metastasis, infarction (bland or septic), resolving hematoma, thrombosed aneurysm, arteriovenous malformation, and other inflammatory conditions (granuloma).[2,62-65] Findings

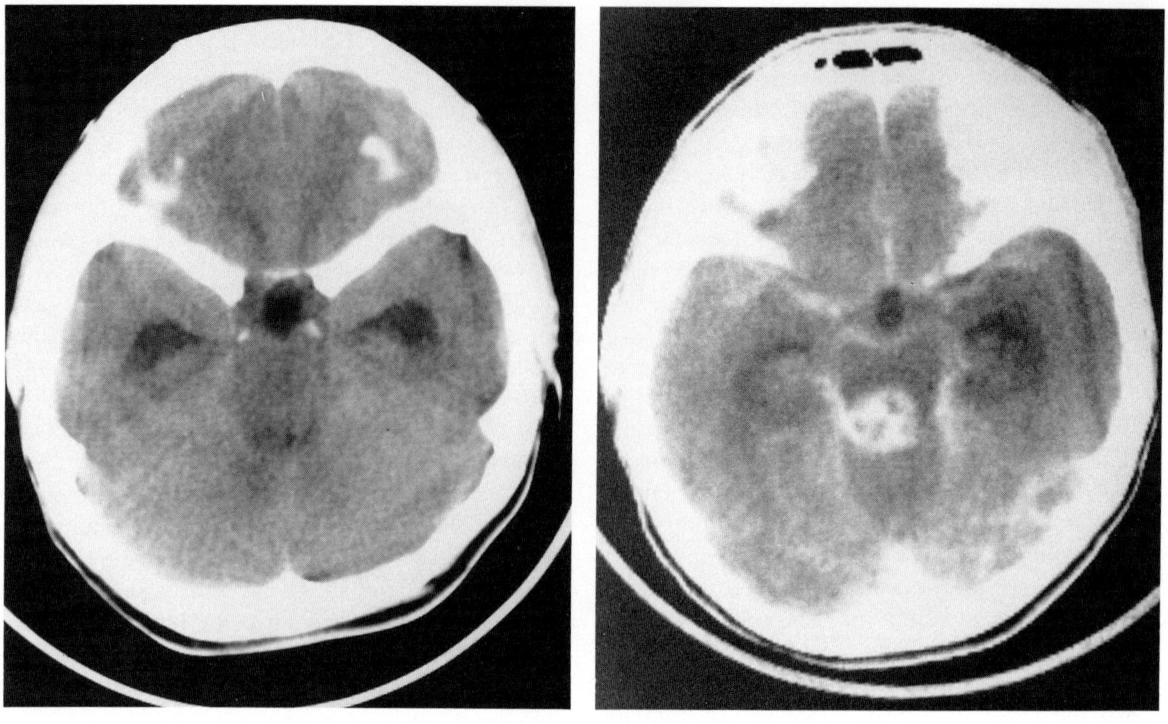

A B

Fig. 22.6. Intraventricular and periventricular nocardial abscess, with obstructive hydrocephalus. (A) Precontrast CT scan demonstrates an ill-defined hypodense area in the region of the upper portion of the fourth ventricle, aqueduct, and midbrain. There is complete obliteration of the perimesencephalic cisterns and enlargement of the third and lateral ventricles. (B) Postcontrast CT shows inhomogeneous enhancement of a rounded mass in the region of the fourth ventricle and aqueduct.

helpful in the differential include the pattern of enhancement, particularly medial thinning of ring enhancement and the presence of daughter rings (Figure 22.7), time course, location, ependymal and/or meningeal enhancement, and the presence of extracerebral-fluid collection (Figure 22.5).[2,7,49]

Daughter abscesses appear as contiguous enhancing rings, often along the medial margin (Figure 22.7). As expected from the experimental model of abscess evolution, various forms of enhancement—such as nodular or solid, incomplete thin ring, or thick and irregular ring—may be observed and have been reported.[49,66] When an abscess ruptures into a ventricle and ependymitis develops, there is coexistent ring enhancement and adjacent ventricular wall enhancement, heralding a poor prognosis.[7]

Edema in the white matter around an abscess is identified by CT in 80–90% of cases,[50] and the volume of edematous white matter is often greater than that of the abscess, thus causing much of the associated mass effect.[7] The false-negative rate for the CT diagnosis of abscess is reported to be only 0–1%.[30,60,67]

The accepted treatment for mature brain abscess is surgical drainage and/or excision, whereas cerebritis and some other types of abscess may be managed medically (antibiotics, steroids).[48,49,52,68] In cases of daughter-abscess formation, intraoperative ultrasound guidance is recommended to ensure that all abscesses are identified and drained (Figure 22.7) For brain-stem abscess, CT-guided stereotactic aspiration has been advocated.[69]

In patients receiving steroid or antibiotic therapy, decreased ring enhnacement of an abscess has been reported.[7,49,61,68,70,71] When an abscess has been successfully treated surgically or medically, serial CT scans will show a decrease in the edema, mass effect, and degree of enhancement with time. A

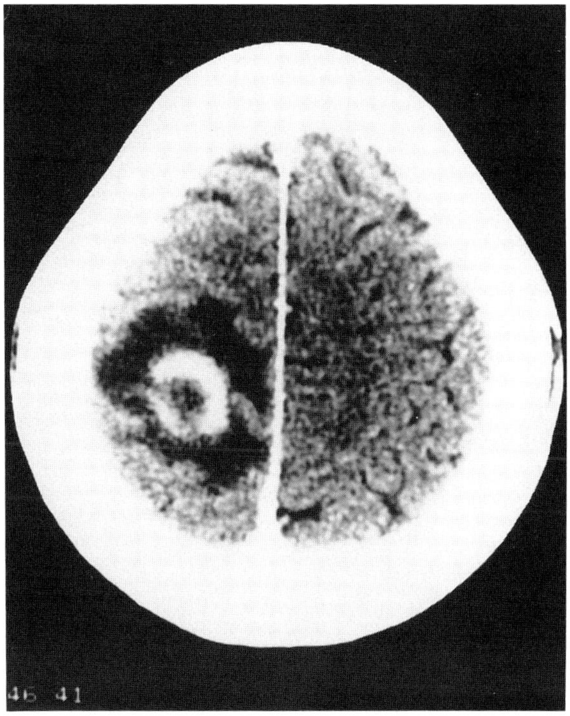

A

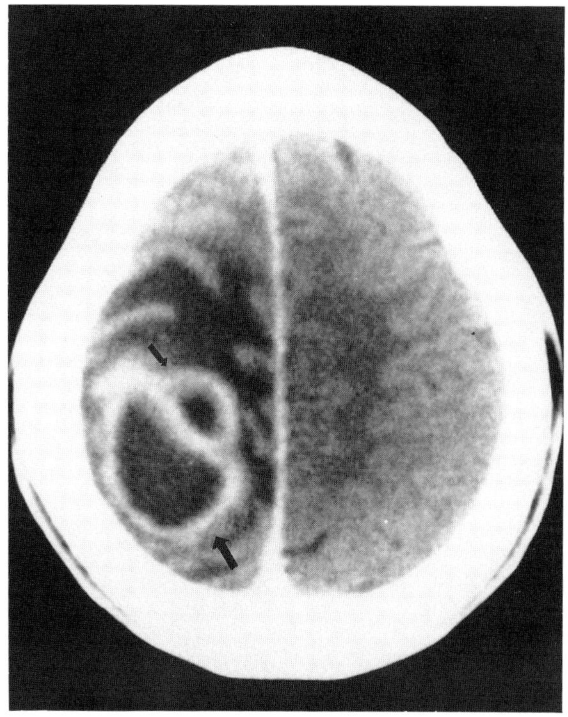

B

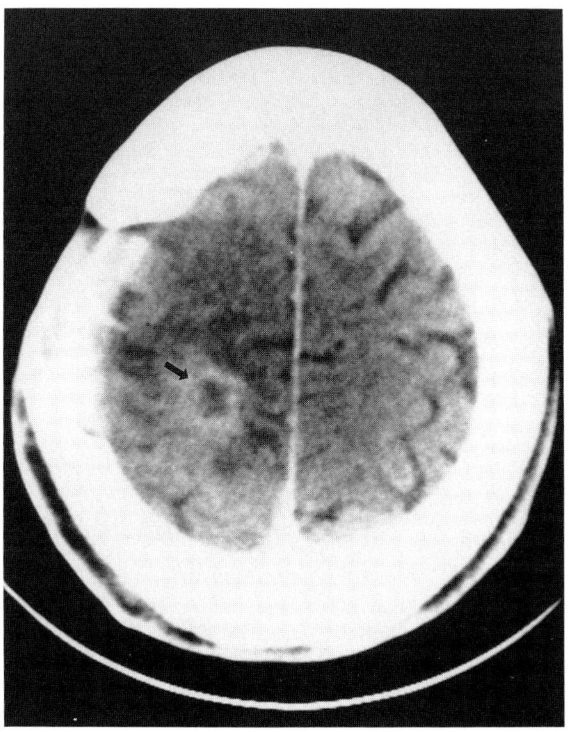

C

Fig. 22.7. Right-parietal-lobe parent and daughter abscesses. A 40-year-old man with severe periodontal disease presented with a focal seizure (involving the left arm), which progressed to a generalized tonic–clonic seizure. (A) Initial postcontrast CT scan shows a 2.5-cm-diameter mass with central hypodensity and thick ring enhancement, as well as surrounding edema, in the right parietal lobe near the gray-matter/white-matter junction. (B) Preoperative, postcontrast CT scan obtained 11 days later shows an increase in size of the original mass (parent abscess, large arrow) and the development of a similar, adjacent mass (daughter abscess, small arrow). The extent of vasogenic edema has increased. (C) Postcontrast CT scan obtained one month after abscess drainage. The larger abscess is no longer present; however, there is persistent ring enhancement at the site (small arrow) of the daughter abscess, despite postoperative IV antibiotic treatment. Anaerobic and aerobic organisms were cultured from the abscess fluid removed at surgery. The daughter abscess was not identified at surgery, and likely was not drained. For this reason, intraoperative ultrasonography is recommended to monitor surgical drainage of intracranial abscesses.

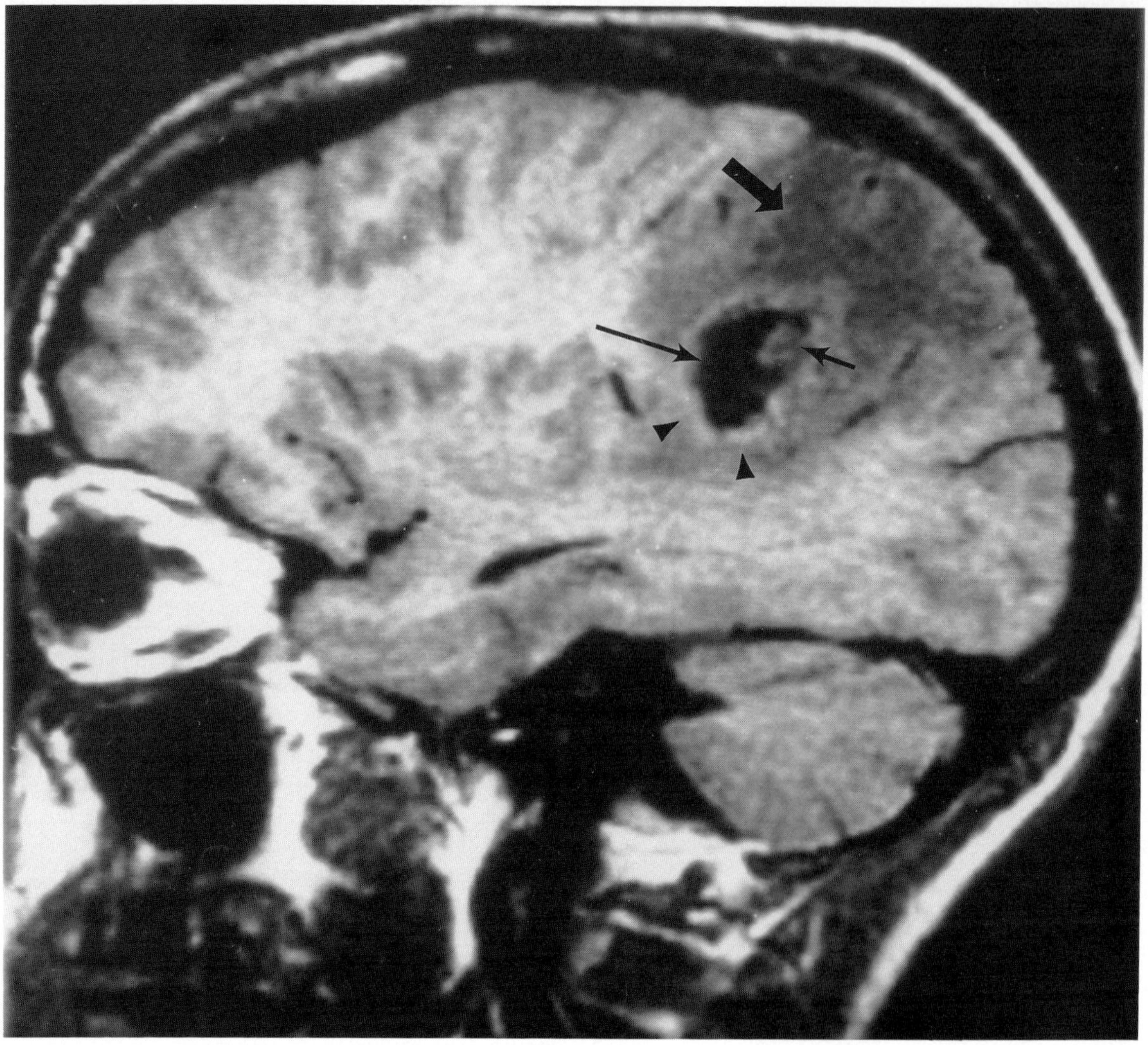

A

Fig. 22.8. Characteristics of pyogenic *(Peptococcus)* bacterial bascess on unenhanced MR scans. (A) Short TR/short TE (600/20) sagittal scan demonstrates a left temporoparietal mass with central, markedly hypointense cavity (long thin arrow), eccentric, slightly hypointense tissue (short thin arrow), irregular iso- to hypointense cavity wall, when compared with normal gray matter. Encircling the cavity wall is a thin hyperintense rim (arrowheads). An extensive surrounding hypointense area represents edematous brain (thick arrow). There is mass effect on the nearby normal brain parenchyma. (B) Long TR/short TE (2,000/30) axial scan shows inhomogeneous intensity within the cavity, with the fluid component (long thin arrow) being slightly more hypointense than the tissuelike component (short thin arrow). Hyperintensity of the cavity wall is separated from that of the surrounding edematous brain (thick arrow) by an iso- to hypointense (relative to gray matter) rim (arrowheads), which corresponds to the hyperintense rim seen in (A). (C) Long TR/long TE (2,000/80) axial scan shows the fluid component (long thin arrow) of the abscess to be markedly hyperintense and the tissuelike component (short thin arrow) to be nearly isointense to gray matter. The abscess rim (arrowheads) is hypointense and separates the iso- to hyperintense cavity wall from the surrounding hyperintense edematous brain (thick arrow). The cavity fluid and the edematous brain appear hyperintense to CSF at TE = 80 msc. (Case courtesy of Dr. Tom Naidich, Baptist Hospital, Miami, Fla.).

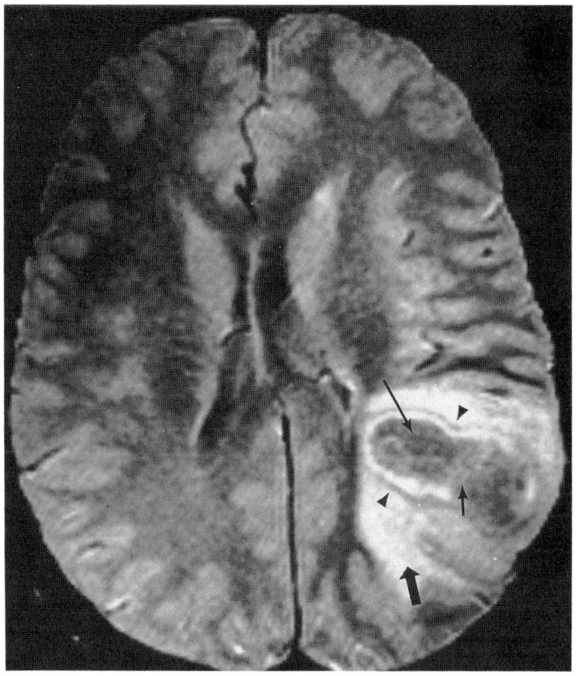

B

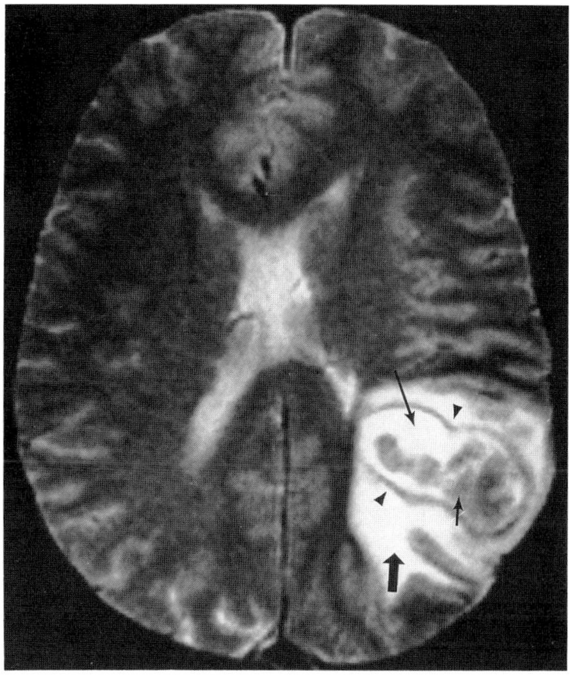

C

Fig. 22.8. *(continued)*

small residual, solidly enhancing lesion may persist even after a full course of antibiotics, but will usually resolve spontaneously within the succeeding three to four months.[49,70] With healing, an area of gliosis remains, and focal calcification is occasionally seen.

Pyogenic abscesses have characteristic MRI features, and frequently these are sufficient to make an accurate diagnosis.[72] In the usual case of a mature abscess with central liquefaction necrosis, the signal intensities on short TR/short TE images have the following order from lowest to highest: CSF ≤ central cavity < surrounding edematous brain < normal brain (gray matter < white matter) (Figure 22.8).[4,72] The order of signal intensities on long TR/long TE images is quite variable, depending on the TE chosen and the protein composition and fluidity of the material in the central cavity. For a TE of 100 ms or less, the order of lowest to highest signal intensities is usually the following: normal brain (white matter < gray matter < CSF < cavity ≤ edematous brain (Figure 22.8).[72] As TE is made longer, the differences in intensity among CSF, cavity fluid, and edema usually become less. This is so because the contribution of T1 relaxation to the signal intensity on long TR images is minimized. The T1 contribution in long TR images is significant at short and intermediate TE, and it is this contribution that gives the central-cavity proteinaceous fluid and the brain edema a higher signal intensity than CSF. Without protein and other macromolecular components, which shorten T1,[45] the cavity fluid should be nearly equal to CSF in signal intensity.

The mature abscess has a rim with distinctive features on unenhanced MR images.[5,72] The rim is iso- to hyperintense to white matter on short TR/short TE images and is usually hypointense on long TR/long TE images (Figure 22.8). A daughter abscess will also have a rim with similar characteristics.[72]

The rim does not show mesial thinning, as the collagen capsule does, nor does it precisely coincide with the enhanced ring seen with iodine-enhanced CT or gadolinium-enhanced MRI.[5] In early studies, the hypointense rim was attributed to collagen or hemorrhage (heme products) in the abscess capsule,[4,5] but more recent work suggests that the rim is hypointense because of localized shortening of T1 and T2 relaxation times by paramagnetic free radicals within phagocytosing macrophages,[5,72] which are heterogeneously distributed in the capsule wall. This hypothesis is supported by the fact that a similar hypointense rim has been observed for granulomas, which are nonhemorrhagic, and for some metastatic foci, which have no evidence pathologically of iron deposition or hemorrhage and yet do have abundant macrophages.[5] Also, as might be expected for phagocytic activity, the hypointense rim resolves with successful surgical or medical treatment of the abscess. It has been suggested that resolution of the hypointense rim may be a better indicator of response to treatment than contrast-enhanced CT (or gadolinium-enhanced MRI), which can show a residual enhancing lesion for months following completion of therapy.[5,49] Other lesions that may have a hypointense rim on long TR/long TE images include evolving hematomas and, infrequently, gliomas.

IV administration of gadolinium-DTPA produces ring enhancement of an abscess capsule on MRI that mimics iodinated contrast enhancement in CT images (Figure 22.9).[72,73] In experimental studies, Grossman and colleagues[73] showed that nonenhanced long TR/long TE images were very sensitive in identifying parenchymal areas of abnormality, while the enhanced short TR/short TE images added specificity by demonstrating the "ring enhancement" that is characteristic of certain lesions. The authors found that gadolinium-enhanced MRI was better than contrast-enhanced CT in detecting small abscesses with necrotic centers and showed ring-enhancing lesions long after the lesions had evolved to nodular enhancement by CT.

As noted earlier, rupture of an abscess into the ventricular system produces ventriculitis, which may be detected by enhancement of the ventricular margins on contrast-enhanced CT. Enhanced MRI

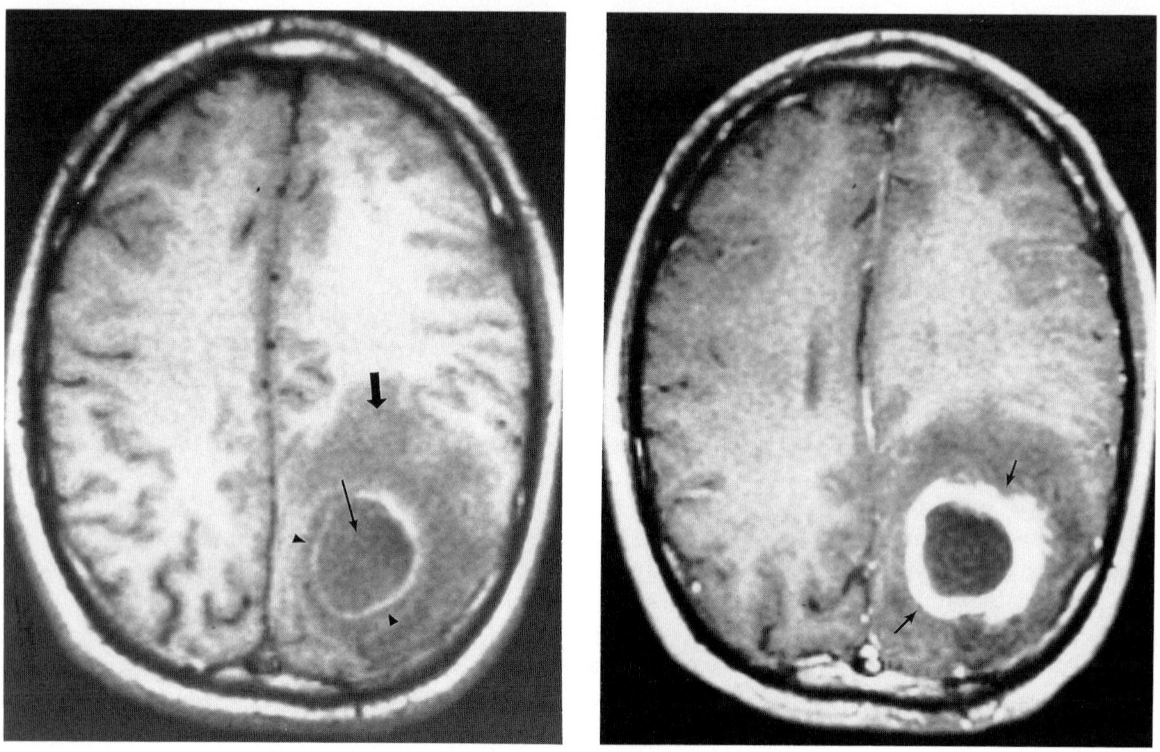

A B

Fig. 22.9. Left-parietal-lobe abscess. A 21-year-old man presented with right homonymous hemianopsia and mild right hemiparesis. Culture of fluid drained from the abscess at surgery grew *Streptococcus viridans*. (A) Pregadolinium short TR/short TE (500/20) scan demonstrates the more hypointense central cavity (long thin arrow), the less hypointense edematous brain (thick arrow), and the thin hyperintense abscess rim (arrowheads). The abscess is centered in the subcortical white matter of the left parietal lobe. (B) Post gadolinium short TR/short TE (500/20) scan shows an enhancing ring (short arrows) around the central cavity. The thin hyperintense rim is within the annular zone of the thick ring. (C) Postcontrast CT shows a thick ring of enhancement nearly identical to that seen by MRI.

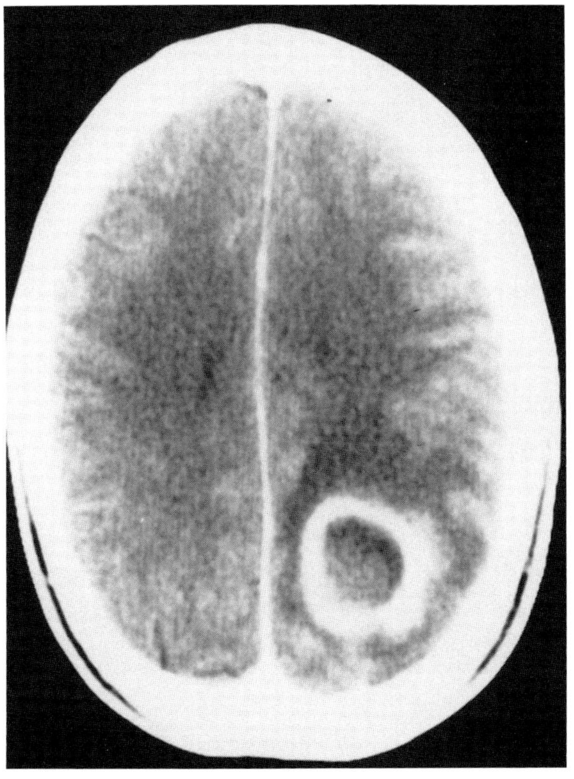

C

Fig. 22.9. *(continued)*

should be at least as sensitive as enhanced CT in detecting this complication. In addition, MRI demonstrates increased signal intensity of purulent intraventricular CSF on both short and long TR images.[4]

Septic Emboli

Septic emboli, often a complication of bacterial endocarditis or systemic infection in a patient with cyanotic congenital heart disease, may result in cerebrovascular occlusion, with the extent of the vascular territory involved dependent on the size of the embolus.[1] There is a range of findings by CT (or MRI) with large emboli producing major arterial branch infarctions, which are seen as areas of low attenuation with patchy and diffuse enhancement in the subacute phase of the infarction,[50] whereas small emboli, which may occlude small arteries and arterioles, produce multiple small abscesses (Figure 22.10) in the region of the gray-matter/white-matter junction, with associated regional edema and mass effect.

Septic embolism may also result in the development of mycotic aneurysms, which are usually located in more peripheral arterial branches than congenital aneurysms, and involve intermediate to small cerebral arteries.[74,75] The mortality rate associated with ruptured mycotic aneurysms is high, and emergency angiography should be performed in patients who are at high risk for developing these aneurysms—and, in fact, in anyone with a history of infection and a CT scan showing subarachnoid or intraparenchymal hemorrhage.[76] During antibiotic therapy, sequential angiograms can be performed to monitor the progression or regression in size of known aneurysms.[76,77]

Spirochetal Infection

Spirochetal diseases of the CNS include syphilis, Lyme disease, leptospirosis, and relapsing fever.[78] Imaging findings for neurosyphilis and Lyme disease are described below.

Based on clinical manifestations, neurosyphilis is divided into early CNS involvement, limited to the meninges, and later involvement, which includes the neuroparenchyma.[78] While most patients with neurosyphilis are asymptomatic, some with early involvement (as early as the secondary stage of systemic infection) will have manifestations of acute syphilitic meningitis or, more often, meningovascular syphilis. Those patients with later parenchymatous involvement may have the better-known forms of tertiary syphilis, general paresis and tabes dorsalis.

Pathologic findings in meningovascular syphilis include widespread thickening of the meninges, meningeal lymphocytic infiltrates, and perivascular lymphocytic infiltrates around small blood vessels.[1] Arteritis may be one of two types: Heubner arthritis, which is more common, and affects large and medium-sized arteries and causes both luminal narrowing and ectasia; or Nissl-Alzheimer arthritis, which affects small vessels and causes luminal narrowing resulting from endothelial and adventitial cell proliferation. Both types of arthritis may result in vessel occlusion, with secondary ischemia and infarction.

Rarely, in the early meningeal phase of neurosyphilis, there is an intense localized inflammatory response that gives rise to a circumscribed mass of granulation tissue known as a gumma.[79] Spirochetes are rarely demonstrated in gummas.[1] Gummas originate from meningeal connective tissue and blood vessels and spread intraparenchymally. Usually, they are located over the cerebral convexity, adhe-

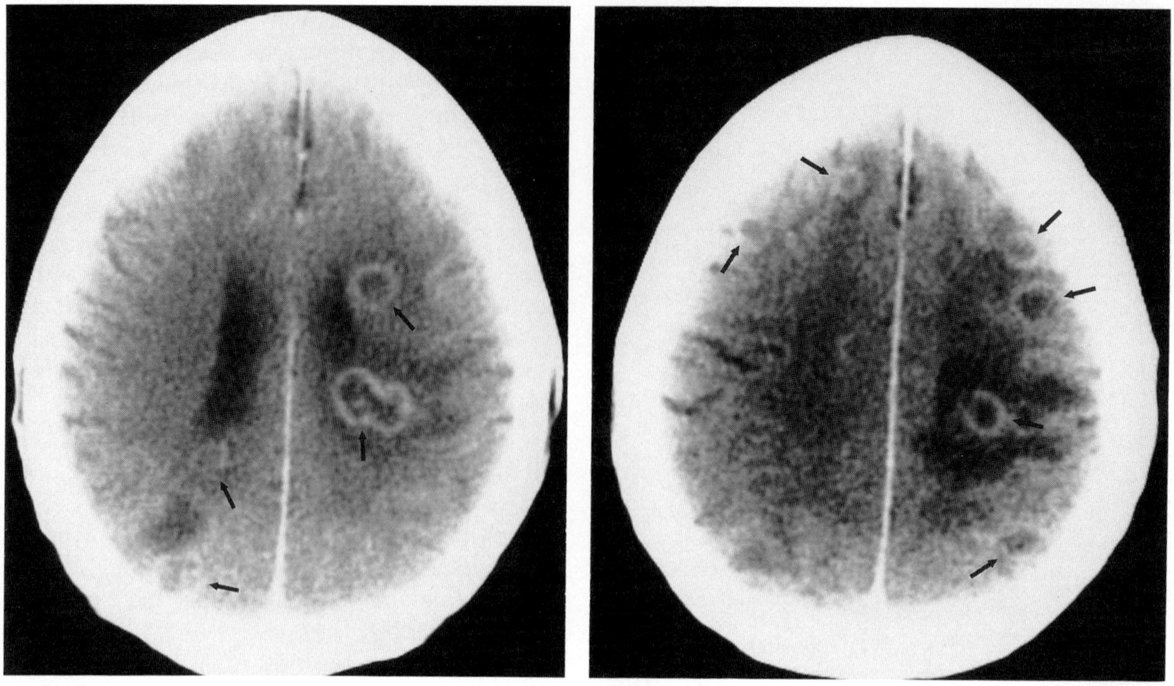

A B

Fig. 22.10. Septic emboli. A 54-year-old man with a history of treated penile carcinoma metastatic to inguinal lymph nodes and of chronic pancreatitis and pseudocysts presented with abdominal pain. During hospitalization, he developed a fever and confusion, and later a right hemiparesis with aphasia. A brain biopsy was performed to rule out metastatic disease. No tumor was found, and instead there were fragments of brain tissue with necrotic material containing extensive polymorphonuclear-cell debris. (A) Postcontrast CT scan demonstrates several ring-enhancing areas (arrows) 1–2cm in their greatest dimension, with adjacent edema, located in the periventricular white matter and at the gray-matter/white-matter junction of both hemispheres. (B) Postcontrast CT scan, at a level 1 cm superior to (A), shows multiple other ring-enhancing lesions (arrows), with associated edema, located peripherally in both hemispheres.

rent to both dura and brain, and are 1 mm to 4 cm in size.[1] They have central caseous or gummatous necrosis, and adjacent vascularity may be marked.

General paresis (paretic dementia) is a chronic meningoencephalitis associated with spirochetes in cortical gray matter that affects the prefrontal cortex and corpus striatum most severely.[1] Opacified leptomeninges, cortical atrophy, and ependymitis are evident morphologically, while microscopically there are degenerative neuronal changes, gliosis, and scattered microglia. Tabes dorsalis is a myelopathy demonstrating atrophic, degenerated, and demyelinated dorsal-nerve roots and posterior spinal columns.

The most common CT abnormality in neurosyphilis in both immunocompetent and immunocompromised patients is diffuse cerebral atrophy.[80,81] In meningovascular syphilis, small infarcts caused by vasculitis appear as multiple small focal hypodensities affecting both gray (cortical and subcortical) and white matter in various arterial distributions, both supratentorial and infratentorial.[82,83] Variable, irregular contrast enhancement may be seen in areas of subacute infarction.[81,82] Transient mild ventricular enlargement has also been observed.[82]

Cerebral angiography shows concentric or asymmetric segmental narrowing of large vessels—especially the supraclinoid internal carotid artery and the proximal horizontal portions of the anterior and middle cerebral arteries—occasionally resulting in a beaded appearance.[82,83] Smaller arteries, such as sylvian branches of the middle cerebral artery, show focal stenosis and dilation. The basilar artery and its branches may exhibit similar findings.[82]

Spin-echo MRI using long TR/long TE sequences is more sensitive than CT in detecting multifocal infarction. In one case, where CT showed only one cortical infarct, MRI demonstrated additional basal ganglia and deep white-matter infarcts, thus suggesting vasculitis.[82]

The CT, MRI, and angiographic findings are nonspecific. The differential diagnosis includes autoimmune vasculitis, infectious basilar meningitis, and drug-induced vasculitis, as well as subarachnoid hemorrhage with vascular spasm.

By CT, a gumma usually appears as a mass with nodular or ring enhancement at the surface of the brain.[81] In one case, though, which proved to be a cerebral gumma, CT showed a right-frontal-lobe hypodense, nonenhancing area with mass effect,[79] Serial CT scans may be used to document complete regression of a presumed gumma with penicillin therapy.[81]

Angiographically, gummas are typically avascular, extraparenchymal masses, with adjacent arteries demonstrating focal dilation and narrowing indicative of vasculitis. However, gummas demonstrating hyperperfusion and a blush, as well as an early draining vein, may be observed.[79]

Lyme disease (Lyme borreliosis) is a multisystem disease that occurs worldwide[84] and is caused by the tick-transmitted spirochete *Borrelia burgdorferi*.[85,86] The skin, joints, heart, and nervous system are primarily affected, and the disease usually occurs in stages, like syphilis.[78] In the modified scheme of Asbrink, it is during stage 2 (disseminated) or stage 3 (persistent) infection (i.e., months to years after the initial tick bite) that neurologic manifestations take place.[86] Approximately 11% of patients with the initial skin lesions (erythema chronicum migrans) subsequently develop neurologic abnormalities, although these may arise without a history of skin involvement.[87-89] The abnormalities generally manifested in stage 2 include aseptic meningitis, cranial neuritis (especially Bell's palsy), motor and sensory radiculitis, mononeuritis multiplex, polyneuritis, myelitis, chorea, and cerebellar ataxia.[86] Those usually manifested in stage 3 include chronic encephalomyelitis, spastic paraparesis, ataxic gait, subtle mental disorders, and dementia.[86,90] Clinically, encephalitis may be acute or chronic, mild or severe.[91]

Since the *B burgdorferi* spirochete has been isolated from CSF, meningitis is thought to result from direct invasion of the CSF, which shows a mild inflammatory response.[85,88] The pathogenesis of parenchymal involvement is less certain. An immune-complex mechanism has been proposed, based on clinical, laboratory, and imaging findings (see below).[89,90,92] However, brain biopsy of a patient with Lyme disease and encephalitis showed a small number of spirochetes, accompanied by an increase in the number of phagocytic microglial cells, with only a minimal inflammatory response.[88] This CNS involvement is reminiscent of tertiary-stage syphilis, although the pathologic equivalents of gumma, meningovascular syphilis, and tabes dorsalis have not been demonstrated in Lyme disease.[88]

Direct spirochetal invasion of peripheral or cranial nerves is suggested by the finding of radicular pain in the dermatome of the tick bite, similar to that seen with herpes zoster. However, pathologically, the spirochetes have not been identified in the lesions, which show predominantly axonal injury with perivascular infiltration of lymphocytes and plasmacytes around epineural blood vessels.[93] Vasculitis, caused by IgM cryoglobulins, has been proposed as a mechanism for mononeuritis multiplex.[89]

CT and MRI findings have been presented for only a few of the reported cases of Lyme disease with neurologic involvement. Often, cranial CT scans are normal, particularly if the patient clinically is in stage 1 or 2.[78] However, CT scans demonstrating multifocal or diffuse, bilateral, periventricular, and deep white-matter hypodense areas, without mass effect, resembling multiple sclerosis (MS) or vascular leukoencephalopathy have been described.[94] In one patient, bilateral thalamic hypodensities were identified on CT.[94] In another patient, there were several bilateral, nonenhancing, hypodense lesions in the white matter of the frontal and temporal lobes as well as in the centra semiovale. Only the right frontal white-matter lesion had associated mass effect, and this resolved in about 1 month.[90]

Spin-echo MRI, obtained in a handful of cases, reportedly shows multiple bilateral periventricular hyperintense areas on long TR images.[88] The lesions are said to resemble MS plaques.[88,94] A hyperintense lesion in the pons was also noted in one of these cases, and correlated with clinical findings.[88]

Granulomatous Disease

CNS tuberculosis (TB) and sarcoidosis, as well as fungal infections, cause a granulomatous inflammatory reaction, which may involve the meninges and/or brain parenchyma.[1] There are two mechanisms for the development of meningitis: (1) rupture of a subependymal or subpial granuloma into the CSF space, which is the favored mechanism in tuberculous leptomeningitis[95]; and (2) penetration of the walls of the meningeal vessels by hematogenously spread, micrometer-sized organisms leading to CSF seeding, as occurs in cryptococcal meningitis.[1,4,5] By either mechanism, the basal meninges are involved early in the course of infection. A thick, gelatinous exudate is characteristically found in the basal cisterns.[95-97] Parenchymal involvement is manifested as granuloma formation, consisting of infectious organisms in a central zone of necrosis, surrounded by reactive epitheloid cells, multinucleated giant cells, and mononuclear inflammatory cells. The "capsule" is often thicker than that of a pyogenic abscess.[13] Granulomas may result from hematogenous spread of systemic disease or from extension of CSF infection into the parenchyma via cortical veins or small penetrating arteries.[1]

Vasculitis resulting directly or indirectly from infection is not uncommon, especially in TB, and may produce severe ischemia and/or infarction. In aspergillosis and mucormycosis, there is direct vessel invasion leading to thrombosis and associated infarction, which is frequently hemorrhagic.

Finally, granulomatous disease often results in hydrocephalus, usually of the communicating type, secondary to blockage of the basal cisterns by inflammatory exudate, but occasionally of the obstructive type, secondary to a focal parenchymal lesion with mass effect or to entrapment of a ventricle caused by granulomatous ependymitis.[1,2,4,95,98]

Tuberculosis

In the United States, less than 0.5% of the cases of TB have CNS involvement. Most of these patients have a clinically detectable form of extracranial TB, but tuberculous meningitis can occur without any evidence of extracranial TB.[95]

The incidence of tuberculous meningitis has been highest in infants and children,[99] but it may be seen at any age, and is among the infections reported in association with the acquired immunodeficiency syndrome (AIDS).[100-102] On plain CT scans, the basal and suprasellar cisterns may be partially or completely obscured by isodense exudate. On contrast-enhanced scans, there is usually diffuse, often intense, enhancement of the basal cisterns, and, less frequently, similar enhancement of the tentorium and sylvian fissures (Figure 22.11).[98,103,104] Associ-

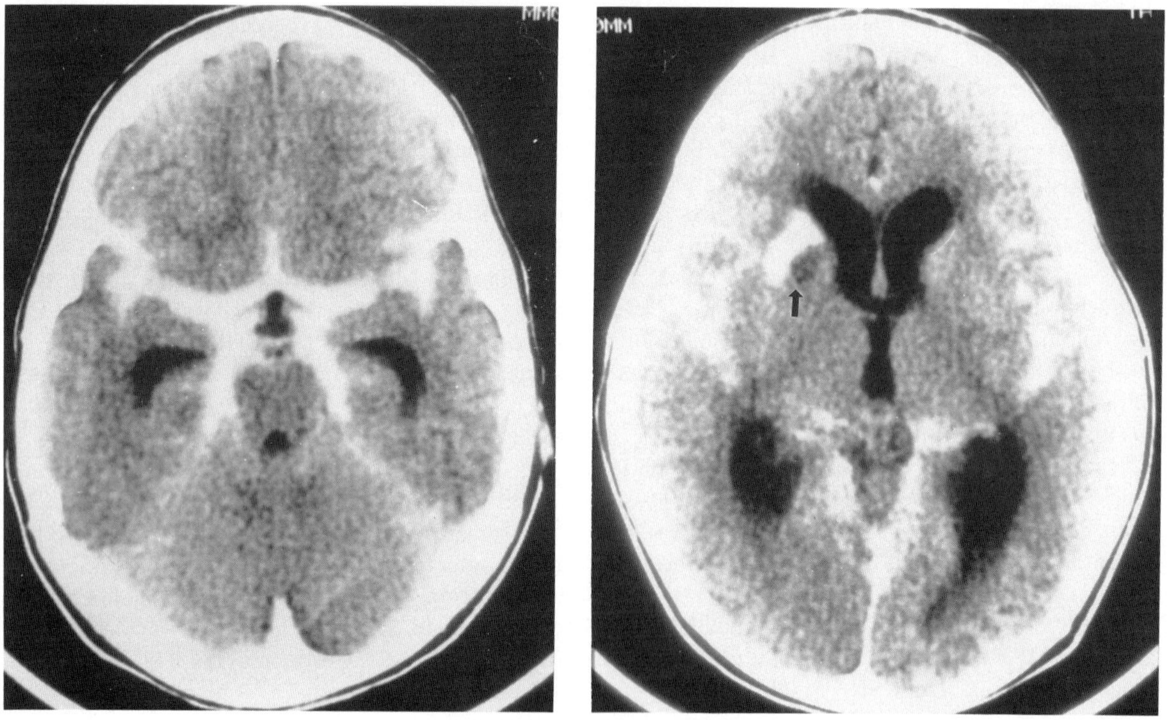

A B

Fig. 22.11. Tuberculous meningitis with communicating hydrocephalus and right basal ganglionic subacute infarct. (A) Postcontrast CT scan demonstrates intense bilateral enhancement of perimesencephalic, suprasellar, and sylvian cisterns. Aqueduct, inferior third ventricle, and frontal horns are enlarged. (B) Postcontrast CT scan at a different level also shows intense bilateral enhancement in the sylvian fissures, retropulvinar, and superior cerebellar cisterns. Subacute infarct (arrow) with peripheral enhancement is seen in the region of the anterior limb of the right internal capsule and caudate head. Faint periventricular hypodensity, best seen anterolateral to the frontal horns, represents interstitial accumulation of CSF.

ated communicating hydrocephalus is detected by CT, as is obstructive hydrocephalus, which is found less frequently.[95] Chronic infection can result in calcification of the basal meninges,[105] which is demonstrated by CT.

Multiplanar MRI, using either short or long TR sequences, is better than CT in demonstrating the distension of the subarachnoid space, which is reported to occur early in tuberculous meningitis.[4] No consistent or characteristic signal abnormalities of the meningeal inflammation or of the exudate in the basal cisterns have been described, although occasionally mild shortening of the T1 and T2 relaxation times relative to CSF has been noted.[5,21] Based on the results of gadolinium enhancement in acute bacterial meningitis, it is to be expected that enhancement of basilar cisterns in tuberculous (or fungal) meningitis will be as extensive as that demonstrated by CT and probably more readily detected. Long TR images (Figure 22.12) demonstrate the bilateral, rather uniform periventricular areas of increased signal intensity, representing interstitial accumulation of CSF due to hydrocephalus (obstructive or communicating).

Tuberculomas are detected by CT in a large minority of cases of tuberculous meningitis.[95] They

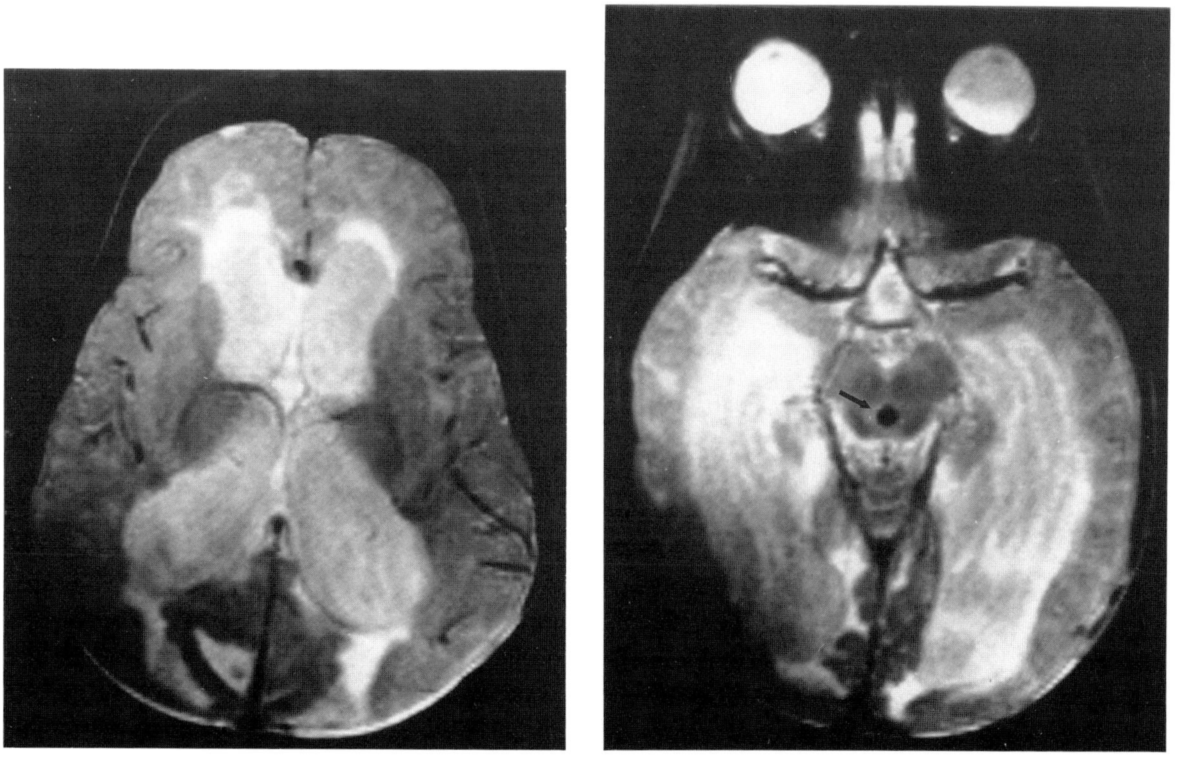

A B

Fig. 22.12. Tuberculous meningitis with evidence of communicating hydrocephalus by routine and ciné MRI. (A) Long TR/long TE (2,400/80) scan shows symmetric enlargement of the lateral ventricles, the expected high signal from CSF, and periventricular areas of higher signal intensity (representing interstitial accumulation of CSF). (B) Long TR/long TE (2,400/80) scan, at a level 2 cm inferior to (A), also demonstrates high-signal CSF in the temporal and occipital horns of the lateral ventricles and in the perimesencephalic cisterns; however, CSF in the aqueduct (arrow) has low signal intensity. This area of low signal is attributed to rapid CSF flow through the aqueduct and is called an area of "signal void." (C) Two frames from a cardiac-gated, gradient-echo (TR/TE = 941/18, with a 10-degree flip angle) aquisition at a fixed sagittal-slice position. A tubular area (arrow) of signal void extending from the posterior third ventricle through the enlarged aqueduct is seen. Areas (arrowheads) of signal void attributable to CSF flow are seen at the outlet of the fourth ventricle and in the premedullary subarachnoid space, consistent with a communicating hydrocephalus. The change in appearance of a signal void area (e.g., through the aqueduct) is due to the pulsatile component of flow, and this is best demonstrated by displaying multiple-gated images in a closed-loop ciné format. Flow void is also seen in major arteries and veins.

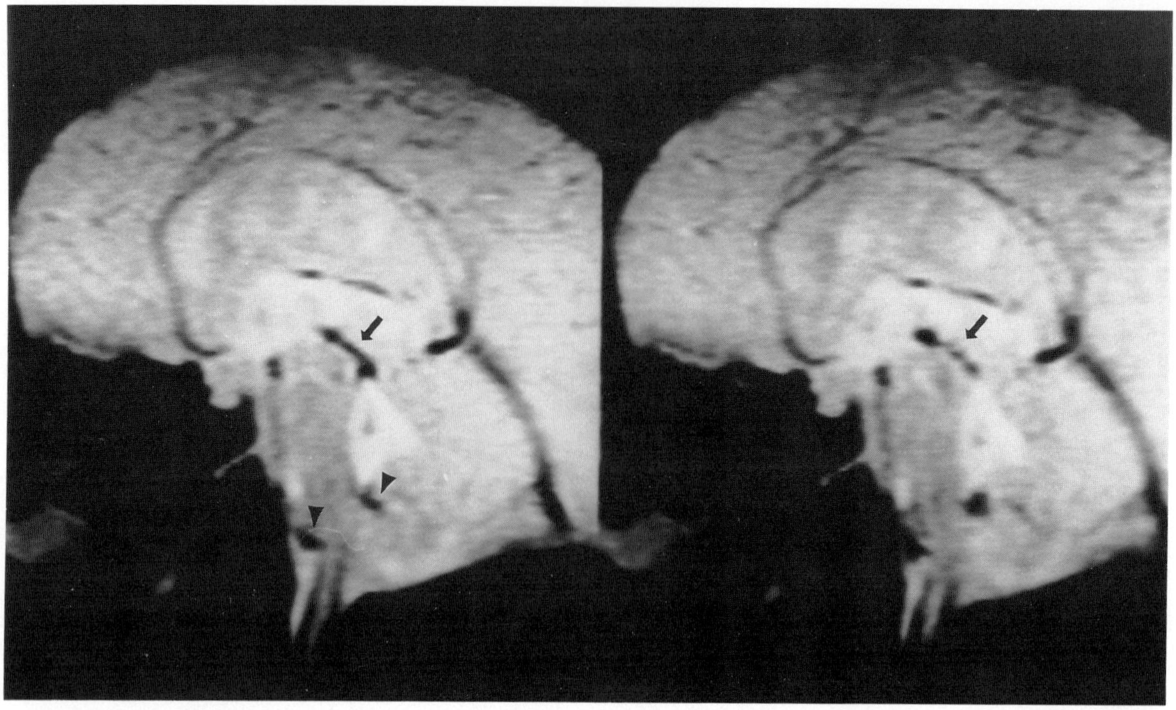

C

Fig. 22.12. *(continued)*

can be located anywhere in the cerebrum or cerebellum, as well as in the subarachnoid, subdural, and epidural spaces. Intraparenchymal granulomas are usually found at the corticomedullary junction and in periventricular regions, as expected for hematogenously disseminated infection.[7,106] Plain CT shows isodense or slightly hyperdense nodules. With IV contrast, these intensely enhance with either a solid nodular (for smaller lesions, usually less than 2 cm) or ring (for larger lesions) configuration.[13,107] Typically, the center of the ring-enhancing lesion is isodense to brain and not hypodense as with pyogenic abscess, whereas the ring is thick, irregularly marginated, and unbroken.[107] The "target sign" with a central nidus of calcification or enhancement within an isodense zone, which is surrounded by the enhancing ring, has been considered characteristic of tuberculoma, although calcification is detected in only 1–6% of tuberculomas.[108]

Low-density edema in the brain surrounding a granuloma may be minimal in smaller lesions, and in general, there is less edema than that surrounding a pyogenic abscess of comparable size.[7,13,109] Edema surrounding tuberculomas is considered to be relatively more prominent in the early stages of granuloma formation.[110]

Extracerebral tuberculomas, adherent to dura along the tentorium or over the convexities, are typically isodense to hyperdense and enhance intensely, resembling *en plaque* meningiomas or dural metastases.[107] While intracerebral tuberculomas are avascular masses angiographically, extracerebral dural-based lesions may show a blush.[111]

The appearance of tuberculomas on long TR/long TE MR images is variable, although often they are hypointense to brain—which, some authors have argued, is due to T2 shortening by paramagnetic free radicals that are produced by macrophages and are heterogenously distributed in the caseous granuloma (Figure 22.13).[5,112] Other authors[110] have argued that T2 shortening is due to increased tissue density, since mature tuberculomas histologically are denser than brain. Any appearance of granulomas as areas of hyperintensity on long TR images has been attributed to central necrosis with liquefaction.

On short TR/short TE images, granulomas are usually isointense to gray matter, and they may have a peripheral, slightly hyperintense rim (perhaps also due to paramagnetic species-shorteining T1).[110] With IV gadolinium, they enhance intensely (Figure 22.14).

TB that involves the brain parenchyma may cause

a focal cerebritis having findings similar to those described earlier for acute pyogenic bacterial infection,[21] or in some cases it may produce an intense localized gyral enhancement.[113] Tuberculous abscess, which is a rare complication,[7,95] has a central area of liquefaction necrosis with pus that appears hyperintense on long TR/long TE images. Its MRI properties are indistinguishable from those of nontuberculous bacterial abscess.[5] Parenchymal infection in TB may occur with or without meningitis.[1]

Extracerebral tuberculomas should be more easily detected with gadolinium-enhanced MRI than with iodine-enhanced CT because of the former's direct multiplanar imaging capability, superb anatomic deliniation on short TR/short TE images, and lack of bone artifact.

Arteries that course through the basal cisterns filled with exudate can become involved directly by the infectious inflammatory infiltrate, indirectly by reactive endarteritis obliterans, or by both processes, with consequent spasm and intimal changes resulting in thrombosis and infarction. Most often, the middle cerebral arteries and their branches are affected, especially the small perforating branches supplying the basal ganglia (Figure 22.11).[2,95] While both CT and MRI can demonstrate ischemic infarcts, MRI is superior in detecting early infarction.[24]

Sarcoidosis

Neurologic manifestations of sarcoidosis are seen in approximately 5% of patients with sarcoid.[114] CNS

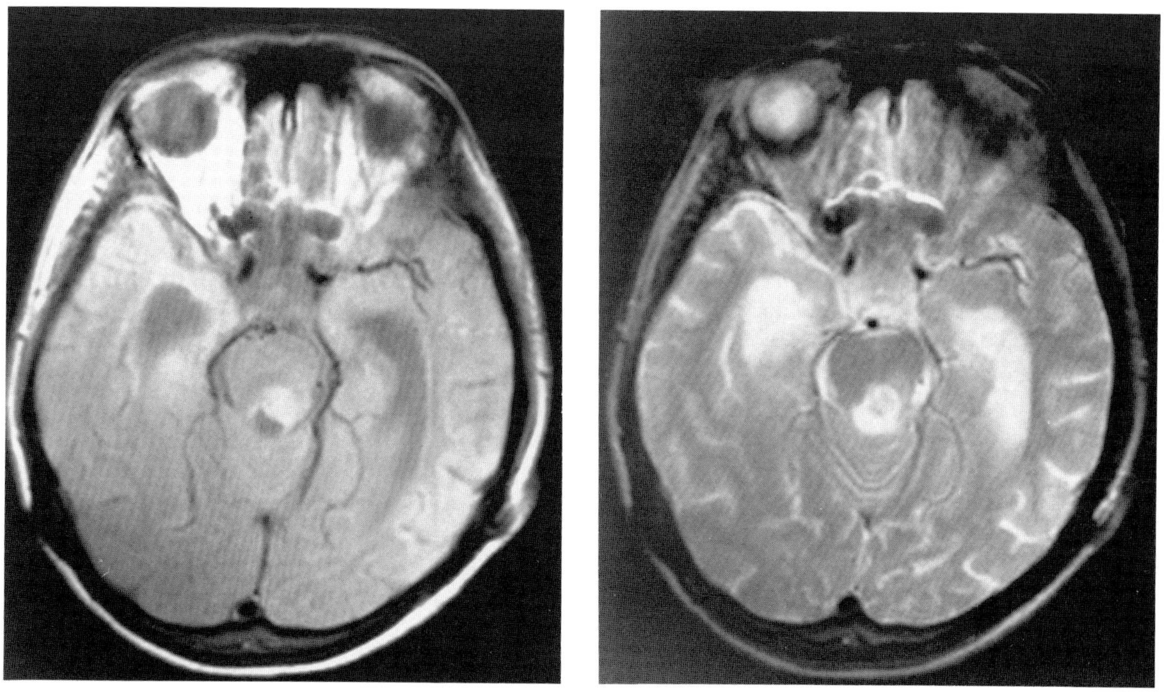

A B

Fig. 22.13. MRI appearance of granulomas on long TR scans. A 17-year-old woman with chronic tuberculous meningitis, hydrocephalus, and multiple granulomas. (A) Long TR/short TE (2,400/20) scan at level of midbrain shows a subependymal mass, hyperintense to CSF and brain, compressing the dilated aqueduct. (B) Long TR/long TE (2,400/80) scan at the same level shows the mass to be hypointense to CSF and approximately isointense to brain parenchyma. This signal-intensity variation is different from that in many tumors and most abscesses that are hyperintense to brain and approach CSF intensity on long TR/long TE scans. (C) Long TR/long TE (2,400/80) scan in the same patient obtained two months after scans (A) and (B). Note the slightly inhomogeneous, isointense (to brain) subependymal masses (representative arrow) around the bodies of the lateral ventricles. Periventricular interstitial accumulation of CSF is seen as increased signal intensity (arrowheads) anterior to the ventricles. (D) Long TR/long TE (2,400/80) right parasagittal scan obtained at the same time as (C) also demonstrates the subependymal isointense nodules (representative arrow) and bilateral periventricular hyperintense areas (arrowheads). Fourth, third, and lateral ventricles are enlarged.

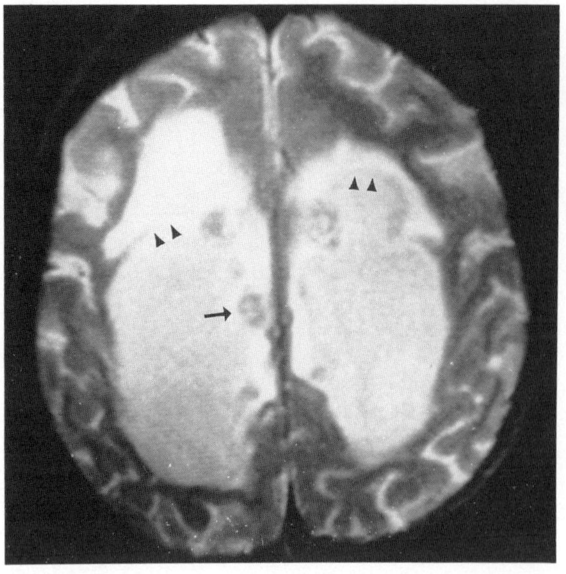

C

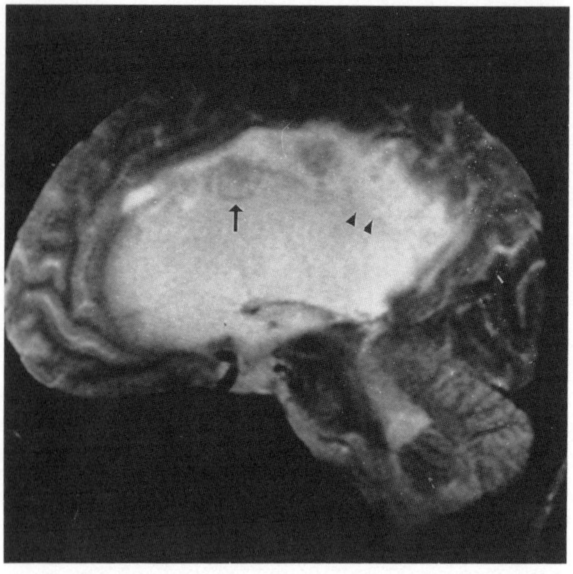

D

Fig. 22.13. *(continued)*

involvement occurs as meningitis and/or parenchymatous disease, which is uncommon.[115] Typically, there is basal or diffuse granulomatous leptomeningitis with secondary involvement of the optic chiasm, hypothalamus, floor of third ventricle, and pituitary gland.[116] Contrast-enhanced CT demonstrates diffuse or focal enhancement of the meninges and underlying brain, indistinguishable from bacterial or fungal meningitis or meningeal carcinomatosis,[98] except for the frequent suprasellar and sellar involvement. Intracerebral granulomatous masses, whether located at the base of the brain or scattered throughout the hemispheres, are slightly hyperdense, well defined, typically nodular, and show a variable, although characteristically minimal, degree of edema on noncontrast CT.[7,116] Following IV contrast administration, they enhance homogeneously.

MRI without gadolinium enhancement is reported to be less sensitive than contrast-enhanced CT in the detection of basilar disease.[117] Gadolinium-enhanced MRI should improve detection of meningeal inflammation (Figure 22.15). With regard to overall detection of intracranial lesions, MRI is more sensitive than CT, and long TR/long TE sequences better demonstrate both hypothalamic involvement and periventricular white-matter changes.[117,118] The signal intensity of granulomatous masses by unenhanced MRI is variable. Most lesions are hyperintense on long TR/long TE images, yet many (including subdural granulomas) are isointense or hypointense (relative to cerebral cortex) on both short and long TR images. Gadolinium-enhanced short TR/short TE scans show marked enhancement of the infiltrating granulomas of the hypothalamus.[5]

Hydrocephalus, communicating or obstructive, is well documented by both CT and MRI. Direct granulomatous involvement, or secondary inflammatory changes, of the cerebral arteries in the basal cisterns or over the convexities, with extension into the Vichow-Robin spaces, can cause vasculitis. Ischemia or infarction, although relatively uncommon, is manifested as multiple hyperintense foci in the white matter and basal ganglia on long TR/long TE images.[5,114] Diffuse periventricular white-matter disease, seen in a minority of cases, appears as hyperintense areas without mass effect on long TR images and is often not detected by CT.[117,118]

CT, MRI, and conventional radiographs of the skull may demonstrate lytic calvarial defects, with nonsclerotic margins, which occasionally arise in cases of sarcoidosis with skeletal involvement.

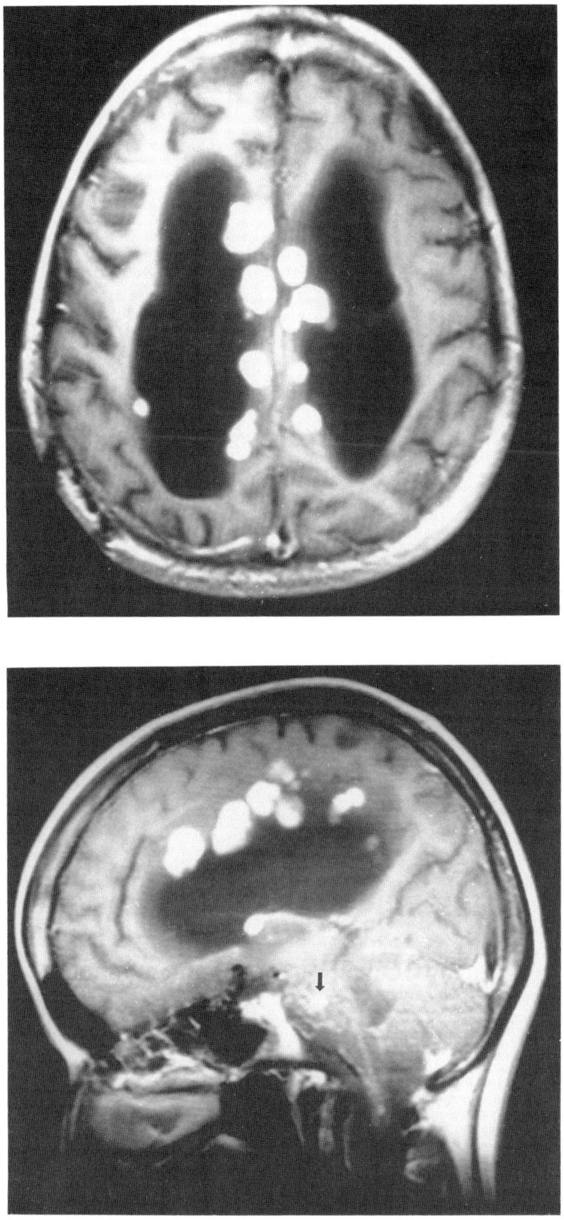

A

B

Fig. 22.14. Gadolinium enhancement of subependymal granulomas in a patient with tuberculous meningitis. (A) Postgadolinium short TR/short TE (700/20) scan corresponding to image (C) in Figure 22.13. There is intense, homogeneous, nodular enhancement of each mass, which facilitates detection and localization. However, note that periventricular-white-matter signal abnormalities are not as well displayed. (B) Postgadolinium short TR/short TE (700/20) scan corresponding to image (D) in Figure 22.13. The intensely enhancing granulomas are again seen, and a brain stem lesion (arrow) is also identified.

Fungal Infection

The fungi that infect the CNS are those that cause systemic or deep mycoses, and they often elicit a granulomatous reaction, with variable degrees of suppuration.[1] Infection in the form of a leptomeningitis and/or focal brain lesion (i.e., granuloma or abscess), as well as associated vasculitis and infarctions, produces CT and MRI findings indistinguishable from those of TB.[5,96] Focal parenchymal lesions can mimic pyogenic abscesses or tumors.[96] CT findings in fungal infection are nonspecific,[119] and they include hydrocephalus, enhancement of the basal cisterns and other CSF spaces (meningitis), solidly enhancing nodules and ring-enhancing lesions (granulomas/abscesses), diffuse and focal areas of low attenuation that may show ill-defined enhancement (vasculitis with infarction or, in the immunocompromised patient, cerebritis/abscess), and mass effect.[2,98,119,120] It has been suggested that ring enhancement of focal lesions represents a walling off of the infection and, as such, implies immunocompetence and a better prognosis for the patient.[119] Scattered areas of low attenuation (in CT scans) or hyperintensity (on long TR/long TE MR scans) in the white matter, without associated mass effect, may result from vasculitis with associated ischemia and infarction.[5] These are indistinguishable from white-matter changes attributable to other causes of vasculitis, infectious demyelination (especially viral), or toxic-anoxic demyelination.[121]

In spite of the general lack of diagnostic imaging specificity for fungal infections, some findings are more commonly associated with certain pathogens. The most frequently encountered systemic mycoses may be divided into those genera that usually infect only immunologically impaired patients *(Aspergillus, Candida, Mucor)* and those that also infect normal hosts (*Cryptococcus, Coccidioides, Histoplasma,* and *Blastomyces*).[96] The former group and *Cryptococcus* are ubiquitous fungi, whereas the remaining genera are geographic, that is, endemic to certain geographic regions.[122]

To aid in the differential diagnosis, a further classification based on the pathogenesis of CNS infection has been suggested.[1] Those fungi that grow in infected tissue as yeast cells *(Cryptococcus, Histoplasma)* are spread hematogenously, reach the microvasculature of the meninges, penetrate the vessel walls, and predominantly cause an acute or chronic leptomeningitis. Less frequently, brain parenchymal lesions, such as granulomas and/or abscesses, are encountered.[1]

In early infection with *Cryptococcus neoformans,* CT scans are often negative, or in immunocompromised patients, have nonspecific changes such as communicating hydrocephalus, dilated CSF spaces, and atrophy.[100,123-127] While meningeal enhancement can occur, it is usually absent.[123,124,127] In advanced or severe cases, there may be obliteration of cortical sulci on plain CT (Figure 22.16). With chronic meningitis, enhancement of the meninges, especially in the basal cisterns, may be evident on contrast-enhanced CT.[7,127] Latent development of subdural hygroma (effusion) has been reported.[7]

Rarely, the brain parenchyma is involved by hematogenous dissemination or by direct spread of the meningeal infection into the cerebral cortex diffusely. In a review of 55 cases of cryptococal intracerebral mass lesions, Fujita and associates[128] found that the lesions were multiple in 35% of patients and were frequently (63% of patients) associated with cryptococal meningitis. The morphologic types of parenchymal lesions include abscess, fibrogranulomatous mass, and a gelatinous mass of cryptococal organisms with minimal or no inflammatory reaction. These lesions can simulate tuberculomas or pyogenic abscesses, and they vary in size to as much as several centimeters in diameter.[128] CT demonstrates poorly marginated hypodense or isodense peripherally located areas, which have variable nodular or ring contrast enhancement, with or without surrounding edema.[128]

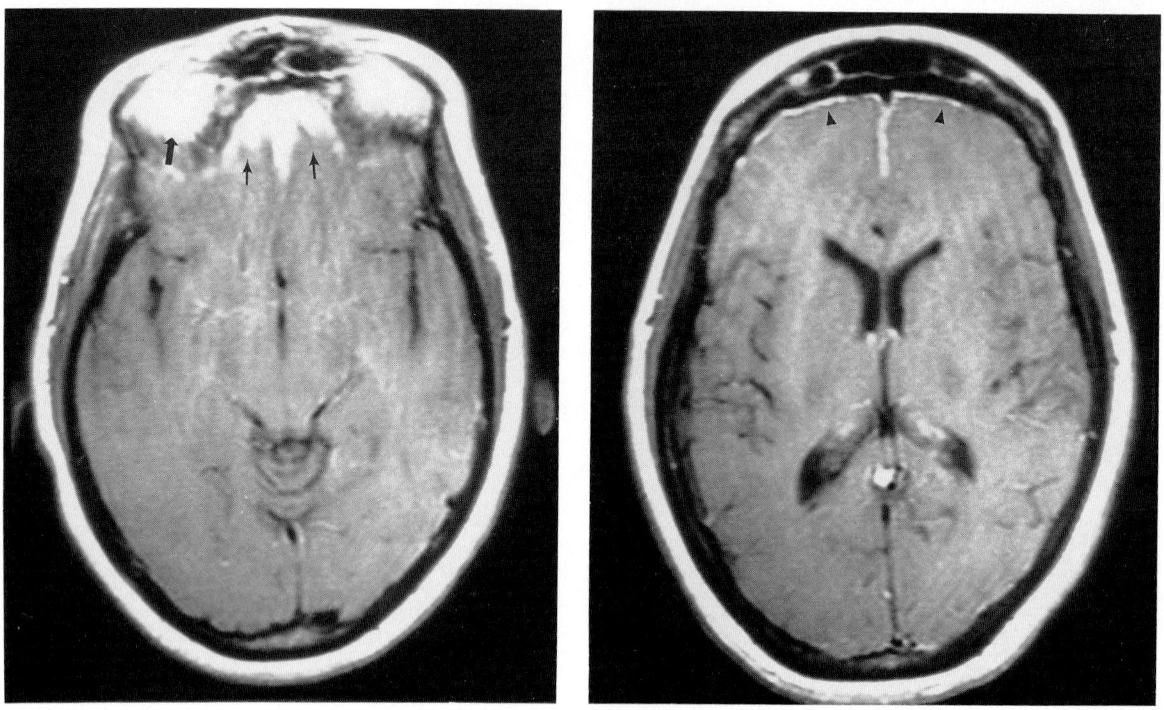

A B

Fig. 22.15. Neurosarcoidosis with meningeal involvement. A 51-year-old black female with a history of biopsy-proved sarcoidosis and no previous neurologic problems presented with seizures on the day of admission to the hospital. Gadolinium-enhanced short TR/short TE scans were obtained 2 days later. (A) Axial scan demonstrates marked bilateral, abnormal enhancement (thin arrows) along the floor of the anterior cranial fossa centrally. The high signal (thick arrow) from fat in the superior aspect of each orbit is identified lateral to the meningeal enhancement. (B) Axial scan, at a level 1.6 cm superior to (A), also shows prominent bilateral meningeal enhancement anterior to the frontal lobes and within the anterior interhemispheric fissure. The thin line of enhancement (arrowheads) anteriorly is easily seen when juxtaposed to the marked hypointensity of the inner table of the frontal bone. Normal enhancement of internal cerebral veins and the vein of Galen is noted. (C) Coronal scan (with slight motion artifact) better delineates the thick, intense enhancement (arrowheads) of the meninges along the planum sphenoidale, cribriform plate, and medial aspect of each orbital roof.

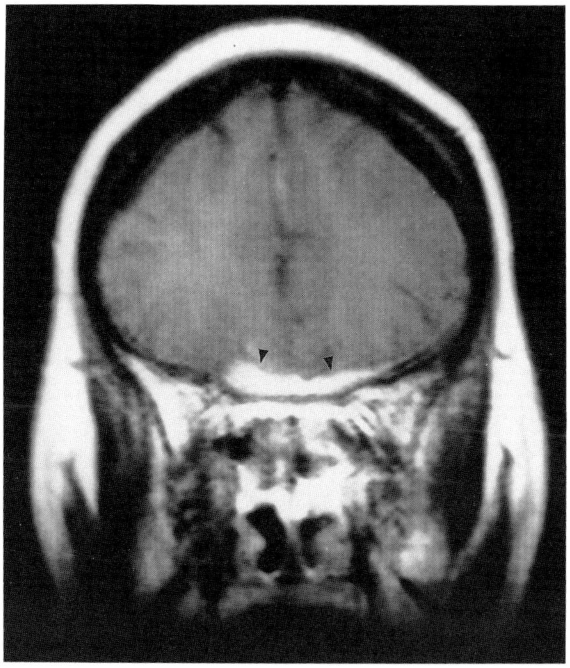

C

Fig. 22.15. *(continued)*

Follow-up scans may demonstrate focal calcification at the site of the lesion.[129] MRI characteristics of the intracerebral mass lesions have not been described.

Infection with *Coccidioides immitis* begins when arthrospores are breathed into the lungs. The organisms appear usually as 40–50-μm-diameter spherules composed of numerous 2–5-μ-diameter yeasts called endospores. When the large spherules rupture, the endospores are released and can be spread hematogenously, infecting the meninges in the same way as do the individual yeast cells of *Cryptococcus* or *Histoplasma*.[1,122] Typically, there is meningeal inflammation with infectious purulent and caseous granulomas, particularly at the base of the brain.[1,7] The most common CT findings are (1) abnormal contrast enhancement of the meningeal surfaces over the convexities and in the basal cisterns, which may be oblitered, distorted, or even hyperdense on the precontrast scan; (2) communicating hydrocephalus; and (3) entrapment of the fourth ventricle, or a part of the third or lateral ventricle, secondary to ependymitis, with development of obstructive hydrocephalus.[98,109,130] Less commonly, focal noncalcified white-matter- or deep-gray-matter-enhancing lesions (representing granulomas), which may be diffusely distributed, are found.[109,130,131] Multiple coccidioidal microabscesses were found throughout the cerebellum in a patient with AIDS and disseminated coccidiodomycosis.[125] Infrequently, focal or diffuse areas of hypodensity in the periventricular and deep white-matter are identified. While the diffuse areas most likely represent transudation of CSF secondary to hydrocephalus, the focal area may represent infarcts secondary to vasculitis.[132] However, vascular occlusions resulting from vasculitis in coccidiodomycosis are considered rare.[130,133]

When skeletal involvement in disseminated coccidioidomycosis includes the calvarium and skull base, destructive lesions, with a variable degree of marginal sclerosis, are detectable by skull films, CT, or MRI.

Those fungi that grow in infected tissue as hyphae only *(Aspergillus, Mucor)* or as pseudohyphae *(Candida)* cause a greater proportion of parenchymal abnormalities relative to meningitis than the fungi that grow as individual yeast cells, since the larger hyphal forms have limited access to the meningeal microcirculation.[1] Hyphal growth results in mycelial colonies capable of invading and obstructing large, medium, and small arteries, leading to infarction, as well as cerebritis. Pseudohyphae, which represent adherent yeast cells and their progeny, are larger than individual cells but smaller than true hyphae. Thus, CNS infection with *Candida* species often results in scattered intraparenchymal granulomatous microabscesses secondary to small-vessel (arteriole) occlusion and tissue breakdown.[4] Clinically, meningitis is also a common feature of CNS candidiasis, and presumably results from penetration of the meningeal microvasculature by individual or small groups of yeast cells.

The CT and MRI findings in candidiasis are nonspecific. On CT, parenchymal lesions are isodense or slightly hypodense and demonstrate a variable degree of ring or nodular enhancement.[100,127] Poorly circumscribed, nonenhancing, hypodense areas have been described for immunosuppressed patients.[119] On MRI, the lesions demonstrate a hypointense center with a surrounding hyperintense zone, representing edema, in long TR/long TE images.[5,100]

Aspergillosis and mucormycosis involving the CNS are marked by several similar findings. Either may result from direct extension of nasal-cavity/paranasal sinus infection or from hematogenous dissemination. CNS aspergillosis (usually *Aspergillus fumigatus* infection) more commonly is due to hematogenous dissemination.[1] When there is direct

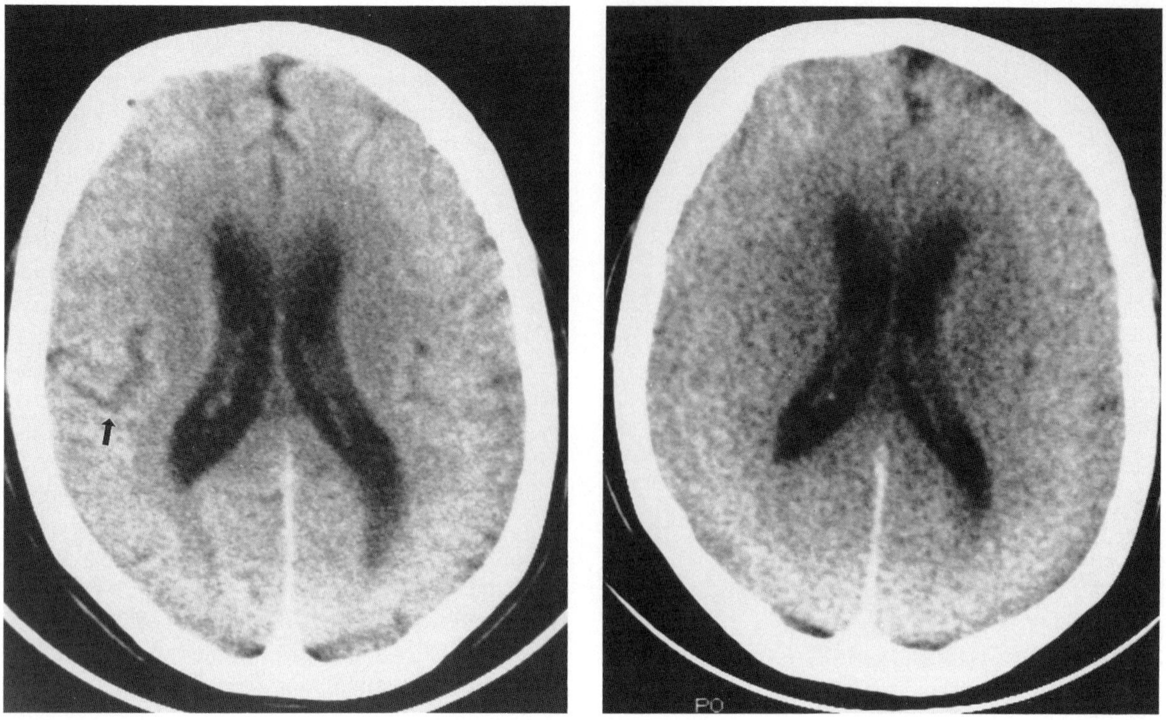

A B

Fig. 22.16. Severe cryptococcal meningitis. A 38-year-old man with AIDS presented with nausea, vomiting, headache, and oral thrush. He was treated for esophageal candidiasis, and his symptoms improved; however, on the fifth day after admission, he became lethargic and then obtunded. (A) Noncontrast CT scan obtained as an emergency on admission. Cortical sulci of frontal and parietal lobes are well seen. The right sylvian fissure (arrow) is more easily seen than the left, at this level. (B) Noncontrast CT scan, at the same level as (A) on the fifth day after admission. The cortical sulci of the frontal and parietal lobes are no longer delineated, although a portion of the anterior interhemispheric fissure still has the low density of CSF. The right sylvian fissure is also no longer seen. The lateral ventricles have not changed significantly in size. On the seventh day after admission, the patient expired. At autopsy, there was evidence of diffuse cryptococcal meningitis with marked involvement of the dura and arachnoid of spinal canal and brain, as well as cryptococcomas in the lungs, kidneys, and lymph nodes.

extension, invasion of the blood vessels, especially the cavernous sinus and circle of Willis, occurs, resulting in angiitis, thrombosis, and infarction.[1] Extension to the subarachnoid space may result in meningitis and meningoencephalitis.[2,4,120,134]

With hematogenous spread, usually from a pulmonary focus, *Aspergillus* hyphae lodge in cerebral vessels, cause occlusion, and grow through the vessel walls, producing hemorrhagic infarction. This converts to septic infarction with associated cerebritis and abscess formation, usually in the distribution of anterior and middle cerebral arteries. These lesions do not generally show granulomatous inflammation histologically.[1] Although an abscess with ring enhancement may be observed, CT often demonstrates poorly circumscribed areas of subtle low attenuation, with or without mass effect, and minimal contrast enhancement, initially focal and later widespread (Figure 22.17).[119,135] CT also depicts subarachnoid hemorrhage resulting from rupture of a mycotic aneurysm or invasion of the anterior or middle cerebral arteries.

CNS mucormycosis is a phycomycosis caused by the genus *Mucor*. It occurs in the uncontrolled diabetic or immunocompromised patient, and is most often of the rhinocerebral (craniofacial) type, with spread of infection along perivascular and perineural channels through the cribriform plate into the frontal lobe or through the orbital apex into the cavernous sinus (Figure 22.18). CT or plain films show bone destruction, often as a late finding.[136,137] Paranasal-sinus involvement appears as mucosal thick-

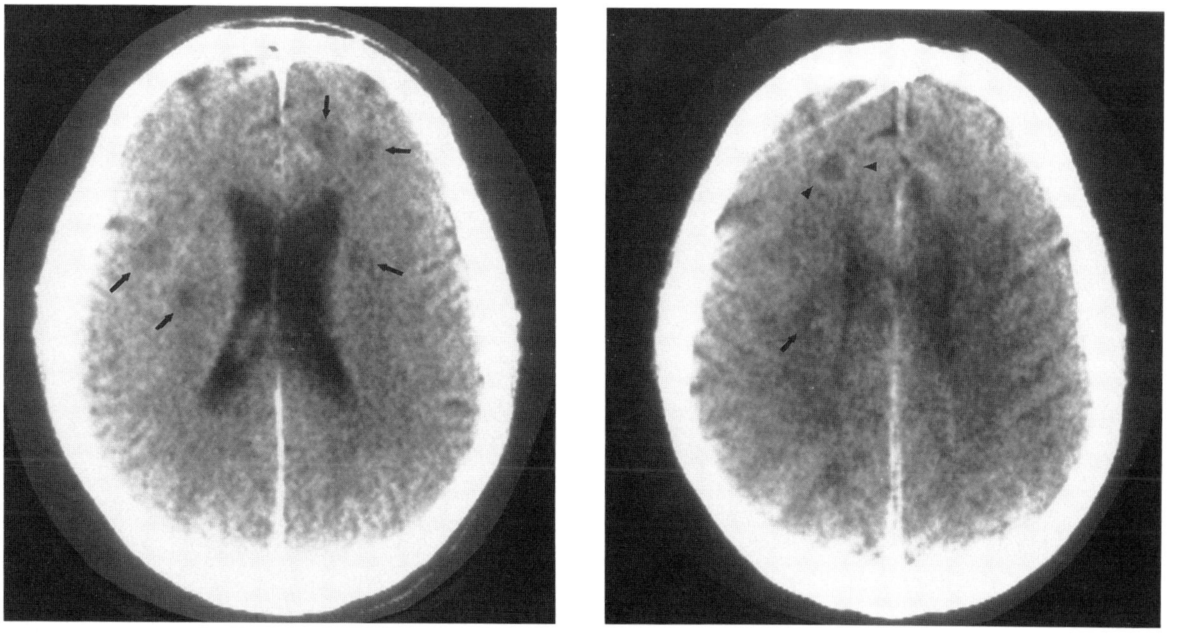

A B

Fig. 22.17. CNS aspergillosis due to hematogenous spread from a pulmonary focus. A 51-year-old immunocompromised man developed pulmonary aspergillosis and multiple brain abscesses (autopsy proven) two months after a renal transplant. (A, and B) Postconstrast CT scans show scattered hypodense rounded areas (arrows) in both hemispheres, primarily located in the distribution of the anterior and middle cerebral arteries. There is no appreciable mass effect associated with these lesions, and only minimal peripheral contrast enhancement (arrowheads). (Case courtesy of Dr. Sean O'Brien, University of Miami/Jackson Memorial Medical Center, Miami, Fla.).

ening, usually without air–fluid levels (Figure 22.18).[137,138] Intracranial mucormycosis causes either infarction or fungal abscess, and usually involves the base of the brain and cerebellum following invasion of the infratemporal fossa or orbit.[137] Intracerebral abscesses appear as hypodense masses with variable peripheral enhancement and little surrounding vasogenic edema.[137] Infarction or abscess formation can be noncontiguous with the primary focus of infection because of vascular dissemination. Distinction between abscess and bland infarct may be difficult. The former is favored if there is cortical sparing, some peripheral ringlike enhancement, minimal surrounding edema, and a distribution not conforming to a vascular territory.[137] Follow-up studies should differentiate between maturing abscess and evolving, bland infarct (Figure 22.18)

Direct invasion or vascular dissemination in mucomycosis may result in a basal meningitis. Exudate involving the fourth ventricle and causing obstructive hydrocephalus demonstrated by CT has been reported.[120,134] CT demonstration of intracranial hemorrhage may warrant subsequent cerebral angiography in order to identify any mycotic aneurysms, which occasionally result from vascular dissemination.[109]

Although there has been limited experience with MRI of CNS aspergillosis and mucormycosis, it is known that MRI is better than CT in evaluating lesions that involve the skull base, especially vascular occlusive lesions. MRI demonstrates both hemorrhagic and nonhemorrhagic infarctions. Sinus inflammation is usually hyperintense on long TR/long TE images. However, aspergillosis may present as a sinonasal mass that is isointense or hypointense (compared with brain) on both long TR/long TE and short TR/short TE images and demonstrates peripheral enhancement with IV gadolinium administration.[46] Direct intracranial extension is well seen on multiplanar long TR/long TE images as intraparenchymal hyperintense areas, or on short TR/short TE, gadolinium-enhanced images as abnormal meningeal or parenchymal enhancement in the same

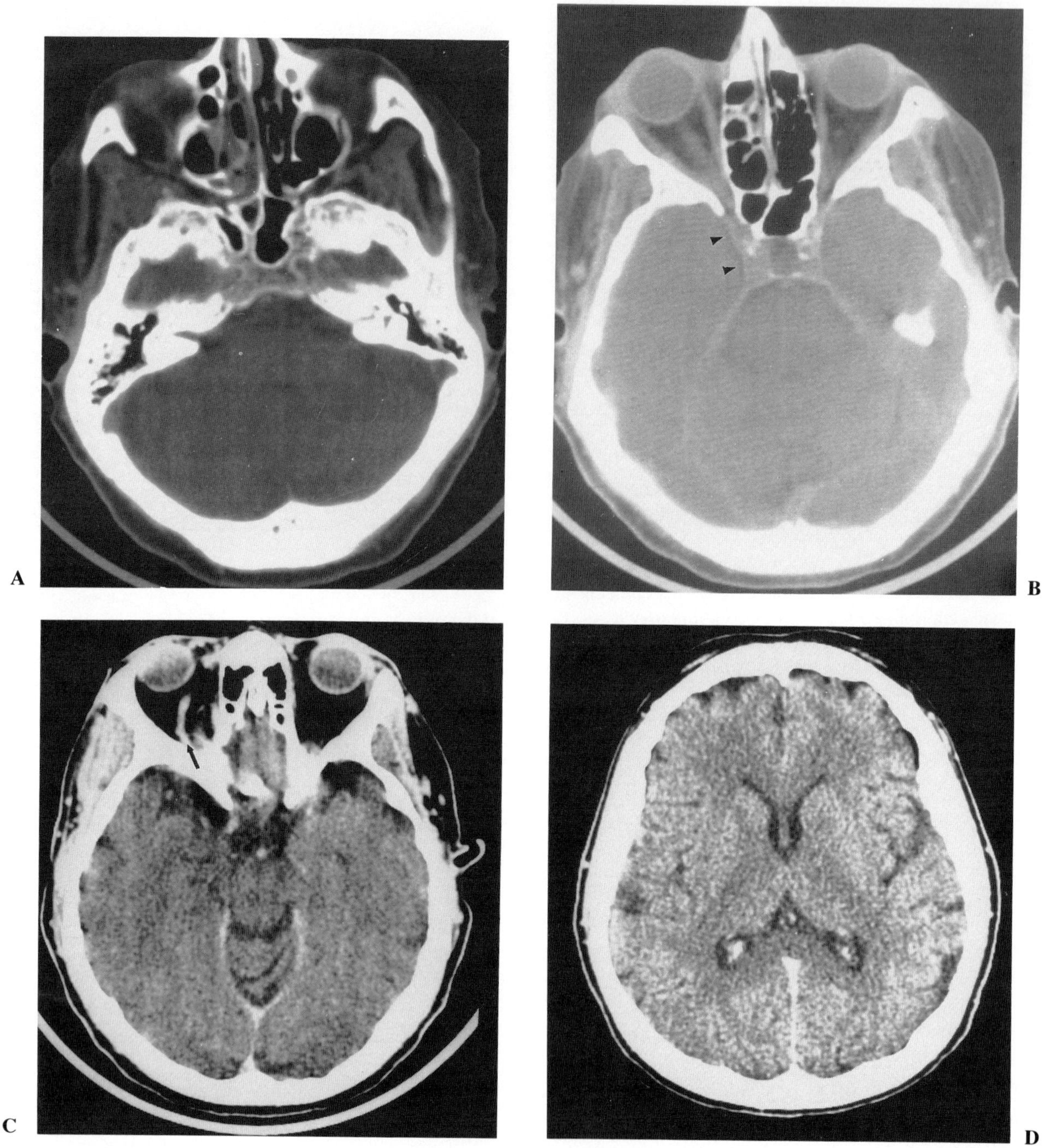

Fig. 22.18. Rhinocerebral mucormycosis with right cavernous sinus thrombosis and subsequent internal carotid-artery infarction. A 71-year-old woman with diabetes mellitus presented with headache, decreased vision and ptosis of the right eye, and palsies of right cranial nerves III, IV, VI, and VI. (A) Postcontrast CT scan obtained on admission shows partial opacification of the right nasal fossa, at the level of the middle turbinate, by soft tissue that extends posteriorly to the sphenopalatine foramen of the pterygopalatine fossa. Right maxillary and ethmoid sinuses are also partially opacified. There is no bone destruction. (B, C) Additional images from the same scan show the right cavernous sinus (arrowheads) to be slightly wider than the left and the right superior ophthalmic vein (arrow) to be minimally enlarged. As in this case, the CT findings of rhinitis, sinusitis, and cavernous sinus invasion may not be striking. (D) On the same CT scan, the brain parenchyma is normal. (E) Noncontrast CT scan obtained 1 week after admission shows a right basal ganglionic infarct. (F) Noncontrast CT scan obtained 3 weeks after admission demonstrates a large infarct involving the complete territories of the right anterior and middle cerebral arteries, with mass effect.

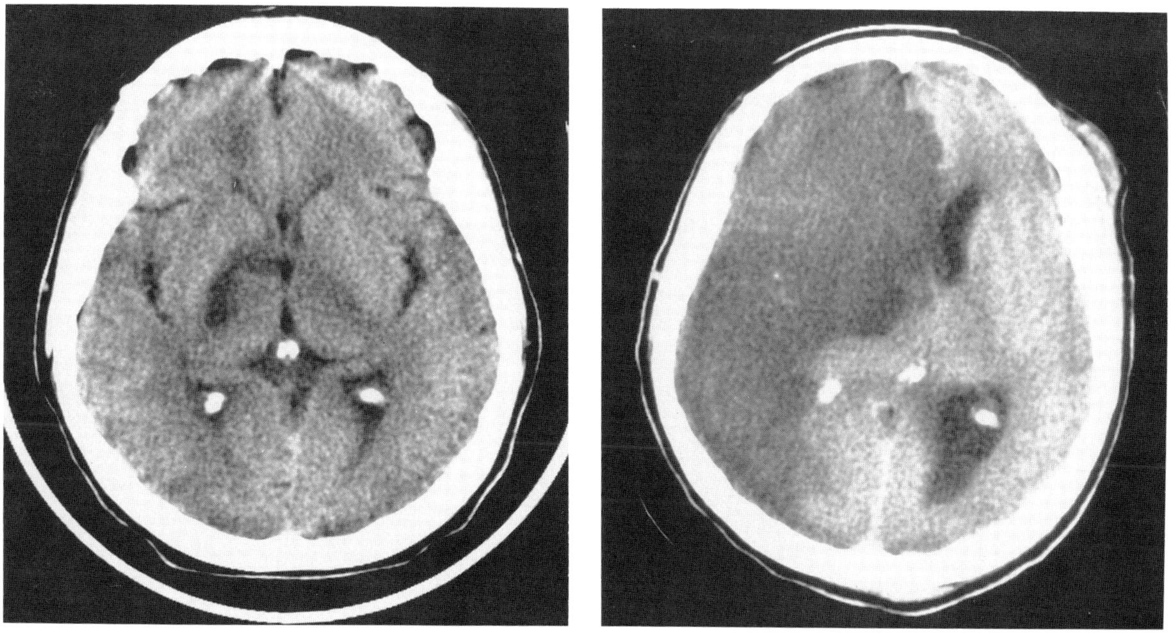
E F

Fig. 22.18. *(continued)*

manner as contrast-enhanced CT, but without the limitations of bone artifacts.

Enzmann and colleagues[119] found that CT underestimated the extent of pathology in patients with widespread fungal disease. It is likely that MRI will give more accurate representation. However, the inability to differentiate various types of fungal disease from one another by CT findings is also true for MRI.

Viral Infection

Whether due to RNA- or DNA-containing viruses, viral infection of the brain usually presents as an encephalitis, a diffuse or multifocal process, often with meningeal involvement (meningoencephalitis), and it may either be acute or result from reactivation of a latent (persistent) virus.[139] While bacterial, fungal, or protozoan infections can cause encephalitis, such diffuse brain involvement is relatively less common.[140]

In the general population, aseptic meningitis is usually due to enterovirus (coxsackieviruses, echoviruses, polioviruses); it occurs less frequently in mumps virus and herpes simplex virus (HSV) infections.[139,141] In AIDS patients, aseptic meningitis is found in association with herpesvirus infections—those attributable to cytomegalovirus (CMV), HSV, and Epstein-Barr virus (EBV)—as well as hepatitis-B virus (HBV) infections.[141] Human immunodeficiency virus type 1 (HIV-1, which was formerly called human T-cell lymphotropic virus type 3, HTLV-3, or lymphadenopathy-associated virus, LAV)[142,143] causes acute or chronic meningitis, as well as subacute encephalitis.[141] Another human retrovirus, HTLV-1, may do the same.

Acute viral encephalitis is usually due to togaviruses (alphavirus and flavivirus genera) and bunyaviruses (California group), both of which have been classified epidemiologically as arboviruses.[144] Encephalitis resulting from reactivation of a latent infection occurs with herpesviruses.[139,145] "Slow" or persistent brain infection, often lasting years, is seen with papovaviruses (JC and simian virus (SV) 40–like viruses), paramyxovirus (morbillivirus), and the viruses causing kuru and Creutzfeldt-Jakob disease (also known as Jakob-Creutzfeldt disease).[139]

Pathologic findings in CNS viral infections are quite variable, ranging from cases with no gross pathology to those with localized hemorrhage and/or necrosis (such as with HSV) to those with diffuse brain congestion and edema, as well as hemorrhage and necrosis (as can occur with HSV and arboviral encephalitides). There is usually some degree of cerebral edema and congestion of meningeal vessels, and not infrequently petechial hemorrhage or congestion in gray or white matter.[139] In general, the major histologic features are those of neuronal degeneration and inflammation.[13]

CT may demonstrate diffuse or multifocal low attenuation involving white and/or gray matter, often with blurring of the gray-matter/white-matter junction.[5] In part, this represents edema, with associated mass effect that becomes more severe as the infection progresses. With sufficient hemorrhage, hyperdense foci appear. Contrast enhancement that is minimal initially may become more prominent later, appearing heterogeneous, often described as "streaky."[13,146] When the acute infection has resolved, there is evidence of atrophy, and dystrophic calcifications may be identified.

MRI demonstrates the inflammatory and neuronal degenerative changes earlier and more accurately.[21,147,148] These appear as scattered or confluent areas of hyperintensity on long TR/long TE images with variable mass effect.[21,149] Focal, subacute hemorrhages are particularly well seen as areas of increased signal on both short TR/short TE and long TR/long TE images.[26] Short or long TR images reveal localized or generalized atrophy occurring in the chronic stage of infection. Most viral encephalitides have these same general features.[11] The more common infections, some of which are distinctive by their location, are discussed more fully below, as are those viral infections frequently associated with acquired immunodeficiency.

Herpesviruses

Herpes-simplex encephalitis may result from CNS infection with either the type 1 (HSV-1) or type 2 (HSV-2) virus. In the neonate, encephalitis is predominantly due to HSV-2 infection acquired during vaginal delivery,[139,150] and often results in severe brain destruction. Initial CT may appear normal or show patchy areas of low attenuation, primarily in the white matter, in both cerebral hemispheres.[151,152] The findings may be difficult to detect, especially in the periventricular white matter, because in the neonate white matter is normally of low density.[151] Early follow-up studies demonstrate a rapid increase in the size of the white-matter low-attenuation areas, as well as finger-like projections of increased attenuation in cortical gray matter.[151,153] Basal ganglia, thalami, and cerebellum may be relatively spared on the early CT scans, but later show abnormal findings.[151] In studies obtained 1 month after onset, there are ventricular enlargement and diffuse, confluent, or multicystic low attenuation (approaching that of CSF) in both hemispheres, representing parenchymal destruction with encephalomalacia and atrophy.[152,153] Later findings also include scattered foci of increased attenuation, consistent with hemorrhage and/or calcification, in the thalamus, periventricular white matter, insular cortex, and centrum semiovale at the corticomedullary junction. Calcifications that may vary from punctate to gyral in shape are recognized as early as 21 days from the onset of symptoms or signs.[151] While Benator and colleagues[152] found no abnormal contrast enhancement on early scans, Noorbehesht and colleagues[151] found minimal, asymmetric enhancement in a meningeal pattern.

There is no preference for temporal-lobe involvement in neonatal HSV encephalitis. The differential diagnosis for the CT findings of infarction, hemmorrhage/calcification, and multicystic encephalomalacia include other viral meningoencephalitides, bacterial encephalitis, hypoxia/anoxia secondary to asphyxia, and twin-to-twin transfusion.[154–156]

In immunocompetent older children and adults, HSV-2 can produce a mild self-limiting meningitis or encephalitis. Encephalitis, though, is predominantly due to reactivation of a latent HSV-1 infection and characteristically involves temporal and inferior frontal lobes, often unilaterally.[139] When untreated, it is usually a fulminant, necrotizing meningoencephalitis. It is thought to result from reactivation of latent infection in the trigeminal ganglion with intracellular spread of virus along those branches of cranial nerve (CN) V that innervate the meninges of the middle and anterior cranial fossa.[139,157]

While CT findings may be abnormal as early as day 2 following clinical presentation, they are usually not present until after day 5, when noncontrast images show poorly defined areas of low density in the anterior/medial temporal lobe with extension to the insula, sparing the lenticular nucleus.[146,158] Both gray and white matter appear involved radiographically, and there is mass effect. Focal hemorrhage, although consistently present at autopsy, may not be detectable. Contrast enhancement in the abnormal low-density areas (Figure 22.19) can be seen as early as day 3, appearing as linear or "streaky,"[146] but is usually not evident until after 1 week, when a gyral or ring pattern of enhancement

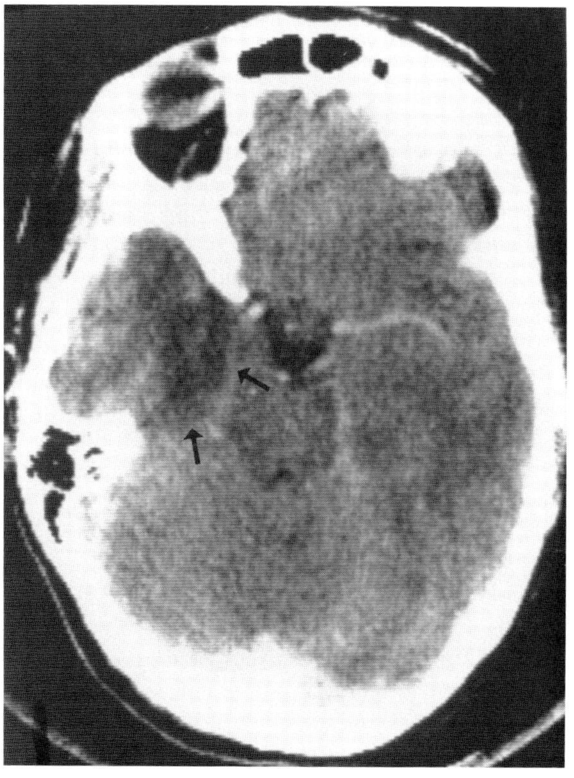

A

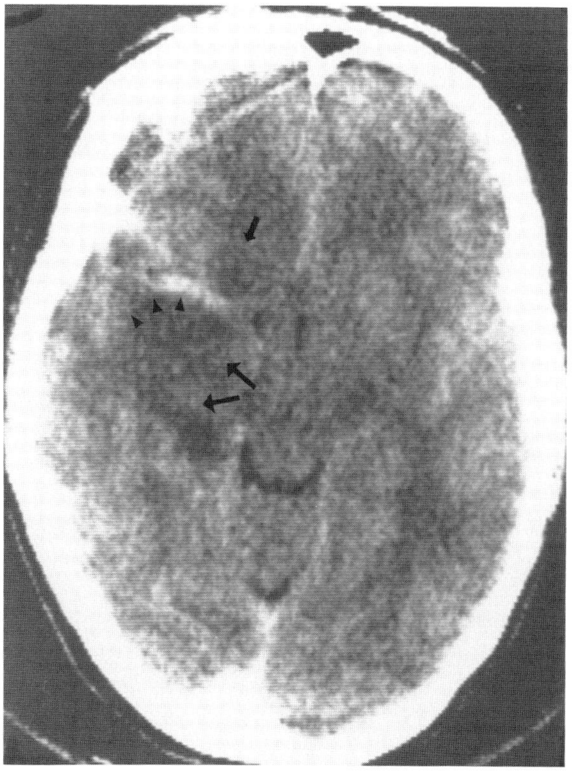

B

Fig. 22.19. Herpes simplex (type 1) encephalitis. An 18-year-old woman had fever and flu-like symptoms for approximately 3 days and then developed headache and a stiff neck. By the fifth day after the onset of symptoms, she was comatose, and a CT scan was obtained. (A, B) Postcontrast CT scans demonstrate a low-density area in the right temporal lobe (long arrows) and posterior frontal lobe (short arrow). There is peripheral enhancement in the sylvian fissure laterally and anteriorly (arrowheads; wider band of enhancement than expected for opacification of middle cerebral artery alone). (Case courtesy of Dr. Jeffery Kochan, University of Miami/Jackson Memorial Medical Center, Miami, Fla.).

is noted in the periphery of the lesion and the region of the sylvian fissure.[158] With more extensive meningoencephalitis, diffuse gyral enhancement results.[159] On follow-up CT scans, there are rapid changes with extension of the low-density zones to include the inferior frontal lobe and the parietal lobe,[158] and bilateral involvement may become apparent. Late in the course of the disease, there is atrophy, with ventricular enlargement secondarily.[159]

Early detection of herpes-simplex encephalitis is important because early treatment with antiviral agents has been shown to improve the patient's prognosis,[160] although many clinicians now institute therapy with acyclovir on an empiric basis without a specific diagnosis because of the relative safety of this agent.[161] MRI is preferred for early detection.[4] Long TR/long TE MR images are more sensitive than CT to the initial pathologic changes in the temporal lobe and inferior frontal lobe, which appear as areas of hyperintensity as early as 2 days following the onset of symptoms or signs.[147] The areas later coalesce and exhibit mass effect. In both the coronal and axial planes, extension from the temporal lobe across the sylvian fissure to the isle of Reil is well seen, as is the sparing of the putamen.[4] There is increased signal intensity in both cortex and white matter, and often MRI demonstrates characteristic bitemporal involvement when CT shows only unilateral infection.[21,147,149] MRI is also better at detecting subacute hemorrhage, which appears as hyperintense foci on both short TR/short TE and long TR/long TE images.[21] Acute hemorrhage may be well shown as a focus of moderate to marked hypointensity on gradient echo images[28] or long TR/long TE spin-echo images.[5,25,26]

Early detection of HSV encephalitis may also be aided by single-photon-emission CT (SPECT) brain scans, following injection of ^{123}I-iodoamphetamine (IMP) or ^{99m}Tc-hexamethylpropyleneamine oxime (HM-PAO). Launes and co-workers[162] have shown markedly increased accumulation of radiotracer in the affected temporal lobes of patients with reportedly negative CT scans as early as 4 to 11 days following the onset of symptoms. However, other investigators[163] have found that CT and SPECT show corresponding abnormalities during this same period.

Rarely, HSV infection may involve the brain-stem secondary to retrograde spread along CN X or CN XII.[164] MRI would be the imaging modality most likely to detect the pathologic changes in cases of brain-stem encephalitis.[165]

In the immunosuppressed patient, the rapidity of disease progression and the severity of the inflammation induced by herpesviruses appear to be inversely related to the degree of immunocompromise,[166] and mild to severe forms of both HSV-1 and HSV-2 encephalitis have been reported.[125] In this regard, Post and colleagues[100] noted that they had not identified a single typical example of necrotizing HSV encephalitis in an AIDS patient, even when culture of brain tissue yielded HSV-1 or HSV-2. Multiple other sites besides temporal lobes may be affected, and concurrent infection with a different pathogen is not uncommon.[125]

CMV infection in the neonate, acquired in utero, results in extensive necrosis of brain parenchyma with focal calcifications and in hydrocephalus.[139] Unenhanced CT demonstrates porencephaly and multiple scattered acreas of parenchymal low density.[2] Ventricular enlargement, which is usually secondary to atrophy, may be markedly asymmetric; however, the possibility of obstruction at the foramen of Monroe, resulting from ependymitis, must also be considered. Characteristically, periventricular calcifications are present.[13] Calcifications are identified in basal ganglia and cortex, but not as frequently as in congenital toxoplasmosis.[2] The differential diagnosis for the CT findings also includes congenital infection with HSV, rubella, polio, and syphilis.

Usually, contrast-enhanced CT does not show periventricular enhancing lesions. However, Post and colleagues[167] reported the case of a 4-month-old infant with immunocompromise and transplacentally acquired HIV infection who initially had only periventricular calcification, but later developed periventricular and deep-white-matter enhancing lesions with edema. Some of the lesions occurred around sites of calcification. Autopsy confirmed that the changes were due to CMV encephalitis, presumably reactivated in the immunocompromised child.

Nearly 90% of adults have antibodies to CMV.[139] In immunocompetent, and most immunocompromised, adults who have reactivation of the latent virus, infection is mild and subclinical.[139,168,169] However, in a minority of immunocompromised individuals, reactivation may produce a necrotizing encephalitis and ependymitis.[170,171] Histologically, white matter is less frequently involved than gray matter or the ventricular ependyma.[172]

CT is not very sensitive in the detection of CMV encephalitis.[170] Reported findings include nonspecific enlargment of ventricles and sulci; diffuse bilateral, periventricular white-matter low density[170,173]; and/or variable ependymal/periventricular enhancement (Figure 22.20), which may be smooth and regular[170] or irregular.[5] Pathologically, necrotic foci of acute encephalitis are observed outside the periventricular region, and a ring-enhancing cerebellar lesion that proved to be a focus of CMV inclusion bodies was reported by Levy.[174]

In cases of CMV ependymitis and encephalitis, long TR/long TE MR images reveal periventricular hyperinstensity that is thick and sometimes nodular, as opposed to a thin band often seen with transependymal resorption of CSF.[5,175] Ramsey and Geremia[176] reported a case in which several periventricular lesions with central hypointensity and surrounding hyperintensity were identified, and these corresponded to cystic areas of enhancement by CT. Gadolinium-enhanced short TR/short TE MR images would be expected to show ependymal and/or periventricular enhancement similar to that observed with contrast-enhanced CT. This pattern of enhancement also is seen with CNS lymphoma, which should be considered in the differential diagnosis for the CT and MRI findings described above.[5,100]

Varicella-zoster virus (VZV) is another herpesvirus that produces latent infection and recurrent expression in adults. Latent virus in the ganglia of the cranial nerves, particularly CN V and CN VII, may reactivate and spread retrograde to the brain stem, producing a localized encephalitis.[145] As noted earlier, brain-stem encephalitis is usually not detected by CT, but MRI may show high intensity in the

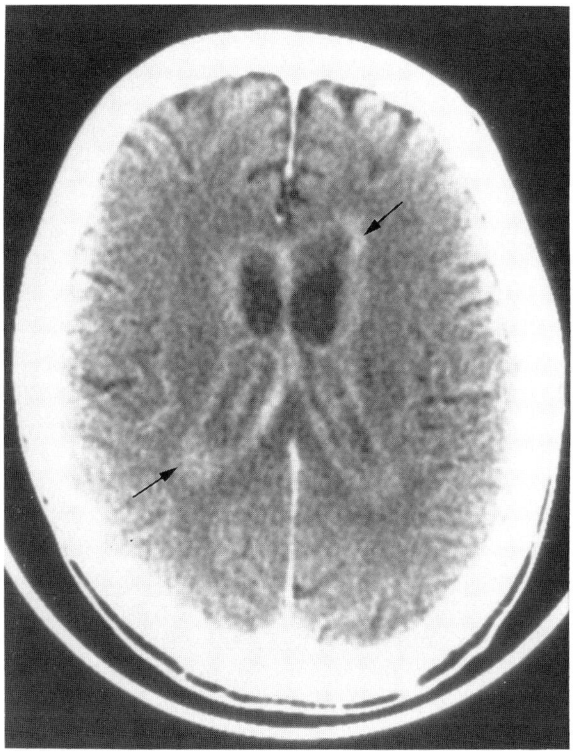

Fig. 22.20. CMV ependymitis and encephalitis. A 40-year-old man with AIDS presented with fever and progressive confusion and lethargy, leading to coma. At autopsy, owl's-eye cells characteristic of CMV were found in the ependyma and subependymal regions. Post-contrast CT scan shows diffuse bilateral ependymal and subependymal/periventricular enhancement (arrows), which is smooth and regular in outline. (Reprinted with permission from Post MJD, Hensley GT, Moskowitz LB, Fishl M: Cytomegalic inclusion virus encephalitis in patients with AIDS: CT, clinical, and pathologic correlation. *AJNR* 1986; 7:275–280.)[170]

brain stem on long TR/long TE images[149] and would better demonstrate any associated brain-stem enlargement.[165]

Diffuse encephalitis associated with VZV infection is rare, and usually develops in immunocompromised patients.[139,145] The white mater is more involved than the gray matter, as in progressive multifocal leukoencephalopathy, and the parenchymal changes may be due to an immune-mediated process rather than, or in addition to, direct brain infection. Long TR/long TE MRI is more sensitive than CT and shows the white-matter changes as areas of hyperintensity. Also, VZV-induced vasculitis with infarction may arise.[145] Zimmerman and colleagues[4] reported a case of herpes-zoster ophthalmitis in which long and short TR images demonstrated bilateral basal ganglia hyperintense foci, representing hemorrhagic infarcts, and arterial digital subtraction angiography showed multiple anterior and middle cerebral-artery stenoses, consistent with vasculitis.

Papovavirus

The JC virus and other SV 40–like oncogenic, human papovaviruses (group B) infect myelin-producing oligodendrocytes, resulting in their alteration and destruction, with associated white-matter demyelination.[139,177] Symptomatic CNS infection is found in immunocompromised patients, specifically 1–4% of AIDS patients,[178] and the disease is termed progressive multifocal leukoencephalopathy (PML). Pathologically, the early lesions of PML are small, are oval or round, and begin in the subcortical white matter and spread to deeper white matter, with sparing of the cortical gray matter.[139] Involvement is most often asymmetric, and lesions may extend across the boundaries of separate vascular distributions.[179] There are demyelination, edema, and reactive astrocytic hyperplasia without necrosis. While lesions may be located anywhere in the CNS, spinal-cord involvement is infrequent. There is a tendency to favor the centrum semiovale posteriority.[13,139]

CT demonstrates low-density area(s) in the subcortical white matter, typically multifocal (Figure 22.21).[180, 181] The lateral margin of the lesion follows the gray-matter/white-matter interface and thus may have a scalloped appearance. The hypodense areas are usually first seen in the parietooccipital white matter, but frontal and temporal white-matter lesions are not uncommon. Characteristically, there is no mass effect or contrast enhancement, although examples of lesions demonstrating mass effect[109,182] and/or peripheral contrast enhancement[109,180] have been reported.

MRI is the study of choice since the lesions represent demyelination and edema. Long TR/long TE spin-echo images are very sensitive to early white-matter changes, and often show asymmetric bilateral involvement missed by CT or more extensive unilateral involvement.[100,175,179] Areas of hyperintensity primarily involve the white matter, distant from the periventricular region, with minimal, if any, gray-matter involvement and no mass effect (Figure 22.22). While the typical pattern of involve-

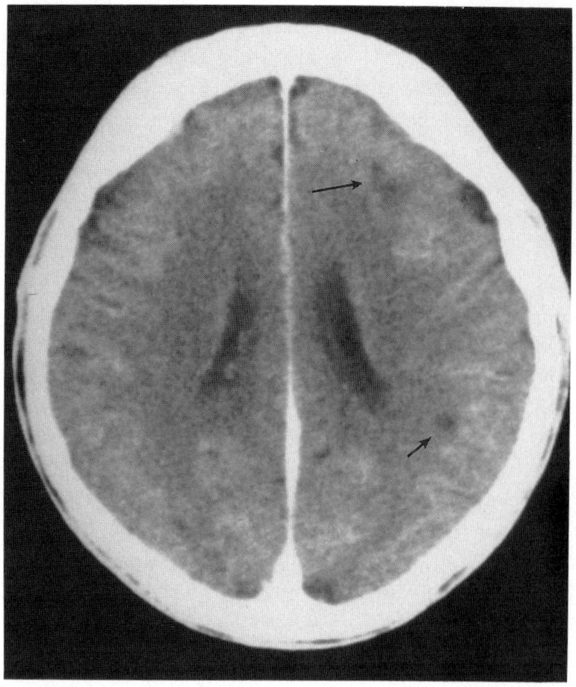

Fig. 22.21. PML in 46-year-old man with AIDS Postcontrast CT scan shows two focal hypodense, nonenhancing areas, without mass effect, in the subcortical white matter of the left hemisphere—one (long arrow) in the frontal lobe and the other (short arrow) in the parietal lobe. At autopsy, these and multiple smaller lesions were identified in the hemispheric white matter and were found to be demyelinated foci with characteristic features of PML.

ment is described as multifocal,[183] the margins of the involved areas are often irregular or poorly defined, and the areas coalesce as the disease progresses, producing a diffuse pattern.[100,184] "Atypical" patterns, which have been observed in a few patients with AIDS, include thalamic[5] and basal ganglia[184] involvement. A biparietal, focally hemorrhagic lesion crossing and enlarging the corpus callosum has also been reported.[184] PML lesions are solely infratentorial in 10% of cases,[175] involving cerebellum and/or brain stem.

Human Retroviruses

Two major groups of human retroviruses have been isolated.[142,143,185–187] The first is the human immunodeficiency virus (HIV), which has two subtypes: HIV-1 (formerly called HTLV-3), which is present on all continents, and HIV-2, which is found mainly in West Africa.[188–190] The second major group includes the human T-cell lymphotrophic virus types 1 and 2: HTLV-1, which can cause T-cell leukemia and lymphoma and neurologic disease,[191] and HTLV-2, which has been isolated from only a handful of leukemic patients in the United States.[1871,191]

Neurologic diseases resulting from direct HIV infection of the CNS include aseptic meningitis, subacute encephalitis, and probably vacuolar myelopathy.[192] In several studies, approximately one third of adult patients with AIDS were found to have subacute (HIV) encephalitis,[125,141,172,193–195] which is clinically manifested as progressive cognitive impairment with behavioral and motor abnormalities (AIDS dementia complex).[196]

In the brain, replicating HIV has been found most often within macrophages and multinucleated giant cells.[192] These cell types, as well as polymorphic microglia, are those most frequently infected by HIV. Astrocytes and oligodroglia are infrequently, and neurons are rarely, infected by HIV. Thus, the characteristic pathologic finding in HIV encephalitis is the presence of multinucleated giant cells, which are scattered throughout the white matter or clustered together in microglial nodules, which themselves are located in cortex and basal ganglia, as well as white matter.[192,197] Initially, the major abnormalities are found in white matter, and as the disease progresses, in the basal ganglia and the cerebral cortex. They also may be found in the brain stem, cerebellum, and spinal cord.[168] In the white matter, there are foci of demyelination, which accompany some of the glial nodules with multinucleated giant cells. Demyelination is a secondary and comparatively late finding, and there is relatively little edema and a paucity of inflammatory cells. The majority of HIV lesions are not seen on gross examination of the brain, although mild to moderate atrophy is apparent.[197]

Early in the course of infection, CT is normal. Later, the most common abnormal CT finding is atrophy, which is mild to moderate, with associated ventricular enlargement.[196,197] Patients who have been followed with serial CT scans over three to six months show a progressive increase in atrophy.[197] The second most common CT finding is the presence of ill-defined low-density areas, representing demyelination, in the supratentorial white matter, with no associated mass effect and no contrast enhancement. This finding was present in 7 of 21 patients studied by Post and co-workers.[197] One case of chronic meningitis with HIV-positive serolo-

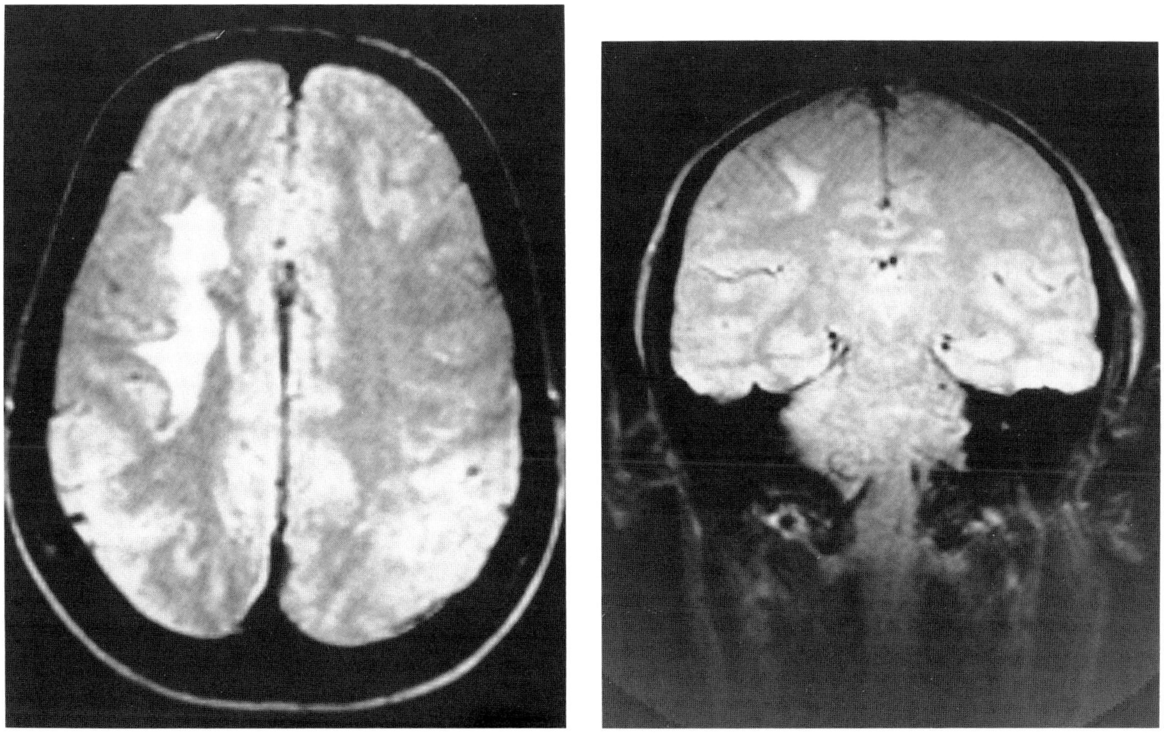

A B

Fig. 22.22. A 38-year-old woman with AIDS presented with left-arm weakness. A brain biopsy showed pathologic changes consistent with PML. Axial (A) and coronal (B) long TR/long TE (2,000/60) images show an elongated, well-defined hyperintense area, without mass effect, in the subcortical white matter of the right frontal and parietal lobes. Note that the lateral margin of the lesion has a scalloped appearance.

gy was reported in the same study, and it showed marked diffuse enhancement of the subarachoid cisterns. Otherwise, contrast enhancement related to HIV infection was not seen.

MRI is more sensitive than CT in detecting the demyelination caused by HIV infection.[196–198] Early findings are usually limited to atrophy.[197] Long TR/long TE images may show hyperintense lesions, without mass effect, in the periventricular white matter and in the centrum semiovale. Post and coworkers[197] observed such lesions in five of seven patients receiving MR scans and noted that the increase in signal intensity in the white matter may be very subtle. The appearance of the lesions varies from scattered, isolated, and unilateral in some patients to large, confluent, and bilateral in others. The extent of involvement roughly parallels the clinical progression of neurologic disease.[197]

Similarly, variability in the size and distribution of white-matter hyperintense lesions on long TR/long TE scans of patients with AIDS dementia complex[196] has been reported (Figure 22.23).[182] The pattern of involvement ranged from less common patchy and punctuate lesions (less than 1 cm in diameter) to diffuse periventricular lesions. A decrease was noted in the size and signal intensity of both diffuse and patchy white-matter lesions in an AIDS patient following AZT (zidovudine, 3'-azido-3'-deoxythymidine, Burroughs Wellcome) therapy. The improvement in the MRI abnormalities correlated with clinical improvement.[183]

Although it has been argued that a diffuse pattern of perventricular-white-matter hyperintensity differentiates HIV encephalitis from the (multifocal) pattern produced by PML,[183] the variability in the size, extent, and distribution of lesions in both HIV and PML brain infections precludes a definite diagnosis by MRI alone.

HTLV-1 is the etiologic agent for adult T-cell leukemia/lymphoma.[186,199] In its natural history and cellular effects,[200] HTLV-1 is distinct from HIV. On the basis of epidemiologic,[201] clinical,[202,203]

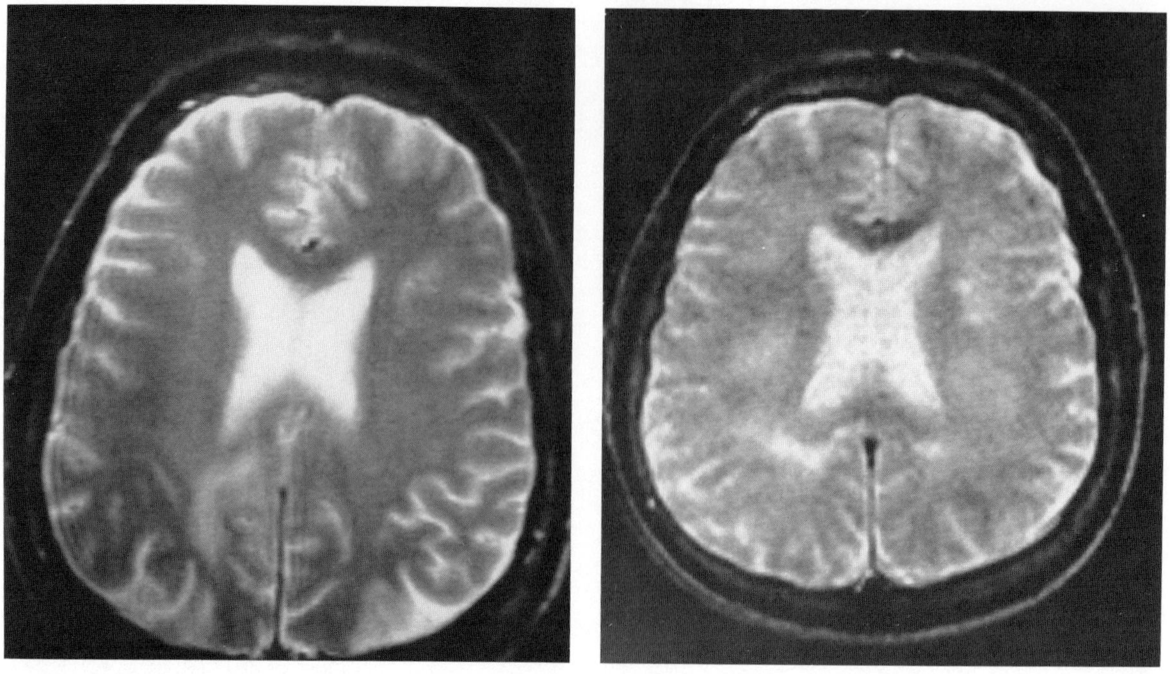

A B

Fig. 22.23. White-matter abnormalities in a 41-year-old HIV-seropositive man with AIDS dementia complex. (A) Initial long TR/long TE (2,400/80) scan at 1.5 tesla demonstrates an elongated, slightly indistinct area of hyperintensity in the right parietooccipital white matter extending from the subcortical region to the periventricular region. There is no mass effect. Mild generalized atrophy is present. (B) Repeat long TR/long TE (2,400/100) scan at 0.5 tesla obtained 2 months later shows additional ill-defined, bilateral, patchy areas of slight hyperintensity, without mass effect, in the deep white matter of both hemispheres.

and neuropathologic reults,[204,205] HTLV-1 is suspected of being the causal agent in tropical spastic paraparesis (TSP) and in HTLV-1-associated myelopathy (HAM).[206] While TSP is clinically similar to certain types of MS, epidemiologic studies[207] and serologic tests,[208,209] although somewhat controversial,[210] argue for a different etiology in these two diseases.[200]

The neuropathologic findings reported for HAM and TSP are similar, and primarily involve the spinal cord, especially the thoracic cord, where capillary proliferation, perivascular cuffing with lymphocytes, demyelination, and axonal loss may be seen.[204,205,211,212] However, widespread inflammatory changes are seen involving the meninges, brain stem, and white matter of the cerebrum and cerebellum, consistent with a chronic meningoencephalomyelitis.[201] Thickening of the media and adventitia of blood vessels in the subarachnoid space, the cord, and the brain suggests a vasculitis as well.[204] While HTLV-1 has been isolated from CSF lymphocytes of a patient with HAM,[213] it is uncertain whether the neuropathologic changes are due to HTLV-1–infected lymphocytes or to true neurotropism of the retrovirus,[200] and analogies have been drawn to HIV infection.[207]

In patients with HAM and TSP, cranial CT scans are normal, although only a few have been reported.[213,214] Long TR/long TE MR images of the brain show discrete punctuate and nodular foci of hyperintensity in the periventricular and subcortical white matter, without mass effect, in approximately 50% of patients, according to limited studies.[203,214–217] However, it has been noted that some of the HTLV-1 patients imaged were over 50 years of age and one had mild hypertension—factors that increase the incidence of white-matter lesions.[218,219]

The white-matter lesions seen in TSP patients

have been described as smaller and fewer than those seen in, or expected for, MS patients with similar clinical deficits and histories,[215,217] although some authors consider the lesions similar (Figure 22.24).[214,220]

Paramyxoviruses

A rare, slow virus infection caused by a measles virus (*Morbillivirus* genus) produces the clinical signs and symptoms of subacute sclerosing panencephalitis (SSPE). In most cases, children and young adults are affected and have had clinical measles, usually before the age of 3.[221] There are classically four stages, progressing from behavioral abnormalities or mental-status changes (stage 1) to loss of cerebral cortical function (stage 4) within one to three years.[222] Diagnosis is based on the clinical manifestations; laboratory findings, including elevated titers of measles antibodies in CSF and serum; and abnormal complexes on the electroencephalogram. Pathologically, gray matter is usually less involved than white matter. In white matter, especially in the centrum semiovale, variable degrees of patchy (early) to diffuse (later) demyelination and gliosis are found.[139] Inflammation is usually minimal. In the gray matter, neuronal loss, gliosis, and perivascular infiltration of lymphocytes occur. Pathologic changes are also found in the basal ganglia, pons, and thalamus.

The CT findings in SSPE vary with the clinical stage. Early, CT is normal or shows diffuse swelling.[223] Later (stages 3 and 4), there is generalized atrophy, with multiple focal hypodense lesions, which do not enhance, in the periventricular and subcortical white matter.[221,224] Infrequently, hypodense, nonenhancing basal ganglionic lesions are detected.[225] Similar basal ganglionic lesions may be produced by mumps virus, another paramyxovirus (see discussion below).[226]

MRI is more sensitive in demonstrating both periventricular and basal ganglionic lesions.[221,227] In stage 2 and 3 patients, diffuse bilateral periventicular-white-matter areas of prolonged T1 and T2 relaxation time, without mass effect, are identified.[10,221–228] In some regions (frontal or occipital), the periventricular changes extend outward to involve the deep and subcortical white matter locally.[221] Well-circumscribed areas having prolonged T1 and T2 may be present in the basal ganglia, especially the putamen.[225] These areas are usually bilateral, either symmetric[225] or asymmetric.[221] Long TR/long TE images are most sensitive and

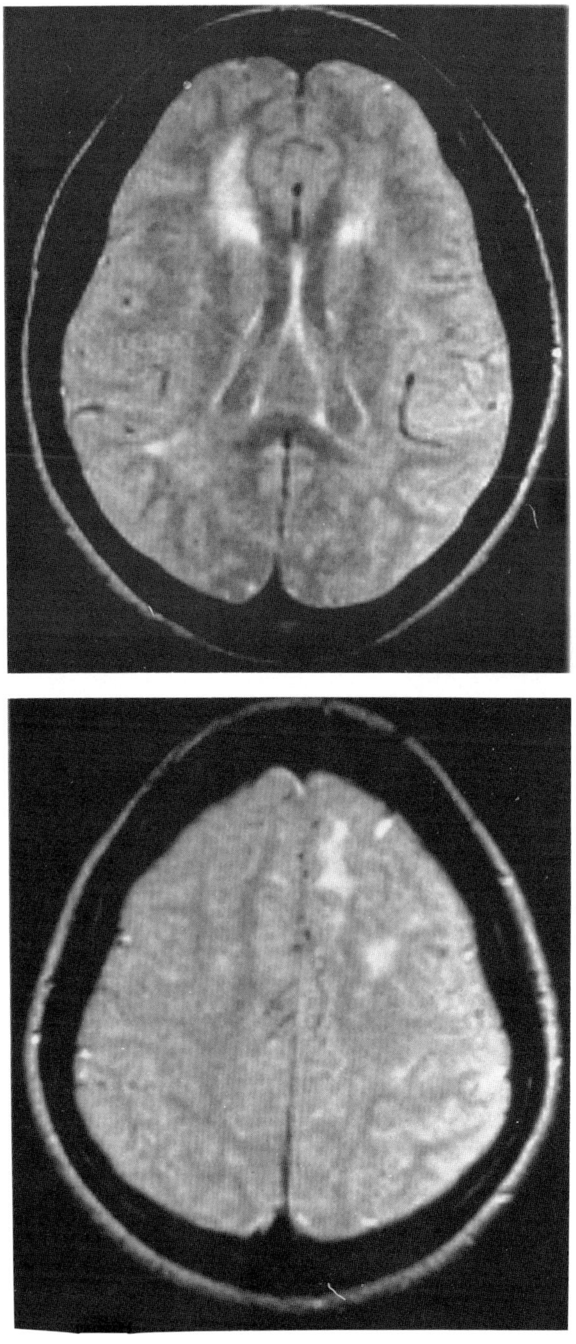

A

B

Fig. 22.24. Progressive TSP in a 30-year-old woman with high serum levels of antibodies to HTLV-1 antigens. Long TR/long TE (2,200/60) scans show scattered bilateral subcortical- and periventricular-white-matter areas of hyperintensity, without mass effect. In other patients who have tested positive for HTLV-1 and have a history of TSP, white-matter lesions are often punctate or nodular in shape (see text). (Case courtesy of Dr. William Sheremata, University of Miami/Jackson Memorial Medical Center, Miami, Fla.)

have demonstrated foci of abnormally increased signal in the cerebellar white matter and in the pons that were undetected by CT. The areas of abnormal MRI signal intensity (or CT density) are thought to represent demyelination and gliosis primarily.[224,229] However, in one case with stage 2 SSPE, areas of high signal in the cerebellar and cerebral white matter, which were identified in an initial study, were found to have decreased in size or disappeared in a follow-up scan obtained 6 months later. These findings were attributed to reversible changes such as inflammation.[221] Atrophy may be the only finding in slowly progressive cases of SSPE.[21]

CNS involvement in mumps virus infection, in the form of aseptic meningitis or meningismus, is common.[230,231] Acute encephalitis is rare, and while there is invasion of the brain parenchyma and infection of neurons, there is little neuronal destruction and inflammation is minimal, primarily involving the gray matter. In cases of severe mumps encephalitis, the clinical findings are more consistent with a postinfectious process, and histologically there are perivenular demyelination and mononuclear perivenular cuffing. The areas of demyelination and inflammation are scattered throughout the cerebral and cerebellar hemipsheres, and are found in the basal ganglia, thalamus, and brain stem.[232] In one case report of mumps encephalitis[233] comparing CT and MRI findings, a patient with an initially normal CT scan was found to have nonenhancing areas of low attenuation in both thalami and the right basal ganglia/internal capsule, with mass effect on a follow-up scan 8 days later. MRI performed at approximately the same time as the second CT showed areas of hyperintensity on long TR/long TE images in the same location as the CT abnormalities, but in addition showed hyperintense areas in cerebellum, midbrain, and right frontal and parietal lobes. The additional lesions correlated better with the patient's symptomatology, and the MRI results helped to rule out herpes-simplex encephalitis, for which the patient was initially treated based on clinical and ^{99m}Tc-glucoheptonate brain-scan results obtained on admission. The imaging findings differ somewhat from those described for acute disseminated encephalomyelitis in which lesions are limited almost exclusively to the white matter (see discussion below).

Creutzfeldt-Jakob disease

Creutzfeldt-Jakob disease (CJD) is a transmissible disease with clinical and neuropathologic characteristics suggestive of a viral infection having a very long incubation period.[139,234] The microscopic neuropathologic feature most important to the diagnosis is spongiform change in the gray matter, cortical as well as subcortical. This is accompanied by loss of neurons with replacement gliosis. White matter is usually not involved, except for secondary Wallerian degeneration.[235,236] The gross appearance of the brain may be normal or show slight diffuse cortical atrophy, slight ventricular enlargement, and in some cases, atrophy of caudate and putamen.

In patients with CJD, serial CT scans during the course of the disease have shown progressive widening of cortical sulci and enlarged lateral ventricles.[237] White-matter abnormalities have not been reported, except in one case where they did not occur earlier than 3 months before death.[238] MRI also has shown only progressive atrophy.[235] However, white-matter involvement has been demonstrated at autopsy, and thus white-matter signal abnormalities should be demonstrable in the terminal stage of the disease. In the initial stages of CJD, the MRI findings are more like those of Alzheimer's disease and the primary degenerative dementias than those of vascular dementia in which periventricular and subcortical white-matter changes are prominent.[219,239]

Acute Disseminated Encephalomyelitis

In acute disseminated encephalomyelitis (ADEM), neurologic symptoms typically begin 5 days to 2 weeks following a viral illness (especially varicella, measles, or rubella) or vaccination, and are often abrupt in onset.[240,241] ADEM may occur without a recognized antecedent. Antemortem diagnosis has been made only infrequently because the symptoms and signs resemble those of primary viral encephalitis, toxic encephalopathy, or acute MS. The hallmark pathologically is multifocal perivenous demyelination, with absence of recoverable virus from the brain, thought to be secondary to complement-mediated endothelial damage.[240,242,243]

Plain and contrast-enhanced CT scans are either normal or have abnormalities that correlate poorly with neurologic deficits.[244] MRI demonstrates patchy areas of high signal intensity on long TR/long TE images in deep and subcortical white matter of the cerebral hemispheres, as well as in the cerebellar white matter, midbrain, and brain stem.[241,245] Characteristically, there are few lesions, asymmetrically distributed and without evidence of hemorrhage, whose locations correlate with the clinical signs and symptoms. The spinal cord may be involved. There is typically no mass effect, although in one reported case, short TR/short TE images showed enlargment of the medulla, in association with a focal hypointense lesion.[241] With high-dose steroid therapy, there is progressive resolution of the MRI signal abnormalities, in conjunction with clinical improvement. The differential diagnosis for the MRI findings includes embolic infarction (which should conform to a vascular distribution), vasculitis (which would not necessarily be limited to white matter), acute hemorrhagic leukoencephalopathy (which would have signal changes consistent with hemorrhage), and MS. MS and ADEM are indistinguishable by plain MRI. It has been suggested that gadolinium-enhanced MRI may distinguish ADEM, in which all lesions would enhance, from MS, in which the active lesions would enhance yet inactive ones would not.[241] However, contrast-enhanced CT has demonstrated a combination of nonenhancing and enhancing lesions in ADEM.[244] In any event, it seems that typical MRI findings, as described above, in combination with the appropriate clinical presentation can confirm a diagnosis of ADEM and obviate more invasive diagnostic studies, as well as indicate the response to therapy.[241]

Parasitic Infection

Toxoplasmosis

Toxoplasma gondii is an obligate intracellular protozoan that can cause diffuse or focal encephalitis, particularly in the fetus infected transplacentally (congenital toxoplasmosis) and in immunocompromised older children and adults. In congenital toxoplasmosis, there is severe brain destruction; abnormal intracranial volume, with either hydrocephalus or microencephaly; and chorioretinitis.[1] Focal lesions are scattered throughout the cerebral hemispheres, usually in the subcortical white matter of frontal and parietel lobes, basal ganglia, ventricular walls, and choroid plexus.[2] These result in focal calcifications, identified by CT, in the neonate and infant. Together with congenital cytomegalic inclusion disease (CMV), toxoplasmosis is the most common cause of intracranial calcifications in children under 1 year of age.[246] In CMV, though, the calcifications are primarily periventricular in location. Other infections that can cause intracranial calcifications in pediatric patients are congenital rubella, syphillis, herpes, and polio. Periependymal and aqueductal granulation tissue may lead to occlusion of the aqueduct.[1] CT demonstrates the resultant dilatation of the third and lateral ventricles. More often, ventricular enlargement is due to severe atrophy.[2]

In the immunologically intact adult, acquired toxoplasmosis is a subclinical and relatively benign infection in which self-limiting lymphadenopathy, and sometimes fever, may occur.[1,247,248] It is a worldwide infection, and the incidence of positive serologic reactions in adults in the United States ranges from 20 to 70%.[1,125] In immunocompromised hosts, the organism may cause a fulminant necrotizing encephalitis, and in AIDS patients, toxoplasma encephalitis has been the most frequently reported opportunistic brain infection.[100,125–127,249]

Pathologically, the focal lesions produced by parenchymal toxoplasma infection have three distinct zones, without a capsule.[249] The central zone is avascular, has a solid and coagulated necrotic center, and contains new organisms. Small-vessel thrombosis and necrosis are characteristic. The intermediate zone is engorged with blood vessels, has fewer areas of necrosis, and contains numerous free extracellular and intracellular tachyzoites, yet very few encysted organisms. Here the inflammatory reaction is intense. In the peripheral zone, vascular changes are few, necrosis is rare, and there are more encysted, and fewer free, organisms than in the intermediate zone. When leptomeningitis is present, it involves only the meninges directly adjacent to the areas of encephalitis. Arteritis of large vessels is absent.

In CT scans without contrast enhancement, the focal lesions either are hypodense or are isodense with surrounding low density, and there is associated mass effect. Optimal contrast enhancement is achieved using the "double-dose delay" (DDD) technique, in which the patient receives approximately 79 g of iodinated contrast by bolus and drip infusion, and then the scan is performed one hour after beginning the infusion.[123] With this technique, most lesions are detected, and they demonstrate ring and/or nodular enhancement (Figure 22.25). Typically, they are located in the cerebral hemispheres at the corticomedullary junction and in the basal ganglia.[249] Much less often, they are located in the cerebellum and brain stem.[100,123] While ring enhancement is usually sharply defined and smooth, large lesions may have irregularly marginated, thick peripheral enhancement. Rarely, subpendymal enhancement is demonstrated.[250] Hemorrhage is atypical.[251] The differential diagnosis of ring-enhancing lesions was described in the section on bacterial abscess; however, in the immunocompromised patient, especially if only one lesion is identified, the possibility of lymphoma must be strongly considered.[100]

Currently, immunocompromised patients who are clinically suspected of having toxoplasma encephalitis and show the characteristic patterns of enhancement described are treated medically with antitoxoplasma medications (pyrimethamine and sulfadiazine).[100] A positive response to treatment can be monitored with serial CT (or MR) scans. Improvement, which is manifested as a decrease in the number and/or size of enhancing lesions, as well as a decrease in edema and mass effect, should be detected within 2–4 weeks (Figure 22.25).[123,125–127,252,253] With continued long-term therapy, scans may return to normal, or may demonstrate residual focal areas of encephalomalacia, occasionally with punctuate calcifications (Figure 22.25), and atrophy. Any interruption in therapy, which must be lifelong, may result in recurrence at the site of a previous lesion and/or the appearance of new lesions, in both cases detectable by the presence of contrast enhancement, often accompanied by surrounding edema and mass effect.[125]

Spin-echo MRI is more sensitive in detecting the presence of new or old toxoplasma lesions than contrast-enhanced CT.[125,251,254] On long TR/long TE images, the lesions have variable intensity. They are either hyperintense and indistinguishable from surrounding edema or are isointense to hypointense (compared with uninvolved brain parenchyma) and

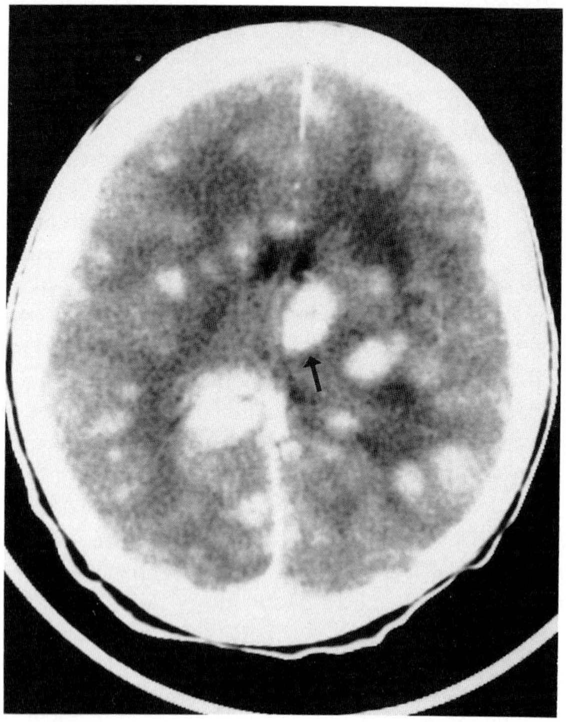

A

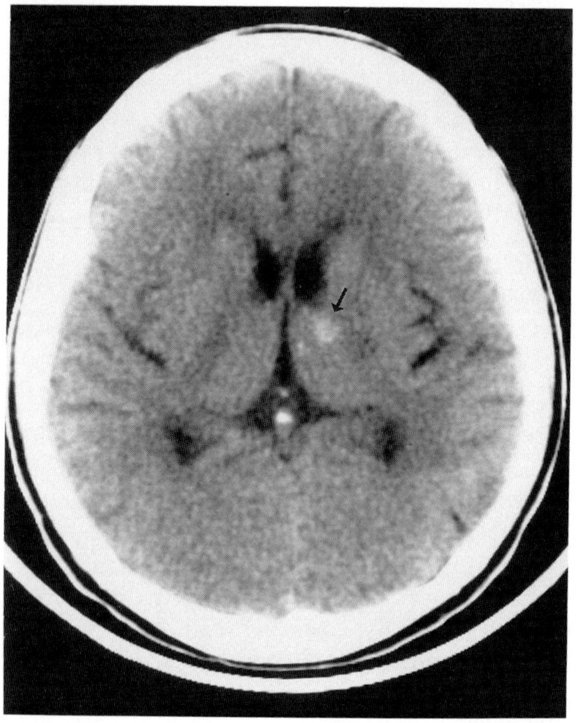

B

Fig. 22.25. Toxoplasmosis, with calcification of a treated thalamic lesion, as demonstrated by CT. (A)DDD postcontrast CT obtained on admission demonstrates multiple bilateral nodular and thick ring-enhancing lesions with edema and diffuse mass effect causing ventricular compression and displacement. Lesions are located in the basal ganglia and scattered throughout both hemispheres, with many at the corticomedullary junction. Note the enhancing lesion (large arrow) in the left thalamus anteriorly. No calcification was present in the precontrast CT. (B) Precontrast CT obtained 3 weeks after the initial CT and after the institution of antitoxoplasma treatment. There is a coarse calcification (small arrow) in the left thalamus anteriorly, at the site of the previously identified enhancing lesion. The edema and mass effect previously seen have resolved. (C)DDD postcontrast CT obtained 3 weeks after (B). There is considerable improvement compared with (A), with fewer and smaller enhancing lesions identified. There is still enhancement of the left thalamic partially calcified lesion (large arrow).

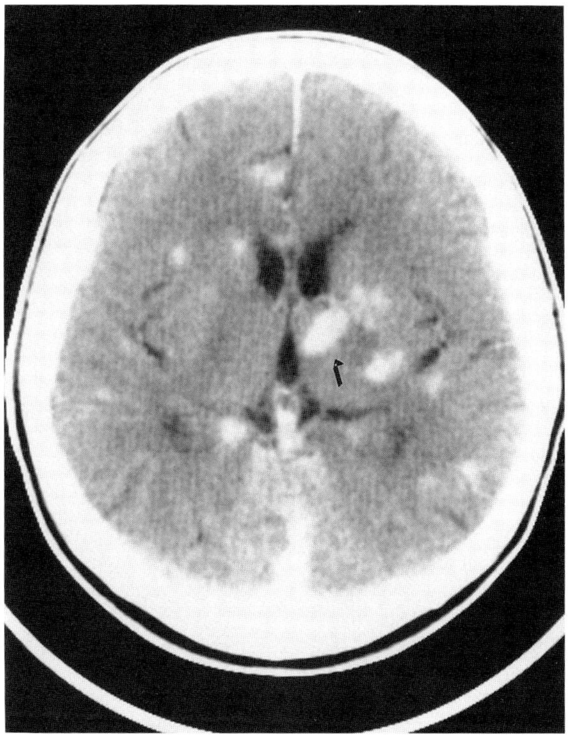

C

Fig. 22.25. *(continued)*

identifiable as a nodular focus surrounded by hyperintense edema (Figure 22.26).[175,254]

Short TR/short TE images demonstrate a focal hypointense area, which, for active lesions, exhibits ring or nodular enhancement (equivalent to contrast-enhanced CT) following IV administration of gadolinium (Figure 22.26). The enhancing lesions are well delineated from surrounding edema.

Treated or healed toxoplasma lesions may calcify, thus being, in whole or in part, decreased in signal intensity on both short and long TR images. This can make detection of the lesions more difficult than with CT.[255] Some lesions, though, appear as punctate hyperintense foci on both short and long TR spin-echo images, perhaps as a result of mineralization that includes paramagnetic ions (e.g., manganese, iron, copper),[255–259] variability in the organization of calcium hydroxyapatite, or subacute hemorrhage.[26] Correlation with CT and serial examinations should permit differentiation between the last and the two former possibilities.

Cysticercosis

Cysticercus infection begins when eggs, rather than larvae, of the pork tapeworm (cestode) *Taenia solium* are ingested by humans and then hatch in the intestine, producing oncospheres, which are the primary larvae.[260] These are distributed hematogenously, primarily involving skeletal muscle and brain. In the brain, the oncospheres develop into secondary larvae, the cysticerci, resulting in neurocysticercosis. When classified by location, four types of neurocysticercosis have been described: parenchymal, meningeal (subarachnoid), intraventricular, and mixed.[261] Whereas most authors consider the brain parenchyma as being the most common location,[109,262,263] others claim that the subarachnoid space is more common.[264–266] The cysticercus is a bladder, or vesicular, larva that is usually 5–20 mm in diameter.[266] The bladder (i.e. cyst wall) envelops, yet is continuous with, the living, solid larva, which is initially bathed in clear fluid. With time, the larva degenerates, and the solid portion of the cyst forms an eccentric round nodule that is usually 2–3 mm (but may be up 8 mm[264]) in diameter and contains the scolex. When the larva dies, the clear cyst fluid becomes turbid and gelatinous.[267] This is the colloid stage of the vesicular form,[267,268] during which time metabolic by-products of the dying larvae are thought to be released, inciting a marked inflammatory reaction.[269,270] Subsequently, the cyst decreases in size, and the cyst membrane thickens. This is the granular nodular stage.[267] In the final, nodular calcified stage, the cyst has completely involuted, and a focal calcification is usually all that remains.

These pathologic findings help to explain the varied appearance of cysticercus lesions by CT and MRI. Kramer and colleagues[268] have outlined a natural history of parenchymal neurocysticercosis, based on serial CT studies, by correlating CT findings with surgical specimens. They found that an acute phase occurs first, during which there is invasion of brain parenchyma by viable bladder larvae and a relatively mild inflammatory response, without formation of a fibrous capsule. In this acute phase, CT or MRI demonstrates a small, focal, nonenhancing area of edema or a small, homogeneously enhancing lesion.[268,271]

Subsequently, there is a chronic phase, with an initial period in which the invaginated living larva is bathed in clear fluid. CT or MRI shows a nonenhancing cystic lesion without edema. Later, in the chronic phase, as the larva dies and by-products are released, there is a more marked host inflammatory response, and a fibrous capsule is formed. Prominent ring enhancement is believed to be second-

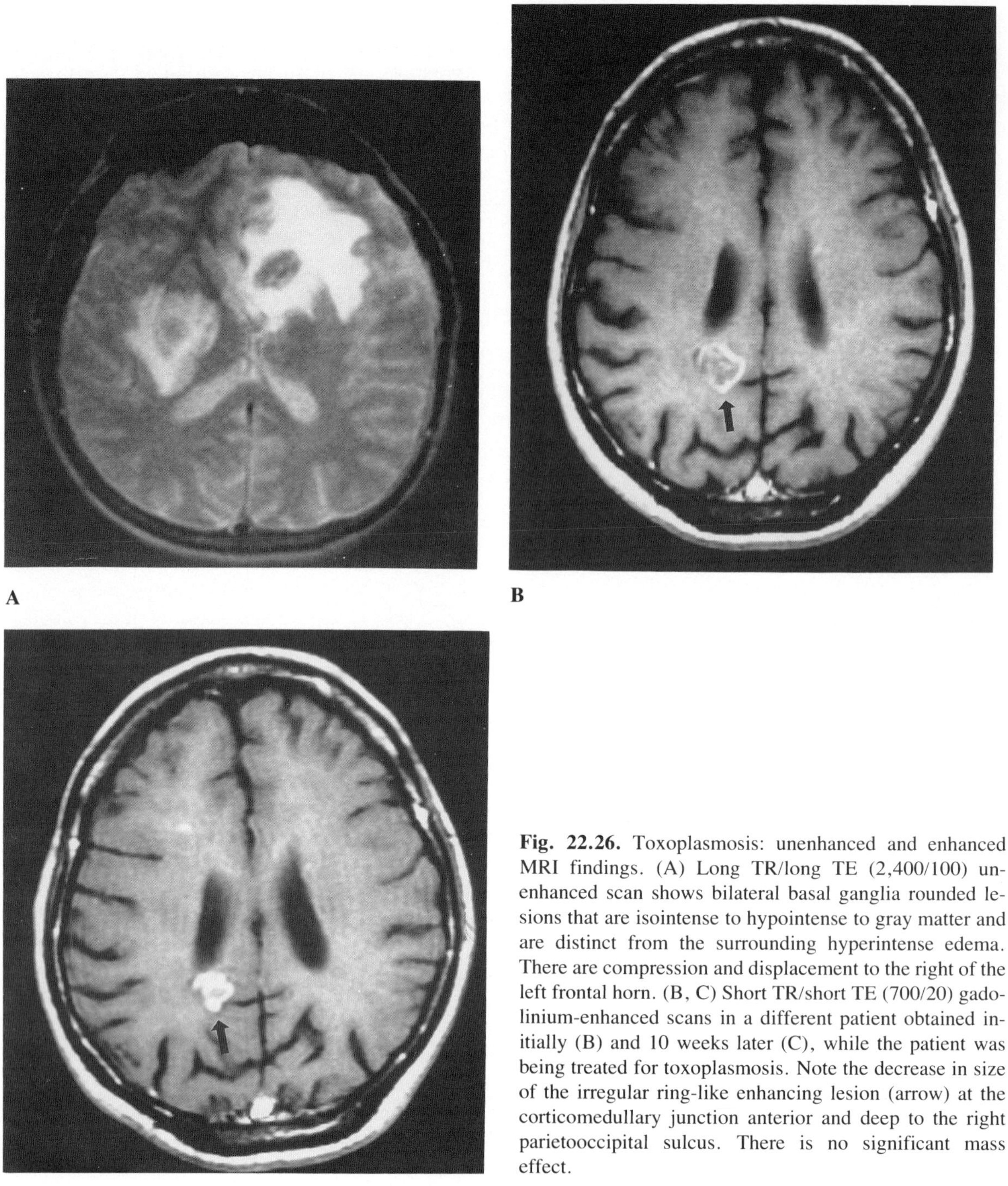

A B C

Fig. 22.26. Toxoplasmosis: unenhanced and enhanced MRI findings. (A) Long TR/long TE (2,400/100) unenhanced scan shows bilateral basal ganglia rounded lesions that are isointense to hypointense to gray matter and are distinct from the surrounding hyperintense edema. There are compression and displacement to the right of the left frontal horn. (B, C) Short TR/short TE (700/20) gadolinium-enhanced scans in a different patient obtained initially (B) and 10 weeks later (C), while the patient was being treated for toxoplasmosis. Note the decrease in size of the irregular ring-like enhancing lesion (arrow) at the corticomedullary junction anterior and deep to the right parietooccipital sulcus. There is no significant mass effect.

ary to formation of the capsule,[270] and a ring-enhancing cystic lesion with surrounding edema becomes evident on CT or MRI scans. With time, the lesion regresses, and there is diminishing edema, although ring enhancement continues (Figure 22.27). Eventually, there is no longer contrast enhancement, and at the site of the lesion, the parenchyma either appears normal or a focal nodular calcification[2] (without or with a surrounding spherical calcification) is seen (Figure 22.27). The time required for an untreated lesion to progress from the acute phase to calcification or disappearance is variable but appears to be on the order of 1 year, based on the results of Kramer and others.[268,272] Cystic lesions, which disappeared and then later were seen as calcified nodules, have been reported.[268]

On CT, parenchymal and intraventricular cysticerci are usually about 1 cm in diameter, and when identified, the 2–4-mm-diameter mural nodule is isotense to hyperintense and may enhance (Figure 22.27).[7,109,262] The parenchymal cystic lesions are hypodense, with attenuation values either equal to or slightly greater than that of CSF,[2,7] and are found primarily in the cerebral gray matter.[13,273] Many apparently intracortical cytisceerci are actually located in a sulcus and can burrow into the cortex (Figure 22.27).[262,264,266]

Intraventricular cysticerci have approximately the same density as CSF.[13] They are lined by a thin membrane, which does not usually enhance. Thus, with CT, they may be suspected only if they cause ventricular distortion or obstruction.[7,273,274] CT scan following the administration of intrathecal contrast has been the procedure of choice in demonstrating these cysts.[275,276]

Cysticercus lesions in the basal subarachnoid cisterns have CT and MRI morphologic characteristics that are different from those in parenchymal and intraventricular locations.[260,262,264,266,267] Here the cysticercus degenerates to form a multilobular cyst ("grapelike cluster"), often several centimeters in size, which lacks a viable scolex. Called a racemose cyst, it is usually located in the cerebellopontine angle and suprasellar cisterns and does not enhance peripherally; its density is equal to that of CSF. Focal cisternal widening suggests its presence, and occasionally there is basal cistern enhancement secondary to granulomatous meningitis.[260,262,264] Intrathecal contrast has been the best method of demonstrating these cysts.[275] A proliferative endarteritis associated with basal cistern cysts has been reported,[264] and angiography may demonstrate arterial narrowing, beading, thrombosis, and infarction resulting from vasculitis.

Because it does not demonstrate the focal nodular calcifications characteristic of cysticercosis as well as does CT, MRI may not be as specific as CT diagnostically. However, MRI appears to be more sensitive in the detection of parenchymal and subarachnoid cysts and perifocal edema.[262] In the early stage of parenchymal cysticercosis (when a viable larva is present inside a cyst), MRI demonstrates the cysticercus lesions as having homogeneous CSF-like intensity on both short and long TR images, except for a mural nodule that is slightly hyperintense to gray matter on the long TR images. The mural nodule is more easily detected by MRI, especially with a long TR/short TE sequence, than by CT.[262] Usually, there is no evidence of surrounding edema in the early stage of infestation.[109,262] Later, as the larva degenerates and dies, long TR images show a surrounding rim of hyperintensity, representing inflammation with edema.[10,262] Also, the cyst itself becomes more hyperintense in the long TR images, so that it may become indistinguishable from surrounding edematous brain tissue. Since the fluid is still relatively hypointense as compared with brain and the mural nodule in short TR images, sometimes these display the cyst better than do the long TR images. In addition, short TR scans optimally demonstrate gadolinium enhancement, and this should further improve the detection and characterization of lesions. After the parasite dies and calcification occurs, MRI may show a focal area of signal void, particularly in gradient-echo images.[255,262]

In the detection of intraventricular cysts, MRI has several advantages over CT, including greater conspicuousness of the mural nodule or scolex, direct coronal and sagittal imaging for evaluation of ventricular distortion, and better visualization of the posterior fossa and fourth ventricle (the most common site of intraventricular cysticerci).[262,264] While the fluid contents of these cysts are isointense to CSF, the mural nodule and wall of the cyst may be seen, and often there is a periventricular rim of hyperintensity representing inflammatory reaction.

The subarachnoid racemose cysts have signal characteristics equivalent to CSF, and since they lack a mural nodule, may be detected only by asymmetric widening of a CSF space or by an inflammatory response in adjacent parenchyma. Com-

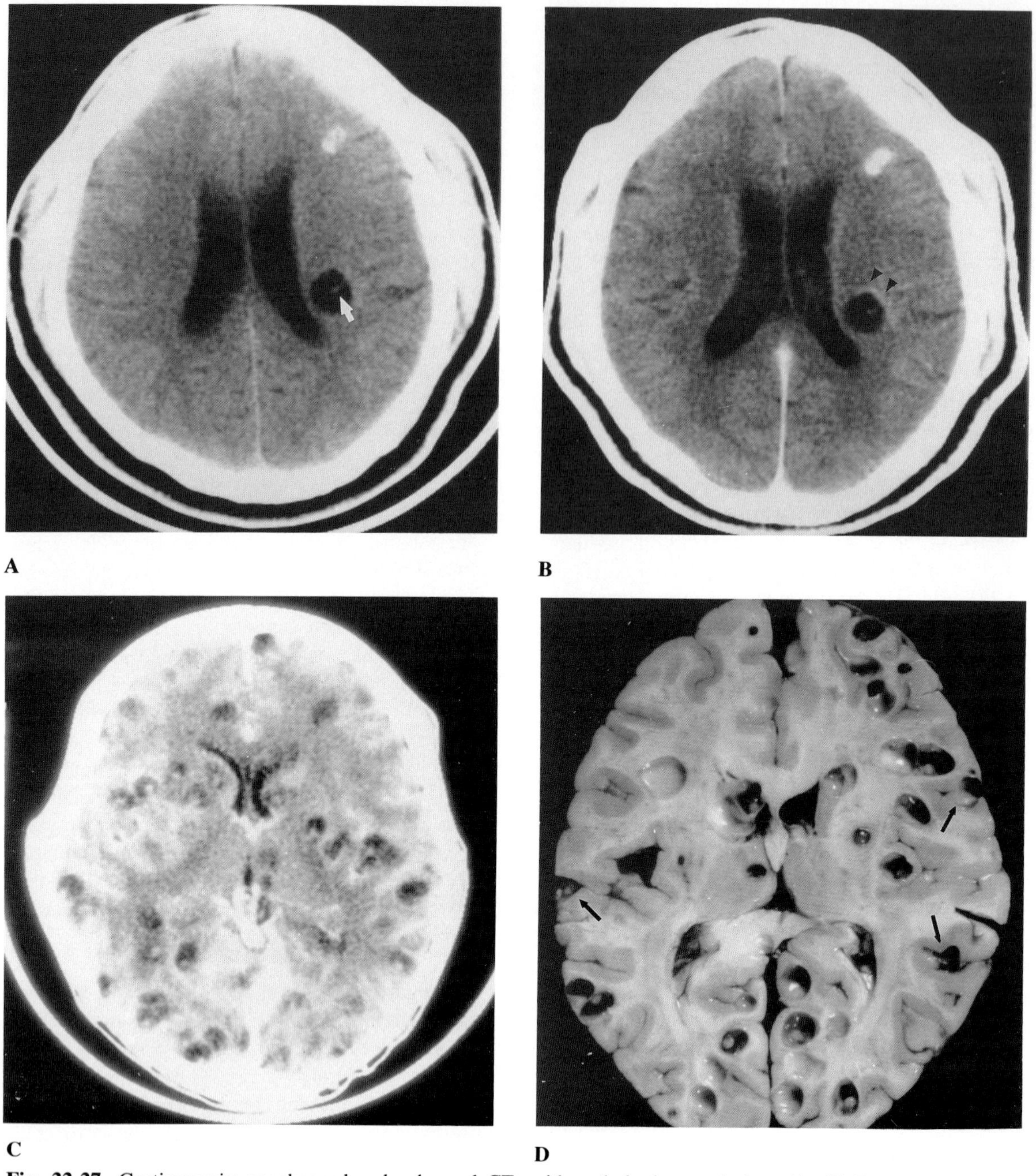

Fig. 22.27. Cysticercosis: unenhanced and enhanced CT, with pathologic correlation. (A, B) Precontrast (A) and postcontrast (B) CT scans showing a left-frontal-lobe coarse, nodular calcification near the corticomedullary junction, and a well-circumscribed, hypodense (equivalent to CSF density) homogeneous mass in the deep white matter lateral to the body of the left lateral ventricle. There is no edema or mass effect. An elongated soft-tissue density (white arrow) extends into the center of this cystic mass and represents the mural nodule. The postcontrast scan demonstrates only minimal partial enhancement (arrowheads) of the cyst wall. There is no enhancement of the mural nodule. (C) Postcontrast CT in a different patient demonstrates mumerous hypodense lesions without and with ring enhancement. In many of the lesions, the mural nodules enhance. The lesions are scattered throughout gray and white matter, with relatively little edema. (D) Pathologic specimen corresponding approximately to the CT (C). Bilateral cystic lesions with mural nodules are identified. The majority of the lesions are located peripherally in gray matter or at the gray-matter/white-matter junction, and some lesions (arrows) project within sulci. (E) Cystericercus cyst with mural nodule, from the same patient as in (C) and (D).

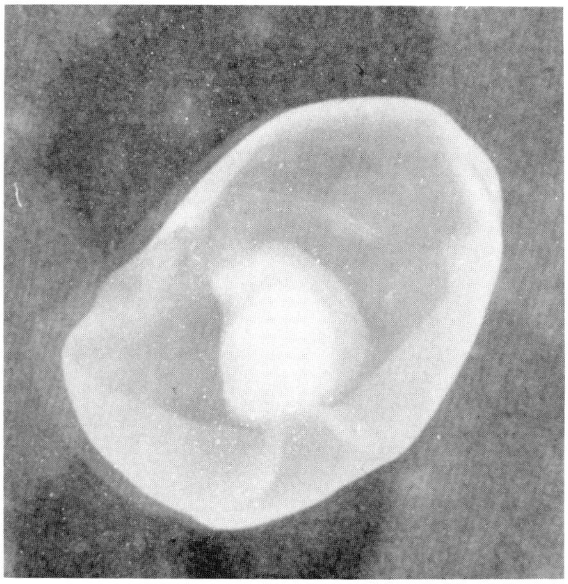

E

Fig. 22.27. *(continued)*

municating hydrocephalus, which can result if there is marked infestation of the subarachnoid space, is well demonstrated by routine or ciné MRI.[23]

Spinal Infection

Spinal infection most often is due to hematogenous seeding from a distant infection, such as in the urinary or respiratory tract. Less often, infection is secondary to prior instrumentation or a surgical procedure.

The common forms of infection are vertebral osteomyelitis and diskitis, paraspinal abscess, epidural abscess, and myelitis. Meningitis was discussed earlier and will be considered only briefly here.

Vertebral Osteomyelitis and Diskitis

Most disk-space infections occur as an extension of vertebral osteomyelitis. The most common early site of osteomyelitis caused by hematogenous spread is the anterior subchondral region of the vertebral body. It is believed that organisms frequently lodge in the low-flow vascular arcades adjacent to the subchondral plate.[277]

These vascular channels do not perforate the end place, except in children, who may have primary infection of the disk. From the subchondral bony end plate, infection spreads to the disk, and accompanying the bone destruction, there is usually a decrease in disk height. The adjacent vertebral body end plate then become involved, so that involvement of two contiguous vertebral bodies almost always represents transdiskal infection rather than multicentric foci.[278] As the infection continues, there may be regenerative changes in the vertebral bodies, more commonly observed in pyogenic infection than in TB.

The characteristic features of vertebral osteomyelitis and diskitis as displayed by plain radiography have been described for tuberculous and pyogenic osteomyelitis.[278–280] In tuberculous osteomyelitis, there is early extension of infection into the disk and destruction of cartilage, detected as narrowing of the disk space.[279] Initially, a poorly marginated, faint lucency involving the end plate may be seen at the edge of the vertebral body.[281] This progresses to irregularity and destruction of the end plate. The most common site of involvement is the lower thoracic and upper lumbar spine. Focal paraspinal soft-tissue thickening (cervical and thoracic spine) or outward bulging of the psoas margin (lumbar spine) is evidence of an associated paraspinal abscess. In serial studies with conventional radiographs or tomograms, the disk space becomes narrower and may disappear, destruction of the vertebral body progresses, and infection extends across the disk to involve the adjacent vertebra.

Usually the posterior arches and articular processes are not involved, so that the vertebral body collapses anteriorly, resulting in an abrupt angular kyphosis, or gibbus (Figure 22.28). Periosteal reaction along the vertebral body margins is uncommon and little, if any, sclerotic reaction is seen.[279]

In spinal TB, two less common radiographic patterns are described.[279] One is the "anterior" pattern in which a vertebra becomes infected by extension from a focus above or below. The infection burrows underneath the anterior logitudinal ligament upward or downward. Irregular erosion or smooth scalloping of the anterior border of the newly involved vertebral body results. There may be little or no vertebral collapse and the disk spaces may be preserved.[279] The other pattern is a "central" type of vertebral osteomyelitis where the primary focus of infection is in the body rather than along a margin and develops as an abscess cavity. The intervertebral disks are not involved as early in this form, and some vertebral collapse may occur before disk changes are detectable.[279]

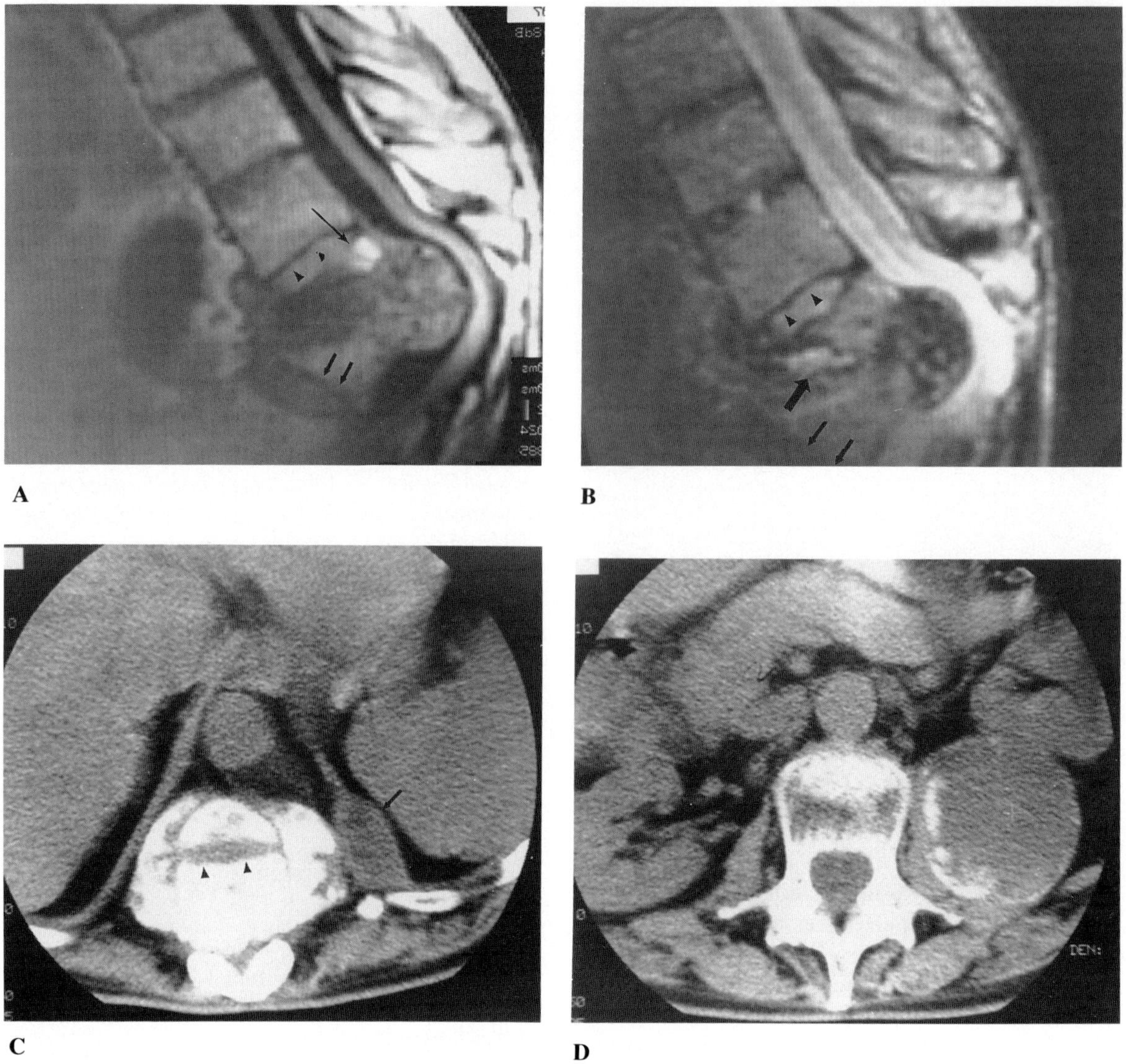

Fig. 22.28. Chronic, tuberculous osteomyelitis of the thoracolumbar spine, with gibbus deformity, cord compression, and left paraspinal abscess. (A, B) Short TR/short TE (700/20) scan (A) and long TR/long TE (2,200/100) scan (B) in the sagittal plane demonstrate destruction of the bodies of T11, T12, and L1, and obliteration of the intervening disk spaces. Most of the upper end plate (arrowheads) of T11 and of the lower end plate (short arrows) of L1 are intact. Preferential destruction and collapse of the vertebral bodies anteriorly lead to kyphotic (gibbus) deformity and posterior displacement of T12, which has been incorporated into a larger calcified mass that protrudes into the canal and impinges on the lower thoracic cord. The patient has had previous laminectomies at T12 and L1. In the T11 body posteriorly, there is a focal area (long thin arrow) with characteristics of a fat island. At the site of destruction anteriorly, though, there is a zone (thick arrow) that has MRI findings consistent with inflammation (see text). (C) Noncontrast CT scan at the T11–T12 level shows the calcified mass protruding into and narrowing the canal, as well as narrowing the neuroforamina. The anterior portion of the T10 body is separated from the mass involving T11 and T12 by the T10–T11 disk space (arrowheads), seen obliquely. The calcified vertebral mass is contiguous with a left paraspinal soft-tissue mass (short arrow). (D) Noncontrast CT scan at the L2 level demonstrates the paraspinal mass, which involves the left psoas muscle and has partial, peripheral calcification.

Hematogenous, pyogenic osteomyelitis is most often due to *S aureus* (Figure 22.29), and the lumbar spine is the usual site of involvement, followed, in order of decreasing frequency, by thoracic spine, sacrum, and cervical spine.[278]

The radiographic findings differ somewhat from those of spinal TB. Plain-film changes are first seen 2–8 weeks after the onset of infection,[282] and the rapid loss of disk height and lysis of adjacent bone favor a pyogenic infection. Occasionally, there is rarefaction or a lytic defect in the end plate without narrowing of the disk space until relatively late (weeks to month after onset).[283] Bone destruction is much less extensive than with TB and usually is confined to contiguous vertebral bodies.[279] Regenerative changes in the form of sclerosis in the vertebral body and periosteal calcification are more pronounced in pyogenic infection. Following antibiotic treatment, the affected disk space may remain relatively intact, or complete bony ankylosis may

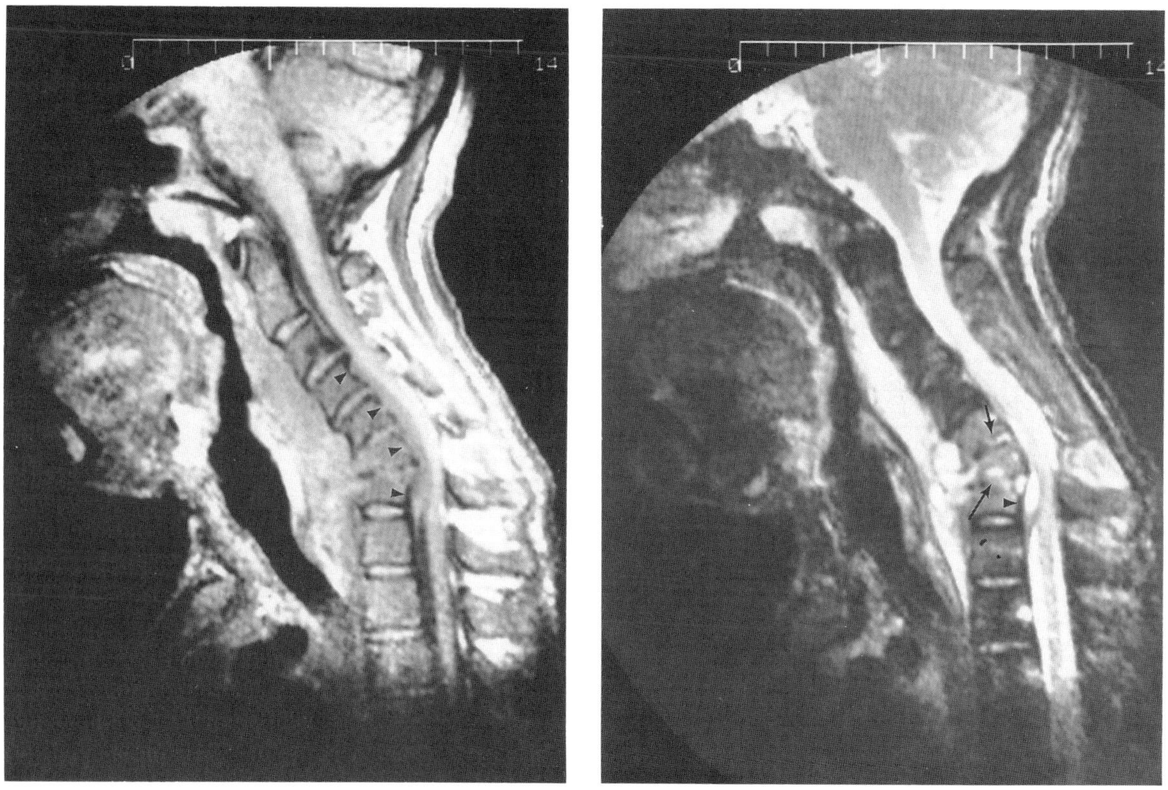

A B

Fig. 22.29. Hematogenous, pyogenic *(S aureus)* osteomyelitis of the cervical spine, with prevertebral and epidural abscess. (A) Short TR/short TE (700/20) sagittal scan demonstrates narrowing and loss of normal signal intensity of the intervertebral disk spaces at C5–6 anteriorly and at C6–7, as well as irregularity of the adjacent end plates. There is collapse, especially anteriorly, of the bodies of C6 and C7, resulting is an abrupt kyphosis. The dural sac and spinal cord are displaced posteriorly and compressed by the nearly homogeneous mass (arrowheads) in the anterior aspect of the canal from C4 to C7–T1, representing an epidural abscess. (B) Long TR/long TE (2,000/100) scan, at the same position as (A), demonstrates diffuse, moderate hyperintensity within the bodies of C5, C6, and C7, representing inflammation/infection. Marked hyperintensity with the C6–7 disk space (long arrow) and the C5–6 disk space (short arrows) represents diskitis, and this hyperintensity extends anteriorly to a multilobulated and diffuse hyperintense area in the prevertebral soft tissues (from C2 to T1–T2). A component (arrowhead) of the epidural mass seen in (A) is also markedly hyperintense and approximates the signal intensity of the prevertebral mass and that of CSF. At surgery, a multiloculated prevertebral abscess and an epidural abscess were identified. (C) Gradient-echo (350/13/10-degree flip angle) axial scan at the C7 level demonstrates the posterior margin (arrowheads) of the epidural abscess. There is diffuse, inhomogeneous hyperintensity in the prevertebral soft tissues (arrows).

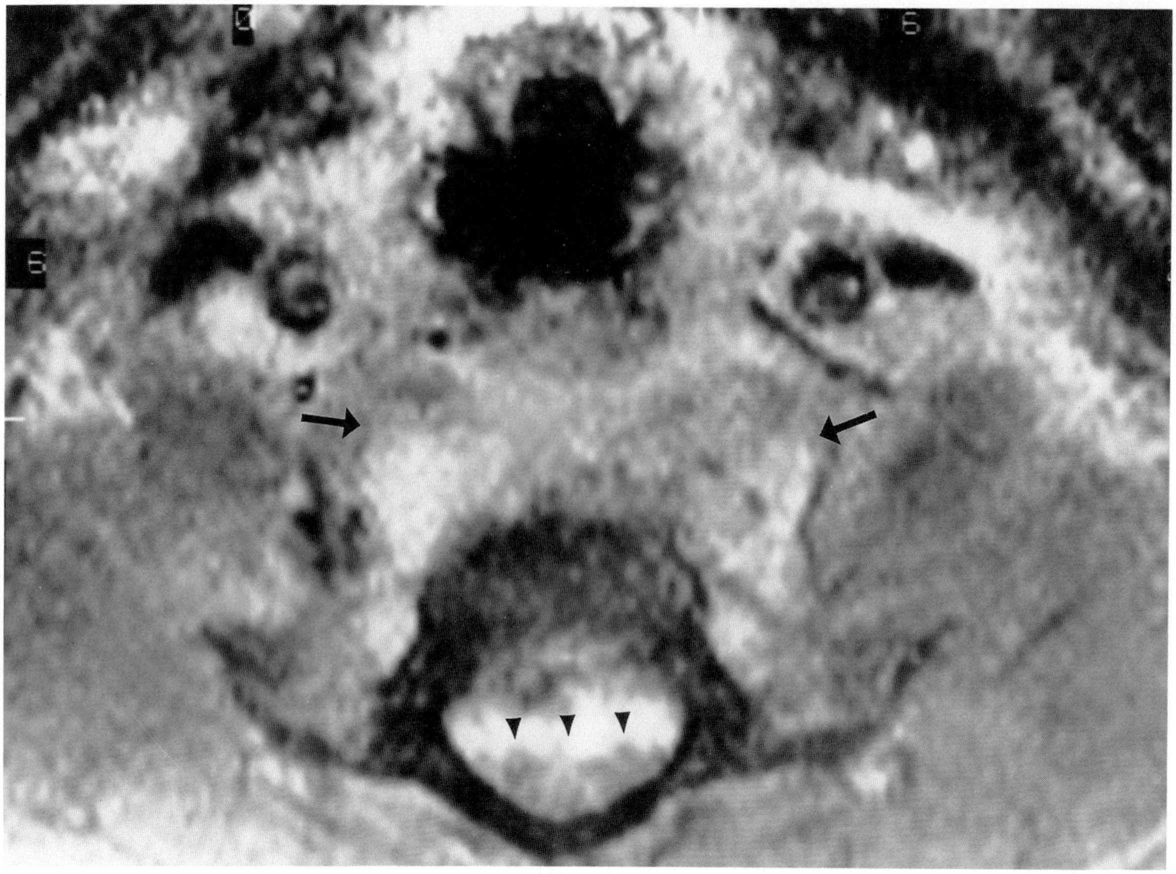

C

Fig. 22.29. *(continued)*

occur. Commonly, there is surrounding osteophytosis. The involved vertebral body may become hyperdense.[278]

There is moderately frequent involvement of the spine in certain fungal infections, including coccidioidomycosis (Figure 22.30), blastomycosis, and actinomycosis. Radiographic findings are similar to those for TB, except that there is a tendency to form sinus tracts.[279] Other fungal infections mimic pyogenic infections.[284,285] Candidiasis involving the spine usually takes place weeks to months following fungemia and should be considered in the workup of immunocompromised patients with back pain and nonspecific findings of vertebral osteomyelitis with diskitis.[286]

Most cases of vertebral osteomyelitis may be diagnosed on the basis of clinical presentation, laboratory analyses, and plain radiographs.[287] Bone and gallium scans are very sensitive in detecting early osteomyelitis, although both may be falsely negative in early infection, especially in spinal TB.[287,288] Increased uptake of radionuclide in bone scans attributable to degenerative disease can make detection of an infectious focus difficult.

CT is more sensitive than plain radiography in detecting osseous and soft-tissue changes and displays bone destruction earlier.[289] It is particularly advantageous in cases where cancellous bone is destroyed, yet cortex is intact. Sequestered avascular bone can often be seen.[283] Involvement of the posterior vertebral elements, which occurs uncommonly in granulomatous disease and only rarely in pyogenic infection, is displayed free of overlying bone and soft tissue by CT.

Compared with conventional radiographs and nuclear-medicine studies, CT better delineates the extent of disease, showing both intra- and paraspinal soft-tissue involvement (Figure 22.28).[287] Paraspinal and epidural abscesses demonstrate edge or ring enhancement on contrast-enhanced CT scans.[280,290] When necessary, CT may be used to guide diagnostic needle aspiration and surgical therapy.

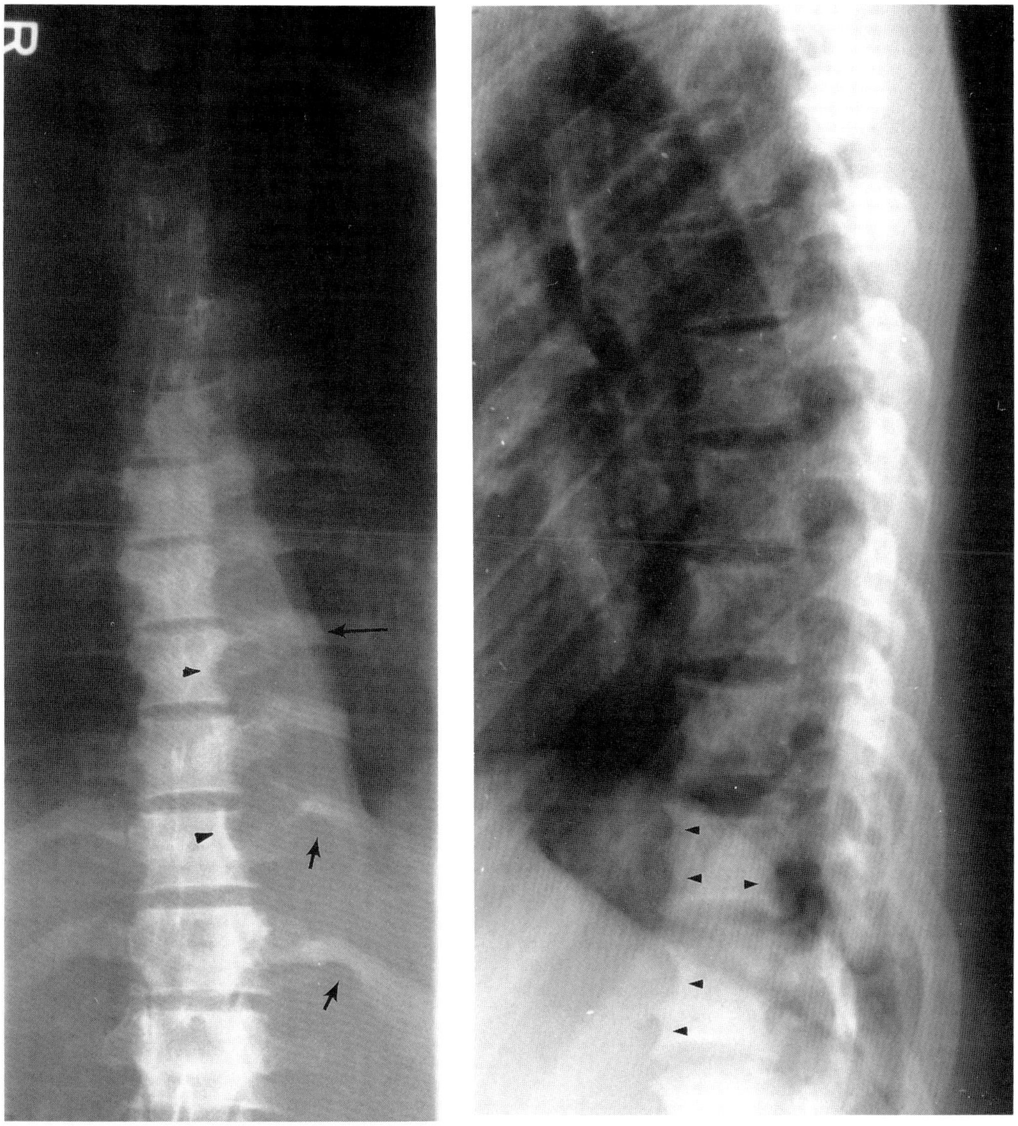

A B

Fig. 22.30. Coccidioidomycosis with paraspinal and epidural abscesses in a 27-year-old woman with a history of chronic meningitis. (A, B) Frontal (left) and lateral (right) radiographs of the thoracic spine demonstrate a left (long arrow) paraspinal soft-tissue mass from T5 to T12, with scalloping (arrowheads) of the anterior, lateral, and posterior margins of the vertebral bodies at multiple levels. Erosion of the posterior portions of several ribs is also evident (short arrows). There are enlarged intervertebral foramina in the lower thoracic spine. (C, D) Short TR/short TE (700/20) scan (C) and long TR/long TE (2,200/120) scan (D) in the midsagittal plane demonstrate the anterior scalloping of the T10 (single white arrowhead) through L1 (double black arrowhead) vertebral bodies, caused by a prevertebral mass, which is of mixed signal intensity on the long TR/long TE images and which elevates the anterior longitudinal ligament. (E) Long TR/long TE midsagittal scan shows that the prevertebral mass extends from the level of T10 (single white arrowhead) cephalad to the level of T7 (double white arrowhead). (F) Long TR/long TE scan in a left parasagittal plane shows communication between the prevertebral component of the abscess seen in (C) and (D) and a left paravertebral component (short arrow) at T11–T12. An elongated, hyperintense collection (long arrows) located in the superficial left paraspinal muscles extends from T12 to L3 and represents another component of the multiloculated abscess. (G) Long TR/long TE axial scan at the T12 level demonstrates the hyperintense prevertebral and left paravertebral components of the abscess, with erosion of the left side of the body of T12 (arrowhead), as well as the component (arrow) extending into the superficial muscles on the left. (H) Ultrasonography in the axial plane at the T12 level shows that both the superficial (arrow) and deeper left paravertebral hyperintense components seen in (E) are cystic, and that they appear to communicate (the patient is prone, and the skin surface is at the top of the image). Fluid obtained from the superficial cystic component by ultrasound-guided, percutaneous needle aspiration contained organisms characteristic of *C immitis*. Incision and drainage of the mass confirmed this finding and revealed acute suppurative and granulomatous inflammation. (I, and J) Comparison of long TR/long TE MR (I) and noncontrast CT (J) axial scans. The prevertebral and

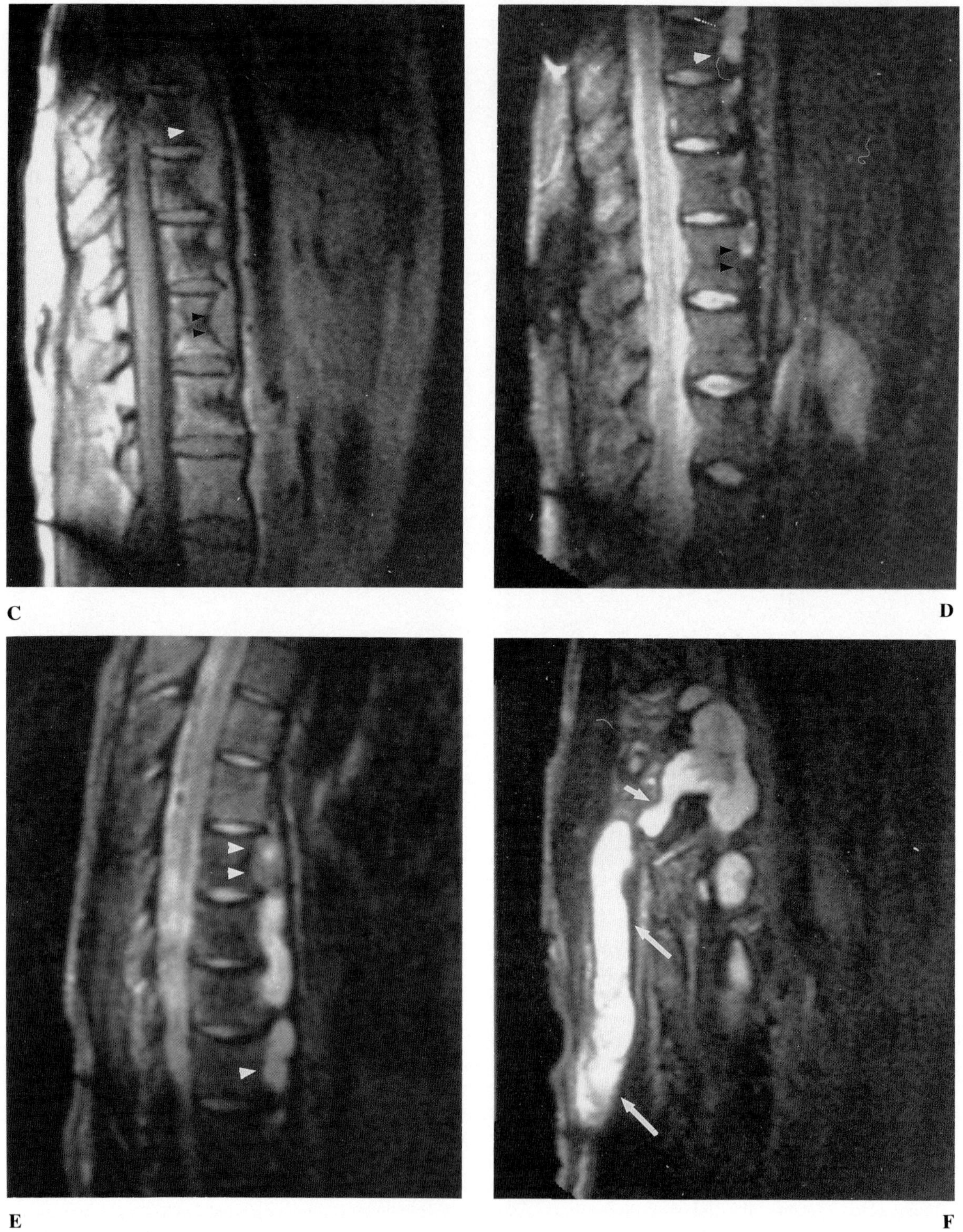

Fig. 22.30 (*continued*) right paravertebral components are markedly hyperintense by MRI and have central hypodensity by CT. The left paravertebral component (arrows) is not as hyperintense by MRI, nor does it have central hypodensity by CT. The scalloping of the body of T9 by the inflammatory masses is well shown by CT.

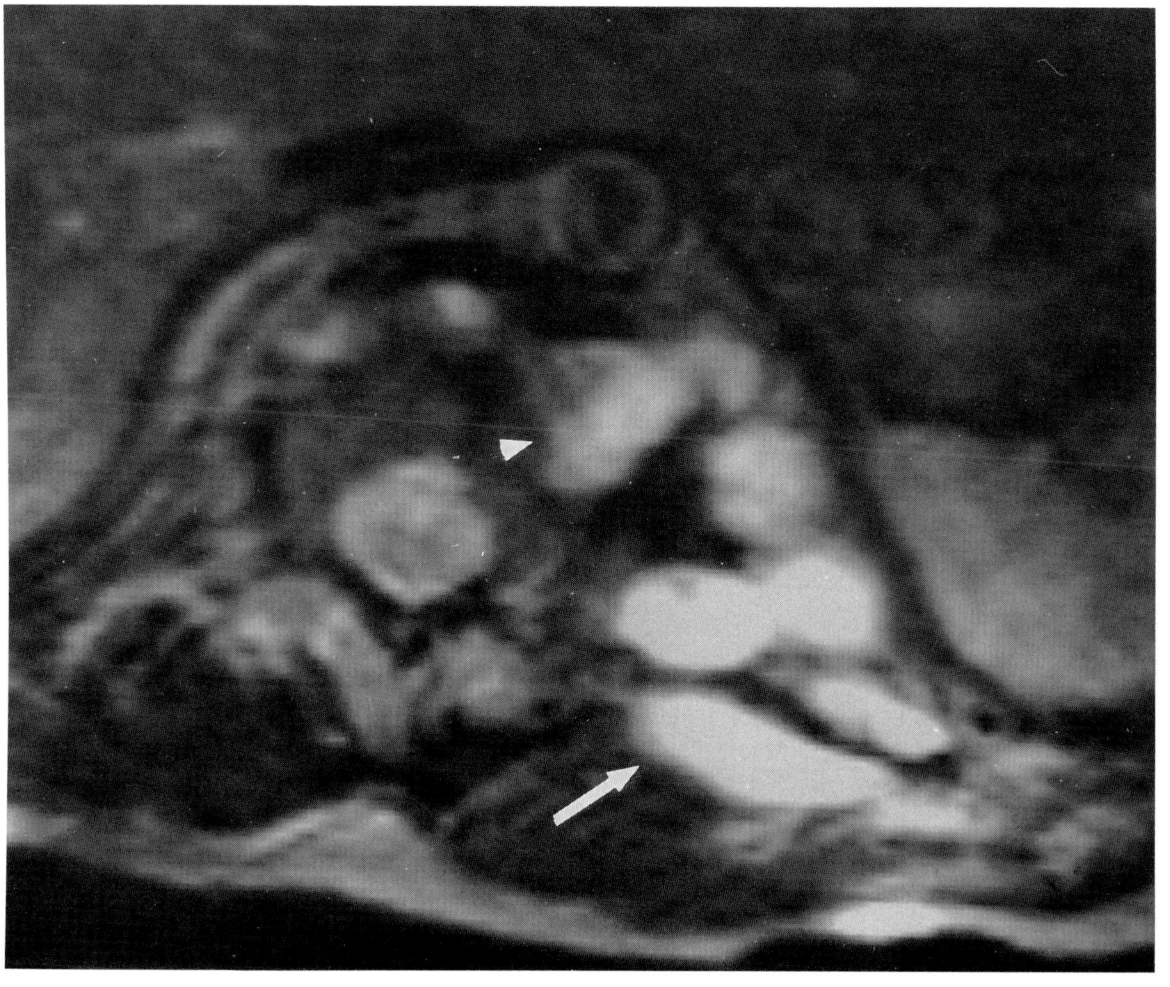

G

Fig. 22.30. *(continued)*

In patients who have had previous surgery[287] or who evidence advanced degenerative changes, where disk-space narrowing and adjacent end-plate sclerosis are shown on plain films, CT can detect a small spinal or paraspinal soft-tissue mass with bone destruction or erosion indicating superimposed infection.[283,290] Sagittal reconstructions from thin-section axial images are quite helpful in demonstrating these erosive changes.

In TB, a paravertebral abscess is usually large and occasionally shows soft-tissue calcification, best identified by CT (Figure 22.28). The presence of a paraspinal abscess usually indicates active disease. In pyogenic spinal infection, a paravertebral abscess is usually smaller and has little, if any, calcification.[290] Fungal infection may also produce a noncalcified paravertebral abscess[286] and have CT features indistinguishable from pyogenic infection.[290]

The accuracy (94%) and sensitivity (96%) of unenhanced MRI in the detection of vertebral osteomyelitis are greater than those of plain films and equal to those of radionuclide (combined bone and gallium) scanning.[291] Plain MRI is less specific (92%) than radionuclide scanning (100%).

The MRI appearance is characteristic.[291] Short TR/short TE images show confluent decreased signal intensity of the vertebral bodies and intervertebral disk space without a discernible margin between the disk and the adjacent vertebral body. On long TR/long TE images, there are abnormal configurations and increased signal intensity of the disk (a streaky linear appearance, or an absence of a

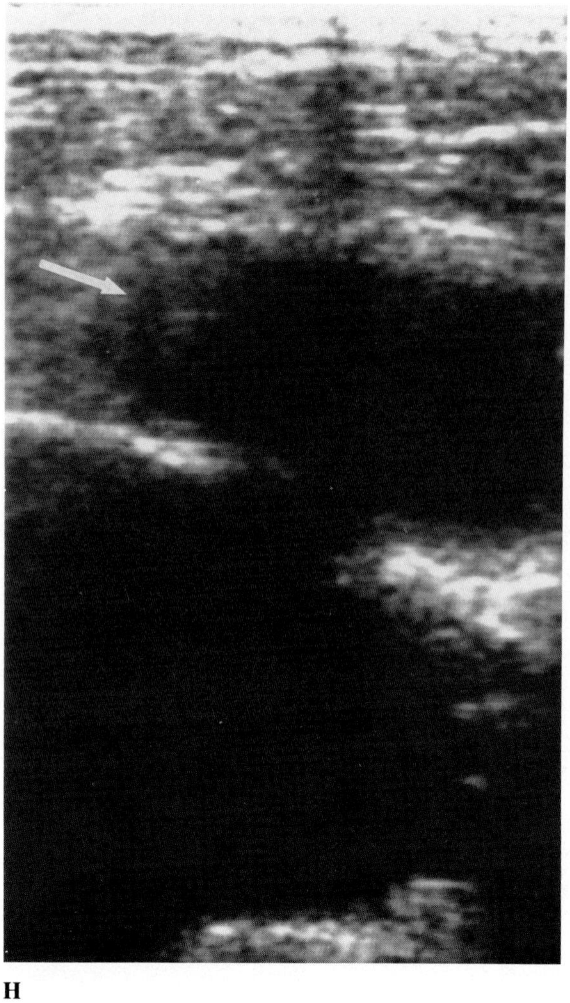

H

Fig. 22.30. *(continued)*

normal low-signal intranuclear cleft in adults over the age of 30),[292] as well as increased signal intensity of the vertebral bodies adjacent to the disk (Figure 22.29). The changes occur earlier than on plain radiographs and about the same time as on radionuclide scans.[291] Antibiotics do not obscure these changes in the early stages of treatment.

Plain MRI can distinguish active vertebral osteomyelitis from two entities commonly encountered in the differential diagnosis on the basis of plain films and/or radionuclide scanning. First, metastatic disease is distinguished by early involvement of the pedicles and by the lack of involvement of the disk space, as on plain films. Second, in severe degenerative disease or previous osteomyelitis at the same site, the disk space is well discerned and usually of low signal intensity on short TR/short TE images, and of decreased, rather than increased, signal intensity in the long TR/long TE images.[291] The vertebral-body margins may be increased or decreased in signal intensity on short and long TR images.

In osteomyelitis, MRI can show asymmetric vertebral-body destruction, with one body markedly destroyed while the adjacent vertebral body is much less affected (Figure 22.28).[293] Long TR/long TE sequences demonstrate paraspinal abscess, as well as prevertebral spread of infection (Figure 22.29), as an area of abnormally increased signal intensity. Similarly, in postdiskectomy patients who develop retrospinal abscess, long TR/long TE images show a collection, extending from the canal to the adjacent soft tissues, that has low signal intensity (but greater than CSF) on short TR/short TE images and high signal intensity on long TR/long TE images.[293]

Gadolinium-enhanced MRI is often valuable in the evaluation of spinal infection, especially when combined with gradient-echo, or long TR/long TE spin-echo, unenhanced MRI.[294] Gadolinium enhancement improves the specificity and accuracy of plain MRI in the detection of vertebral osteomyelitis and diskitis by showing definitive enhancement in the disk space on short TR/short TE images.[294] Normally, the intervertebral disk, vertebral body, ligamentum flavum, and adjacent muscles and fat have negligible contrast uptake, although the epidural venous plexus, as well as dorsal-nerve-root ganglia and nerve roots that have left the subarachnoid space, may enhance.[295]

The infected disk may show a central low signal with thick or thin peripheral enhancement, or broad dense enhancement throughout most of the disk space that corresponds to the pattern of increased signal on the long TR/long TE images. Sagittal views are the best projection for visualizing enhancement in the infected disk space. Delayed images following contrast enhancement are less helpful than immediate ones.[294] In patients undergoing IV antibiotic therapy, there is a relative decrease in the abnormal enhancement in the disk space, and resolution of abnormal enhancement correlates with clinical resolution of infection.[294]

Gadolinium-enhanced MRI, especially with coronal imaging, is particularly useful for demonstrating extension of disk-space infection into the paravertebral soft tissues. In both pyogenic[294] and tuberculous[296] spinal infection, there is enhancement of the disk space and adjacent paraspinal soft tissues, indicating active infection that may be biopsied by either MRI or CT guidance. Enhanced MRI usually

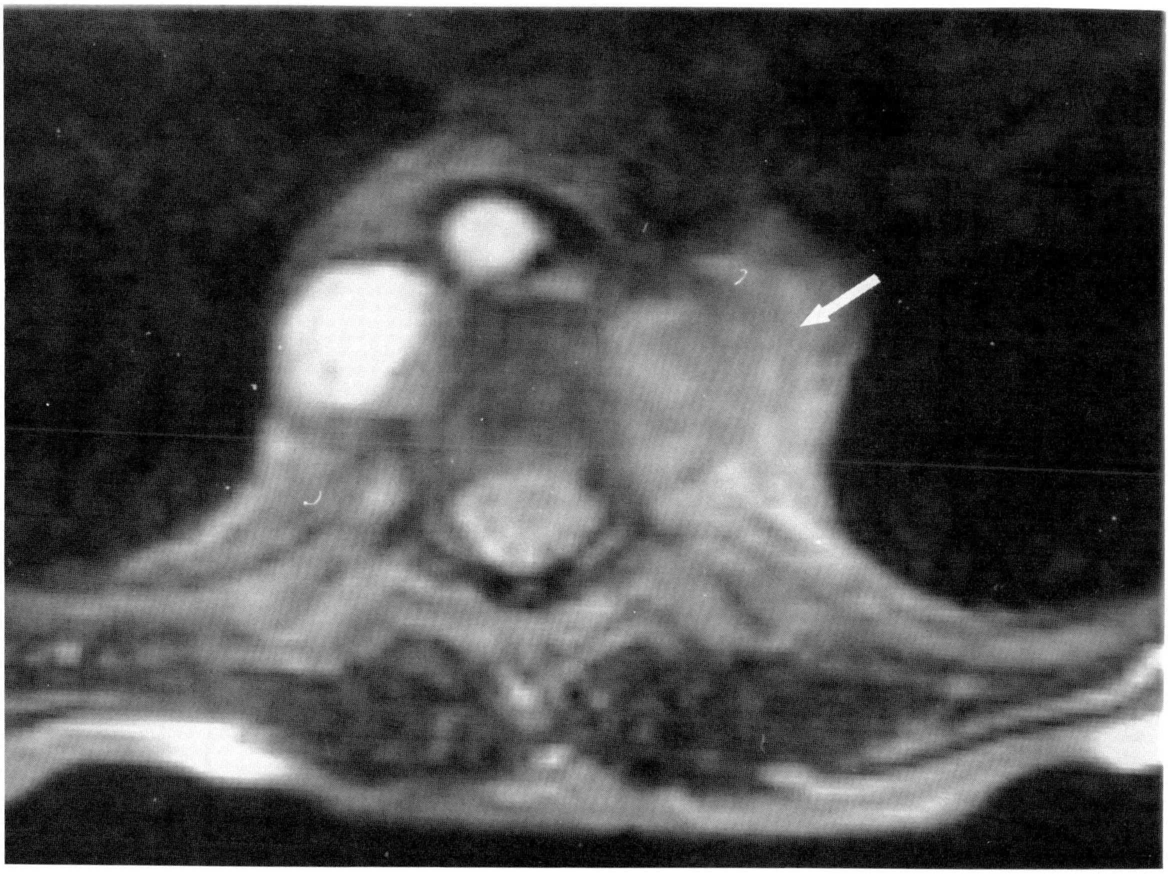

I

Fig. 22.30. *(continued)*

cannot differentiate pyogenic infection from fungal infection, or, in many cases, from mycobacterial infection.[294] While extension of infection under the anterior longitudinal ligament and erosion of the anterior portions of the vertebral bodies, characteristic of TB, are easily seen, calcifications detectable by CT are often missed by MRI.

Epidural Abscess

While an epidural abscess is usually a complication of vertebral osteomyelitis and diskitis, it may occur without vertebral involvement.[291,294] Epidural spread of infection is usually manifested as a subacute growth of inflammatory granulation tissue with microabscesses extending several levels above and below the site of vertebral involvement.[287] When the epidural (or intradural) compartment is the primary source of infection, a more fulminant, purulent abscess can be seen.[297]

Plain radiographs do not show evidence of epidural abscess, except in unusual cases of chronic infection with scalloping of the posterior margins of the vertebral bodies or neuroforaminal enlargement (Figure 22.30).

High-resolution CT often can demonstrate abnormal intraspinal soft tissues without the need for IV enhancement, except when the normal anatomy is considerably distorted by previous surgery, previous arachnoiditis, or extensive disease. However, in patients with neurologic deficit, and in those in whom surgical intervention is planned, intrathecal contrast should be used. High-resolution CT following myelography (CT myelography) accurately depicts the extent of an extradural mass compressing the contrast-filled subarachnoid sac. The extent of involvement is frequently much greater than the length of the infected vertebral bodies and intervertebral disk space.[287] High-resolution CT myelography occasionally has proved superior to plain MRI in demonstrating epidural abscess (see below).[293]

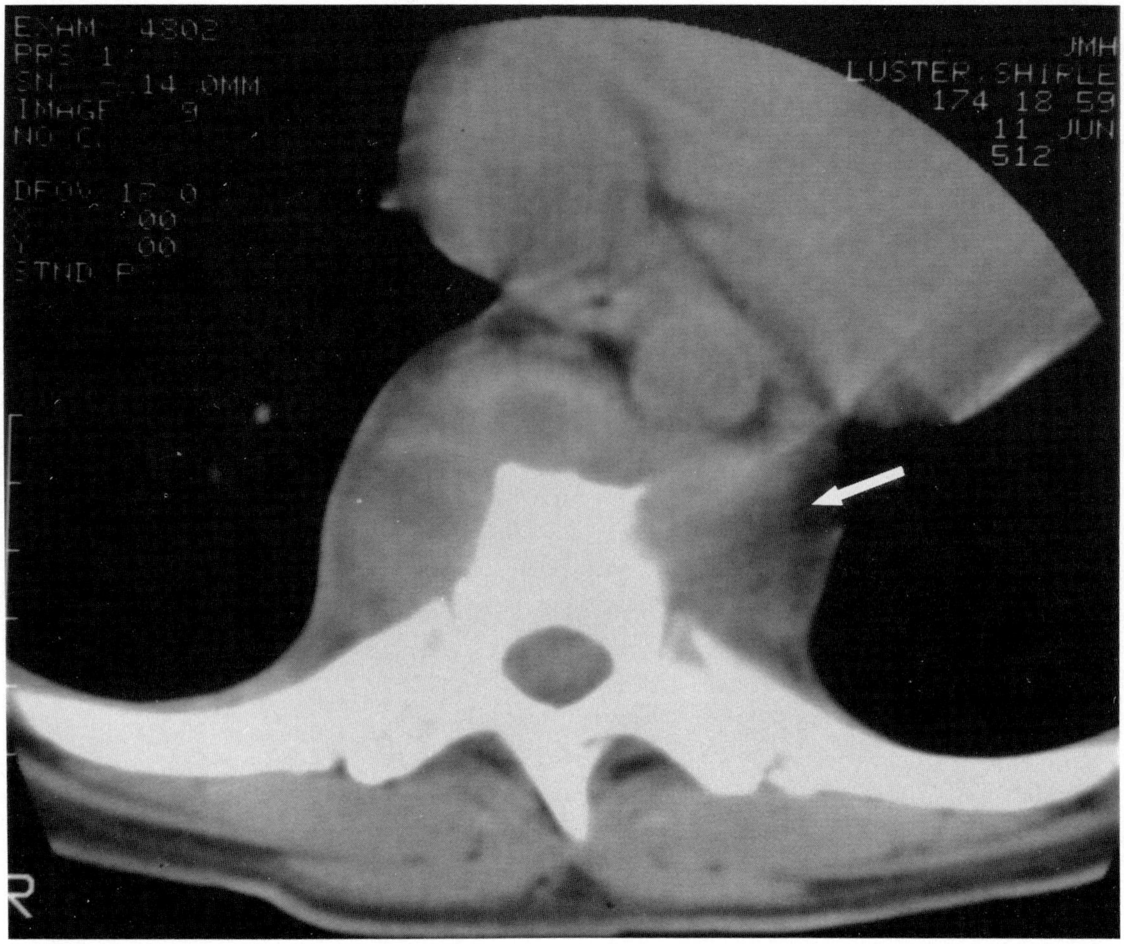

J

Fig. 22.30. *(continued)*

The appearance on plain MRI of an epidural abscess is variable. Usually it appears as a clearly identifiable extradural mass with high signal intensity on long TR/long TE spin-echo images (Figure 22.29) or gradient-echo images. However, in some cases, especially in patients with concomitant meningitis, an extensive inhomogeneous collection of mixed signal intensity is seen, and detection of the epidural abscess separate from the subarachnoid space is difficult.[293] This problem can often be resolved by short TR/short TE images obtained before and after IV gadolinium administration. The initially isointense to hypointense epidural mass usually enhances markedly and homogeneously, distinguishing it from low-signal CSF within the thecal sac and from adjacent uninvolved soft tissue and bone. Occasionally, intraspinal enhancement is quite inhomogenous, and delineation of epidural abscess separate from meningitis remains difficult. The differential diagnosis for gadolinium enhancement of intradural structures includes leptomeningeal tumor[298] and chronic arachnoiditis.[295,299]

In cases of epidural abscess accompanied by meningitis, intraoperative spinal ultrasonography has proved valuable and is recommended.[293] Epidural abscess appears as an echogenic mass compressing the dural sac, while meningitis is seen as abundant echogenic material distending the sac and replacing the normal anechoic CSF.

Myelitis

In patients with pyogenic or granulomatous spinal infection, with or without epidural abscess, plain MRI using spin-echo long TR/long TE sequences or gradient-echo sequences may detect a diffuse increased signal in the cord secondary to either edema, ischemia, infarction, or direct infection.[293,294,300,301]

Infectious or parainfectious myelitis is an uncommon complication of viral infection. The presentation may be acute, with transverse spinal involvement, or subacute and progressive, with diffuse involvement. Acute transverse myelitis has been etiologically associated with viral diseases such as measles, varicella, and typhoid, as well as with smallpox vaccinations, [302] Its occurrence in patients with AIDS reportedly is rare, and can result from herpesvirus infections,[141,303] as can ascending myelitis.[125] Myelitis may be due to either a primary viral infection or, more commonly, a secondary, immune-mediated mechanism.

Pathologic abnormalities in transverse myelitis involve both gray and white matter. Hyperemia, perivascular lymphocytic infiltration, and demyelination, sometimes extensive, are found. The thoracic cord is most commonly affected.[141]

Most radiographic studies in the past have been limited to routine myelography. Eighty percent of patients with acute transverse myelitis have normal examinations. In the remaining 20%, diffuse cord swelling with or without myelographic block is the most frequent abnormal finding. High-resolution CT myelography also demonstrates diffuse cord swelling, which in two reported cases extended from C 4 to T4 and from C6 to T5, with subtotal block at T5.[304] Plain MRI in these same patients also showed diffuse swelling, yet there was no evidence of increased signal intensity on the long TR/long TE images. The differential diagnosis of fusiform cord swelling, as demonstrated by CT myelography, includes syringohydromyelia, hematomyelia, and intramedullary neoplasm. Each of these possibilities would have different and specific findings by plain and gadolinium-enhanced MRI.[305,306]

Of the human retrovirus infections, HTLV-1 primarily involves the spinal cord,[206] and HIV infection is associated with vacuolar myelopathy.[192] Some of the histopathologic changes in these two conditions are similar—demyelination, axonal loss, and vacuolation in the white matter involving especially the posterior and lateral colums of the thoracic cord.[192,201,205,207] Myelography and CT are normal.[175,204,213,214] MRI of the cervical and thoracic spine in a few HTLV-1–antibody-positive patients without[215] and with[217] TSP has not demonstrated any signal abnormalities of the cord, but this may be due in part to technical limitations. In advanced cases of either HTLV-1 or HIV, cord atrophy should be evident.

Myelopathy or myelitis is a feature of spirochetal infection of the CNS. Tabes dorsalis is a tertiary form of neurosyphilis associated with atrophic, degenerated, and demyelinated posterior spinal columns.[1] In Lyme disease with progressive encephalomyelitis, there is predominatly axonal injury with demyelination of both proximal and distal nerve segments.[93] Also, Lyme disease may present with transverse myelitis.[78] To our knowledge, no typical spinal MRI features in these infections have been described or correlated with the pathologic changes.

References

1. Parker JC Jr, Dyer MC: Neurologic infections due to bacteria, fungi, and parasites, in Doris RL, Roberston DM (eds): *Textbook of Neuropathology*. Baltimore, Williams & Wilkins, 1985, pp. 632–703.
2. Post MJD, Hoffman TA: Cerebral inflammatory disease, in Rosenberg RN (ed): *The Clinical Neurosciences;* Heinz ER (assoc ed.): vol. 4, *Neuroradiology*. New York, Churchill Livingstone, 1984, pp 525–594.
3. Swartz MN, Dodge PR: Bacterial meningitis—review of selected aspects. *N Engl J Med* 1965; 272:725–731, 779–787, 842–848, 898–902, 954–960, 1003–1010.
4. Zimmerman RA, Bilaniuk LT, Sze G: Intracranial infection, in Brant-Zawadzki M, Norman D (eds): *Magnetic Resonance Imaging of the Central Nervous System*. New York, Raven Press, 1987, pp 235–257.
5. Sze G, Zimmerman RD: The magnetic resonance imaging of infections and inflammatory diseases. *Radiol Clin North Am* 1988;26:839–859.
6. Waggener JD: The pathophysiology of bacterial meningitis and cerebral abscesses: an anatomical interpretation. *Adv Neurol* 1974;6:1–17.
7. Lee SH: Infectious diseases, in Lee SH, Rao KCVG (eds): *Cranial Computed Tomography*. New York, McGraw-Hill Book Co, 1983, pp 505–546.
8. Bilaniuk LT, Zimmerman RA, Brown L, et al: Computed tomography in meningitis. *Neuroradiology* 1978;16:13–14.
9. Centeno RS, Winter J, Bentsen JR, Kneeland WF: CT evaluation of *Haemophilus influenzae* meningitis with clinical and pathological correlation. *Comput Radiol* 1983;7:243–249.
10. Enzmann DR: *Imaging of Infections and Inflammations of the Central Nervous System: Computed Tomography, Ultrasound, and Nuclear Mag-*

netic Resonance. New York, Raven Press, 1984, pp 188–233.
11. Cockrill HH Jr, Dreisbach J, Lowe B, et al: Computed tomography in leptomeningeal infection. *AJR* 1978;130:511–515.
12. Goldberg HI: Stroke, in Lee SH, Rao KCVG (eds): *Cranial Computed Tomography*. New York, McGraw-Hill Book Co, 1983, pp 631–640.
13. Newton TH, Norman D, Alvord EC, et al: The CT scan in infectious diseases of the CNS, in Norman D, Korobkin M, Newton TH (eds): *Computed Tomography*. San Francisco, University of California Press, 1977, pp 719–740.
14. Zimmerman RA, Patel S, Bilaniuk, LT: Demonstration of purulent bacterial intracranial infections by computed tomography. *Am J Roentgenol* 1976; 127:155–165.
15. Stovring J, Snyder RD: Computed tomography in childhood bacterial meningitis. *J Pediatr* 1980; 96:820–823.
16. Schultz P, Leeds NE: Intraventricular septations complicating neonatal meningitis. *J Neurosurg* 1973;38:620–626.
17. Naidich TP, McLone DG, Tamanouchi Y: Periventricular white matter cysts in a murine model of gram-negative ventriculitis. *AJNR* 1983;4:461–465.
18. Zimmerman RA, Bilaniuk LT, Gallo E: CT of the trapped fourth ventricle. *Am J Roentgenol* 1978; 130:503–506.
19. Nelson JD, Watts CC: Calcified subdural effusion following bacterial meningitis. *Am J Dis Child* 1969;117:730–733.
20. Zimmerman RD, Leeds NE, Danziger A: Subdural empyema: CT findings. *Radiology* 1984;150:417–422.
21. Sze G: Infections and inflammatory diseases, in Stark DD, Bradley WG Jr (eds): *Magnetic Resonance Imaging*. St. Louis, CV Mosby Co, 1988, pp 316–343.
22. Mathews VP, Kuharik MA, Edwards MK, et al: Gd-DTPA-enhanced MR imaging of experimental bacterial meningitis: evaluation and comparison with CT. *AJNR* 1988;9:1045–1050.
23. Quencer RM, Hinks RS, Post MJD, Calabro G: Intracranial flow of cerebrospinal fluid: qualitative and quantittive evaluation with cine MR imaging. *Radiology* 1989;173(P):115.
24. Brandt-Zawadzki M, Kucharczyk W. Vascular disease: ischemia, in Brandt-Zawadzki M, Norman A (eds): *Magnetic Resonance Imaging of the Central Nervous System*. New York, Raven Press, 1987, pp 221–234.
25. Gomori JM, Grossman RI, Goldberg H, et al: Intracranial hematomas: imaging by high field MR. *Radiology* 1985;156:99–103.
26. Barkovich AJ, Atlas SW: Magnetic resonance of intracranial hemorrhage. *Radiol Clin North Am 1988;26:801–820*.
27. Bradley WG Jr, Waluch V: Blood flow: magnetic resonance imaging. *Radiology* 1985;154:443–450.
28. Atlas SW, Mark AS, Fram EK, Grossman RI: Vascular intracranial lesions: applications of gradient-echo MR imaging. *Radiology* 1988;169:455–461.
29. Weingarten K, Zimmerman RD, Becker RD, et al: Subdural and epidural empyemas: MR imaging. *AJNR* 1989;152:615–621.
30. Blaquiere RM: The computed tomographic appearances of intra- and extracerebral abscesses. *Br J Radiol* 1983;56:171–181.
31. Danziger A, Price H, Schechter MM: An analysis of 113 intracranial infections. *Neuroradiology* 1980; 19:31–34.
32. Moseley IF, Kendall BE: Radiology of intracranial empyemas, with special reference to computed tomography. *Neuroradiology* 1984;26:333–345.
33. Bannister G, Williams B, Smith S: Treatment of subdural empyema. *J Neurosurg* 1988;55:82–88.
34. Smith HP, Hendrick EB: Subdural empyema and epidural abscess in children. *J Neurosurg* 1983; 58:392–397.
35. Carter BL, Bankoff MS, Fisk JD: Computed tomographic detection of sinusitis responsible for intracranial and extracranial infections. *Radiology* 1983;147:739–742.
36. Luben MG, Whelan MA: Recent diagnostic experience with subdural empyema. J Neurosurg 1980; 52:764–771.
37. Wetterling T, Schonle PW, Bardosi A, Holzgraefe M: Acute subdural and subgaleal empyema. *Neurochirurgia* 1987;30:149–151.
38. Kaufmann DM, Leeds NE: CT in the diagnosis of intracranial abscess. *Neurology* 1977;27:1069–1073.
39. Grinelli VS, Bentson JR, Helmer E, Winter J: Diagnosis of interhemispheric subdural empyema by CT. *J Comput Assist Tomogr* 1977;1:99–105.
40. Sadhu VK, Handel SF, Pinto RS, Glass TF: Neuroradiologic diagnosis of subdural empyema and CT limitations. *AJNR* 1980;1:39–44.
41. Dunker RO, Khakoo RA: Failure of computed tomographic scanning to demonstrate subdural empyema. *JAMA* 1981;246:1116–1118.
42. Macchi PJ, Grossman RI, Gomori JM, et al: High field MR imaging of cerebral venous thrombosis. *J Comput Assist Tomogr* 1986;10:10–15.
43. McMurdo SK, Brant-Zawadzki M, Bradley WG, et al: Dural sinus thrombosis: study using intermediate field strength MR imaging. *Radiology* 1986;161:83–86.
44. Som PM, Shapiro MD, Biller HF, et al: Sinonasal tumors and inflammatory tissues: differentia-

tion with MR imaging. *Radiology* 1988;167:803–805.
45. Som PM, Dillon WP, Fullerton GD, et al: Chronically obstructed sinonasal secretions: observations on T1 and T2 shortening. *Radiology* 1989;172:515–520.
46. Shapiro MD, Som PM: MRI of the paranasal sinuses and nasal cavity. *Radiol Clin North Am* 1989; 27:447–475.
47. Enzmann DR, Britt RH, Yeager AS: Experimental brain abscess evolution: computed tomographic and neuropathologic correlation. *Radiology* 1979;133: 113–122.
48. Zimmerman RA, Bilaniuk LT, Shipkin PM, et al: Evolution of cerebral abscess: correlation of clinical features with computed tomography: a case report. *Neurology* 1977;27:14–19.
49. Whelan MA, Hilal SK: Computed tomography as a guide in the diagnosis and follow-up of brain abscesses. *Radiology* 1980;135:633–671.
50. Nielsen H, Gyldenstadt C: CT in the diagnosis of cerebral abscess. *Neuroradiology* 1977;12:207–217.
51. Claveria LE, DuBoulay GH, Moseley IF: Intracranial infections: investigations with C.A.T. *Neuroradiology* 1976;12:59–71.
52. Enzmann DR, Britt RH, Placone R: Staging of human brain abscess by computed tomography. *Radiology* 1983;146:703–708.
53. Alvord EC Jr, Shaw CM: Infectious, allergic, and demyelinating diseases of the nervous system, in Newton TH, Potts DG (eds): *Radiology of the Skull and Brain: Anatomy and Pathology*, vol 3. St. Louis, CV Mosby, 1977, pp 3088–3172.
54. Moore GA, Thomas CM: Infections including abscesses of the brain, spinal cord, intraspinal and intracranial lesions. *Surg Ann* 1974;6:413–417.
55. Samson DS, Clark K: A current review of brain abscess. *Am J Med* 1973;54:201–210.
56. Heineman HS, Braude AI: Anaerobic infection of the brain: observations on 18 consecutive cases of brain abscess. *Am J Med* 1963;35:682–697.
57. Morgan H, Wood MW: Cerebellar abscesses: a review of 7 cases. *Surg Neurol* 1975;3:93–96.
58. VanDellen JR, Bullock R, Postma MH: Cerebellar abscess: the impact of computed tomographic scanning. *Neurosurgery* 1987;21:547–550.
59. Stevens EA, Klorman D, Kramer RA, et al: CT brain scanning in intraparenchymal pyogenic abscesses. *AJR* 1978;130:111–114.
60. Price H, Danziger A: The role of computed tomography in the diagnosis and management of intracranial abscess. *Clin Radiol* 1978;29:571–577.
61. New RJ, Davis KR, Ballantine HT Jr: Computed tomography in cerebral abscess. *Radiology* 1976; 121:641–646.
62. Coularu CM, Seshul M, Donaldson J: Intracranial ring lesions: can we differentiate by computed tomography? *Invest Radiol* 1980;15:103–112.
63. Piszczor M, Thornton G, Bia FJ: The evaluation of contrast-enhancing brain lesions: pitfalls in current practice (clinical conference). *Yale J Biol Med* 1985;58:19–27.
64. Dobkin JF, Healton EB, Dickson PC, Brust JC: Nonspecificity of ring enhancement in "medically cured" brain abscess. *Neurology* 1984:34:139–144.
65. Salzman C, Tuazon CU: Value of the ring-enhancing sign in differentiating intracerebral hematomas and brain abscesses. *Arch Int Med* 1987;147: 951–952.
66. Chin LC, Jensen JC, Cornell SH, et al: Computerized tomography of brain abscess. *CT* 1977; 1:33.
67. Shaw MDM, Russell JA: Value of computed tomography in the diagnosis of intracranial abscess. *J Neurol Neurosurg Psychiatry* 1977;40:214–220.
68. Rosenblum ML, Hoff JT, Norman D, et al: Nonoperative treatment of brain abscesses in selected high risk patients. *J Neurosurg* 1980;52:217–225.
69. Nauta HJ, Contreras FL, Weiner RL, Crofford MJ: Brain stem abscess managed with computed tomography-guided stereotactic aspiration. *Neurosurgery* 1987;20:476–480.
70. Robertheram EB, Kessler LA: Use of computerized tomography in nonsurgical management of brain abscess. *Arch Neurol* 1979;36:25–26.
71. Quartey GR, Johnston JA, Rozdilsky B: Decadron in the treatment of cerebral abscess. *J Neurosurg* 1976;45:301–310.
72. Haimes AB, Zimmerman RD, Morgello S, et al: MR imaging of brain abscesses. *AJR* 1989; 152:1073–1085.
73. Grossman RI, Joseph PM, Wolf G, et al: Experimental intracranial septic infarction: magnetic resonance enhancement. *Radiology* 1985;155:649–653.
74. Frazee JG, Cahan LD, Winter J: Bacterial intracranial aneurysms. *J Neurosurg* 1980;53:633–641.
75. Bohmfalk GL, Story JL, Wissinger J:, et al: Bacterial intracranial aneurysm. *J Neurosurg* 1978;48: 369–382.
76. Moskowitz MR, Rosenbaum RE, Tyler HA: Angiographically monitored resolution of cerebral mycotic aneurysms. *Neurology* 1974;24:1103–1108.
77. Cantu RC, LeMay M, Williamson HA: The importance of repeated angiography in the treatment of mycotic embolic intracranial aneurysms. *J Neurosurg* 1966;25:189–193.
78. Pachner AR: Spirochetal diseases of the CNS. *Neurol Clin* 1986;4:207–222.
79. Kaplan JG, Sterman AB, Horoupian D, et al: Luetic

meningitis with gumma: clinical, radiographic, and neuropathologic features. *Neurology* 1981;31:464–467.
80. Ihmeidan IH, Post MJD, Katz D, et al: Radiographic findings in HIV+ patients with neurosyphilis. *AJNR* 1989;10:896.
81. Godt P, Stoeppler L, Wischer U, Schroeder HH: The value of computed tomography in cerebral sphilis. *Neuroradiology* 1979;18:197–200.
82. Holland BA, Perrett LV, Mills CM: Meningovascular syphilis: CT and MR findings. *Radiology* 1986;158:439–442.
83. Holmes MD, Brant-Zawadzki MM, Simon RP: Clinical features of meningovascular syphilis. *Neurology* 1984;34:553–556.
84. Schmid GP: The global distribution of Lyme disease. *Rev Infect Dis* 1985;7:41–50.
85. Steere AC, Grodzicki RL, Kornblatt AN, et al: The spirochetal etiology of Lyme disease. *N Engl J Med* 1983;308:733–740.
86. Steere AC: Lyme disease. *N Engl J Med* 1989; 321:586–596.
87. Steere AC, Broderick TF, Malawista SE: Erythema chronicum migrans and Lyme arthritis: epidemiologic evidence for a tick vector. *Am J Epidemiol* 1978;108:312–321.
88. Pachner AR, Duray P, Steere AC: Central nervous system manifestations of Lyme disease. *Arch Neurol* 1989;46:790–795.
89. Reik L Jr, Burgdorfer W, Donaldson JO: Neurologic abnormalities in Lyme disease without erythema chronicum migrans. *Am J Med* 1986;81:73–78.
90. Reik L Jr, Smith L, Khan A, Nelson W: Demyelinating encephalopathy in Lyme disease. *Neurology* 1985;35:267–269.
91. Finkel MF: Lyme disease and its neurologic complications. *Arch Neurol* 1988;45:99–104.
92. Steere AC, Pachner AR, Malawista SE: Neurologic abnormalities of Lyme disease: successful treatment with high-dose intravenous pencillin. *Ann Intern Med* 1983;99:767–772.
93. Vallat JM, Hugon J, Lubeau M, et al: Tick-bite meningoradiculoneuritis: clinical, electrophysiologic, and histologic findings in 10 cases. *Neurology* 1987;37:749–753.
94. Kohler J, Kasper J, Kern U, et al: Borrelia encephalomyelitis. *Lancet* 1986;2:35.
95. Sheller, JR, Des Prez RM: CNS tuberculosis. *Neurol Clin* 1986;4:143–158.
96. Lyons RW, Andriole VT: Fungal infections of the CNS. *Neurol Clin* 1986;159–170.
97. Salaki JS, Louria DB, Chmel H: Fungal and yeast infections of the central nervous system: a clinical review. *Medicine* 1984;63:108–132.
98. Enzmann DR, Norman D, Main F, Newton TH: CT of granulomatous basal arachnoditis. *Radiology* 1976;120:341–344.
99. Pfeutze KH, Radner DB (eds): *Clinical Tuberculosis: Essentials of Diagnosis and Treatment.* Springfield, Ill, Charles C Thomas, 1966, p 104.
100. Post MJD, Berger JR, Hensley GT: The radiology of central nervous system disease in acquired immunodeficiency syndrome, in Taveras JM, Ferrucci JT (eds): *Radiology: Diagnosis—Imaging—Intervention,* vol 3. Philadelphia, J B Lippincott, 1986, pp 1–26.
101. Bishburg E, Sunderam G, Reichman LB, Kapila R: Central nervous system tuberculosis with the acquired immunodeficiency syndrome and its related complex. *Ann Intern Med* 1986;105:210–213.
102. Sellwyn PA, Harted D, Lewis VA, et al: A prospective study of the risk of tuberculosis among intravenous drug users with human immunodeficiency virus infection. *N Engl J Med* 1989; 320:545–550.
103. Casselman ES, Hasso, AN, Ashual S, et al: Computed tomography of tuberculous meningitis in infants and children. *J Comput Assist Tomogr* 1980;4:211–216.
104. Armitsu T, Jabbari B, Buckler RE, et al: Computed tomography in a verified case of tuberculous meningitis. *Neurology* 1979;29:384–386.
105. Lorber J: Intracranial calcification following tuberculous meningitis in children. *Acta Radiol* 1958; 50:204–210.
106. Rovira, M, Romero F, Torrent O, Ibarra: Study of tuberculosis by CT. *Neuroradiology* 1980;19:137–141.
107. Welchman JM: Computerized tomography of intracranial tuberculomata. *Clin Radiol* 1979;30:567–573.
108. Whelan MA, Stern J: Intracranial tuberculoma. *Radiology* 1981;138:75–81.
109. Rodriguez-Carbajal J, Palacios E, Naidich TA: Infectious and parasitic disorders—supratentorial, in Taveras JM, Ferrucci JT (eds): *Radiology: Diagnosis—Imaging—Intervention* vol 3. Philadelphia, J B Lippincott, 1986, pp 1–22.
110. Gupta RK, Jena A, Sharma DK, et al: MR imaging of intracranial tuberculomas. *J Comput Assist Tomogr* 1988;12:280–285.
111. Shiga H, Ysgishita A, Akiyama T: The neuroradiologic findings in a case of cerebral tuberculoma. *Neuroradiology* 1979;17:279–281.
112. Zimmerman RD, Becker RD, Devinsky O, et al: Magnetic resonance features of cerebral abscesses and other intracranial inflammatory lesions. *Acta Radiol* (suppl) 1986;369:754.
113. Jinkins JR: Focal tuberculous cerebritis. *AJNR* 1988;9:121–124.
114. Stern BJ, Krumholz A, Johns C, et al: Sarciodosis and its neurological manifestations. *Arch Neurol* 1985;42:909–917.

115. Leeds NE, Zimmerman RD, Elkin CM, et al: Neurosarcoidosis of the brain and meninges. *Sem Roentgenol* 1985;20:387–392.
116. Kumpe DA, Rao KCVG, Garcia JH, Heck AF: Intracranial neurosarcoidosis. *J Comput Assist Tomogr* 1979;3:324–330.
117. Hayes WS, Sherman JL, Stern BJ, et al: MR and CT evaluation of intracranial sarcoidosis. *AJNR* 1987; 8:841–847.
118. Ketonen L, Oksanen U, Kuuliala I: Preliminary experience of magnetic resonance imaging in neurosarcoidisis. *Neuroradiology* 1987;29:127–129.
119. Enzmann DR, Brant-Zawadzki M, Britt RH: CT of central nervous system infections in immunosuppressed patients. *AJNR* 1980;1:239–243.
120. Michael MA: Cerebral phycomycosis. *J Comput Assist Tomogr* 1979;3:417–420.
121. Holland BA: Diseases of white matter, in Brant-Zawadzki M, Norman D (eds): *Magnetic Resonance Imaging of the Central Nervous System*. New York, Raven Press, 1987, pp 259–277.
122. Kobayashi GS: Fungi, in Davis BD, Dulbecco R, Eisen HN, Ginsbert HS (eds): *Microbiology*. New York, Harper & Row, 1980, pp 817–850.
123. Post MJD, Kursunoglu SJ, Hensley GT, et al: Cranial CT in acquired immunodeficiency syndrome: spectrum of diseases and optimal contrast enhancement technique. *AJNR* 1985;6:743–754.
124. Elkin CM, Leon E, Grennell SL, Leeds N: Intracranial lesions in the acquired immunodeficiency syndrome. Radiological (computed tomographic) features. *JAMA* 1985;253:393–396.
125. Levy RM, Bredesen DE, Rosenblum ML: Neurological manifestations of the acquired immunodeficiency syndrome (AIDS): experience at UCSF and review of the literature. *J Neurosurg* 1985;62:475–495.
126. Whelan MA, Kricheff LL, Handler M, et al: Acquired immunodeficiency syndrome: cerebral computed tomographic manifestations. *Radiology* 1983; 149:477–484.
127. Kelly WM, Brant-Zawadzki M: Acquired immunodeficiency syndrome: neuroradiologic findings. *Radiology* 1983;149:485–491.
128. Fujita NK, Reynard M, Sapico FL, et al: Cryptococcal intracerebral mass lesions. *Ann Intern Med* 1981;94:382–388.
129. Britt, RH, Enzmann DR, Remington JS: Intracranial infection in cardiac transplant recipients. *Ann Neurol* 1981;9:108–119.
130. Dublin AB, Phillips HE: Computed tomography of disseminated cerebral coccidoidomycosis. *Radiology* 1980;135:361–368.
131. McGahan JP: Classic and temporary imaging of coccidioidomycosis. *Am J Roentgenol* 1981;136: 393–404.
132. Kobayaski RM, Coel M, Niwayama G, et al: Cerebral vasculitis in coccidioidal meningitis. *Ann Neurol* 1977;1:281–284.
133. Ferris EJ: Arteritis, in Newton TH, Potts DG (eds): *Radiology of the Skull and Brain,* vol 2, St. Louis, Mosby, 1974, pp 2566–2597.
134. Sweeney PJ, Hahn JF, McHenry MC, et al: Mucormycosis presenting as positional nystagmus and hydrocephalus. *J Neurosurg* 1980;52:270–272.
135. Grossman RI, Davis KR, Taveras JM, et al: Computed tomography of intracranial aspergillosis. *J Comput Assist Tomogr* 1981;5:646–650.
136. Sazo, A, Wilner HI, Metes JJ: Craniofacial mucormycosis: computed tomographic and angiographic findings in two cases. *Radiology* 1981;139:623–629.
137. Gamba JL, Woodruff WW, Djang WT, Yeates AE: Craniofacial mucormucosis: assessment with CT. *Radiology* 1986;160:207–212.
138. Centeno AS, Bentson Jr, Mancuso AA: CT scanning in rhinocerebral mucormycosis and aspergillosis. *Radiology* 1981;140:383–389.
139. Leestma JE: Viral infections of the nervous system, in Davis RL, Robertson DM (eds): *Textbook of Neuropathology*. Baltimore, Williams & Wilkins, 1985, pp 704–787.
140. Donat JF, Rhodes H, Groover RV, Smith TF: Etiology and outcome in 42 children with acute nonbacterial meningoencephalitis. *Mayo Clin Proc* 1980;55:156–160.
141. Briton CB, Miller JR: Neurologic complications of acquired immune deficiency syndrome (AIDS). *Neur Clin* 1984;2:315–339.
142. Barre-Sinoussi F, Chermann JC, Rey F, et al: Isolation of a T-lymphotropic retrovirus from a patient at risk for acquired immune deficiency syndrome (AIDS). *Science* 1983;22:868–871.
143. Gallo RC, Salahuddin SZ, Popovic M, et al: Frequent detection and isolation of cytopathic retroviruses (HTLV-III) from patients with AIDS and at risk for AIDS. *Science* 1984;224:500–503.
144. Rennels MB: Arthropod-borne virus infections of the central nervous system. *Neuro Clin* 1984;2:241–254.
145. Tenser RB: Herpes simplex and herpes zoster. Nervous system involvement. *Neurol Clin* 1984;2:215–240.
146. Zimmerman RD, Russell EJ, Leeds NE, Kaufman D: CT in the early diagnosis of herpes simplex encephalitis. *AJR* 1980;134:61–66.
147. Schroth G, Kretzschmar K, Gawehn J, Voight K: Advantages of magnetic resonance imaging in the diagnosis of cerebral infections. *Neuroradiology* 1987;29:120–126.
148. Tarr RW, Edwards KM, Kessler RM, et al: MR of mumps encephalitis: comparison with CT evaluation. *Pediatr Radiol* 1987;17:59–62.

149. Davidson HD, Steiner RE: Magnetic resonance imaging of infections of the central nervous system. *AJNR* 1985;6:499–504.
150. Whitley RJ, Hutto C: Neonatal herpes simplex virus infections. *Pediatr Rev* 1985;7:119–126.
151. Noorbehesht B, Enzmann DR, Sullender W, et al: Neonatal herpes simplex encephalitis: correlation of clinical and CT findings. *Radiology* 1987;162:813–819.
152. Benator, RM, Magill HL, Gerald B, et al: Herpes simplex encephalitis: CT findings in the neonate and young infant. *AJNR* 1985; 6:539–543.
153. Herman TE, Cleveland RH, Kushner DC, Taveras JM: CT of neonatal herpes encephalitis. *AJNR* 1985;6:773–775.
154. Wolpe JJ: Neurology of the newborn, in Shaffer AJ, Markowitz M (eds): *Major Problems in Clinical Pediatrics,* Philadelphia, Saunders, 1981, pp 508–515.
155. Yoshioka H, Kadomoto Y, Mino M et al: Multicystic encephalomalacia in liveborn twin with stillborn macerated co-twin. *J Pediatr* 1979;95:798–800.
156. Stannard MW, Jimenez JF: Sonographic recognition of multiple cystic encephalomalacia. *AJNR* 1983; 4:1111–1114.
157. Damasio AR, Van Hoesen GW: The limbic system and the localization of herpes simplex encephalitis. *J Neurol Neurosurg Psychiatry* 1985;48:297–301.
158. Davis JM, Davis KR, Kleinman GN, et al: Computed tomography of herpes simplex encephalitis, with clinico-pathological correlation. *Radiology* 1978;129:409–416.
159. Enzmann DR, Ranson B, Norman P, et al: Computed tomography of herpes simplex encephalitis. *Radiology* 1978;129:419–425.
160. Whitley RJ, Soong SJ, Dolin R, et al: Adenine arabinoside therapy of biopsy proven herpes simplex encephalitis: National Institute of Allergy and Infectious Diseases collaborative antiviral study. *N Engl J Med* 1977;197:289–294.
161. Whitley RJ, Cobbs CW, Alford CA Jr, et al: Diseases that mimic herpes simplex encephalitis. *JAMA* 1989;262:234–239.
162. Launes J, Nikkinen P, Lindroth L, et al: Diagnosis of acute herpes simplex encephalitis by brain perfusion single photon emission computed tomography. *Lancet* 1988;1:1188–1191.
163. Nara T, Nozaki H, Hishimoto H: SPECT in diagnosis of herpes simplex encephalitis (letter to editor). *Lancet* 1988;2:516.
164. Roman-Campos A, Toro G: Herpetic brainstem encephalitis. *Neurology* 1980;30:981–985.
165. Furman JM, Brownstone PK, Balch RW. Atypical brainstem encephalitis: magnetic resonance imaging and oculographic features. *Neuroradiology* 1985; 35:438–440.
166. Price R, Chernik NL, Horta-Barbosa L, Posner JB: Herpes simplex encephalitis in an anergic patient. *Am J Med* 1973;54:222–228.
167. Post MJD, Curless RG, Gregorios JB, et al: Reactivation of congenital cytomegalic inclusion disease in an infant with HTLV-III associated immunodeficiency: a CT-pathologic correlation. *J Comput Assist Tomogr* 1986;10:533–536.
168. Navia BA, Cho E-S, Petito CK, Price RW: The AIDS dementia complex: II. Neuropathology. *Ann Neurol* 1986;19:525–535.
169. Bale JF Jr: Human cytomegalovirus infection and disorders of the nervous system. *Arch Neurol* 1984;41:310–320.
170. Post MJD, Hensley GT, Moskowitz LB, Fishl M: Cytomegalic inclusion virus encephalitis in patients with AIDS: CT, clinical, and pathologic correlation. *AJNR* 1986;7:275–280.
171. Reichert CM, O'Leary TJ, Levens DL, et al: Autopsy pathology in the acquired immune deficiency syndrome. *Am J Pathol* 1983;112:357–382.
172. Petito CK, Cho E-S, Lemann W, et al: Neuropathology of acquired immunodeficiency syndrome (AIDS): an autopsy review. *J Neuropathol Exp Neurol* 1986;45:635–646.
173. Snider WD, Simpson DM, Nielsen S, et al: Neurological complications of acquired immune deficiency syndrome: analysis of 50 patients. *Ann Neurol* 1983;14:405–418.
174. Levy RM, Pons VG, Rosenblum ML: Central nervous system mass lesions in the acquired immunodeficiency syndrome (AIDS). *J Neurosurg* 1984;61:9–16.
175. Sze G, Brant-Zawadzki MN, Norman D, Newton HT: The neuroradiology of AIDS. *Sem Roentgenol* 1987;22:42–53.
176. Ramsey RG, Geremia GK: CNS complications of AIDS: CT and MR findings. *AJR* 1988;151:449–454.
177. Brooks BR, Walker DL: Progressive multifocal leukoencephalopathy. *Neurol Clin* 1984;2:299–313.
178. Krupp LB, Lipton RB, Swerdlow ML, et al: Progressive multifocal encephalopathy: clinical and radiographic features. *Ann Neurol* 1985;17:344–349.
179. Guilleux M-H, Steiner RE, Young IR: MR imaging in progressive multifocal leukoencephalopathy. *AJNR* 1986;7:1033–1035.
180. Heinz ER, Drayer BP, Haenggeli CA, et al: Computed tomography in white matter disease. *Radiology* 1979;130:371–378.
181. Carroll BA, Lane B, Norman D, Enzmann D: Diagnosis of progressive multifocal leukoencephalopathy by computed tomography. *Radiology* 1977; 122:137–141.
182. Cunningham ME, Kishore RPS, Rengachry SS, Preskorn S: Progressive multifocal leukoencephalo-

pathy presenting as a focal mass lesion in the brain. *Surg Neurol* 1977;8:448–450.
183. Olsen WL, Longo FM, Mills CM, Norman D: White matter disease in AIDS: findings at MR imaging. *Radiology* 1988;169:445–448.
184. Mark AS, Atlas SW. Progressive multifocal leukoencephalopathy in patients with AIDS: appearance on MR images. *Radiology* 1989;173:517–520.
185. Clavel F, Guetard D, Brun-Uezinet F, et al: Isolation of a new human retrovirus from West African patients with AIDS. *Science* 1986;233:343–346.
186. Poiesz BJ, Ruscetti FW, Gazdar AF, et al: Detection and isolation of type-C retrovirus particles from fresh and cultured lymphocytes of a patient with cutaneous T-cell lymphoma. *Proc Natl Acad Sci USA* 1980;77:7415–7419.
187. Kalyanaraman US, Sarngadharan MG, Robert-Guroff M, et al: A new subtype of human T-cell leukemia virus (HTLV-II) associated with a T-cell variant of hairy cell leukemia. *Science* 1982;218: 571–573.
188. Clavel F, Mansinho K, Chamaret S, et al: Human immunodeficiency virus type 2 infection associated with AIDS in West Africa. *N Engl J Med* 1987;316:1180–1185.
189. Cortes E, Detels R, Aboulafia D, et al: HIV-1 and HIV-2, and HTLV-1 infection in high-risk groups in Brazil. *N Engl J Med* 1989;320:953–958.
190. Curran JW, Morgan WM, Hardy AM, et al: The epidemiology of AIDS: current status and future prospects. *Science* 1985;229:1352–1357.
191. Rosenblatt JD, Chen ISY, Wachsman W: Infection with HTLV-I and HTLV-II: evolving concepts. *Sem Hematol* 1988;25:230–246.
192. Petito CK: Review of central nervous system pathology in human immunodeficiency virus infection. *Ann Neurol* 1988;23 (suppl):S54–S57.
193. Moskowitz LB, Hensley GT, Chan JC, et al: The neuropathology of acquired immune deficiency syndrome. *Arch Pathol Lab Med* 1984;108:867–872.
194. Snider WD, Simpson DM, Nielsen S, et al: Neurological complications of acquired immune deficiency syndrome: analysis of 50 patients. *Ann Neurol* 1983;14:403–418.
195. Ho DD, Rota TR, Schooley RT: Isolation of HTLV-III from cerebrospinal fluid and neural tissue of patients with neurologic syndromes related to the acquired immunodeficiency syndrome. *N Engl J Med* 1985;313:1493–1497.
196. Navia BA, Jordan BD, Price RW: The AIDS dementia complex: I. clinical features. *Ann Neurol* 1986;19:517–524.
197. Post MJD, Tate LG, Quencer RM, et al: CT, MR, and pathology in HIV encephalitis and meningitis. *AJNR* 1988;9:469–476.
198. Gartner S, Markovits P, Markovits DM, et al: Virus isolation from and identification of HTLV-III/LAV-producing cells in brain tissue from a patient with AIDS. JAMA 1986;256:2365–2371.
199. Yoshida M, Miyoshi I, Hinuma Y: Isolation and characterization of retrovirus from cell lines of human adult T-cell leukemia and its implication in the disease. *Proc Natl Acad Sci (USA)* 1982;79:2031–2035.
200. Editorial: HTLV-I comes of age. *Lancet* 1988; 1:217–219.
201. Roman GC: The neuroepidemiology of tropical spastic paraparesis. *Ann Neurol* 1988;23(suppl): S113–S120.
202. Osame M, Igata A, Matsumoto M, et al: HTLV-I-associated myelopathy: a report of 85 cases. *Am Neurol* 1987;22:116.
203. Vernant JC, Maurs L, Gessain A, et al: Endemic tropical spastic paraparesis associated with human T-lymphotropic virus type I: a clinical and seroepidemiological study of 25 cases. *Ann Neurol* 1987;21:123–130.
204. Akizuki S, Nakazato O, Higuichi Y, et al: Necropsy findings in HTLV-I-associated myelopathy. *Lancet* 1987;1:156–157.
205. Piccardo P, Ceroni M, Rodgers-Johnson P, et al: Pathological and immunological observations on tropical spastic paraparesis in patients from Jamaica. *Ann Neurol* 1988;23(suppl):S156–S160.
206. Roman GC, Osame M: Identity of HTLV-I-associated tropical spastic paraparesis and HTLV-I-associated myelopathy. *Lancet* 1988;1:651.
207. Rodgers-Johnson P, Morgan O StC, Mora C, et al: The role of HTLV-I in tropical spastic paraparesis in Jamaica. *Ann Neurol* 1988;23(suppl):S121–S126.
208. Kuroda Y, Shibasaki H, Sato H, Okochi K: Incidence of antibody to HTLV-I is not increased in Japanese MS patients. *Neurology* 1987;37:156–158.
209. Madden DL, Mundon FK, Tzan NR, et al: Antibody to human and simian retrovirus, HTLV-I, HTLV-II, HIV, STLV-III, and SRV-I not increased in patients with multiple sclerosis. *Ann Neurol* 1988;23(suppl): S171–S173.
210. Koprowski H, DeFreitas EC, Harper ME, et al: Multiple sclerosis and human T-cell lymphotropic retroviruses. *Nature* 1985;318:154–160.
211. Montgomery RD, Cruickshank EK, Robertson WB, McMenemey WH: Clinical and pathological observation on Jamaican neuropathy. *Brain* 164;87:425–462.
212. Mani KS, Mani AJ, Montgomery RD: A spastic paraplegic syndrome in South India. *J Neurol Sci* 1969;9:179–199.
213. Hirose S, Uemura Y, Fujishita M, et al: Isolation of HTLV-I from cerebrospinal fluid of a patient with myelopathy. *Lancet* 1986;2:397–398.
214. Tournier-Lasserve E, Gout O, Gessain A, et al: HTLV-I brain abnormalities on magnetic resonance

imaging, and relation with multiple sclerosis. *Lancet* 1987;2:49–50.
215. Mattson DH, McFarlin DE, Mora C, Zaninovic V: Central-nervous-system lesions detected by magnetic resonance imaging in an HTLV-I antibody positive symptomless individual. *Lancet* 1987;2:49.
216. Miller DH, Newton MR, Rudge P, Cruickshank K: Magnetic resonance imaging in HTLV-I antibody positive patients. *Lancet* 1987;2:514.
217. Newton M, Miller D, Rudge P, et al: Antibody of human T-lymphotropic virus type I in West-Indian-born UK residents with spastic paraparesis. *Lancet* 1987;1:415–416.
218. Miller DH, Newton MR, Rudge P, Cruickshank K: Magnetic resonance imaging in HTLV-I antibody positive patients. *Lancet* 1987;2:514.
219. Bowen BC, Barker WB, Lowenstein DA, et al: MR signal abnormalities in memory disorder and dementia. *AJNR* 1990;11:283–290.
220. Sheremata WA, Quencer R, Gatti E, et al: Magnetic resonance imaging (MRI) of tropical spastic paraplegia. *Neurology* 1987;37(suppl):322.
221. Tsuchiya K, Yamauchi T, Furui S, et al: MR imaging vs CT in subacute sclerosing panencephalitis. *AJNR* 1988;9:943–946.
222. Jabbour JT, Garcia JH, Lemmi H, et al: SSPE: a multidisciplinary study of eight cases. *JAMA* 1969; 207:2248–2254.
223. Pedersen H, Wulff CH: Computed tomographic findings of early subacute sclerosing panencephalitis. *Neuroradiology* 1982;23:31–32.
224. Duda EE, Huttenlocker PR, Patronas NJ: CT of subacute sclerosing panencephalitis. *AJNR* 1980; 1:35–38.
225. Woodard KG, Weinberg PE, Lipton HL: Basal ganglia involvement in subacute sclerosing panencephalitis: CT and MR demonstration. *J Comput Assist Tomogr* 1988;12:489–491.
226. Goutiere F, Alcardi J: Acute neurological dysfunction associated with destructive lesions of the basal ganglia in children. *Ann Neurol* 1982;12:328–332.
227. Takemoto K, Koizumi Y, Kogame S, et al: Magnetic resonance imaging of subacute sclerosing panencephalitis. *Jpn Clin Radiol* 1986;31:999–1004.
228. Case records of the Massachusetts General Hospital (case 25-1986). *N Engl J Med* 1986;314:1689–1700.
229. Schoeman JF, Bezing K-LV, Hewlett RH: Correlative clinical, neuroradiological and pathological findings in subacute sclerosing panencephalitis. A report of 5 cases. *S Afr Med J* 1982;62:447–450.
230. Koskinienmi M, Donner M, Petty O: Clinical appearance and outcome in mumps encephalitis in children. *Acta Paediatr Scand* 1983;72:603–609.
231. Jubelt B. Enterovirus and mumps virus infections of the nervous system. *Neurol Clin* 1984;2:187–207.
232. Donohue WL, Playfair FD, Whitaker L: Mumps encephalitis: pathology and pathogenesis. *J Pediatr* 1955;47:395–412.
233. Tarr RW, Edwards KM, Kessler RM, Kulkarni MV: MRI of mumps encephalitis: comparison with CT evaluation. *Pediatr Radiol* 1987;17:59–62.
234. Bendheim PE: The human spongiform encephalopathies. *Neurol Clin* 1984;2:281–298.
235. Kovanen J, Erkinjuntti T, Iivanainen M, et al: Cerebral MR and CT imaging in Creutzfeldt-Jakob disease. *J Comput Assist Tomogr* 1985;9:125–128.
236. Park TS, Kleinman GM, Richardson EP: Creutzfeldt-Jakob disease with extensive degeneration of white matter. *Acta Neuropathol* 1980;52:239–342.
237. Rao CVGK, Brennan TG, Garcia JH: Computed tomography in the diagnosis of Creutzfeldt-Jakob disease. *J Comput Assist Tomogr* 1977;1:211–215.
238. Macchi G, Abbamondi AL, Di Trapani G, Sbriccoli A: On the white matter lesions of the Creutzfeldt-Jakob disease. Can a new subentity be recognized in man? *J Neurol Sci* 1984;63:197–206.
239. Erkinjuntti T, Sipponen JT, Iivanainen M, et al: Cerebral NMR and CT imaging in dementia. *J Comput Assist Tomogr* 1984;8:614–618.
240. Alford EC: Acute disseminated encephalomyelitis and "allergic" neuroencephalopathies, in Vinken PJ, Bruyn GW (eds): *Handbook of Clinical Neurology*, vol 9. New York, American Elsevier, 1980, pp 501–571.
241. Atlas Sw, Grossman RI, Goldberg HI, et al: MR diagnosis of acute disseminated encephalomyelitis. *J Comput Assist Tomogr* 1986;10:798–801.
242. Carpenter S, Sampert PW: Post-infectious perivenous encephalitis and acute hemorrhagic encephalitis, in Minkler J (ed): *Pathology of the Nervous System*, vol 3. New York, McGraw-Hill, 1968, pp 2260–2269.
243. Hart MN, Earle KM: Hemmorhagic and perivenous encephalitis: a clinical-pathological review of 38 cases. *J Neurol Neurosurg Psychiatry* 1975;38:585–591.
244. Lukes SA, Norman D: Computed tomography in acute disseminated encephalitis. *Ann Neurol* 1983; 13:567–572.
245. Dunn V, Bale JF Jr, Zimmerman RA, et al: MRI in children with postinfectious disseminated encephalomyelitis. *Mag Res Imag* 1986;4:25–32.
246. Harwood-Nash DC, Fitz CR: Neuroradiology in infants and children, vols 1, 2, 3. St. Louis, CV Mosby, 1976, pp 152–155, 461–608, 855–901.
247. Krick JA, Remington JS. Current concepts in parasitology. Toxoplasmosis in the adult—an overview. *N Engl J Med* 1978;298:550–553.
248. Remington JS: Toxoplasmosis in the adult. *Bull NY Acad Med* 1978;50:211–527.

249. Post MJD, Chan JC, Hensley GT, et al: Toxoplasma encephalitis in Haitian adults with acquired immunodeficiency syndrome: a clinical-pathologic-CT correlation. *AJNR* 1983;4:155–162.
250. Cohen W, Koslow M: An unusual CT presentation of cerebral toxoplasmosis. *J Comput Assist Tomogr* 1985;9:384–385.
251. Levy RM, Rosenbloom S, Perrett LV: Neuroradiology findings in AIDS: a review of 200 cases. *AJNR* 1985;7:833–839.
252. Horowitz SL, Bentsen JR, Benson F, et al: CNS toxoplasmosis in acquired immunodeficiency syndrome. *Arch Neurol* 1983;40:649–652.
253. Handler M, Ho V, Whelan M, Budzilovich G: Intracerebral toxoplasmosis in patients with acquired immunodeficiency syndrome. *J Neurosurg* 1983; 59:944–1001.
254. Post MJD, Sheldon JJ, Hensley GT, et al: Central nervous system disease in acquired immunodeficiency syndrome: prospective correlation using CT, MR imaging, and pathologic studies. *Radiology* 1986;158:141–148.
255. Atlas SW, Grossman RI, Hackney DB, et al: Calcified intracranial lesions: detection with gradient-echo-acquisition rapid MR imaging. *AJNR* 1988; 9:253–259.
256. Engelstad BL, Wolf GL: Contrast agents, in Stark DD, Bradley WG Jr (eds): *Magnetic Resonance Imaging*. St. Louis, C V Mosby, 1988, pp 161–181.
257. Scotti G, Scialfa G, Tampiere D, Landoni L: MR imaging in Fahr disease. *J Comput Assist Tomogr* 1985;9:790–792.
258. Duckett S, Galle P, Escourolle R, et al: Presence of zinc, aluminum, magnesium in striopalledodentate (SPD) calcifications (Fahr's disease): electron probe study. *Acta Neuropathol* 1977;38:7–10.
259. Dozik M, Kulczycki J: Laser-spectrographic analysis of the cation content in Fahr's syndrome. *Arch Psychiatr Nervenkr* 1970;225:135–142.
260. Marquez-Monter H: Cysticercosis, in Marcial-Rojas (ed): *Pathology of Protozoal and Helminthic Diseases with Clinical Correlation*. Baltimore, Williams & Wilkins, 1971, pp 592–617.
261. Carbajal JR, Palacios E, Azar-Kia B, et al: Radiology of cysticercosis of the central nervous system including computed tomography. *Radiology* 1977; 125:127–131.
262. Suss RA, Maravilla KR, Thompson J: MR imaging of intracranial cysticercosis: comparison with CT and anatomopathologic features. *AJNR* 1986;7:235–242.
263. Byrd SE, Locke GE, Biggers S, Percy AK: The computed tomographic appearance of cerebral cysticercosis in adults and children. *Radiology* 1982;144:819–823.
264. Lotz J, Hewlett R, Alheit B, Bowen R: Neurocysticercosis: correlative pathomorphology and MR imaging. *Neuroradiology* 1988;30:35–41.
265. Cardenas JC: Cysticercosis of the nervous system: pathologic and radiologic findings. *J Neurosurg* 1962;19:635–640.
266. Rabiela-Cerrantes MT, Rivas-Hernandez A, Rodriques-Ebarra J, et al: Anatomopathological aspects of human brain cysticercosis, in Flisser A, Williams K, Larralde C, et al (eds): *Cysticercosis: Present State of Knowledge and Perspectives*. New York, Academic Press, 1982, pp 179–200.
267. Escobar A: The pathology of neurocysticercosis, in Palacios E, Rodriquez-Carbajal J, Taveras JM (eds): *Cysticercosis of the Central Nervous System*. Springfield, Ill, Charles C Thomas, 1983, pp 27–54.
268. Kramer LD, Locke GE, Byrd SE, Daryabagi J: Cerebral cysticercosis: documentation of natural history with CT. *Radiology* 1989;171:459–462.
269. Nowak TV, Murphy S: Cerebral cysticercosis. *Wisc Med J* 1978;77:32–34.
270. Case records of the Massachusetts General Hospital (case 40—1970). *N Engl J Med* 1977;297:773–780.
271. Jankowski R, Zimmerman RD, Leeds NE: Cysticercosis presenting as a mass lesion at the foramen of Monro. *J Comput Assist Tomogr* 1979;3:694.
272. Minguetti G, Ferreira M: Computed tomography in neurocysticercosis. *J Neurol Neurosurg Psychiatr* 1983;46:936–942.
273. Benston JR, Wilson GH, Helmer E, et al: Computed tomography in intracranial cysticercosis. *J Comput Assist Tomogr* 1977;1:464–471.
274. Dublin AB, French BN: Cysticercotic cyst of the septum pellucidum. *AJNR* 1980;1:205–206.
275. Zee CS, Segall HD, Apuzzo MLJ, et al: Unusual neuroradiological features of intracranial cysticercosis. *Radiology* 1980;137:397–407.
276. Zee C-S, Tsai FY, Segall HD, et al: Entrance of metrizamide into an intraventricular cysticercosis cyst. *AJNR* 1981;2:189–191.
277. Stauffer RN: Pyogenic vertebral osteomyelitis. *Orthop Clin North Am* 1975;6:1015–1027.
278. Resnick CS, Resnick DL: Pyogenic osteomyelitis and septic arthritis, in Taveras JM, Ferrucci JT (eds): *Radiology: Diagnosis—Imaging—Intervention,* vol 5. Philadelphia, JB Lippincott, 1986, pp 1–11.
279. Juhl JH: Paul and Juhl's essentials of roentgen interpretation (4th ed). Philadelphia, Harper & Row, 1981, pp 275–278.
280. Palacios E, Rodriguez-Carbajal J: Inflammatory and parasitic processes of the spinal canal, in Taveras JM, Ferrucci JT (eds): *Radiology: Diagnosis—Imaging—Intervention,* no 13. Philadelphia, JB Lippincott, 1986, pp 1–6.
281. Bonakdar-pour A, Gaines VD: The radiology of

osteomyelitis. *Orthop Clin North Am* 1983;14:21–23.
282. Malawski SK: Pyogenic infection of the spine. *Int Orthop (SICOT)* 1977;1:125–131.
283. Lifeso RM: Value of computed tomographic scanning in infectious disease of the spine, in Post MJD (ed): *Computed Tomography of the Spine*. Baltimore, Williams & Wilkins, 1984, pp 738–764.
284. Mawk JR, Erickson DL, Chou SN, et al: Aspergillus infections of the lumbar disc spaces. Report of three cases. *J Neurosurg* 1983;58:270–274.
285. Buruma OJ, Kraane H, Kunst MW: Vertebral osteomyelitis and epidural abscess due to mucormycosis. A case report. *Clin Neurol Neurosurg* 1979;81:39–44.
286. Pennisi AK, Davis DO, Wiesel S, Moskovitz P: CT appearance of *Candida* diskitis. *J Comput Assist Tomogr* 1985;9:1050–1054.
287. Burke DR, Brant-Zawadzki M: CT of pyogenic spine infection. *Neuroradiology* 1985;27:131–137.
288. Mettler FA Jr, Guiberteau MJ: Essentials of nuclear medicine imaging (2nd ed). Orlando, Fla, Grune & Stratton, 1986, p 261.
289. Golimbu C, Firooznia H, Rafi M: CT of osteomyelitis of the spine. *AJR* 1984;142:159–163.
290. Whelan MA, Schonfeld S, Post MJD, et al: Computed tomography of nontuberculous spinal infection. *J Comput Assist Tomogr* 1985;9:280–287.
291. Modic MT, Feiglin DH, Piraino DW, et al: Vertebral osteomyelitis: assessment using MR. *Radiology* 1985;157:157–166.
292. Aguila LA, Piraino DW, Modic MT: Magnetic resonance-imaging of the intranuclear cleft. *Radiology* 1985;155:155–158.
293. Post MJD, Quencer RM, Montalvo BM, et al: Spinal infection: evaluation with MR imaging and intraoperative US. *Radiology* 1988;169:765–771.
294. Post MJD, Quencer RM, Eismont FJ, Green BA: Gadolinium-enhanced MR: its value in the detection and diagnosis of spinal infection. *AJNR* 1989;10:881.
295. Sze G: Gadolinium-DTPA in spinal disease. *Radiol Clin North Am* 1988;26:1009–1024.
296. de Roos A, van Persijn van Meerten EL, Bloem JL, Bluemm RG: MRI of tuberculous spondylitis. *AJR* 1986;147:79–82.
297. Waldvogel FA, Vasey H: Osteomyelitis: the past decade. *N Engl J Med* 1980;303:360–370.
298. Sze G, Abramson A, Krol G, et al: Gadolinium-DPTA in the evaluation of intradural extramedullary spinal disease. *AJNR* 1988;9:153–163.
299. Dillon WP, Norman D, Newton TH, et al: Intradural spinal cord lesions: Gd-DPTA-enhanced MR imaging. *Radiology* 1989;170:229–237.
300. Baker AS, Ojemann RG, Swartz MN, Richardson EP Jr: Spinal epidural abscess. *N Engl J Med* 1975;293:463–478.
301. Feldenzer JA, McKeever PE, Schaberg DR, et al: Experimental spinal epidural abscess: a pathological model in the rabbit. *Neurosurgery* 1987;20:859–867.
302. Miller HG, Stanton JB, Gibbons JD: Para-infectious encephalomyelitis and related syndromes. A critical review of the neurological complications of certain specific fevers. *Q J Med* 1956;25:427–505.
303. Kincaid JC: Myelitis and myelopathy, in Baker AB, Baker LH (eds): *Clinical Neurology,* Vol 3. Philadelphia, Harper & Row, 1989, pp 1–36.
304. Merine D, Wang H, Kumar AJ, et al: CT myelography and MR imaging of acute transverse myelitis. *J Comput Assist Tomogr* 1987;11:606–608.
305. New PFJ, Shoukimas GM: Thoracic spine and spinal cord, in Stark DD, Bradley WG (eds): *Magnetic Resonance Imaging*. St. Louis, CV Mosby, 1988, pp 632–665.
306. Sze G, Krol G, Zimmerman RD, Deck MDF: Intramedullary disease of the spine: diagnosis using gadolinium-DTPA-enhanced MR imaging. *AJNR* 1988;9:847–858.

23
Evaluation of Cerebrospinal Fluid

ROBERT E. VAN SCOY

Spinal-fluid examination is usually diagnostic and necessary in patients with meningitis, is frequently nondiagnostic and sometimes dangerous in patients with encephalitis, and is nondiagnostic and hazardous in patients with brain abscess. Thus, the decision to do a spinal tap in a patient suspected of having a central-nervous-system (CNS) infection requires careful judgment.

Once the decision has been made to obtain cerebrospinal fluid (CSF), further consideration is needed to decide which tests should be conducted on the precious sample of fluid. Communication between the clinician and the laboratories, especially the microbiology laboratory, is very helpful.

Cerebrospinal Fluid

CSF is a clear, colorless, metabolically active fluid that fills the subarachnoid spaces and has many important functions.[1] The subarachnoid space is between the two innermost layers of the meninges—the pia mater and the arachnoid (collectively called the leptomeninges). The pia mater is adherent to the brain and spinal cord, and the arachnoid more loosely covers the brain and spinal cord. Where these two layers are widely separated, cisterns are formed, such as the cisterna magna between the cerebellum and medulla. The dual, outer, tough, dense meningeal layers, called the dura mater, are adherent to the skull. In the vertebral area, the outer layer becomes the periosteum and the inner dural layer loosely encases the spinal cord. The space between these two layers is the epidural space. The inner or spinal dural layer is penetrated by the needle during a spinal tap.

The volume of CSF is about 125–150 mL, which is produced mostly in the choroid plexus at the rate of 500–600 mL per day. The CSF serves as a cushion and as a vector for diffusion of metabolites into and out of the brain, and it has an excretory role for drugs and metabolic products.

Some normal CSF values are shown in Table 23.1.

Contraindications and Indications

Relative contraindications to spinal-fluid examination include the presence of papilledema, focal central neurologic deficits, or bleeding diatheses. Computed tomography (CT) should be done in cases of papilledema and focal central neurologic deficits. After the CT findings and the clinical presentation are considered, the need for spinal-fluid evaluation may be determined to outweigh the risk. If so, only a small amount of CSF should be removed. A significant bleeding diathesis should be corrected before CSF is obtained.

Infection in the tissue that the needle would traverse is considered an absolute contraindication.

Complications

The complications of spinal taps (Table 23.2) were reviewed in an excellent article by Marton and Gean.[4]

Following a spinal tap, headache occurs when one is sitting or standing, but it usually is relieved by lying down. It may last for several days. The use of

Table 23.1 Normal CSF values.[a]

Pressure	
65–195 mm H_2O	
Patient should be extended from the flexed position	
Changes with position, blood pressure, venous return, Valsalva maneuver	
Cell count[b]	
Adults: 0–5 mononucleated cells	
5–10, borderline	
>10, abnormal	
0 eosinophils	
Protein[c]	
0–45 mg/dL	
(Ventricular, 6–15 mg/dL; cisternal, 15–25 mg/dL)	
Glucose	
Ratio of CSF to blood glucose, ≥ 0.6	
Takes 2–4 hrs to equilibrate	
If blood glucose concentration is high, then ratio decreases (for example, if blood glucose concentration is 700 mg/dL, the ratio is about 0.4)	
In diabetics with high blood glucose concentration, ratio of <0.3 may correlate best with meningitis.[2]	
(Ventricular, 6–18 mg/dL higher than lumbar CSF)	

[a]For normal values in neonates, see Sarff et al.[3]
[b]Correct for blood in CSF as follows: true CSF leukocytes = measured CSF leukocytes − blood leukocytes × CSF erythrocytes/blood erythrocytes.
[c]Correct CSF protein − serum protein × CSF erythrocytes/blood erythrocytes.

a 20-gauge or smaller needle is thought to reduce the incidence. In one study,[5] the incidence of headache after a spinal tap was found to be 0.5% when subjects were prone for several hours and 36.5% if they were supine.

Brain herniation is the most feared complication. If there is clinical evidence of a mass lesion or increased intracranial pressure, careful reassessment of the need for CSF examination is necessary.

Much of the information on the complications of spinal tap has been obtained from series that included disorders other than infectious diseases, so care in interpretation is indicated.

Table 23.2. Complications of spinal tap.

Complication	Percent
Headache	10–25
Immediate painful paresthesias	13
Persistent paresthesias	<1
Local hematoma	0.2
In patients with coagulation deficits	≤7
Meningitis	Very low
Herniation with elevated intracranial pressure	Unknown
If papilledema	Perhaps 1.2
If no papilledema	Perhaps 12
In subarachnoid hemorrhage	Perhaps 11

Procedure

The procedure and its possible complications should be discussed with the patient or with an appropriate relative in a manner that provides maximum assurance.

Before performing the tap, an assistant should help position the patient in the lateral recumbent position, with the back perpendicular to the table. The patient should be curled into a ball with knees, hips, and back flexed. A 20-gauge or smaller needle then is directed exactly perpendicular to the back. It is common to feel a snapping sensation as the needle penetrates the dura. Frequent removal of the stylet allows for checking for CSF flow. When CSF flow is obtained, the pressure is measured with a manometer. When the needle is properly placed, the pressure should vary by 5–10 mm H_2O with respiration.[1] Even if the opening pressure is elevated, adequate fluid should be withdrawn. Removal of fluid for study does not pose a major risk, as does the subsequent CSF leak from the dural puncture. When the opening pressure is elevated, the fluid should be removed slowly and the pressure monitored. If the pressure reaches one half that of the opening level, no more fluid should be removed.

An alternative position for the procedure is to have the patient sit with the neck and thoracic spine in full flexion, which may improve the identification of the posterior spinous processes and midline. This approach may be helpful for patients who have severe scoliosis or ankylosing spondylitis or are severely obese.[6]

The fluid should be processed immediately. If it absolutely cannot be, it should not be refrigerated because *Neisseria meningitis* is fragile and will die in the cold. Some bacteria will replicate at 37°C, so storage at incubation temperatures is preferable when processing is delayed.

The human immunodeficiency virus (HIV) causes aseptic meningitis and predisposes to other causes of meningitis. Therefore, the persons doing and assisting with spinal taps are advised to avoid recapping needles and to dispose of them in an appropriate punctureproof container. The universal procedures for handling body fluids should be observed.

Tests

Selection of Tests

It is necessary to decide exactly which tests should be done. Although one wants to perform all essential tests, excessive tests not only increase the cost but also reduce the frequently scarce volume needed for vital cultures. Therefore, discretion is important. Powers[7] reviewed the medical charts of 104 adults who underwent lumbar puncture in a university hospital emergency department. Fungal element testing was negative each of the 72 times it was done, cultures for fungi and tuberculosis were uniformly negative, and all immunologic tests had negative results. The average cost of CSF tests in this series was $325. Careful evaluation of the epidemiologic characteristics of the patient and of the diagnosis in question would likely diminish the use of unnecessary testing.

CSF Pressure

The CSF pressure may be increased by congestive heart failure, meningitis, superior vena caval obstruction, thrombosis of the intracranial venous sinus, acute elevation of serum osmolality, impaired reabsorption of CSF, or an intracranial mass lesion.

Alternatively, low pressure occurs in association with dehydration, shock, chronic serum hyperosmolality, dural tears (from trauma, including previous spinal taps), neurosurgical procedures, subdural hematomas in elderly patients, spinal subarachnoid block, and barbiturate intoxication.

The Queckenstedt and Tobey-Ayer tests[8] sometimes are used to evaluate CSF pressure, but they rarely are indicated in the emergency evaluation of meningitis. The Queckenstedt test is performed by occluding the jugular veins bilaterally for 10 seconds. The result is normal if the CSF pressure increases 150 mm H_2O and then returns to baseline in 15–20 seconds. The result is positive if there is no elevation; this suggests herniated disks, vertebral fractures, extradural abscesses, or neoplastic adhesion. The Tobey-Ayer test involves unilateral compression of a jugular vein when contralateral lateral sinus obstruction is suspected. These tests should not be done if CSF pressures are elevated or if cerebrovascular disease is suspected.

Gross Appearance

As CSF is normally clear and colorless, the sample should be compared with clear water. Centrifuged CSF supernatant may be pink to yellow in subarachnoid hemorrhage. This color disappears in about 8–10 days, but bilirubin xanthochromia may take 2–4 weeks to disappear.

Cultures

This chapter addresses CSF evaluation, but it should be recalled that blood and other appropriate substances should be cultured before administering antimicrobial agents. These cultures include not only bacterial blood cultures in cases of suspected bacterial meningitis but also blood or other cultures for fungi, *Brucella,* viruses, and *Mycobacteria* in selected cases. A detailed discussion of one approach to microbiologic processing of spinal fluid was published by Washington.[9]

Bacterial Cultures

If the spinal-fluid sample is bloody after the Gram stain has been prepared, the remaining sample is centrifuged at 2,000 rpm for 10 minutes. The spinal fluid then is aspirated in a syringe and forced through a 0.45-μm filter, and the "upstream" surface of the filter is placed face down on a chocolate-blood-agar medium, slid across the agar for a short distance, and tamped down on the surface. The sediment may be used for thioglycolate, chocolate-blood-agar, and blood-agar inoculation. If the CSF is nonbloody, the thioglycolate is inoculated before the filter procedure is carried out. The specimens are incubated at 35°C with 5–10% CO_2.

Viral Cultures

If the laboratory does not perform needed viral culturing, several milliliters of CSF should be frozen at –70°C in a sterile, secure container and shipped in dry ice to the appropriate regional laboratory. Medical Research Council-5 cells (MRC-5) and a rhesus-monkey kidney (RMK) medium are used.

Patients infected with HIV present several special circumstances. As mentioned above, the risk of acquiring this infection requires that needles and body fluids from all patients be handled with particular care. HIV infection has been associated with asymptomatic and symptomatic spinal-fluid abnormalities from HIV encephalitis or meningitis early and late in the course of the disease. Abnormalities include increased protein, increased cells, positive cultures for the HIV virus, and oligoclonal bands.[10,11] The severity of immunosuppression in the acquired immunodeficiency syndrome (AIDS) may cause a diminished inflammatory reaction to opportunistic infections in the spinal fluid.

Fungal Cultures

CSF cultures are routinely negative for *Coccidioides immitis*. Multiple cultures for other fungi—such as *Cryptococcus neoformans, Histoplasma capsulatum, Blastomyces dermatitidis,* and *Sporothrix schenckii*—may be necessary before positive results are obtained. Ventricular or cisternal fluid may improve the possibility of positive cultures in fungal meningitis such as blastomycosis.[12,13] A large volume of CSF, perhaps 10 ml, is beneficial for a higher chance of isolation. If less than 0.5 ml is available, an inhibitory mold agar medium should be inoculated by dropping the fluid in different spots on the medium. If more fluid is available, it should be filtered as described above.

Mycobacterial Cultures

Mycobacterial cultures also may be positive only if multiple, large-volume (10-ml) specimens of CSF are obtained. Cultures may be negative in 20% of cases, but even if positive, the results are too late for early, effective treatment to be instituted. BACTEC bottles are inoculated, as are 7H10/7H11 biplates. Large specimens are centrifuged and the sediment suspended in 1.5–2.0 ml and divided evenly for these three media. Multiple, large samples are preferred when possible.

Brucella

If brucellosis is suspected, the laboratory should be notified so that both blood and CSF cultures can be processed appropriately. CSF cultures for *Brucella* frequently are negative in cases of *Brucella* meningitis. Blood cultures or blood and CSF serologic tests in combination with the clinical picture of subacute meningitis are the usual methods by which the diagnosis is made.

Anaerobes

Similarly, culture for anaerobes might be considered if the patient has an adjacent head and neck infection or some other clue to the possibility of anaerobic infection. When anaerobic infection is suspected, the CSF should be sent in an anaerobic container. If it is not received in this type of container, the laboratory should notify the physician of the less than optimal situation and process the sample immediately.

The laboratory routinely should differentiate *Corynebacteria* from *Listeria monocytogenes,* which tends to be found in patients with cellular (T-lymphocyte) immunosuppression. *Listeria* organisms are motile at 20–25°C, a trait that differentiates them from *Corynebacteria* organisms, which are common among spinal-fluid and blood-culture contaminants. Fluorescent antibody testing also distinguishes *Listeria* from *Corynebacteria*.

Other Cultures

Cultures for certain organisms such as *Leptospira* might be reasonable only in very unusual circumstances. Culture for other organisms, including *Rickettsia* and *Treponema pallidum,* might be available only on a research basis or in special laboratories.

Glucose

Several disorders are associated with a diminished CSF glucose concentration (Table 23.3).[14] The CSF/serum glucose ratio is usually 0.6 or more, but this ratio usually decreases as the serum glucose concentration increases. It takes about 2–4 hours for the CSF glucose value to equilibrate to the serum glucose value.

Protein

Because the CSF protein level may be increased by many different disorders (Table 23.4), an elevated

Table 23.3. Causes of decreased CSF glucose concentration.

Bacterial meningitis	Insulinoma
Tuberculous meningitis	Hypoglycemia
Fungal meningitis	Neoplasms
Certain viral meningitides	Subarachnoid hemorrhage
Herpes simplex	Chemical meningitis
Herpes zoster-varicella	Amebic meningitis
Lymphocytic choriomeningitis	Sarcoidosis of meninges
Mumps	Trichinosis
Neurosyphilis	

Table 23.4. Causes of increased CSF protein concentration.

Infectious diseases	Noninfectious inflammation
Endocrine disorders	Cerebrovascular disorders
Certain medicines	Elevated serum proteins
Multiple sclerosis	
Subacute sclerosing panencephalitis	
Disorders decreasing absorption of CSF or obstructing flow	

value in itself is not helpful in diagnosis, except to indicate that an abnormality is present.

Leukocyte Count and Differential Count

General rules regarding an increased leukocyte count are helpful (see "Classic Patterns"), as is learning the details of the many exceptions.[15,16] A predominance of neutrophils is associated with bacterial meningitis, but it may be seen early in viral, tuberculous, and fungal meningitis. However, 10% of patients with bacterial meningitis will have fewer than 50% neutrophils, whereas 10% of viral-meningitis cases may have more than 50% neutrophils. In the latter instance, they generally will become mononuclear within 12 hours. Patients with bacterial meningitis usually have more than 500 cells/mm^3, and those with the viral form have fewer than 100 cells/mm^3. However, low cell counts have been found with *Haemophilus influenzae, Neisseria,* and overwhelming streptococcal pneumonia infections. Table 23.5 lists causes of CSF leukocytosis.

Table 23.5. Causes of CSF leukocytosis.

Neutrophils	*Lymphocytes*
Bacterial meningitis	Tuberculous meningitis
Early viral meningitis	Fungal meningitis
Early tuberculous meningitis	Viral meningitis
Early fungal meningitis	Sporochetal meningitis
Amebic meningoencephalitis	Syphilis
Subdural empyema (occasionally)	Lyme disease
Cerebral abscess with rupture into ventricle	Leptospirosis
?Brain abscess—early stage	Partially treated bacterial meningitis
Blood in CSF	*Listeria monocytogenes*
Posthemorrhagic infarct	Measles, SSPE[a]
Subarachnoid hemorrhage	Multiple sclerosis
Injected chemical meningitis	Polyneuritis
Antimicrobials, antimetabolites, anesthetics, contrast media	Temporal arteritis
Dermoid, craniopharyngioma release of material into CSF	Alcohol abuse
Repeated spinal taps	Periarteritis nodosa
Mollaret's meningitis	Guillain-Barré syndrome
Behćet's syndrome	Intravenous drug abuse
Hypersensitivity meningitis	*Eosinophils*
Sulfonamides, tolmetin, ibuprofen, isoniazid	Infections
	Bacterial
	Viral
	Fungal
	Rocky Mountain spotted fever
	Parasitic

[a]Subacute sclerosing panencephalitis.

Stains

Gram Stain

The Gram stain may be positive in approximately 60–90% of patients with bacterial meningitis. It is nearly 100% specific when administered by well-trained observers.

Acridine Orange

This stains nucleic acid of bacteria orange against a yellow-to-green background. It has been reported to be positive in 100% of cases of untreated bacterial meningitis when the Gram stain was positive in only 75%. However, it is not a differential stain and so is useful only if the Gram stain is negative.

India Ink

The India-ink stain is a negative stain used to identify *C neoformans* and its frequently prominent capsule. Although it is popular, its use is inappropriate because the cryptococcal antigen test is very rapid, more sensitive, and more specific. Also, erythrocytes and other cells have been misidentified as *Cryptococcus* by nonexpert examiners.

Acid-Fast Test

If a pellicle forms, the organisms are more likely to be trapped in it, so this portion of the sample should be stained. Perhaps fewer than 25% of acid-fast smears are positive in cases of tuberculous meningitis.

Wet Mount for Amebae

In suspected cases of amebic meningitis, amebic organisms may be seen. The most experienced observer should be called upon to examine the slide.

Bacterial Antigen Tests

Counterimmunoelectrophoresis

In this test, CSF and known antibodies to suspected pathogens are placed in wells in an agar plate and electric current is applied to stimulate more rapid migration. A precipitin line is formed in approximately 30 minutes where antigen from the CSF meets antibody between the wells. The test is perhaps most useful in cases of previously treated bacterial meningitis because it depends on the presence only of antigen and not of viable organisms. False-positive results have occurred because of cross-reactions from antigens of other bacteria. False-negative results also may be seen in very early meningitis, in certain bacterial types, or when antibody quality is poor. Bloody CSF samples should be centrifuged before performing counterimmunoelectrophoresis. The reported positive rates include the following[17]: *Neisseria* meningitis, 50–90%; *Streptococcus pneumoniae,* 50–100%; *H influenzae* B, 80%; and group B streptococcus, 60–90%.

Enzyme-Linked Immunoassay

Although techniques have been developed for detecting antigen by this test, they have not yet been widely adopted.

Latex Agglutination

Latex particles are coated with antibody to known antigens in this test, and agglutination occurs when the antigen is present in the specimen. The test has been remarkably successful with *C neoformans* and is used widely to detect bacterial antigens. Although it is more sensitive than counterimmunoelectrophoresis for pneumococcal meningitis and meningococcal meningitis, it may not be as specific as a result of nonspecific agglutination. However, it is quicker and technically easier.

Serology

Rickettsial

Rickettsial serologic tests (such as for Rocky Mountain spotted fever) may be helpful for confirming a suspected diagnosis, but they are usually done too late to permit appropriate treatment.

Serum tests for *Brucella,* agglutination, or enzyme-linked immunoassay may be diagnostically adequate in the predisposed patient with subacute meningitis.

Fungal

A complement-fixation test that is positive for *C immitis* is diagnostic of CNS infection, except in rare cases of parameningeal infection, being positive in approximately 95% of cases. Because the cultures are positive in perhaps only a third of cases, the serologic test is critical.[18] The cryptococcal "serologic" test is a test for the presence of cryptococcal capsular antigen in the CSF, which is found in more than 95% of cases, but essentially is never present if cryptococcal meningitis is not present, if there is no contamination with blood, and if the antibody reagent is of good quality.

Sporotrichosis meningitis may be diagnosed by slide latex agglutination test or enzyme immunoassay in the absence of positive cultures.[19] Histoplasma meningitis also has been diagnosed by serologic testing.[20]

Viral

Serum acute and convalescent viral serologic tests are helpful for documenting the cause of certain viral CNS infections such as arbovirus and lymphocytic choriomeningitis virus infections. A fourfold increase in the CSF/serum viral serology ratio of the suspected virus may be helpful, especially when compared with a reference virus. Specific CSF immunoglobulin classes, including IgM, may aid in the diagnosis of viral infections.[21,22] However, the development of DNA probes for viral and other microbial antigens seems a more promising technique because antigen would be present earlier in the illness than would antibodies.

Syphilis Tests

Virtually all patients with CNS syphilis show positive results on serum fluorescence treponemal antibody (FTA) tests. Although CSF FTA and reagin tests in combination with cell counts may not be as sensitive, they increase the specificity.[4] Some authors recommend treating the asymptomatic patient who has a positive result on serum FTA testing without doing a spinal tap. The symptomatic patient probably should have a spinal-fluid examination to increase the specificity and to look for evidence of other disease. Infection with HIV may cause difficulties in interpreting CSF serologic results, as well as in treating syphilis.

Table 23.6. Causes of low glucose concentration and predominance of polymorphonuclear neutrophils.

Common cause
Bacterial meningitis
Less common causes
Viral meningitis, in early phase only[a]
Certain parameningeal infections[a]
Embolic infarction[a]
Amebic meningoencephalitis
Tuberculous meningitis, in very early stage[a]
Acute hemorrhagic leukoencephalitis
Chemical meningitis: for example, contrast media, material from dermoids and craniopharyngiomas
Mollaret's meningitis
Behçet's syndrome
Drug induced[a]

[a]Usually glucose value is normal.

Table 23.7. Causes of low glucose concentration and predominance of lymphocytes.

Common causes
Tuberculous meningitis
Fungal meningitis
Neoplastic meningitis
Less common causes
Partially treated "pyogenic meningitis"
L monocytogenes, Leptospira, syphilis
Viral meningitis (10% mumps, less often in lymphocytic choriomeningitis and echovirus meningitis)
Sarcoid meningitis

Table 23.8. Causes of normal glucose concentration and predominance of lymphocytes.

Common causes
Viral meningitis and encephalitis
Postinfectious encephalomyelitis
Less common causes
"Pyogenic meningitis," partially treated
Parameningeal infections
Fungal and tuberculous meningitis (early)
Parasitic diseases such as toxoplasmosis, trichinosis, cysticercosis
Neoplastic meningitis
Harada's syndrome and Vogt-Koyanagi syndrome
Lupus erythematosus
Primary cerebral granulomatous arteritis
Migrainous syndrome

Table 23.9. Causes of normal glucose concentration, predominance of polymorphonuclear neutrophils, negative Gram stain.

Parameningeal infection
Epidural abscess
Subdural empyema
Brain abscess
Bacterial endocarditis
Migrainous syndrome

Cytology

The complex and rapidly developing area of identifying specific tumors by various histologic and monoclonal antibody techniques is outside the scope of this chapter.

Miscellaneous Tests

Several other tests have been proposed to help differentiate various causes of meningitis or other CNS infections. Although they may have been shown to give statistically different results in comparing one diagnosis with another, their clinical value when the other, more routine tests are not helpful is debatable. The lactic-acid value is higher in bacterial than in viral meningitis, but this differentiation is usually possible with routine testing, and false results have occurred.

The lactate dehydrogenase concentration is also higher in bacterial than in viral meningitis, but high levels also have been described in nonbacterial meningeal reactions.

The limulus lysate assay is positive in perhaps 90% of gram-negative meningitis cases and thus might help differentiate *Escherichia coli* meningitis from group B streptococcus neonatal meningitis. However, the clinical usefulness of this test as compared with the combination of Gram stain, counterimmunoelectrophoresis, and latex agglutination tests remains in question.

Classic Patterns

Certain patterns of CSF findings have been described[15] that have common and uncommon causes (Tables 23.6 to 23.9).

References

1. Conly JM, Ronald AR: Cerebrospinal fluid as a diagnostic body fluid. *Am J Med* 1983;75 (special issue) 1B:102–108.
2. Powers WJ: Cerebrospinal fluid to serum glucose ratios in diabetes mellitus and bacterial meningitis. *Am J Med* 1981;71:217–220.
3. Sarff LD, Platt LH, McCracken GH Jr: Cerebrospinal fluid evaluation in neonates: comparison of high-risk infants with and without meningitis. *J Pediatr* 1976;88:473–477.
4. Marton KI, Gean AD: The spinal tap: a new look at an old test. *Ann Intern Med* 1986;104:840–848.

5. Brocker RJ: Technique to avoid spinal-tap headache. *JAMA* 1958;168:261–263.
6. Bannister R: *Brain's Clinical Neurology,* 6th ed. London, Oxford University Press, 1985.
7. Powers RD: Emergency department lumbar puncture: clinical application and utility of laboratory testing. *Am J Emerg Med* 1987;5:516–520.
8. Dougherty JM, Roth RM: Cerebral spinal fluid. *Emerg Med Clin North Am* 1986;4:281–297.
9. Washington JA: *Laboratory Procedures in Clinical Microbiology,* 2nd ed. New York, Springer Verlag, 1985.
10. Hollander H, Stringari S: Human immunodeficiency virus-associated meningitis: clinical course and correlations. *Am J Med* 1987;83:813–816.
11. Appleman ME, Marshall DW, Brey RL, et al: Cerebrospinal fluid abnormalities in patients without AIDS who are seropositive for the human immunodeficiency virus. *J Infect Dis* 1988;158:193–199.
12. Kravitz GR, Davies SF, Eckman MR, et al: Chronic blastomycotic meningitis. *Am J Med* 1981;71:501–505.
13. Gonyea EF: The spectrum of primary blastomycotic meningitis: a review of central nervous system blastomycosis. *Ann Neurol* 1978;3:26–39.
14. Fishman RA: *Cerebrospinal Fluid in Disease of the Nervous System*. Philadelphia, WB Saunders Co, 1980.
15. Swartz MN, O'Hanley P: Central nervous system infections, in Rubenstein E, Federman DD (eds): *Scientific American Medicine,* vol 3. New York, Scientific American, 1987, pp 1–28.
16. Yarki A, Puthuran P: Value of second lumbar puncture in confirming a diagnosis of aseptic meningitis. *Arch Neurol* 1979;36:581–582.
17. Kaplan S: Antigen detection in cerebrospinal fluid—pros and cons. *Am J Med* 1983;75 (special issue) 1B:109–118.
18. Bouza E, Dreyer JS, Hewitt WL, et al: Coccidioidal meningitis: an analysis of thirty-one cases and review of the literature. *Medicine* 1981;60:139–172.
19. Scott EN, Kaufman L, Brown AC, et al: Serologic studies in the diagnosis and management of meningitis due to *Sporothrix schenckii*. *N Engl J Med* 1987;317:935–940.
20. Plouffe JF, Fass RJ: Histoplasma meningitis: diagnostic value of cerebrospinal fluid serology. *Ann Intern Med* 1980;92:189–191.
21. Forsberg P: Studies on immunoglobulins and specific antibodies in central nervous system infections. *Acta Neurol Scand* 1986;73 (suppl):6–76.
22. Forsberg P, Fryden A, Link H, Örvell C: Viral IgM and IgG antibody synthesis within the central nervous system in mumps meningitis. *Acta Neurol Scand* 1986;73:372–380.

Index